DYSPHAGIA

Clinical Management in Adults and Children

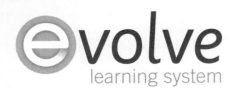
learning system

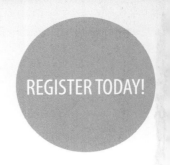
REGISTER TODAY!

To access your free Evolve Resources, visit:

http://evolve.elsevier.com/Groher/dysphagia/

Evolve Student Learning Resources for Groher & Crary: *Dysphagia: Clinical Management in Adults and Children*, second edition, offers the following features:

- **Video Clips**

  More than 50 video clips that highlight selected content within chapters and critical thinking cases on Evolve.

- **Bonus Full-Length Video**

  An introduction to adult swallowing disorders.

- **Critical Thinking Cases**

  Provide opportunities for students to test their application and critical thinking skills.

- **Glossary**

  Serves as a valuable reference tool for students beginning their studies in this specialty area.

ELSEVIER

DYSPHAGIA
Clinical Management in Adults and Children

Michael E. Groher, PHD, FASHA
Professor
Truesdail Center for Communicative Disorders
University of Redlands
Redlands, California

Michael A. Crary, PHD, FASHA
Professor, Speech-Language Pathology
Director, Swallowing Research Laboratory
Department of Communication Sciences and Disorders
University of Central Florida
Orlando, Florida

ELSEVIER

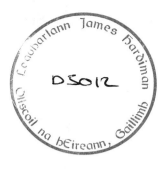

ELSEVIER

3251 Riverport Lane
St. Louis, Missouri 63043

DYSPHAGIA: CLINICAL MANAGEMENT IN ADULTS
AND CHILDREN, SECOND EDITION

ISBN: 978-0-323-18701-5

Notices

Knowledge and best practice in this field are constantly changing. As new research and experience
broaden our understanding, changes in research methods, professional practices, or medical treatment may
become necessary.

Practitioners and researchers must always rely on their own experience and knowledge in evaluating
and using any information, methods, compounds, or experiments described herein. In using such
information or methods they should be mindful of their own safety and the safety of others, including
parties for whom they have a professional responsibility.

With respect to any drug or pharmaceutical products identified, readers are advised to check the most
current information provided (i) on procedures featured or (ii) by the manufacturer of each product to be
administered, to verify the recommended dose or formula, the method and duration of administration, and
contraindications. It is the responsibility of practitioners, relying on their own experience and knowledge
of their patients, to make diagnoses, to determine dosages and the best treatment for each individual
patient, and to take all appropriate safety precautions.

To the fullest extent of the law, neither the Publisher nor the authors, contributors, or editors assume
any liability for any injury and/or damage to persons or property as a matter of products liability,
negligence or otherwise, or from any use or operation of any methods, products, instructions, or ideas
contained in the material herein.

Library of Congress Cataloging-in-Publication Data
Groher, Michael E., author.
  Dysphagia : clinical management in adults and children / Michael E. Groher, Michael A. Crary.—Second
edition.
    p. ; cm.
  ISBN 978-0-323-18701-5
  I. Crary, Michael A., 1952- , author. II. Title.
  [DNLM: 1. Deglutition Disorders. WI 250]
  RC815.2
  616.3′23—dc23

2015009495

Content Strategy Director: Penny Rudolph
Content Development Manager: Jolynn Gower
Senior Content Development Specialist: Brian Loehr
Marketing Manager: Brittany Clements
Publishing Services Manager: Hemamalini Rajendrababu
Project Manager: Kiruthiga Kasthuriswamy
Designer: Ashley Miner

Printed in United States of America

Last digit is the print number: 9 8 7 6 5 4 3 2

Working together
to grow libraries in
developing countries

www.elsevier.com • www.bookaid.org

Contributors

Second Edition

PAMELA DODRILL, PHD, CCC-SLP
Feeding & Swallowing Team
Department of Otolaryngology & Communication
    Enhancement
Boston Children's Hospital
Boston, Massachusetts

Developmental Therapy Team
Department of Pediatric Newborn Medicine
Brigham & Women's Hospital
Boston, Massachusetts

First Edition

JO PUNTIL-SHELTMAN, BCS-S
Board Certified Specialist in Swallowing and Swallowing
    Disorders
Speech-Language Pathologist
Dixie Regional Medical Center
St. George, Utah

HELENE M. TAYLOR, MA, CCC-SLP, CLE
Speech-Language Pathologist
Dysphagia and Craniofacial Clinic Team Member
Primary Children's Medical Center
Salt Lake City, Utah

This book is dedicated to the individuals who have influenced our own work, many of whom were pioneers in the development and support of the multidisciplinary concept of dysphagia management. The clinical and translational research that each has provided has built the foundation for a subspecialty that undoubtedly will continue to grow and benefit the patients we treat:

Joan Arvedson, Ian Cook, Nick Diamant, Olle Ekberg, Michael Feinberg, Susan Langmore, George Larsen, Maureen Lefton-Greif, Jeri Logemann, Arthur Miller, Robert Miller, JoAnn Robbins, Reza Shaker

And to the members of the first multidisciplinary dysphagia team at a major teaching hospital, Johns Hopkins:

Jim Bosma, David Bucholtz, Martin Donner, Bronwyn Jones, Haskins Kashima, Patti Linden, Bill Ravich

And finally, to those who represent a new generation of clinical scientists, many of whom have influenced our efforts and others with whom we have worked directly. These individuals and many others whose work we have read and respect will continue to provide us with important insights:

Margareta Bülow, Susan Butler, Giselle Carnaby, Julie Cichero, Ichiro Fujishima, Maggie Lee Huckabee, Paula Leslie, Rosemary Martino, Gary McCulloch, Bonnie Martin-Harris, Cathy Pelletier, David Smithard, Catriona Steele, Koji Takahashi, and more.

Clinical science can be a slow science. It requires not only dedication to time and effort, but true commitment to the patients who will eventually benefit from these efforts. Clinical science is not without setbacks, pitfalls, and flaws. So to those who engage in clinical science in the name of helping others, we attempt to remember the words of two prominent world citizens, and we apologize if we convey their words incorrectly:

First they ignore you,
then they laugh at you, then they argue with you, then you win.
Mahatma Gandhi

It is common sense to take a method and try it.
If it fails, admit it frankly and try another.
But above all, try something.
Franklin D. Roosevelt

With best wishes to all,
M. G. & M. C.

Preface

Welcome to the second edition of *Dysphagia: Clinical Management in Adults and Children!* As in any new field of endeavor, information accumulates rapidly and subsequently changes our perspectives. This is a good thing in the clinical sciences; we continue to add to our understanding of a problem, in this case, swallowing disorders in children and adults. First and foremost we have updated each chapter to reflect new understandings. Access to imaging materials and critical thinking cases on Evolve has improved. Critical thinking cases that have proven so valuable in classroom discussions remain, and new ones to highlight different aspects of patient management have been added. We are pleased to welcome Pamela Dodrill, PhD, to the list of contributing authors. Pamela has recently moved to Boston Children's Hospital from the Royal Children's Hospital in Brisbane, Australia, where she spent 12 years as the senior speech-language pathologist on the dysphagia team. She has published numerous papers on pediatric swallowing issues and is a frequent presenter on this topic at international meetings.

Our focus continues to be for the clinician who wants to establish a basic and comprehensive foundation in managing infants, children, and adults with swallowing disorders. The emphasis is on the processes of providing diagnostic and treatment services for persons with dysphagia, and on the research that supports those services. Because of the comprehensive approach, some details of diagnosis and treatment will not be fully appreciated after the first reading by novice clinicians, but will be useful for journeyman clinicians. It is our opinion that the organization of this text will be an aid to the professor who is providing instruction in dysphagia management at a basic and advanced level. Aids in teaching include access to an extensive library of swallowing examinations (on the companion Evolve website); a liberal use of short, clinically based examples of a myriad of problems associated with dysphagia; critical thinking case examples (Clinical Corner boxes in the chapters); and cases that require students to analyze their own decision-making skills as they integrate historical, clinical, and imaging results using a series of prompts that probe their problem-solving skills (on the Evolve website). Unfamiliar terms have been highlighted in bold and defined in an accompanying glossary. In addition, we have tried to infuse our own biases and insights with anecdotal stories (Practice Notes in the chapters) given to us by the hundreds of patients we have treated.

The Table of Contents has been revised based on feedback from practicing clinicians and professors involved in the care of infants and children. In the prior edition material relevant to infants and children was embedded in chapters that also addressed adults. In this edition, infants and children have been assigned a separate section (Part III, chapters 12-15). We hope that this reorganization might facilitate teaching and the comprehension of concepts related to this specific patient group.

It is our opinion that dysphagia management is best taught by illustrating approaches to problem solving. To this end we have tried to avoid being prescriptive in favor of an emphasis on discovering available options for care and in weighing the risks and benefits of those options. Too often prescriptive approaches in clinical care take away one's options to solve patient care problems.

The successful management of persons with dysphagia is accomplished only through the cooperation of numerous specialists (see Chapter 1). Although it is well known that a multidisciplinary approach with these patients is best, this approach also may suffer from failure to coordinate care. Often, the coordination of that care is accomplished by the speech-language pathologist. In this text we have emphasized the role of the speech-language pathologist. The roles of other disciplines are explained largely in the clinical case presentations within each chapter.

Ultimately, this is a text that highlights the problems of persons with dysphagia and how professionals might ameliorate their swallowing difficulties. It will become apparent that swallowing difficulty may be secondary to a large number of medical and sometimes nonmedical (psychogenic) disorders, and that swallowing problems are more than a physiologic change in the swallowing mechanism. The text takes the perspective that being unable to swallow normally might result in major consequences to one's medical and psychological health. Secondary medical problems such as aspiration pneumonia, undernutrition, and dehydration may predispose the patient to other complications such as immunocompromise, mental confusion, or death. Because of this, dysphagia specialists must develop a strong background of general medical knowledge. The reader should be able to understand or be alerted to key medical concepts relating to the dysphagic circumstance within each chapter, but may have to go beyond this text for more detailed explanations of some concepts.

Being unable to ingest one's favorite foods safely, or being unable to eat normally in public, understandably will affect one's quality of life with the potential for secondary episodes of depression, anxiety, and social withdrawal. Preparation of special diets is time consuming and in some cases economically challenging. In short, our lifestyles frequently revolve around mealtimes. Interruptions to these normal routines are potentially devastating. Therefore treatments are geared not only to the restoration of physiologic function, but ultimately to a state of psychosocial normalcy that was disturbed as a result of a failure to swallow normally. Care of persons with dysphagia should be viewed as an attempt to rehabilitate lost function as well as prevent future medical complications by retaining learned rehabilitative strategies.

Managing persons with dysphagia has become a subspecialty for many health care professionals. For the speech-language pathologist it is a specialty that has emerged only within the last 30 years. As clinicians have become more familiar with the issues involved in the care of dysphagic persons, clinical and basic science investigators have helped answer and ask questions that have helped improve the quality of that care. Many of these efforts have come together in a journal *(Dysphagia)* devoted exclusively to dysphagia; a research society that meets annually (the Dysphagia Research Society); and the largest special interest division, number 13 (Dysphagia), within the American Speech-Language-Hearing Association. There also has been a steady increase of texts with contributions from many disciplines aimed at the pathologic condition, diagnosis, and treatment of persons with swallowing disorders. It is our hope that this text will not only add to that number, but also inspire those researchers and clinicians interested in dysphagia to continue the quest to improve the lives of persons with swallowing disorders.

Contents

CHAPTER 1

Dysphagia Unplugged

Michael E. Groher and Jo Puntil-Sheltman

To view additional case videos and content, please visit the evolve website.

CHAPTER OUTLINE

OBJECTIVES

1. Define *dysphagia* and its ramifications.
2. Discuss the epidemiology of dysphagia.
3. Discuss the medical and social consequences of dysphagia.
4. Provide an overview of the clinical management of dysphagia.
5. Discuss the role of persons who manage dysphagia.
6. Discuss the types of settings in which dysphagic patients might be seen and how this might affect their management.

WHAT IS DYSPHAGIA?

Dysphagia takes its name from the Greek root phagein, meaning to ingest or engulf. Combined with the prefix dys-, it connotes a disorder of or difficulty with swallowing. It is correctly pronounced with a long or short *a*. The final syllable, "ja," requires a hard pronunciation rather than the soft "dja" to avoid confusion with the communicative language disorder, *dysphasia* (see Practice Note 1-1).

Taber's Cyclopedic Medical Dictionary[1] defines five subcategories of dysphagia:

1. Constricta: narrowing of the pharynx or esophagus
2. Lusoria: esophageal compression by the right subclavian artery
3. Oropharyngeal: difficulty with propulsion from the mouth to the esophagus
4. Paralytica: Paralysis of muscles of mouth, pharynx, or esophagus

PRACTICE NOTE 1-1

While acting as a consultant to a food production company, I asked them what they thought the extent of their market would be, indicating that to my knowledge we only had gross estimates of how many persons with dysphagia would benefit from specialized foods. They told me that they had been working with a firm that did an extensive analysis on this topic and had prepared a detailed report on the potential market. I asked them to send me a copy because I was interested in data that documented the **incidence** of dysphagia in the United States. Two weeks later I received a package with a copy of the data. To my surprise, there were at least 15 pages of references. On closer inspection of the first page, I noticed that the firm they had hired had used the key word *dysphasia*, not *dysphagia*. I broke the news to them that what they had paid for was an extensive review of the literature on language disorders after neurologic injury, not swallowing disorders. What a difference a single letter can make!

BOX 1-1   SUMMARY OF CONDITIONS THAT MAY CONTRIBUTE TO DYSPHAGIA

Neurologic Diagnoses
Stroke
Traumatic brain injury
Dementia
Motor neuron disease
Myasthenia gravis
Cerebral palsy
Guillain-Barré syndrome
Poliomyelitis
Infectious disorders
Myopathy

Progressive Disease
Parkinsonism
Huntington's disease
Progressive supranuclear palsy
Wilson's disease
Age-related changes

Connective Tissue/Rheumatoid Disorders
Poly- and **dermatomyositis**
Progressive systemic sclerosis
Sjögren's disease
Scleroderma
Overlap syndromes

Structural Diagnoses
Any tumor involving the alimentary tract

Iatrogenic Diagnoses
Radiation therapy
Chemotherapy
Intubation or **tracheostomy**
Postsurgical cervical spine fusion
Postsurgical coronary artery bypass grafting
Medication-related

Other or Related Diagnoses
Severe respiratory compromise
Psychogenic condition(s)

5. Spastica: Dysphagia from spasm of the pharynx or esophagus

In clinical practice, only *oropharyngeal dysphagia* from this list is used with any frequency.

Interestingly, medical students learn that dysphagia is a swallowing problem primarily associated with disease of the esophagus. However, when used properly the term should refer to a swallowing disorder that involves any one of the three stages of swallowing: oral, pharyngeal, or esophageal. Some might extend the term to the stomach or lower gastrointestinal tract as primary disorders in these structures such as the stomach may secondarily affect other parts of the gastrointestinal tract such as the esophagus. It is not a primary medical diagnosis but rather a **symptom** of underlying disease and therefore is described most often by its clinical characteristics (**signs**). Complaints such as coughing and choking during or after a meal, food sticking, **regurgitation**, **odynophagia**, drooling, unexplained weight loss, and nutritional deficiencies all may be associated with dysphagia. Because dysphagia is a symptom of underlying disease that is not necessarily specific to the swallowing tract, it can be associated with varied diagnoses. These diagnoses are summarized in Box 1-1. Throughout this text, most of these diagnoses will receive individualized attention. See Chapter 7 for a full discussion of symptoms and signs associated with dysphagia.

Dictionary-based definitions of dysphagia imply that it is the result of a physiologic change in the muscles needed for swallowing. Physiologic change often leads to the two hallmarks of dysphagia: delay in the propulsion of a **bolus** as it transits from the mouth to the stomach or misdirection of a bolus. Misdirection can be defined as bolus material entering the upper airway or lungs, or material that enters the mouth, pharynx, or esophagus during swallowing attempts but fails to reach the stomach. In these circumstances, classification of dysphagia by either clinical or imaging examination seems warranted and straightforward.

However, not all patients with physiologic abnormalities of the swallowing mechanism show obvious delay in bolus flow or misdirection of bolus flow. The question that may arise for the clinician (and often for the researcher who has selected a cohort of patients with dysphagia) is the degree of severity of physiologic changes in the swallowing musculature needed before a patient is classified as having dysphagia. For instance, physiologic changes in the swallowing musculature have been described in older persons[2]—such as reduction in tongue strength or esophageal motility—both of which may delay the delivery of food or liquid to the stomach. However, only when such changes result in perceptible changes in eating habits or associated medical complications such as **undernutrition** or **aspiration pneumonia** is a person classified as truly having dysphagia. Because swallowing is a dynamic process, persons may not exhibit signs and symptoms of dysphagia with every swallow and every bolus type. In these cases, they may be considered to be at risk for dysphagia or, alternatively, operationally defined as dysphagic. It is also possible that the swallowing musculature is normal but the patient is not alert enough to use that musculature because of his or her decompensated medical condition. In such cases it is assumed that attempts to swallow would result in dysphagic complications. In these cases, the patient may be classified as at risk for dysphagia. Patients may demonstrate abnormalities of behavior that interfere with the normal swallowing process; these may cause dysphagic signs and symptoms or put the patient at risk for dysphagia. Therefore dysphagia is defined not only by abnormalities of the mechanics of the swallowing musculature, but also by the consequences of failure, or potential failure, of that musculature owing to factors not always specifically related to swallow mechanics. For this reason the authors prefer the definition of dysphagia offered by Tanner[3]: "Dysphagia: [an] impairment of emotional, cognitive, sensory, and/or motor acts involved with transferring a substance from the mouth to stomach, resulting in failure to maintain **hydration** and nutrition, and posing a risk of choking and aspiration" (p. 16).

A swallowing disorder should be distinguished from a feeding disorder. A *feeding disorder* is impairment in the process of food transport outside the alimentary system. A feeding disorder usually is the result of weakness or incoordination in the hand or arm used to move the food from the plate to the mouth. In the United Kingdom and the United States a feeding disorder, particularly in the context of infants and children, may be the same as a swallowing disorder. Persons with feeding disorders (motor transfer problems) also may be dysphagic, such as those with cerebral palsy whose neurologic disability affects both feeding (motoric transfer) and swallowing. It is not known whether a feeding disorder that might require assistance with food transport also affects the subsequent act of swallowing, perhaps by interfering with timing of swallowing events.

A swallowing disorder also is to be distinguished from an eating disorder such as **anorexia** or **bulimia** nervosa. Whereas patients with dysphagia, bulimia, and anorexia may have difficulty with poor appetite, changes in dietary selections, and problems with the oral preparation of the bolus, patients with bulimia and anorexia rarely have demonstrable changes in or complaints of swallowing difficulty.[4]

INCIDENCE AND PREVALENCE

The incidence of a disorder is the reported frequency of new occurrences of that disorder over a long time (usually at least 1 year) in relation to the population in which it occurs. The prevalence of a disorder is the number of cases in a population during a shorter, prescribed period, usually in a specific setting. Exact measures of the incidence and prevalence of swallowing disorders in large and various populations are impossible because of differences in accepted definitions of dysphagia, the setting in which it is measured (acute, rehabilitation, **chronic**), and differences in the measurement tools across studies to detect it.[5] For instance, asking a patient if she or he has a swallowing disorder to determine the prevalence is a very different method of detection compared with the use of an imaging examination such as **videofluoroscopy**. Most demographic data that are reported relating to swallowing disorders are prevalence data. The importance of knowing the prevalence of a disorder can help guide clinicians in the detection of that disorder and therefore helps plan how resources might be devoted to that disorder. For instance, if an examiner knew that a certain abnormality was found in less than 1% of that population, the examiner may not spend time looking for that abnormality because its expected frequency of occurrence would be low. If, however, a particular abnormality was found in more than 50% of the persons with a particular disorder, the examiner would be alerted to expect the occurrence of deficits associated with that disorder. Therefore if the data suggested that 50% of patients who have had an acute stroke could have dysphagia, and that 20% of that group might have **silent aspiration**, an examiner would expect that half of the patients with acute stroke would have swallowing impairment and about half of those are at high risk for silent aspiration. Furthermore, pneumonia develops in 37% of acute stroke patients with aspiration.[6] Knowledge of these prevalence data provides valuable assistance to medical personnel who initially screen for and manage the medical complications after acute stroke (see Chapters 3 and 7).

The American Speech-Language-Hearing Association (ASHA) estimates that 6 to 10 million Americans show some degree of dysphagia, although it is not known how these estimates were made.[7] Kuhlemeier[8] reported that the incidence of reported dysphagia in the state of Maryland rose from 3 in 1000 in 1979 to 10 in 1000, probably as a result of better reporting methods. Using these estimates, approximately 25,000 persons in Maryland in 1989 had dysphagia as either a primary or secondary diagnosis.

Prevalence by Setting

Estimates of prevalence of dysphagia vary by setting because certain age groups (older adults and premature newborns) and diagnoses (neurogenic) are more likely to demonstrate dysphagia. For instance, patients entering a **rehabilitation setting** may not have as many accompanying medical problems and dysphagia as those entering a nursing home. Conversely, infants born prematurely may have many medical problems that may secondarily result in dysphagia. In a survey of the entire population of an acute general hospital, fewer patients with dysphagia would be found in the general population compared with a survey of a special section of that hospital, such as the stroke unit.

Community

Estimates of the prevalence of dysphagia among older persons living in the community range from 16% to 22%.[9,10] One study reported on the prevalence of dysphagia in a younger cohort (14- to 30-year-olds) living in the community who had been referred for complaints of dysphagia.[11] In this selected group, 70% had demonstrable pathologic conditions that accompanied their symptoms.

Acute and Chronic Geriatric Care

Of the 211 patients admitted to an acute geriatric unit in Singapore, the prevalence of dysphagia was 29% on admission and 28% at discharge.[12] In a nursing home in Maryland (chronic care), as many as 60% of residents had a combination of swallowing and feeding difficulty.[13] A similar number (53%) was found in a chronic care facility in Spain,

two urban nursing homes in South Korea, and in eight nursing homes in Portugal.[14-16] One study found that when feeding and swallowing difficulty were combined, as many as 87% of the residents in a home for the aged were at risk for inadequate oral intake.[17] Follow-up data of nursing home residents with oropharyngeal dysphagia indicate a mortality rate of 45% at 1 year.[18]

Acute General Hospitals

Using the Fleming Index of Dysphagia, a tool to identify dysphagia, Layne et al.[19] found that nearly one third of their patients had a diagnosis consistent with dysphagia. These findings were nearly 18% higher than those provided by Groher and Bukatman,[20] who reported a 13% prevalence rate in similar settings. The discrepancy in prevalence was explained by the fact that patients who were dehydrated in the study by Layne et al. were classified as dysphagic, whereas this was not a marker for dysphagia used in the collection of the Groher and Bukatman data.

Acute Rehabilitation Unit

Of 307 consecutive admissions to an acute rehabilitation facility, one third of patients were dysphagic.[21] Of this group, half had dysphagia as a result of a stroke, followed by traumatic brain injury (20%), spinal cord injury and brain tumor (7%), and progressive neurologic disease (5%). On admission, the patients with the most severe dysphagia were those with traumatic brain injury, followed by stroke. The least severe dysphagia occurred in those with brain tumors.

Special Populations

Some primary medical diagnoses are more likely to precipitate dysphagic symptomatology, such as diseases that affect the central and peripheral nervous system and disorders affecting the structures of the alimentary tract, such as cancer. An estimated 300,000 to 600,000 persons in the United States each year are affected by dysphagia from neurologic disorders alone; most cases occur after a stroke.[5] If these data are reliable, dysphagia is a common symptom after a stroke.

Stroke

Prevalence reports of dysphagia after stroke depend on when in the course of recovery the detection of a swallowing impairment was made. For instance, in acute stroke (less than 5 days after onset) the prevalence of dysphagia may be as high as 50%, whereas 2 weeks after stroke only 10% to 28% of patients may be dysphagic. Recognizing these discrepancies, Smithard et al.[22] provided follow-up of 121 (untreated) acute stroke patients for 6 months using a clinical dysphagia examination and videofluoroscopy to detect swallowing deficits. Immediately after stroke, 51% were believed to be at risk for aspiration. After 7 days, only 27% were still considered to be at risk. At 6 months, 3% of the survivors had persistent difficulty, whereas 3% who previously were not dysphagic were now considered at risk. These results suggest that early detection is important in preventing dysphagic complications and that a significant number of patients will improve without intervention specific to their dysphagia. Similarly, comparable prevalence figures for dysphagia on admission (43% to 51%) were found by Gordon et al.[23] and Mann et al.,[24] although the latter group noted a higher prevalence of dysphagic symptoms at 6 months (50%) than other studies with prevalence rates that ranged from 3% to 9%.[22,24] Daniels et al.[25] found that 36 (65%) of 55 patients with acute stroke had dysphagia. Of these 36, more than half aspirated. Of these, two thirds did so silently, suggesting that events of aspiration could be detected only by videofluoroscopy, not the bedside examination. In long-term follow-up, 94% of these patients returned to oral intake. Interestingly, the presence or absence of silent aspiration did not discriminate between patients who returned to successful oral feeding. After analyzing prevalence reports from two large stroke databases, Gonzalez-Fernandez et al.[26] found a significantly higher prevalence of dysphagia in Asians when compared with Whites and Blacks (see Clinical Corner 1-1).

Head and Neck Cancer

Surprisingly, there have been no large studies of the prevalence or incidence of swallowing disorders in unselected patients after treatment for head and neck cancer, although it is well known that dysphagia is a frequent complication. Dysphagia can result from the removal of tissue, with subsequent sensory and motor loss, and the effects of radiation therapy and chemotherapy. Before patients in their

---

CLINICAL CORNER 1-1: SEVERE DYSPHAGIA

L. G. was admitted to the hospital for a left brain stroke. On admission he was nonresponsive and a nasogastric feeding tube was placed to provide nutrition and hydration. As his responsiveness improved, the nasogastric feeding tube was removed and he began oral feeding. As he fed himself, it was noted that he choked on most attempts and dysphagia was suspected. The clinical evaluation noted a weak tongue and poor laryngeal elevation. The imaging examination showed signs of tracheal aspiration. The diagnosis of dysphagia secondary to stroke was confirmed.

Critical Thinking
1. Why might a **nasogastric tube** be placed on admission?
2. Should the nasogastric tube have been removed? Why do you think it was removed?

---

study received treatment, Pauloski et al.[27] found that 59% had symptoms consistent with dysphagia. In a large multi-center treatment trial of patients with laryngectomies who were treated with either surgery and radiation or radiation and chemotherapy, approximately 33% had some type of swallowing-related difficulty at 2-year follow-up.[28] Using a questionnaire, Maclean et al.[29] noted that 71% of their 197-person sample reported some difficulty with their swallowing. In a series of 46 patients treated by **supraglottic laryngectomy**, 60% had dysphagia after their hospital stay.[30] In 21 patients following supraglottic laryngectomy using a transoral carbon dioxide laser approach, most experienced dysphagia with aspiration after 2 weeks, but it significantly decreased at 12-month follow-up.[31] In a mixed group of 87 head and neck cancer patients who were at least 1 year posttreatment, oropharyngeal dysphagia was present in 50.6%, mostly to solids.[32] Fifty-one percent of patients reported a decrease in their quality of life because of their swallowing disability. Evidence suggests that patients with pharyngeal tumor **resections** and those with tumors involving the tongue base are more likely to have dysphagia.[33]

Head Injury

Dysphagia is common after severe head injury. Data report that the incidence of dysphagia ranges from 4.5% (9 of 199) of consecutive admissions in an **acute care setting**[34] to an incidence of 78% (31 of 40) in a similar setting.[35] Discrepancies in reporting may be attributable to the initial severity of the injury and the method used to detect and define dysphagia. Incidence data are available for patients who survive head injury and enter a rehabilitation setting; the incidence ranges from 27% to 30%[34,36] to 42% (218 of 524).[37] In a mixed group (type of injury and time after onset), Lazarus and Logemann[38] found that approximately half of the patients they examined with videofluoroscopy showed evidence of dysphagia. Among patients with head injuries entering a rehabilitation setting, Winstein[36] found that 27% were dysphagic on admission to rehabilitation and that only 6% were dysphagic after 5 months of rehabilitation. Of 62 consecutive patients receiving outpatient rehabilitation, Yorkston et al.[35] reported that 13% remained dysphagic. In general, the more severe the initial injury, the higher the incidence of dysphagia. In a retrospective review of 219 patients admitted for head injury who were suspected of dysphagia, logistic regression revealed that those who were older, tracheotomized, and aphonic were more likely to enter the next level of care with a feeding tube than those who did not evidence these findings.[39] Some patients remain comatose and are unable to eat, whereas others require extensive neurosurgical procedures with prolonged intubation and mental status changes, all of which may preclude attempts at oral ingestion. However, once patients enter the rehabilitation setting, their chances of returning to oral feeding are good.

Progressive Neurologic Disease

Progressive neurologic diseases that frequently result in dysphagia include **Parkinson's disease** and its variants, **amyotrophic lateral sclerosis** (ALS), **multiple sclerosis** (MS), and myasthenia gravis; diseases of systemic rheumatic origin such as dermatomyositis, polymyositis, **rheumatoid arthritis** (RA), scleroderma, and **Sjögren's syndrome**; and variants of dementing syndromes such as Alzheimer's and frontotemporal disease. Systemic rheumatic disorders are far rarer than Parkinson's disease or MS but merit consideration in a discussion of dysphagia and neurologic disease. Because of the progressive nature of these disease processes, the point in disease progression at which dysphagic symptoms occur is never certain. For instance, some patients report dysphagia as the initial symptom of the disease, whereas others may never mention dysphagia. In general, however, as disease severity increases, so does dysphagia. Complications from dysphagia, particularly those that threaten pulmonary function, may lead to aspiration pneumonia and death (see Chapter 6).

Parkinson's Disease. Although dysphagia secondary to Parkinson's disease appears to be common, accurate measurements are restricted by subject selection bias and dysphagia detection methods. However, most authors agree that dysphagia occurs in at least 50% of patients with Parkinson's disease.[40-42] In 72 patients with Parkinson's disease of varying severity, Leopold and Kagel[43] found that as many as 82% reported swallowing difficulty. Using the Unified Parkinson's Disease Rating Scale, a scale that acquires data by self-report, Walker et al.[44] found that 32% of their patient sample complained of dysphagia. In patients with early stage disease, Sung et al.[45] found manometric abnormalities on both liquid and more viscous bolus types with disruptions of esophageal motility during repetitive swallowing tasks. Interestingly, the esophageal abnormalities were present even before overt manifestations of dysphagia were present. That patients with Parkinson's disease may not be accurate reporters of dysphagic symptoms is well-known. Kalf et al.[46] performed a meta-analysis using 12 studies to establish the prevalence of dysphagia associated with Parkinsonism. One third of the patients sampled complained of dysphagia, whereas more than 80% had objective demonstrations of its presence. The prevalence of dysphagia may be higher in patients with Parkinson's disease who also have significant dementia.[47]

Amyotrophic Lateral Sclerosis. When ALS affects the **bulbar musculature**, dysphagia may be one of the first symptoms of the disease. In studies of patients with ALS at first diagnosis, 25% to 30% have evidence of bulbar symptomatology.[48,49] It can be assumed that at least one third of patients with a diagnosis of ALS will have some difficulty swallowing, particularly as the disease progresses.[50] Known characteristics of disease progression that affect the bulbar musculature result in progressively severe dysphagia symptomatology.[51]

Multiple Sclerosis. Hartelius and Svensson[52] found that more than 33% of a large series of patients with MS had either chewing or swallowing problems. Dysphagic complaints in patients receiving follow-up care in an outpatient clinic ranged between 30% and 40%.[53] Similar to those with ALS, not all patients with MS will have dysphagia unless the bulbar musculature is involved, and symptoms are more likely to appear as the disease progresses. After evaluating 143 consecutive patients with primary and secondary progressive MS, Calcagno et al.[54] confirmed dysphagic symptoms in 34%. Their study showed a positive relation between dysphagia and disease severity and between dysphagia and brainstem involvement. After surveying 309 patients with MS, DePauw et al.[55] found that 24% had chronic swallowing difficulty and another 5% admitted to transitory difficulty. As patients became more disabled according to a scale of disability measurement, the prevalence of dysphagia increased to 65%.[55]

Myasthenia Gravis. In selected populations of patients with myasthenia gravis, approximately one third will be dysphagic.[56] The prevalence of dysphagia depends largely on the extent of muscle fatigue and other medical complications such as respiratory impairment secondary to an acute exacerbation of muscle weakness.

Muscular Dystrophy. There are no published reports of the prevalence of dysphagia in muscular dystrophy, although there are reports of swallowing dysfunction secondary to peripheral oropharyngeal and esophageal muscle weakness in those with oculopharyngeal, Duchenne, and myotonic muscular dystrophy.[57-59]

Polymyositis and Dermatomyositis. Oh et al.[60] documented the prevalence of dysphagia in those inflammatory diseases affecting muscle. Of the 783 patients studied, 62 were dysphagic. Oropharyngeal dysphagia was present in 18 with dermatomyositis, and 9 with **polymyositis**. As with other progressive neurologic conditions, with these disorders the course and response to medical therapy may differ; therefore the presence of dysphagia is variable. Because of their predilection to involve the **proximal muscle**, swallowing can be affected in these disorders. Multiple disorders of pharyngeal function following videofluoroscopic swallowing studies were noted in a small group of patients with polymyositis (6), dermatomysitis (4), and **inclusion body myositis**.[61]

Rheumatoid Arthritis. Geterude et al.[62] found that 8 of 29 patients with RA had complaints of dysphagia. In a series of 31 patients with dysphagia and RA, Ekberg et al.[63] documented pharyngeal dysfunction in 20.

Scleroderma. As many as 90% of patients with scleroderma have swallowing-related complaints.[64] Accompanying **erosive esophagitis** was found in 60% of 53 patients with scleroderma.[65] In these patients, dysphagia was always an accompanying complaint. In patients with scleroderma, dysphagic complaints usually are confined to the esophagus, although secondary effects on the oral and pharyngeal stages resulting from esophageal dysmotility should be considered.

Sjögren's Syndrome. As many as 75% of patients with Sjögren's syndrome have dysphagia.[66] The potential of this syndrome to involve all stages of swallowing function is well known.

Dementia. Alagiakrishnan et al.[67] did a **systematic review** of the prevalence of dysphagia in dementia. Nineteen studies met the review criteria. Prevalence ranged from 13% to 57%, developing in the later stages of those with frontotemporal dementia and in earlier stages in those with Alzheimer's disease (see Clinical Corner 1-2).

Developmental Disability. Leslie et al.[68] discussed the need to document the true prevalence of dysphagia in those with developmental disorders to highlight the need for appropriate intervention. They could find only estimates of prevalence ranging from 36% in the community to 73% who were inpatients. After studying those patients referred for dysphagia evaluations, Chadwick and Jolliffe[69] concluded that the prevalence of those with dysphagia and concomitant mental or physical disability was 8.1%. Observations of adults with Down syndrome living in a residential facility who were eating a regular diet revealed that 56.5% were at risk for respiratory infection based on overt signs of cough during the meal.[70] Smith et al. found a similar prevalence in a younger group of hospitalized patients with Down syndrome (mean age 7.45). Those with significant neurologic delay or tracheostomy were more likely to be at risk for dysphagia.[71]

Mental Illness. Few prevalence data have been recorded on patients with mental illness who may show signs of dysphagia. Noting this omission, Aldridge and Taylor[72] completed a systematic review in an attempt to document prevalence and treatment interventions. Ten studies met the inclusion criteria documenting those with dysphagia or those who expired from choking asphyxiation. Adults with mental illness in one study were 43 times more likely to die from organic mental illness compared with the general population. Six studies revealed a range of prevalence of dysphagia from 9% to 42%. None of the studies provided data on treatment intervention or outcomes (see Clinical Corner 1-3).

Phagophobia. Phagophobia, or the fear of swallowing, may be associated with psychogenic etiologic factors such as panic disorders, posttraumatic stress disorder, social phobia, or obsessive compulsive disorders. Those with phagophobia usually describe their problem as the sensation that they are unable to swallow in the absence of any documented sensory or motor abnormality. Baijens et al.[73] reviewed 12 published studies that attempted to establish the prevalence and treatment of the disorder. Most had serious methodologic flaws with low levels of evidence that made it too difficult to establish reliable prevalence statistics.

Premature Infants. The incidence of infants born prematurely in the United States has increased to more than 12%

CLINICAL CORNER 1-2: MEDICATION RISK

M. M. was admitted to the burn unit with severe burns to the head, neck, and upper torso. Because of associated pain he was heavily sedated. As his condition improved and before he was allowed to eat orally, a request for a swallowing evaluation was made because it was noticed he was not swallowing his secretions well. The evaluation of swallowing revealed normal strength of the swallowing musculature; however, he was disoriented and could not maintain his alertness level for more than 30 seconds. Because of his poor mental status and alertness level, he was not allowed to eat and was considered to be at risk for dysphagia.

Critical Thinking

1. How might medications contribute to dysphagia?
2. Could poor mental status result in choking? Give some examples.

CLINICAL CORNER 1-3: PSYCHIATRIC DIAGNOSIS

L. T. was admitted to the psychiatry unit with symptoms of acute schizophrenia. When eating, it was noted he would take excessive time to finish, with intermittent choking episodes. The speech pathologist who evaluated him for signs and symptoms of dysphagia found that the oropharyngeal swallowing musculature was intact. As she watched the patient eat, she noted a rapid feeding rate with inappropriate bite sizes. She also noted excessive talking while eating, and the choking episodes occurred during these talking periods. The patient was classified as dysphagic as a result of emotional and behavioral abnormalities.

Critical Thinking

1. What other types of behavioral disorders might contribute to dysphagia?
2. Why did this patient choke while eating and talking?

of all live births and 18% of African-American births.[74] A growing concern has been the incidence of emotional and neurodevelopmental disabilities in the very low birth weight population (less than 26 weeks' gestation). Estimates indicate that as many as 90% of low birth weight infants may be prone to disorders of feeding.[75]

Spinal Cord Injury. In a study that evaluated the use of clinical versus imaging studies in adults with tetraplegia, Shem[76] and colleagues reported that 38% of the 39 patients who were enrolled had evidence of oropharyngeal dysphagia. Four subjects were diagnosed with aspiration.

CONSEQUENCES OF DYSPHAGIA

Because dysphagia frequently accompanies many medical diagnoses, it is important to appreciate its potential effect on patient care. It is well recognized that dysphagia is a symptom of disease, but it also has the potential to secondarily precipitate morbidity and mortality. As such, its influence on health can be substantial. Additionally, it can affect the patient's overall quality of life.

Medical Consequences

A potential complication of patients with oropharyngeal dysphagia is aspiration pneumonia. The treatment of aspiration pneumonia is costly, and it is associated with increased length of stay in the hospital,[77] greater disability at 3 and 6 months,[77,78] and poorer nutritional status during hospitalization.[77] One study[77] found an increased mortality risk in stroke patients for whom swallowing was considered unsafe at 6 months' follow-up, whereas another study did not find this relation at 3 months.[78] Dehydration is a frequent adjunct in those with dysphagia after stroke.[77-79] Dehydration can lead to increased mental confusion and generalized organ system failure, both of which lead to greater decompensation of swallowing.[80] Dysphagia may lead to undernutrition, which adversely affects energy levels (ability to sustain a swallow), and if severe or chronic, compromises the immune system. Compromise to the immune system potentially delays healing and increases susceptibility to infection, sepsis, and death.[80]

Psychosocial Consequences

Oral ingestion of food and liquid is a pleasurable activity for most people. Social interactions often revolve around sharing a meal. "Let's have lunch, are you free for dinner, or can we meet for an early breakfast?" Having a piece of wedding cake, being offered an hors d'oeuvre at a party, enjoying a midnight snack, and going to one's favorite restaurant are all examples of common situations that

---

CLINICAL CASE EXAMPLE 1-2

A request for services was sent to the speech pathologist to evaluate a 70-year-old man for suspected dysphagia. He had lived in the nursing home for 2 years after a left brain stroke that left him with **aphasia** and poor mobility. He spent most of his day sitting in a wheelchair or in bed watching TV and was beginning to show evidence of **decubitus ulcers** on his coccyx. The nurses reported he was showing increased disinterest in his soft mechanical diet and was choking at most meals on his liquids. He rarely finished a meal. A review of his medical record revealed a consultation from the dietitian who noted that his **albumin** was 3.0 g/dL, he had lost 5% of his body weight in the past 2 weeks, and he was **hypernatremic.** Based on these parameters the dietitian concluded that the patient was undernourished and dehydrated and wondered if his previous history of dysphagia was contributory. The patient was examined in bed. He was able to follow one-step commands and name simple objects but was not oriented to time or place. During the examination the patient fell asleep every minute and the speech pathologist had to continually awaken him to maintain his attention and cooperation. An examination of his oral peripheral speech mechanism revealed a mild right facial weakness but otherwise was normal. Test swallows with various food items were delayed but without overt coughing. Tests with liquids revealed numerous choking episodes. Based on his physical examination and the results of his laboratory tests, it was concluded that his swallow may improve if he were properly hydrated and nourished, and that it was unlikely that hydration and nourishment could be accomplished by mouth because his alertness level was poor. Furthermore, his nutritional and hydration requirements would have to be elevated because of fluid loss from the decubitus ulcers. It also was likely that his ulcers would not heal unless his protein stores were improved. For this reason, a **nasogastric tube** was recommended with regular reevaluation of his laboratory values and mental status to make recommendations for possible return to oral feeding. It was hypothesized that, because he had been eating normally before this acute change, the dysphagia was most consistent with a change in metabolic status and not related to a change in his neurologic presentation.

---

require the ability to swallow. Swallowing difficulty therefore may limit the extent to which a person might socialize, leading to major changes in a normal lifestyle (see Practice Note 1-2). Fear of overt choking episodes and the associated discomfort might contribute to social isolation and accompanying depression. Spouses and family members are equally affected because of the potential social limitations dysphagia may precipitate. Even making subtle changes in dietary preferences to compensate for dysphagia

PRACTICE NOTE 1-2

I first met George at the New York Hospital in the out-patient clinic. He obviously was a man of means as he told stories of extensive travel. His swallowing evaluation that day revealed it was not safe for him to eat orally because of a specific muscle weakness, and a **gastrostomy** tube was recommended. He was noticeably upset by this recommendation. Because he was only 35 years old, we suspected that this might put an end to his life as a world traveler; however, George was not convinced. After his gastrostomy was placed, to my surprise he told me he had made arrangements for a 3-week trip to Spain and Portugal. He had arranged to ship cases of formula for his tube to each hotel on his travel itinerary before his departure. When he arrived in Spain, his formula was waiting. Normally he would have dined on bouillabaisse and fresh fish with a fine Chablis. Instead, he self-administered six cans of a liquid formula per day into his gastrostomy tube and continued to enjoy the ambience of Europe. He was determined not to let his severe pharyngeal dysphagia interfere with other aspects of his life.

may lead to feelings of discontent. Eating may no longer be pleasurable. It becomes an activity performed only for nourishment. The need for special preparations at mealtime provides additional stress. Special dietary supplements may be costly, often posing financial burdens.

Clinical Management

The care of patients in whom dysphagia is suspected usually begins with a basic process of identification in an attempt to answer the question of whether dysphagia is present. This process can be the result of a simple screening, such as watching a patient eat or drink small amounts of food. Such a screening might be done after a patient has had an acute neurologic event such as a stroke. Some patients begin to eat without screening because the risk factors for dysphagia are not present. An example might be a patient who has not had any swallowing difficulty in the past but required a feeding tube immediately after an operation for medical purposes and who has been cleared by the physician to return to oral ingestion. As the patient returns to eating, either the medical staff or the patient notices swallowing difficulty. Outpatients may report to their general practitioner that they are having swallowing difficulty. In all these situations a clinical evaluation of swallowing will be initiated.

Clinical Examination

The clinical evaluation should include a thorough review of the medical and psychosocial history (see Chapter 7). This is followed by a physical evaluation that includes a screening of mental status, an evaluation of the musculature of the head and neck, and, if appropriate, trial swallows of liquid, semisolid, and solid materials. If the clinical examination fails to adequately explain the patient's symptoms or requires more in-depth visualization of any phase of the swallowing sequence, an imaging study may be necessary. The clinical indicators for use of imaging assessment techniques have been published by ASHA.[81]

Imaging Examination

Imaging the **aerodigestive tract** most commonly is done by barium x-ray studies, direct visualization, and measurement of pressures within the aerodigestive tract during swallowing attempts. The most common x-ray technique that assesses the oral, pharyngeal, and cervical esophageal phases of swallowing is the modified barium swallow (videofluoroscopy). ASHA provides a statement of guidelines for speech-language pathologists (SLPs) who perform this procedure.[82] A standard barium swallow (**esophagram**) may be used to evaluate the esophagus. Direct visualization of the pharyngeal, laryngeal, and esophageal compartments is done by **endoscopy**. Guidelines for the performance and interpretation of the endoscopic evaluation of swallowing by SLPs are provided by ASHA.[83] Patient preparation and positioning for each of these studies vary according to focus of the anatomic region being examined. Pressure measurements during swallowing (**manometry**) are more routinely done for clinical purposes in the esophagus than in the mouth or pharynx. A full discussion of these and other instrumental techniques used in the evaluation of swallowing is provided in Chapter 8.

Treatment Options

Ideally, the clinical and imaging evaluations will lead to a treatment plan. The goal of most treatment plans is to ensure that the patient can consume enough food and liquid to remain nourished and hydrated and that the consumption of these materials does not pose a threat to airway safety resulting in aspiration pneumonia. If treatment is indicated, four main areas are considered: behavioral, dietary, medical, and surgical. These options may be applied as compensatory, rehabilitative, or preventive interventions (see Chapters 9, 10, and 15 for full discussion of each).

Behavioral interventions include engaging the patient in some change in swallowing behavior. Changes may take the form of simple compensations, such as a change in posture or eating rate; in rehabilitative strategies, such as teaching a patient a new way to swallow; or in strengthening muscles. Dietary interventions might include modifications of texture, taste, or volume. Medical interventions may include a change in medication negatively affecting mental status and swallow or the placement of a nasogastric feeding tube. Surgical interventions might include mobilization of a weak vocal fold or the placement of a gastrostomy tube. Combinations of these options are common; however, the timing of each intervention is patient dependent. A full discussion of treatment planning, including options and details of rationale and use, is presented in Chapters 9, 10, and 15.

WHO MANAGES DYSPHAGIA?

Patients who have disruptions in swallowing potentially involve many members of the medical community. Those whose dysphagia is related to the head and neck may see an otolaryngologist, dentist, SLP, or neurologist. To further define the disorder, these specialists often need the services of a radiologist. Those whose swallowing disorder may be of esophageal origin may require the services of a gastroenterologist. If the swallowing disorder is related to an acute respiratory condition, a patient may be under the care of a pulmonologist, pulmonary physical therapist, and respiratory therapist. If the swallowing disorder is related more to the process of feeding, an occupational therapist frequently is involved. If the swallowing disorder results in compromise to the nutritional system, a dietitian is consulted. While the patient is in the hospital, the nurse frequently is involved in the identification and treatment of the patient's swallowing disorder. In short, patients with swallowing disorders require the attention of many specialists who must work in concert to achieve swallowing safety and nutritional stability. The prominence of individual roles at any given time depends on the patient presentation.

Ideally, health care professionals who are concerned about the patient's swallowing safety and nutritional adequacy will work together toward the mutual goal of improving the patient's swallowing performance. Coordination of effort is important if timely results are to be achieved. Some medical centers have designated swallowing teams and swallowing team leaders. In many hospitals, the SLP assumes the role of swallowing team leader. The role each specialist plays on the team varies across settings. For instance, some gastroenterologists diagnose and treat swallowing problems that involve the esophagus, but disorders of the esophagus are not their special interest. Specific interest in the swallowing-impaired patient also varies. For instance, few radiologists have a specific interest in patients who report dysphagia. The result of this variance in interest and focus is that not all swallowing disorder teams are the same, and in some cases not all potential members are represented.

Speech-Language Pathologist

SLPs have taken a leading role in the management of patients with dysphagia related to poor oral and pharyngeal swallowing mechanics. In most centers, they coordinate the swallowing team and are frequently the first professional to perform a history and physical examination that is specific to oropharyngeal dysphagia. Based on these data they consult other members of the dysphagia team, obtain approval from the patient's attending physician for any additional testing or referrals, and integrate the rehabilitative components of the dysphagia treatment program. Only within the past 20 years have specific practice guidelines for managing dysphagia by SLPs been developed. These include an outline of the knowledge and skills needed to treat oropharyngeal dysphagia and the need to understand the esophageal components of swallowing to make appropriate medical referrals.[84]

SLPs were evaluating and treating articulation disorders of children with cerebral palsy as early as the 1940s. Because of the decompensation of the oromotor system in children with cerebral palsy, both speech and swallowing were affected; however, treatments specific to swallowing were not a routine part of care by the SLP. Working in a medical setting studying patients with Parkinson's disease in the late 1960s, Dr. Jeri Logemann found that videofluoroscopy was ideally suited to study patients' speech and swallowing skills. Soon this technique was used to study the effects of cancer in the head and neck on swallowing performance, and in 1976 at the American Speech and Hearing Association National Convention she presented one of the first papers by an SLP on the diagnosis and treatment of swallowing disorders after surgical procedures for cancer in the head and neck. That the paper was accepted at the convention was a monumental achievement because there was no recognized category for a paper on swallowing, and evaluating and treating patients with swallowing disorders was not within the accepted scope of practice for an SLP. This radical departure from the traditional role of the SLP raised more than a few eyebrows (see Practice Note 1-3).

PRACTICE NOTE 1-3

I well remember the reaction of ASHA in the 1970s and early 1980s to the acceptance of the role of the SLP in managing patients with dysphagia. It was the "new guard" versus the traditionalists. Letters to the editor flew back and forth, most arguing that this area of practice was potentially life threatening and SLPs did not have the medical background necessary to be competent. Treating patients with dysphagia labeled one as borderline heretic with threats of a breach of ethics. Today, patients with dysphagia dominate the caseloads of SLPs working in medical settings, and children with dysphagia are being managed in the public school setting. And both ASHA and the medical community have embraced the role of the SLP in these efforts.

As Logemann was beginning her distinguished career in dysphagia management, Dr. George Larsen, also working in a medical setting with adults, began to develop treatments specific to patients with neurogenic swallowing disorders. Because so many of his patients with speech and language disorders had accompanying swallowing dysfunction, he began to search the literature for relevant treatment approaches. He discovered a literature full of descriptions of how a person swallows but no mention of how to treat the impairment. Using his background in neurology and physiology, he began to develop treatment approaches and reported them in the literature. He wrote about appropriate postures[85] and the need for some patients to bring the swallowing sequence under volitional control.[86] He was convinced that the most successful approaches would result from a team effort, and he described the use of trained feeding volunteers as part of the process.[85] The momentum to evaluate and treat swallowing disorders in children and adults grew throughout the 1980s. The momentum was sustained by the publication of two texts by SLPs summarizing empirical evidence supporting the role of the SLP and emphasizing the need for collaboration among various medical professionals.[87,88] Both texts have undergone revisions. Today, SLPs have assumed a leadership role in providing care to children and adults with oropharyngeal dysphagia. SLPs are at the forefront of providing the research and educational components that support their clinical efforts. Miller and Groher[89] have described a more detailed history of the involvement of the SLP in the management of swallowing disorders (see Clinical Corner 1-4).

CLINICAL CORNER 1-4: ELECTRICAL STIMULATION

Dr. Miller and I followed Dr. Larsen to a patient with occult hydrocephalus who could not initiate a swallow. Results of examination of his oral peripheral mechanism were normal, and Dr. Larsen suggested that we needed to stimulate laryngeal elevation. The following day we watched in disbelief as Dr. Larsen approached the patient with a probe tip wrapped in gauze, dipped in saline solution, and attached to a primitive facial nerve stimulator. As he applied the electric current to the thyroid notch, a swallow was initiated and the patient continued to swallow without the assistance of the stimulation. Our collective elation that "treatment" could be so easy was quickly dampened when Dr. Larsen warned it could be dangerous to use such a technique with every patient because it could trigger **laryngospasm** and death. We learned two things that day: not all treatments are for every patient, and some treatments carry accompanying risk.

Critical Thinking
1. Why might an electrical current facilitate swallowing?
2. Name other types of medical treatments that carry risk.

Otolaryngologist

The otolaryngologist is skilled in the evaluation of the upper digestive tract. In particular, the use of endoscopy by otolaryngologists for direct visualization of the structures of the nasopharynx, oropharynx, pharynx, and larynx adds information relative to the structural, sensory, and motor aspects of the pharyngeal stage of swallowing. In patients with head and neck cancer who require surgery, otolaryngologists provide surgical and postsurgical management. In this regard, they must be sensitive not only to issues of cancer control, but also to the preservation of speech and swallowing functions. The otolaryngologist may be involved with the surgical placement and removal of a patient's **tracheostomy tube**. Because these tubes may interfere with normal swallowing, these specialists work with the dysphagia team to remove the tubes as soon as medically feasible.

Gastroenterologist

The gastroenterologist who participates on the swallowing disorders team usually has a special interest in the esophagus. Because primary esophageal disorders that precipitate dysphagia can have secondary effects on the pharyngeal and oral stages of swallowing, it is important to include the gastroenterologist in the evaluation of the patient who may appear to only have symptoms that relate to the oral or pharyngeal stages of swallowing (see Chapter 5). The gastroenterologist is familiar with the management of **gastroesophageal reflux disease (GERD),** or heartburn, a symptom that may be related to dysphagia. The gastroenterologist may use special sensors that measure the amount of acid content in the alimentary tract using a test called **24-hour pH monitoring**. The gastroenterologist may use manometry, or combined impedance and manometrics to measure esophageal motility and prescribe medications to improve esophageal motility or to control GERD. The use of esophageal endoscopy to make visual observations of the esophageal mucosa to rule out a stricture or cancer is a role of the gastroenterologist. The gastroenterologist is responsible for the nonsurgical placement of a feeding tube in the stomach called a **percutaneous endoscopic gastrostomy** tube.

Radiologist

The radiologist who may be a regular member of the swallowing disorders team often has a special interest in the gastrointestinal tract. Radiologists provide both dynamic (videofluorographic) and static (plain films) imaging of the aerodigestive tract and lung fields. Often these studies provide the diagnostic information that guides swallowing treatment. Special tests such as computed tomography performed after static images of the aerodigestive tract are done by a radiologist. The SLP frequently works in conjunction with the radiologist in performing the modified barium swallow (see Chapter 8). The interpretation of the modified barium swallow study is often done concurrently by the SLP and the radiologist.

Neurologist

Because the majority of patients with oropharyngeal dysphagia have swallowing impairment as a result of neurologic disease, the neurologist has an important role in the identification and subsequent management of swallowing problems. It is critical that patients with symptoms of dysphagia without a known cause be considered for evaluation by the neurologist. Some neurologic diseases that precipitate dysphagia can be treated with medication. Finding a cause also is important in providing the patient with an explanation for the dysphagia and in providing a prognosis for future complications.

Dentist

Patients with dysphagic symptoms may be identified first by the dentist during routine dental care. Of particular interest to the dentist are any oral-stage manifestations of swallowing disorders, such as problems with chewing, bolus formation, or dental disorders such as **osteoradionecrosis** that would make swallowing painful. The dental **prosthodontist** is skilled at making appliances for the oral cavity that can facilitate swallowing in patients who have had oral structures removed because of cancer. In Japan, the dentist is often the team leader in the care of patients with dysphagia. Dental hygienists may play a role by providing oral care that limits the presence of oral pathogen formation. If colonized, such pathogens when aspirated may precipitate pneumonia and secondary lung infection.

Nurse

The nurse has 24-hour responsibility for monitoring the patient's swallowing problem. Monitoring the amount of intake and recording it in the medical record is an important role for the nurse. Not only do nurses often identify problems during eating in patients in whom dysphagia is not suspected, but they also provide the guidance necessary to help the patient with identified dysphagia use recommended swallowing strategies. Other responsibilities include administering tube feedings, maintaining good oral hygiene, and assigning volunteers to assist selected patients at mealtime.

Dietitian

The dietitian assesses the patient's nutritional and hydration needs and monitors the patient's response to those needs.

Because dysphagia frequently affects a patient's nutrition and hydration status, and because the result of poor nutrition and hydration affects a patient's overall medical stability, it is important to involve the dietitian in the care plan for patients with dysphagia. Because dietitians frequently monitor mealtime activities, they may be the professional who initially detects a swallowing disorder. If specialized dysphagic diets are ordered for the patient, the dietitian may communicate with the food service to ensure that the special diet is prepared properly. If a patient is unable to eat orally, the dietitian may make a recommendation for a tube feeding. Guidelines for the amount and rate of tube feeding frequently are recommended by the dietitian. As patients return to oral feeding the SLP and dietitian closely monitor intake. As oral feeding improves, the dietitian adjusts the amount of tube feeding to appropriate levels.[90]

Occupational Therapist

The occupational therapist is skilled in retraining the patient to self-feed. If the patient is unable to self-feed because of weakness or incoordination, the occupational therapist needs to be involved in the patient's care. Special adaptive feeding devices, such as a **plate guard** or built-up utensils for easier grasping, are ordered by the occupational therapist to assist the patient in achieving feeding independence. In some medical centers, the SLP and occupational therapist work closely with infants in the neonatal intensive care unit (NICU).

Neurodevelopmental Specialist

The NICU setting can influence the infant's brain development and organization as well as the parent-infant relationship. The neurodevelopmental specialist (NDS) is keenly aware of this relationship and will tailor the infant's care to individual needs. An NDS may be a speech pathologist or occupational therapist who has specialized in assisting the premature infant in developmental growth by fostering supportive care during the infant's nervous system development. Neurodevelopmental care includes, but is not limited to, proper infant positioning to support neurodevelopmental tone and maturation. Often it is important to regulate to tolerance the infant's visual, tactile, and auditory stimulation. Feeding is one of the most difficult tasks in which a premature infant can succeed. The NDS provides continued assessment regarding the timing and safety of the infant's oral feedings by breast or bottle. The NDS also monitors the infant's physiologic and behavioral responses to the environment and fosters a positive outcome.

Pulmonologist and Respiratory Therapist

Although the pulmonologist may not be a regular member of the dysphagia team, patients of pulmonologists frequently have swallowing disorders that require management by the swallowing team. Patients with respiratory disorders that require tracheostomy and **ventilatory** support (respirators) often have accompanying swallowing difficulty. Working with the respiratory therapist and pulmonologist to improve pulmonary toilet is an important step toward **decannulation**. Removing a patient's respiratory supports often is a prerequisite for improving the swallowing response.

CLINICAL CASE EXAMPLE 1-3

The SLP was called by the thoracic surgeon to the intensive care unit for a consultation. Her patient had just undergone **cardiac** bypass surgery and had respiratory complications requiring the placement of a tracheostomy tube. The patient was now medically stable and was ready to resume oral feeding. The SLP consulted with the respiratory therapist, who mentioned that the patient still required some oxygenation by facial mask for short periods during the day. After noting those times, the SLP returned when the mask was not in use because it might potentially interfere with the evaluation. On physical evaluation the patient had reduced tongue strength and could make a weak, breathy voice only when the tracheotomy tube was occluded. She had a nasogastric tube in place for nutritional purposes. During the evaluation the dietitian came in and told the SLP that the patient was not tolerating the feeding given by nasogastric tube and that it would be beneficial for the patient to begin to eat orally because some of those complications could be avoided. The SLP gave the patient small amounts of ice chips and water, as well as gelatin and pudding. The patient showed delayed swallowing of all materials and a weak cough on the liquids. The SLP believed that the patient might be at risk for aspiration because of pharyngeal weakness that may have involved the true vocal fold. She believed an imaging study that would allow her to observe the pharyngeal stage of swallow would be appropriate and that swallowing endoscopy would be the test of choice because it could be accomplished at the patient's bedside. She received approval for the study from the consulting physician and the test was performed the same day. Swallowing endoscopy revealed that during the coughing episodes the patient was protecting her airway; however, there appeared to be some weakness in the left true vocal fold. She recommended that the patient start a special dysphagic diet and communicated that to the dietitian, who made the arrangements. The otolaryngologist was consulted for his opinion on whether any intervention would be appropriate for the vocal fold weakness. The SLP designed specific swallowing instructions and shared them with the patient and nursing staff. This case is a good example of how many disciplines can be involved in caring for a patient who has dysphagia.

LEVELS OF CARE

The prevalence, cause, and type of swallowing disorder that might be encountered depend in part on the setting in which the patient is seen. Correspondingly, the role of each professional may be different, or access to some medical specialties may not be available. For instance, it is rare for a gastroenterologist to have a full-time appointment in a nursing home facility or that a radiologist would be on staff in that facility. Traditionally, levels of care are divided into five categories: acute, **subacute**, rehabilitation, **skilled nursing**, and **home health**.

Acute Care Setting

In a survey of two acute care hospitals, Groher and Bukatman[20] found the prevalence of swallowing-related disorders to be 13%. The majority of these patients were found in the intensive care units and the neurology and neurosurgery units. Owing to the acute nature of their illness, patients in the acute care setting frequently have multiple medical complications, require intubation tubes connected to ventilators, have tracheostomy tubes in place, require feeding tubes for nutrition, and have frequent changes in their physical and mental status. Because their stay in the hospital may be short (2 to 5 days), their swallowing needs must be addressed rapidly. Frequently there is not sufficient time or patient cooperation because of mental status to order sophisticated laboratory tests. In this circumstance, the clinician may have to rely on the history and clinical evaluation to make a diagnosis and establish a treatment plan. If an instrumental evaluation is recommended, care must be given to scheduling. If the patient is able to cooperate with laboratory testing and is a candidate to proceed for further rehabilitation, his or her future care is facilitated if the acute care clinician can document the swallowing disorder with an imaging technique such as videofluoroscopy or endoscopy.

Neonatal Intensive Care Unit

Children born prematurely often must stay in the hospital for extended periods in the NICU. Specialized interventions for premature newborns such as improved systems of delivering respiratory support have resulted in higher survival rates of low birth weight infants. In the 1980s, the concept of integrated developmental care was introduced to minimize the potential for emotional and neurodevelopmental disorders after discharge. This type of care emphasizes the coordinated efforts of nurses, physicians, therapists, and other care providers toward common goals, with each discipline supporting the other. This type of care also recognizes issues of parent–child separation and the atypical environment of a hospital on the child's development.

More recently, infants admitted to the NICU are managed by "cluster care." Before the availability of cluster care, infants received medical care at any hour during the day. However, the cluster care concept allows infants to sleep for 3 hours, after which time they are awakened for all their care, including feeding, diaper changes, and needed tests. Cluster care allows the infant to regularize his or her schedule, similar to what would occur outside the hospital environment.

Subacute Care Setting

Patients admitted to subacute care usually are not ready for a strenuous rehabilitation program. They may require additional medical monitoring but not the type of costly care of an acute admission associated with intensive care. If a swallowing treatment goal was formulated in the acute setting, the action plan to achieve that goal is implemented in the subacute unit. For instance, if the goal was to try to wean a patient from the tracheostomy tube as a way to ensure swallowing safety, the swallowing team would work toward that goal. If a patient continued to require tube feeding after leaving the acute care unit, a goal of the swallowing team in the subacute unit might be to begin restoring oral **alimentation**. Patients may stay in the subacute unit from 5 to 28 days. After this admission, they may be discharged home, to a rehabilitation facility, or to a **skilled nursing facility**.

Rehabilitation Setting

Patients who enter rehabilitation settings usually are judged to have the physical stamina needed to complete a full day of tasks oriented toward restoring lost function. In most cases, the patient also will be able to learn new information. For those with swallowing impairment, it may mean they need to learn or solidify their learning of new swallowing strategies. The role of the speech pathologist is to teach the patient swallowing strategies (see Chapters 10 and 15). This may include special maneuvers or postures. It also may entail specialized diets. Frequently, the goal in the rehabilitation setting as it pertains to swallowing is to return the patient to a dietary level that is as near to normal as possible while ensuring swallowing safety. Swallowing safety may be defined as the maintenance of nutrition and hydration without medical complications. Not only is it considered medically unsafe for a patient to get food or fluid in the lungs, but it is also unsafe to not get sufficient nutrition and hydration to maintain normal bodily functions. For instance, lack of proper nutrition and hydration can lead to excessive fatigue, mental status changes, poor wound healing, anorexia, and a greater chance of developing infections. After a 1-month period of successful rehabilitation, the patient usually is discharged home. Those in whom medical complications develop during rehabilitation or who do not improve to a level of partial independence may be discharged to a skilled nursing facility.

Skilled Nursing Facility

Patients who enter skilled nursing facilities usually have either not responded to attempts at rehabilitation, are not candidates for rehabilitation after their acute hospitalization, are too ill to be at home, or have chronic medical conditions that require monitoring in a structured environment. The prevalence of swallowing disorders in this setting has been reported to be as high as 60%.[13] The high prevalence in this setting is because the patients have multiple medical problems that predispose them to dysphagia. The majority, for instance, may have a neurologic disease that has compromised the swallowing musculature or has interfered with the cortical controls needed to complete the swallowing sequence. Their swallowing disorders are chronic. Some patients will have seen some recovery in their dysphagia, whereas others will continue to rely on tube feedings. For those who recover, it is important to help them maintain their skills. Those who must rely on tube feedings after their hospital stay will require reevaluation for the possibility of returning to oral feeding. For some, returning to oral alimentation will not be possible. Because of the potential for patients in this setting to be medically fragile, it is easy to decompensate their swallowing skills by a slight change in medical status, rather than a new, major event such as stroke. An example of this phenomenon might be a patient who is not swallowing a sufficient amount of liquids, who may then develop a urinary tract infection that results in a fever with generalized fatigue, anorexia, and a disinterest in eating. In this situation, the patient may not be ingesting enough calories to be able to sustain the strength needed to produce a safe swallow throughout the entire meal. As a consequence of fatigue, the patient is more likely to show signs of dysphagia.

Another example might be a patient who has been eating well but whose medications were changed. The unwanted side effect from the medication change could negatively affect the nervous system to create a problem with motor movement, and swallowing is secondarily affected. For example, medications that create sedative effects are capable of decompensating an already fragile swallow by slowing motor movement and interfering with the cortical controls necessary to complete an entire meal. The potential for fluctuations in metabolism in this patient population often make it difficult to establish a single factor that precipitated the dysphagia.

It is known that patients in skilled nursing facilities usually are in older age cohorts. Not only do they endure the effects of diseases that result in dysphagia commonly found in older persons (e.g., stroke, Parkinson's disease), but they also have impairments in swallowing as a result of the aging process. Change in taste perception and in the strength and speed of the swallowing muscles are examples of these alterations. The speech pathologist working in the skilled nursing facility is kept busy managing the large number of patients with swallowing disorders. Many patients with dysphagia are able to eat safely only if they are at the proper dietary level and only if they are following the recommended feeding strategies. Any change in baseline metabolism or any new neurologic insult may decompensate their swallowing skills so that they are at risk for developing medical complications. Many times the focus of therapeutic effort for the SLP working in the skilled nursing facility is one of prevention—attempting to keep patients as safe as possible while eating, even in the circumstance of suspected dysphagia. Such preventive efforts not only may require direct intervention with behavioral and dietary treatment strategies, but also entail monitoring of mealtime activities to ensure that patients who are at risk of aspiration are following the prescribed dysphagia treatment plan.

Often the mental or physical status of patients in the skilled nursing environment interferes with their ability to cooperate with a formal dysphagia evaluation. Clinicians must rely on a combination of the medical history and detailed observations of each meal to establish the treatment plan. If the patient is not eating orally, the clinician often must rely on the physical examination and on his or her judgment of how well the patient managed attempts at oral ingestion as part of that examination. The examination will be limited further by poor access to modified barium swallow studies or other laboratory investigations. Transportation of patients to receive these tests presents another challenge because chronically ill patients are difficult to move.

The chronic medical conditions of patients in skilled nursing facilities often are life threatening. For this reason, patients and their families may execute an **advance directive** (see Chapter 11). The advance directive is a statement executed by the patient or family (if they hold medical power of attorney) of their desires and wishes regarding their medical care in life-threatening situations, such as whether the patient would want to be resuscitated for cardiac arrest. Part of this directive may pertain to their wishes to sustain nutrition, especially when the support for nutrition may involve feeding tubes. Patients may elect to not be fed by a feeding tube despite the risk of aspiration and life-threatening pneumonia. In these cases, the role of the swallowing clinician is to recommend the safest mode of ingestion, making sure that the patient and family understand the potential risks.

Home Health

Patients who have left the hospital or the rehabilitation setting for home may require additional monitoring or direct

---

CLINICAL CORNER 1-5: INTERDISCIPLINARY COOPERATION

An 86-year-old man who had been living in a nursing home was admitted to the hospital with a suspected right brain stroke. He was confused on admission, and the attending physician did not think it was safe for him to eat orally so a nasogastric tube was placed. At the nursing home he was eating a modified soft diet because his teeth were in poor repair. He had a past history of GERD and **Barrett's esophagitis**. After 2 days a swallowing evaluation was ordered before he was allowed to resume oral feeding.

Critical Thinking

1. How many medical disciplines might become involved with this patient? Who and why?
2. What are the chances that he will be dysphagic based on his history? Are age and prior living setting considerations in this case? How might these facts affect the diagnosis and treatment?
3. Are there any special issues revolving around which side of the brain was injured that might relate to dysphagia?

---

treatment from therapists who perform their responsibilities in the patient's home environment. Patients who are unable to swallow should receive regular reevaluations for attempts at oral feeding unless oral feeding is contraindicated by the medical care team. Most often, the clinician responsible for managing the swallowing disorder in the home environment is ensuring that the patient is following the swallowing strategies or has improved to a point at which consideration should be given to changing the dietary level. These changes often are made in consultation with the patient and family and are based on the physical examination and observations of eating (review Clinical Corner 1-5).

TAKE HOME NOTES

1. Dysphagia is a symptom of a disease, not a primary disease. It is characterized by a delay or misdirection of something swallowed as food moves from the mouth to the stomach. It has both medical and psychosocial consequences on a patient's quality of life.
2. A *feeding disorder* usually refers to the process of food transport. An eating disorder may not be related to a swallowing disorder.
3. The prevalence of dysphagia is highest in patients with neurologic disease.
4. Patients in acute care intensive care units and those in skilled nursing facilities tend to be at highest risk for dysphagia.
5. There may not be a clear link between dysphagic symptoms and the patient's primary medical diagnosis in patients who reside in skilled nursing facilities.

6. Patients in skilled nursing facilities are medically fragile, and their swallowing response can be easily decompensated by fatigue or an acute medical condition such as an infection.
7. Aspiration of liquid and food is the consequence of those materials entering the airway below the level of the vocal folds.
8. Aspiration of liquid or food may or may not produce a lung infection known as aspiration pneumonia.
9. Respiratory impairments such as those requiring an endotracheal tube or tracheostomy tube also interfere with swallowing.
10. The SLP frequently is the coordinator of the swallowing team and therefore needs to have an understanding of each team member's perspective of the dysphagic patient. Many specialists could become involved in the care of a patient with dysphagia.
11. The evolution of the NICU has provided advanced technologies to maintain survival for infants as young as 23 weeks' gestational age. The feeding specialist in the NICU often is skilled in neurodevelopmental studies.

REFERENCES

1. *Taber's cyclopedic medical dictionary*, Philadelphia, 1993, F.A. Davis.
2. Achem SR, Devault KR: Dysphagia in aging. *J Clin Gastroenterol* 39:357, 2005.
3. Tanner DC: *Case studies in communicative sciences and disorders*, Columbus, OH, 2006, Pearson Prentice Hall.
4. Barofsky I, Fontaine KR: Do psychogenic dysphagia patients have an eating disorder? *Dysphagia* 13:24, 1998.
5. Agency for Health Care Policy and Research: *Diagnosis and treatment of swallowing disorders (dysphagia) in acute-care stroke patients (evidence report/technology assessment No. 8)*, Rockville, MD, 1999, Agency for Health Care Policy and Research.
6. Doggett DL, Tappe KA, Mitchell MD, et al: Prevention of pneumonia in elderly stroke patients by systematic diagnosis and treatment of dysphagia: an evidence-based comprehensive analysis of the literature. *Dysphagia* 16:279, 2001.
7. American Speech-Language-Hearing Association: *Ad Hoc Committee on Dysphagia Report,* April: 57, 1987. Available at www.asha.org.
8. Kuhlemeier K: Epidemiology and dysphagia. *Dysphagia* 9:209, 1994.
9. Bloem BR, Lagaay AM, van Beek W, et al: Prevalence of subjective dysphagia in community residents aged over 87. *Br Med J* 300:721, 1990.
10. Lindgren S, Janzon L: Prevalence of swallowing complaints and clinical findings among 50-70 year old men and women in an urban population. *Dysphagia* 6:187, 1991.
11. Lundquist A, Olsson R, Ekberg O: Clinical and radiologic evaluation reveals high prevalence of abnormalities in young adults with dysphagia. *Dysphagia* 13:202, 1998.
12. Lee A, Sitoh YY, Lien PK, et al: Swallowing impairment and feeding dependency in the hospitalized elderly. *Ann Acad Med Singapore* 28:371, 1999.
13. Siebens H, Trupe E, Siebens A, et al: Correlates and consequences of eating dependency in the institutionalized elderly. *J Am Geriatr Soc* 34:192, 1986.
14. Guijarro Silveira LJ, Garcia VD, Fernandez NM, et al: Disfagia orofaringea en ancianos ingresados en una unidad de convalecencia. *Nutr Hosp* 26:501, 2011.
15. Park YH, Hae-Ra H, Faan BMO, et al: Prevalence and associated factors of dysphagia in nursing home residents. *Geriatr Nurs (Minneap)* 34:212, 2013.
16. Nogueira D, Reis E: Swallowing disorders in nursing home residents: how can the problem be explained? *Clin Interv Aging* 8:221, 2013.
17. Steele CM, Greenwood C, Ens I, et al: Mealtime difficulties in a home for the aged: not just dysphagia. *Dysphagia* 12:43, 1997.
18. Croghan JE, Burke EM, Caplan S, et al: Pilot study of 12 month outcomes of nursing home patients with aspiration on videofluoroscopy. *Dysphagia* 9:141, 1994.
19. Layne KA, Losinski DS, Zenner PM, et al: Using the Fleming Index of Dysphagia to establish prevalence. *Dysphagia* 4:39, 1989.
20. Groher ME, Bukatman R: The prevalence of swallowing disorders in two teaching hospitals. *Dysphagia* 1:3, 1986.
21. Cherney LR: Dysphagia in adults with neurologic disorders: an overview. In Cherney LR, editor: *Clinical management of dysphagia in adults and children*, Gaithersburg, MD, 1994, Aspen.
22. Smithard DG, O'Neill PA, England R, et al: The natural history of dysphagia following a stroke. *Dysphagia* 12:188, 1997.
23. Gordon C, Langton HR, Wade DT: Dysphagia in acute stroke. *Br Med J* 295:411, 1987.
24. Mann G, Hankey GJ, Cameron D: Swallowing function after stroke—prognosis and prognostic factors at 6 months. *Stroke* 30:744, 1999.
25. Daniels SK, Brailey K, Priestly DH, et al: Aspiration in patients with acute stroke. *Arch Phys Med Rehabil* 79:14, 1998.
26. Gonzalez-Fernandez M, Kuhlemeier KV, Palmer JB: Racial disparities in the development of dysphagia after stroke: analysis of the California (MIRCal) and New York (SPARCS) inpatient databases. *Arch Phys Med Rehabil* 89:1358, 2008.
27. Pauloski BR, Rademaker AW, Logemann JA, et al: Pretreatment swallowing function in patients with head and neck cancer. *Head Neck* 22:474, 2000.
28. Hillman RE, Walsh MJ, Wolf GT, et al: Functional outcomes following treatment for advanced laryngeal cancer. *Ann Otol Rhinol Laryngol* 107:2, 1998.
29. Maclean J, Cotton S, Perry A: Dysphagia following total laryngectomy: the effect on quality of life, functioning, and psychological well-being. *Dysphagia* 24:314, 2009.
30. Beckhardt RN, Murray JG, Ford CN, et al: Factors influencing functional outcome in supraglottic laryngectomy. *Head Neck* 16:232, 1994.
31. Roh JL, Kim DH, Park CI: Voice, swallowing and quality of life in patients after transoral laser surgery for supraglottic carcinoma. *J Surg Oncol* 98:184, 2008.
32. Garcia-Peris P, Paron L, Velasco C, et al: Long-term prevalence of oropharyngeal dysphagia in head and neck cancer patients: impact on quality of life. *Clin Nutr* 26:710, 2007.
33. McConnel FM, Logemann JA, Rademaker AW, et al: Surgical variables affecting postoperative swallowing efficiency in oral cancer patients: a pilot study. *Laryngoscope* 104:87, 1994.
34. Field LH, Weiss CJ: Dysphagia with head injury. *Brain Inj* 3:19, 1989.

35. Yorkston KM, Honsinger MJ, Matsuda PM, et al: The relationship between speech and swallowing disorders in head-injured patients. *J Head Trauma Rehabil* 4:1, 1989.

36. Winstein CJ: Neurogenic dysphagia: frequency, progression, and outcome in adults following head injury. *Phys Ther* 63:1992, 1983.

37. Cherney LR, Halpern AS: Recovery of oral nutrition after head injury in adults. *J Head Trauma Rehabil* 4:42, 1989.

38. Lazarus C, Logemann JA: Swallowing disorders in closed head trauma patients. *Arch Phys Med Rehabil* 68:79, 1987.

39. Mandaville A, Ray A, Robertson H, et al: A retrospective review of swallow dysfunction in patients with severe traumatic brain injury. *Dysphagia* 29:310, 2014.

40. Lieberman AN, Horowitz L, Redmond P, et al: Dysphagia in Parkinson's disease. *Am J Gastroenterol* 74:157, 1980.

41. Edwards LL, Pfeiffer RF, Quigley EMM, et al: Gastrointestinal symptoms in Parkinson's disease. *Mov Disord* 6:151, 1991.

42. Bushmann M, Dobmeyer SM, Leeker L, et al: Swallowing abnormalities and their response to treatment in Parkinson's disease. *Neurology* 39:1309, 1989.

43. Leopold NA, Kagel MC: Prepharyngeal dysphagia in Parkinson's disease. *Dysphagia* 11:14, 1996.

44. Walker RN, Dunn JR, Gray WK: Self-reported dysphagia and its correlates within a prevalent population of people with Parkinson's disease. *Dysphagia* 26:92, 2011.

45. Sung HY, Kim JS, Lee KS, et al: The prevalence and patterns of pharyngoesophageal dysmotility in patients with early stage Parkinson's disease. *Mov Disord* 25:2361, 2010.

46. Kalf JG, de Swart BJM, Bloem JM, et al: Prevalence of oropharyngeal dysphagia in Parkinson's disease: a meta-analysis. *Parkinsonism Relat Disord* 18:311, 2011.

47. Bine JE, Frank EM, McDade HL: Dysphagia and dementia in subjects with Parkinson's disease. *Dysphagia* 10:160, 1995.

48. Caroscio JT, Mulvihill MN, Sterling R: Amyotrophic lateral sclerosis: its natural history. *Neurol Clin* 5:1, 1987.

49. Mulder DS: *The diagnosis and treatment of amyotrophic lateral sclerosis*, Boston, 1980, Houghton Mifflin.

50. Fattori B, Grosso M, Bongioanni P, et al: Assessment of swallowing by oropharyngoesophageal scintigraphy in patients with amyotrophic lateral sclerosis. *Dysphagia* 21:280, 2006.

51. Hillel AD, Miller RM: Bulbar amyotrophic lateral sclerosis: patterns of progression and clinical management. *Head Neck* 11:51, 1989.

52. Hartelius L, Svensson P: Speech and swallowing symptoms associated with Parkinson's disease and multiple sclerosis: a survey. *Folia Phoniatr Logop* 46:9, 1994.

53. Restivo DA, Marchese-Ragona R, Patti F: Management of swallowing disorders in multiple sclerosis. *Neurol Sci* 4:338, 2006.

54. Calcagno P, Ruoppolo G, Grasso M, et al: Dysphagia in multiple sclerosis—prevalence and prognostic factors. *Acta Neurol Scand* 105:40, 2002.

55. DePauw A, Dejaeger E, D'hooghe B, et al: Dysphagia in multiple sclerosis. *Clin Neurol Neurosurg* 104:345, 2002.

56. Murray JP: Deglutition in myasthenia gravis. *Br J Radiol* 35:43, 1962.

57. Restivo DA, Marchese R, Staffieri A, et al: Successful botulinum toxin treatment of dysphagia in oropharyngeal myotonic dystrophy. *Gastroenterology* 199:1416, 2000.

58. Nozaki S, Umaki Y, Sugishita S, et al: Videofluorographic assessment of swallowing function in patients with Duchenne muscular dystrophy. *Clin Neurol (Rinsho Shinkeigaku)* 47:407, 2007.

59. Bellini M, Biagi S, Stasi C, et al: Gastrointestinal manifestation in myotonic muscular dystrophy. *World J Gastroenterol* 12:1821, 2006.

60. Oh TH, Brumfield TH, Hoskin KA, et al: Dysphagia in inflammatory myopathy: clinical characteristics, treatment strategies, and outcome in 62 patients. *Mayo Clin Proc* 82:441, 2007.

61. Langdon CP, Mulcahy K, Shepherd K, et al: Pharyngeal dysphagia in inflammatory muscle diseases resulting from impaired suprahyoid musculature. *Dysphagia* 27:408, 2012.

62. Geterude A, Bake B, Bjelle A: Swallowing problems in rheumatoid arthritis. *Acta Otolaryngol* 111:1153, 1991.

63. Ekberg O, Redlund-Johnell I, Sjoblom KG: Pharyngeal function in patients with rheumatoid arthritis. *Acta Radiol* 28:35, 1987.

64. Fulp SR, Castell DO: Scleroderma esophagus. *Dysphagia* 5:101, 1990.

65. Zamost BJ, Hirschber J, Ippoliti AF, et al: Esophagitis in scleroderma: prevalence and risk factors. *Gastroenterology* 92:421, 1987.

66. Grande L, Lacima G, Ros E, et al: Esophageal motor function in primary Sjögren's syndrome. *Am J Gastroenterol* 88:378, 1993.

67. Alagiakrishnan K, Bhanji RA, Kurian M: Evaluation and management of oropharyngeal dysphagia in different types of dementia: a systematic review. *Arch Gerontol Geriatr* 56:1, 2013.

68. Leslie P, Crawford H, Wilkinson H: People with a learning disability and dysphagia: a Cinderella population. *Dysphagia* 24:103, 2009.

69. Chadwick DD, Jolliffe J: A descriptive investigation of dysphagia in adults with intellectual disabilities. *J Intel Disabil Res* 53:29, 2009.

70. Smith CH, Teo Y, Simpson S: An observational study of adults with Down syndrome eating independently. *Dysphagia* 29:52, 2014.

71. O'Neill AC, Richter GT: Pharyngeal dysphagia in children with Down syndrome. *Otolaryngol Head Neck Surg* 149:146, 2013.

72. Aldridge KJ, Taylor NF: Dysphagia is a common and serious problem for adults with mental illness: a systematic review. *Dysphagia* 27:124, 2012.

73. Baijens LWJ, Koetsenruijter K, Pilz W: Diagnosis and treatment of phagophobia: a review. *Dysphagia* 28:260, 2013.

74. Martin JA, Hamilton BE, Sutton P, et al: *Births: final data for 2002* (National Vital Statistics Report, vol 52, no 10), Hyattsville, MD, 2003, National Center for Health Statistics.

75. Arvedson J, Brodsky L: *Pediatric swallowing and feeding: assessment and management*, ed 2, San Diego, 1993, Singular.

76. Shem KL, Castillo K, Wong SL, et al: Diagnostic accuracy of bedside swallow evaluation versus videofluoroscopy to assess dysphagia in individuals with tetraplegia. *Phys Med Rehabil* 4:283, 2012.

77. Smithard DG, O'Neill PA, Park C, et al: Complications and outcome after acute stroke. Does dysphagia matter? *Stroke* 27:1200, 1996.

78. Kidd D, Lawson J, Nesbitt R, et al: The natural history and clinical consequences of aspiration in acute stroke. *Q J Med* 88:409, 1995.

79. DePippo KL, Holas MA, Reding MJ, et al: The Burke Dysphagia Screening Test. *Stroke* 24:173, 1993.

80. Andreoli TE, Carpenter CCJ, Griggs RC, et al: *Cecil essentials of medicine*, ed 6, Philadelphia, 2004, WB Saunders.

81. American Speech-Language-Hearing Association: *Clinical indicators for instrumental assessment of dysphagia: guidelines, ASHA 2002 Desk Reference*, Rockville Pike, MD, 2002, ASHA.

82. American Speech-Language-Hearing Association: Guidelines for speech-language pathologists performing videofluoroscopic swallowing studies. *ASHA Suppl* 24:178, 2004.

83. American Speech-Language-Hearing Association: *The role of the speech-language pathologist in the performance and interpretation*

of endoscopic evaluation of swallowing, technical report, Rockville Pike, MD, 2005, ASHA.

84. American Speech-Language-Hearing Association: Knowledge and skills for speech-language pathologists providing services to individuals with swallowing and/or feeding disorders. *ASHA Suppl* 22:81, 2002.

85. Larsen GL: Rehabilitation of dysphagia: mechanica, paralytica, pseudobulbar. *J Neurosurg Nurs* 8:14, 1976.

86. Larsen GL: Rehabilitation for dysphagia paralytica. *J Speech Hear Disord* 37:187, 1972.

87. Logemann JA: *Evaluation and treatment of swallowing disorders*, San Diego, 1983, College-Hill Press.

88. Groher ME, editor: *Dysphagia: diagnosis and management*, Stoneham, MA, 1984, Butterworth.

89. Miller RM, Groher ME: Speech-language pathology and dysphagia: a brief historical perspective. *Dysphagia* 8:180, 1993.

90. Heiss CJ, Goldberg L, Dzarnoski M: Registered dietitians and speech-language pathologists: an important partnership in dysphagia management. *J Am Dietetic Assn* 110:1291, 2010.

CHAPTER 2

Normal Swallowing in Adults

Michael E. Groher

To view additional case videos and content, please visit the evolve website.

OBJECTIVES

1. Define the key anatomic structures involved in swallowing.
2. Define the groups of muscles that participate in swallowing.
3. Define the peripheral and central neurologic controls for swallowing.
4. Discuss the key physiologic components that occur when moving a bolus from the mouth to the stomach.
5. Discuss how normal swallowing is affected by bolus type and delivery.
6. Describe swallowing associated with normal aging.

Normal swallowing includes an integrated, interdependent group of complex feeding behaviors emerging from interacting cranial nerves of the brainstem and governed by neural regulatory mechanisms in the medulla, as well as in sensorimotor and limbic cortical systems. Healthy individuals simultaneously perform the sequential sensory and motor patterns of mastication and swallowing with little effort and conscious awareness. For purposes of simplification, such sensory-guided discriminatory feeding and sensory-cued, stereotyped swallowing behaviors usually are divided into four stages (Practice Note 2-1): (1) the oral preparatory stage, in which food is masticated in preparation for transfer; (2) the oral stage, which entails the transfer of material from the mouth to the oropharynx; (3) the pharyngeal stage, in which material is transported away from the oropharynx, around an occluded **laryngeal vestibule**, and through a relaxed cricopharyngeus muscle into the upper esophagus; and (4) the esophageal stage, in which material is transported through the esophagus into the gastric cardia. An additional stage of swallowing that precedes the oral stage has been proposed by Leopold and Kagel,[1] who argue that visual appreciation of the bolus before its placement in the oral cavity may send a cognitive message that may help stimulate saliva during bolus preparation.

Knowledge of the anatomic and physiologic aspects of this interdependent group of voluntary and involuntary behaviors requires detailed study if the goal is to rehabilitate persons with dysphagia, which may be caused by a wide array of neurologic and structural impairments resulting from injury or disease affecting the central nervous system, cranial nerves, and muscles.

PRACTICE NOTE 2-1

A single bolus of varying texture and size can be chewed and swallowed while a person holds a conversation, and at the same time a beverage may be imbibed while various portions of the more solid food are held in the mouth. With relaxation of the pharyngeal constrictors, a sword can be passed from the pharynx through the cricopharyngeal muscle (not recommended without practice) and, with effort, a person can swallow solids while standing on his or her head!

NORMAL ANATOMY

The oral cavity extends from the lips anteriorly to the nasopharynx posteriorly and contains the tongue, gums, and teeth. The oral cavity is separated from the nasal cavity by the bony palate and velum (soft palate). It is composed of a highly mobile lower jaw, or mandible, consisting of a U-shaped body containing important ridges for muscle attachments. The upper jaw, or maxilla, meets the zygomatic or cheek bone and is adjoined by the L-shaped palatine bones, lying posterior to the nasal cavity. The perpendicular part of the palatines forms the back of the nasal cavity, whereas the horizontal part forms the back of the bony palate. The velum and posterior nasopharyngeal wall seal and open communication between the nasal and oral cavities during swallowing and respiratory behaviors, respectively. The nasopharynx lies above the velum, and the oropharynx lies posterior to the mouth. The pharynx extends below to the esophagus; its inferior portion is called the hypopharynx and is separated from the esophagus by the cricopharyngeal muscle (Figure 2-1). The cartilaginous larynx lies anterior to the hypopharynx at the upper end of the trachea, suspended by muscles attached to the hyoid bone. The cricoid cartilage lies above the trachea, with the thyroid cartilage above it. Both are suspended from muscles attached to the hyoid bone, which itself is suspended between the jaw, tongue, and sternum by suprahyoid and infrahyoid musculature.

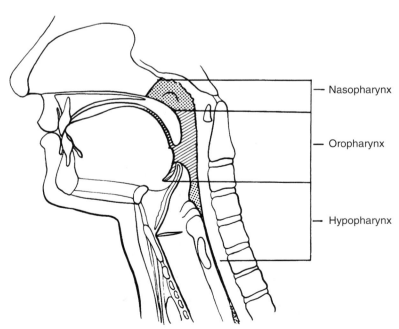

— Nasopharynx

— Oropharynx

— Hypopharynx

FIGURE 2-1   Lateral view of the anatomy of the head and neck with demarcations of three major regions: nasopharynx, oropharynx, and hypopharynx.

The respiratory system is protected during pharyngeal swallow by occlusive muscular constriction of the laryngeal vestibule and downward displacement of the epiglottis. The true vocal cords are at the inferior margin of the **laryngeal ventricle** and are attached anteriorly at the thyroid cartilage and posteriorly at the arytenoid cartilages. The vestibular (false) vocal folds separate the ventricle and the vestibule. The epiglottis extends from the base of the tongue into the pharyngeal cavity.

The valleculae are lateral recesses at the base of the tongue on each side of the epiglottis. The piriform sinuses are lateral recesses between the larynx and the anterior hypopharyngeal wall (Figure 2-2). These recesses serve as important anatomic landmarks in the videoradiographic assessment of pharyngeal swallow. Figure 2-3 shows a lateral view of the key anatomic structures in the region of the head and neck.

Oral Preparatory Stage

The mandibular branch of the trigeminal nerve (cranial nerve [CN] V) innervates the principal muscles for chewing behaviors. The primary muscles of chewing are the masseter, temporalis, and pterygoid muscles, which attach to the sphenoid wing of the temporal bone. The masseter closes the jaw while the temporalis moves it up, forward, or backward (Table 2-1). The medial pterygoid muscles work bilaterally to elevate the mandible while they shift the jaw to the opposite side unilaterally. The lateral pterygoid muscles work together, pulling down or forward while moving the jaw or chin to the opposite side unilaterally. Both sets of pterygoid muscles cooperate to grind in mastication.

The facial nerve (CN VII) innervates lower facial muscles attached to the maxillae and mandible of the skull. These include the buccinator muscles, which compress the lips and flatten the cheeks in the movement of food across the teeth (Table 2-2). The buccinator fibers blend with those of the orbicularis oris, the sphincter of the lips.

The hypoglossal nerve (CN XII) innervates the tongue, which contains four separate intrinsic muscle masses that have different effects on the shape, contour, and function of the tongue.

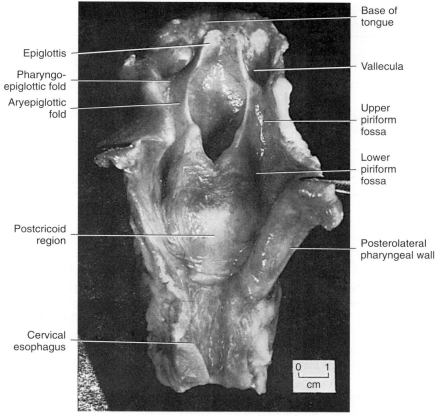

Epiglottis

Pharyngo-epiglottic fold

Aryepiglottic fold

Base of tongue

Vallecula

Upper piriform fossa

Lower piriform fossa

Postcricoid region

Posterolateral pharyngeal wall

Cervical esophagus

0   1
cm

FIGURE 2-2   Anatomic specimen of the pharyngeal compartment as it surrounds the airway. The bolus flows into the **vallecular spaces** and around the epiglottis inferiorly into the piriform fossa before entering the esophagus.

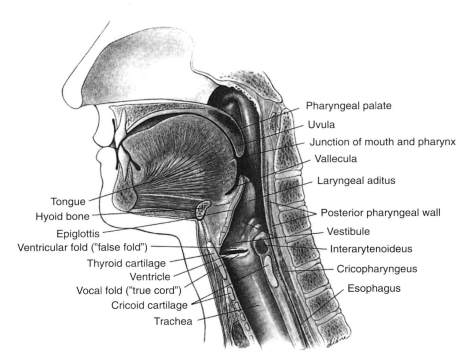

FIGURE 2-3 Lateral view of the anatomy of the head and neck pertinent to swallowing. (From Bosma JF, Donner MW, Tanaka E et al: Anatomy of the pharynx, pertinent to swallowing, *Dysphagia* 1:24, 1986.)

TABLE 2-1 Muscles of Mastication

Muscle	Origin	Insertion	Nerve	Action
Temporalis	Temporal fossa of skull	Ramus and coronoid process of mandible	Trigeminal	Elevates or closes mandible; retracts mandible
Masseter	Zygomatic arch	Ramus of mandible	Trigeminal	Elevates or closes mandible
Medial pterygoid	Palatine bone, lateral pterygoid plate, tuberosity of maxilla	Ramus of mandible	Trigeminal	Elevates or closes mandible
Lateral pterygoid	Great wing of sphenoid and lateral pterygoid plate	Neck of condyle of mandible	Trigeminal	Depressor or opener of mandible; protrudes mandible; permits side-to-side movement of mandible

Oral/Pharyngeal Stage

The pharyngeal cavity of the neck, which is suspended from the base of the skull and anchored to the top of the sternum, is formed by 26 pairs of **striated muscles** innervated by six cranial and four cervical nerves. The horseshoe-shaped hyoid bone in the neck serves as a fulcrum that provides a mechanical advantage for pharyngeal musculature associated with swallowing behaviors of the posterior tongue, pharynx, and larynx.

In the nasopharynx, five muscles adjust the position of the velum with respect to the food bolus: the palatoglossal and levator veli palatini muscles (pharyngeal plexus and accessory nerve), which elevate the soft palate and seal the nasopharynx; the tensor veli palatini (mandibular branch of the trigeminal nerve), which tenses the palate and dilates the orifice of the eustachian tube; the palatopharyngeal muscle (pharyngeal plexus and spinal accessory nerve), which depresses the soft palate, approximates the palate or pharyngeal folds, and constricts the pharynx; and the muscularis uvula (spinal accessory nerve), which shortens the soft palate (Table 2-3).

The hypoglossal (CN XII), trigeminal (CN V), and facial (CN VII) nerves innervate the suprahyoid group of muscles. The hypoglossal nerve supplies the geniohyoid, which draws the hyoid bone up and forward, depressing the jaw, and the trigeminal nerve supplies the mylohyoid, which elevates the hyoid bone and tongue and depresses the jaw

TABLE 2-2 Muscles of the Face

Muscle	Origin	Insertion	Nerve	Action
Orbicularis oris	Neighboring muscles, mostly buccinators; has many layers of tissue around the lips	Skin around lips and angles of the mouth	Facial	Closes, opens, protrudes, inverts, and twists lips
Zygomaticus minor	Zygomatic bone	Orbicularis oris in upper lip	Facial	Draws upper lip upward and outward
Levator labii superior	Below infraorbital foramen in maxilla	Orbicularis oris in upper lip	Facial	Pulls up or elevates upper lip
Levator labii superior alaeque nasi	Process of maxilla	Skin at mouth angle, orbicularis oris	Facial	Raises angle of the mouth
Zygomaticus major	Zygomatic bone	Fibers of the orbicularis oris, angle of the mouth	Facial	Draws upper lip upward; draws angle of mouth upward and backward; the smiling muscle
Levator anguli oris	Canine fossa of maxilla	Lower lip near angle of the mouth	Facial	Pulls up corners of mouth
Depressor anguli oris	Outer surface and above lower border of mandible	Skin of cheek, corner of mouth, lower border of mandible	Facial	Draws lower lip down; draws angle of mouth down and inward
Depressor labii inferior	Lower border of the mandible	Skin of lower lip, orbicularis oris	Facial	Depresses lower lip
Mentalis	Incisor fossa of mandible	Skin of chin	Facial	Pushes up lower lip; raises chin
Risorius	Platysma, fascia over the masseter skin	Angle of mouth, orbicularis oris	Facial	Draws corners or angle of mouth outward; causes dimples; gives expression of strain to face
Buccinator	Alveolar process of maxilla, buccinators ridge of mandible	Angle of mouth, orbicularis oris	Facial	Flattens cheek; holds food in contact with teeth; retracts angles of the mouth

TABLE 2-3 Muscles of the Palate

Muscle	Origin	Insertion	Nerve	Action
Levator veli palatini	Apex of temporal bone	Palatine aponeurosis of soft palate	Vagus and accessory	Raises soft palate
Tensor veli palatini	Fossa of sphenoid bone	Palatine aponeurosis of soft palate	Trigeminal	Stretches soft palate
Palatoglossus	Undersurface of soft palate	Side of tongue	Vagus and accessory	Raises back of tongue during the first stage of swallowing
Palatopharyngeus	Soft palate	Pharyngeal wall	Vagus and accessory	Shuts off nasopharynx during second stage of swallowing
Uvulae	Posterior nasal spine and palatine aponeurosis	Into uvula to form its chief bulk or content	Vagus and accessory	Shortens and raises uvula

(Table 2-4). The digastric muscles contain anterior and posterior bellies. The anterior belly is innervated by the mandibular branch of the trigeminal nerve (CN V) and depresses the jaw or raises the hyoid bone, whereas the posterior portion is innervated by the facial nerve (CN VII) and elevates or retracts the hyoid. The facial nerve (CN VII) innervates the stylohyoid muscle, which elevates the hyoid bone during swallowing. In addition, the hyoglossus and the genioglossus serve as laryngeal elevators, as well as extrinsic tongue muscles, and are designed to depress the tongue or help elevate the hyoid bone when the tongue is fixed. The accessory nerve (CN XI), in association with the hypoglossal (CN XII) nerve, innervates the styloglossus, which draws the tongue up and back during swallowing. The glossopharyngeal (CN IX) and accessory (CN XI) nerves also cause the palatoglossus to raise the back of the

TABLE 2-4 Suprahyoid Muscles

Muscle	Origin	Insertion	Nerve	Action
Mylohyoid (anterior belly digastric)	Inner surface of mandible	Upper border of hyoid bone	Trigeminal	Elevates tongue and floor of mouth; depresses jaw when hyoid bone is in fixed position
Digastric (anterior belly)	Intermediate tendon by loop of fascia to hyoid bone	Lower border of mandible	Trigeminal	Raises hyoid bone if jaw is in fixed position; depresses jaw if hyoid bone is in fixed position
Geniohyoid	Mental spine of mandible	Hyoid bone	Cervical (C1 and C2) through hypoglossal	Draws hyoid bone forward; depresses mandible when hyoid bone is in fixed position
Stylohyoid	Stylohyoid process of temporal bone	Body of hyoid at greater cornu	Facial	Elevates hyoid and tongue base
Hyoglossus	Greater cornu of hyoid	Into tongue sides	Hypoglossal	Tongue depression
Genioglossus	Upper genial tubercle of mandible	Hyoid, inferior tongue, and tip of tongue	Hypoglossal	Protrusion and depression
Styloglossus	Anterior border of styloid process	Into side of tongue	Hypoglossal	Elevates up and back
Palatoglossus	Anterior surface of soft palate	Dorsum and side of tongue	Glossopharyngeal, vagus, and accessory	Narrows fauces and elevates posterior tongue

tongue and lower the velum. The styloglossus and palatoglossus raise the back of the tongue and lower the sides of the soft palate.

The vagus nerve (CN X) and the spinal accessory nerve (CN XI) innervate the muscular pharynx, whose superior, middle, and inferior constrictor muscles constitute its external circular layer and work together to transport a bolus of food toward the esophagus during swallowing. Three other muscles constitute the internal longitudinal layer of the pharynx: the palatopharyngeus, stylopharyngeus, and salpingopharyngeus. The stylopharyngeus (glossopharyngeal nerve) elevates the pharynx, and to some extent the larynx, during swallowing, and the salpingopharyngeus (accessory nerve and pharyngeal plexus) draws the lateral walls of the pharynx up. The palatopharyngeus muscle draws the velum down.

The cricopharyngeal muscle is an important single muscle that lies at the transition level between the pharynx and the esophagus. Functionally, it is separate from both the pharynx and the esophagus and acts as a sphincter, relaxing during passage of the bolus from the pharynx into the esophagus. It is innervated by both pharyngeal branches of the vagus and sympathetic fibers from the middle and inferior cervical ganglia. The key muscles used in the oral and pharyngeal stages of swallowing are shown in Figure 2-4.

Esophageal Stage

The esophagus is a distensible tube, approximately 21 to 27 cm (10 inches) long, connecting the pharynx (at C6) and

stomach (at T12). It is separated from the pharynx by the pharyngeal esophageal segment (PES) and from the stomach by the lower esophageal sphincter (LES). Under resting conditions, the esophageal **lumen** is collapsed, creating a potential space that can easily distend up to 3 cm to accommodate swallowed air, liquids, or solids. The esophagus is lined with a protective, stratified, squamous epithelium that covers an inner layer of circular fibers and an outer layer of longitudinal fibers. At its proximal end (upper fourth) the muscle is striated, whereas the distal two thirds are composed of **smooth muscle**. The middle third, in the region of the aorta, is a combination of smooth and striated muscle. As it courses through the thorax at the level of the carina, the esophagus runs lateral and posterior to the left ventricle of the heart, creating a natural bend as it courses anteriorly toward the diaphragmatic hiatus. After passing the diaphragmatic hiatus, it connects to the body of the stomach at the level of the LES. The smooth muscle of the LES is arranged in a specialized spiral configuration as it joins the inner oblique muscle zone of the stomach. The relation of the esophagus to the heart and tracheobronchial tree, as well as its path through the diaphragmatic hiatus, is shown in Figure 2-5.

NORMAL PHYSIOLOGY

Many studies have examined the normal aspects of the oropharyngeal swallow sequence. The rationale usually given for such studies is that clinicians must be able to

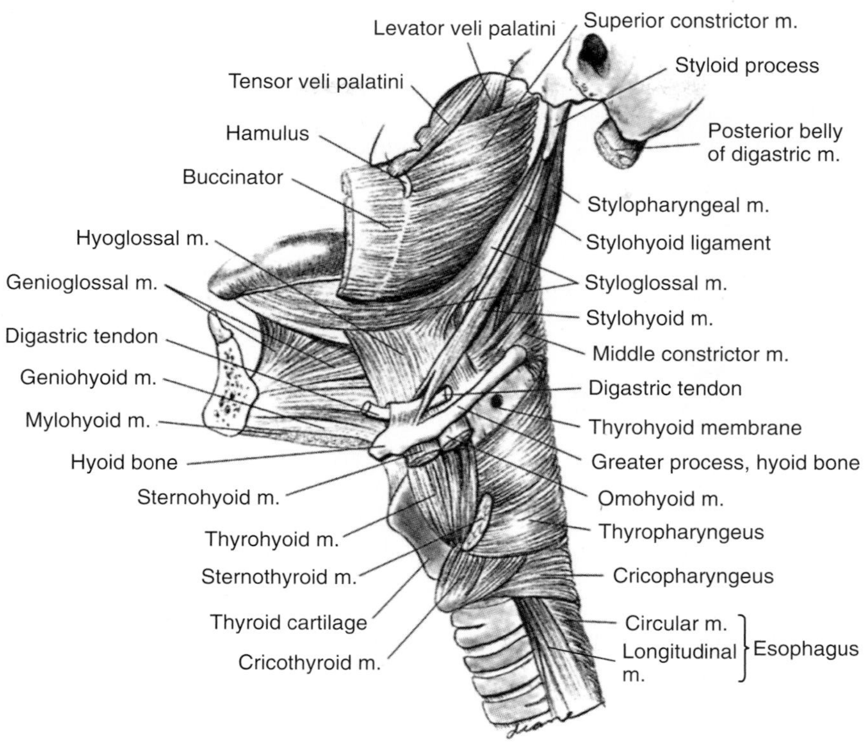

FIGURE 2-4   Lateral view of the key muscles of the head and neck used in swallowing. (From Bosma JF, Donner MW, Tanaka E et al: Anatomy of the pharynx, pertinent to swallowing, *Dysphagia* 1:24, 1986.)

compare normative data with patient data to determine whether an abnormality exists. Although this approach to detection has heuristic appeal, studies of the normal swallow have revealed significant variability among normal (healthy) subjects, particularly in the oral preparatory and oral stages of swallowing.[2-5] Part of this variability is attributable to subject selection, bolus type, and the tools used to measure swallow performance. Other variability seems inherent in the swallowing process. It appears that the mechanism for swallowing must be variable to accommodate the variations of bolus type and amount for successful ingestion in different circumstances of eating, such as eating while talking, in varied environments, and at various rates. The astute clinician will not ignore those aspects of normal swallow performance that have been empirically evaluated but should also be imminently cognizant of placing a person's functional swallow in the context of his or her swallowing complaint, past medical history, and the results of physical and instrumental examinations. Busy clinicians often make timing comparisons to normal values based on real-time observations with particular attention to changes in timing as it might affect actual invasion or potential threat to the airway.

Normal swallowing performance depends on the rapid transfer of the bolus from the oral cavity to the stomach. A liquid bolus may pass through the pharynx within 2 seconds and enter the stomach in less than 5 seconds. Efficient movement is accomplished by the strength of the neuromuscular contraction exerted on the bolus and on the forces of gravity. Efficient bolus movement is accomplished when coordinated neuromuscular contractions and relaxations create zones of high pressure on the bolus and zones of negative pressure below the level of the bolus. Some parts of the swallowing chain, such as the esophagus, remain under negative pressure because of their location. Creating zones of high and low pressure is largely accomplished by the coordination and strength of the swallowing valves: lips, velum, airway closure, and the PES opening and closing. A patent nasal airway also may be important (Practice Note 2-2). The tongue provides the initial positive driving force. The tongue's posterior deflection provides the basis for laryngeal elevation by applying traction to the hyoid bone. Efficient (i.e., timely and strong) laryngeal elevation helps create a negative zone of pressure in the pharynx, particularly in the region of the PES. This allows the bolus to move rapidly, and therefore safely, from a zone of high pressure into a zone of negative pressure. Moving from a zone of high pressure into another zone of high pressure caused by a pathologic condition (e.g., muscle weakness or incoordination) inhibits bolus flow and results in **stasis** and residue that may be aspirated into the airway.

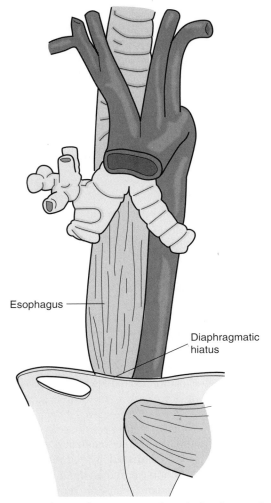

Esophagus

Diaphragmatic
hiatus

FIGURE 2-5   The esophagus courses through the chest cavity and through a hiatus in the diaphragm, ending at the level of the stomach.

PRACTICE NOTE 2-2

Try experiencing the effects of an open valve (the lips) and a closed nasal passage on your own swallowing performance. First swallow your saliva as usual. Then try to swallow your saliva with your lips open, noticing the differences in effort expended. Do the same thing with the nose open and then pinch the nostrils closed and swallow.

Oral Preparation

Food or liquid in the mouth stimulates taste, temperature, and pressure (touch) receptors. The primary receptors of taste are located on the tongue, on the hard and soft palate, in the pharynx, and in the supralaryngeal region. The receptors are activated by saliva. Saliva is produced by the activation of the submandibular, submaxillary (autonomic

aspects of CN VII), and parotid glands (autonomic aspects of CN IX). Activation of these glands is achieved by the actions of the jaw, tongue, and hyoid bone during bolus preparation and by the inherent taste of the bolus. The primary sensory receptors on the dorsum of the tongue responsible for the perception of salt, sweet, sour, and bitter are activated by saliva. In addition to facilitating taste and bolus formation, saliva is important in the maintenance of adequate oral hygiene by controlling microorganisms, in the regulation of the acidity levels in the stomach and esophagus because of its bicarbonate composition, and in the breakdown of carbohydrates. The number of times a person swallows saliva in 1 hour can vary between 18 and 400 and largely depends on the rate of salivary flow.[6]

Sensations of taste are carried by the chorda tympani branch of CN VII on the anterior two thirds of the tongue and through the greater petrosal branch on the hard and soft palate. Taste on the posterior third of the tongue is mediated by CN IX. Sensations of taste are sent to the nucleus tractus solitarii (NTS) in the medulla of the brainstem (see sections on neurologic controls), where they are transmitted to the sensorimotor cortex by the thalamus. Taste receptors in the region of the **laryngeal aditus** are carried to the NTS by the superior laryngeal branch of CN X. Appreciation of taste depends largely on smell. Smell sensations are carried by direct stimulation of the nasal cavity and by smell elicited by chewing, during which odors travel posteriorly into the nasopharynx. Interpretation of smell is ultimately accomplished through the thalamus to the frontal and temporal cortices by information carried by CN I. Information (memories) relating to smell may be stored in the **hippocampus**. Although it is clear that certain peripheral mechanisms are important in the elicitation of swallow, their exact role in normal and dysphagic subjects remains unclear.[7] For instance, interruptions by anesthetic injections in some of the key peripheral sensory input channels do not interfere with the motor swallow response.[7]

The coordinated action of the tongue and jaw moves a bolus laterally onto the molar table for deformation. Further deformation is accomplished by variable contacts of the tongue to the hard palate. Although the tongue may play a large role in containing the bolus in the oral cavity before swallow, evidence indicates that during solid bolus mastication, material is allowed to collect in the vallecular recesses at the tongue base before swallow initiation.[5] The ultimate role of the tongue is to manipulate, shape, hold, and then transfer the bolus into the oropharynx, signaling the onset of the oral stage of swallow as the swallowing sequence transitions into the pharyngeal stage with the passage of the bolus through the oropharyngeal port. The exact nature of the sensory cues that signal a bolus is ready for swallowing is not completely understood; however, studies have shown that the superior laryngeal nerve (SLN) branch of the vagus is important in swallow initiation[8] and in the sensory protective mechanisms of the upper airway.[9] After studying 266 normal subjects who swallowed varying types of boluses ranging from buttered bread to cake to carrots, and peanuts, Engelen et al.[10] concluded that masticatory performance when preparing a bolus is more dependent on the bolus characteristic than on oral physiology. The mechanics of bolus preparation can be appreciated with videofluoroscopy. The first images are taken as the patient faces the camera and chews a piece of cracker (Video 2-1). The undulating and varied movements of the tongue and jaw are apparent. In the lateral view, the tongue can be seen touching the hard palate as material is pushed toward the tongue base, filling the valleculae before the swallow (Video 2-2).

Oral Stage

Once the bolus is prepared, the tongue tip is elevated to occlude the anterior oral cavity at the alveolar ridge, and the bolus is held against the hard palate. The edges of the tongue dorsum contain the bolus laterally. The tongue tip and dorsum appear to work longer in containment activity than the posterior tongue after the oral stage is initiated; however, the posterior tongue is more responsible for delivering the bolus into the pharynx.[11] Before—but almost simultaneous with—the first posterior movement of the tongue, respiration ceases (see following section on respiration), followed by arytenoid cartilage approximation precipitating true vocal fold adduction. Retraction of the tongue is primarily accomplished by extrinsic tongue muscles: digastricus (CN V), mylohyoid (CN V), and the geniohyoid (CN XII). The tongue base applies positive pressure to the tail of the bolus by its contact with the velum and posterior pharyngeal wall, which allows the bolus to move rapidly through the pharynx into an open PES. As the tongue propels the bolus posteriorly, the palatopharyngeal folds are pulled medially to form a slit through which the bolus can pass. The levator veli palatini muscles help elevate the velum to seal the nasopharyngeal opening. The combined action of the tongue's contact to the velum and posterior pharyngeal wall and sealing the nasopharynx contribute to the maintenance of positive pressure on the bolus as it moves toward zones of negative pressure in the hypopharynx. By the tongue's connections to the hyoid bone, and the hyoid bone's connections to the thyroid and cricoid cartilages, the larynx is pulled up and forward, resting under the tongue base that now partially covers the opening to the airway. Using 13 formalin-fixed cadaver sections, Pearson et al.[12] concluded that the geniohyoid muscle was most active in the anterior displacement of the hyoid bone, whereas the mylohyoid was most responsible for superior movement. As the larynx rises, the cartilaginous epiglottis makes its descent over the top of the airway, completing an elaborate system of airway protection that

allows the bolus to be directed toward the esophagus rather than into the trachea. The extent of epiglottic descent depends on anterior hyoid displacement, tongue base retraction force, and bolus size.[13] Rapid and complete laryngeal elevation (2 to 3 cm on average) aids in creating negative pressure in the region of the hypopharynx. As the bolus enters the pharynx, it is divided by the vallecular spaces at the level of the tongue base, helping deflect it away from the airway as an additional component of airway protection.

Respiration and Swallow

Protection of the upper airway through the oropharyngeal phase of swallowing is crucial to swallowing safety. Respiration and swallowing are linked by their anatomy (common conduits of mouth and pharynx) and their neuroanatomic relations in the medulla of the brainstem. This relation is expressed functionally because respiration is inhibited by swallowing, and disorders of respiration often affect swallow safety (see Chapter 6). The period of airflow inhibition (swallow apnea) in most normal adults begins before the onset of the oral stage of swallow.[14,15] During mastication, respiratory patterns are modified from normal tidal patterns; however, apnea does not occur until the bolus collects at the vallecular level.[16] A short exhalation cycle precedes shallow apnea. As the tail of the bolus passes through the PES, the larynx descends and respiration continues on the exhalation cycle slightly before the PES closes.[15] Exhalation is accompanied by a buildup of subglottic pressure that separates the vocal folds. This release of pressure is heard as an audible burst by using a stethoscope placed at the laryngeal level.[17] This burst of exhalation is considered a protective feature in case any swallowed material is lodged in the upper airway. This explosion of exhaled air is encouraged with the Heimlich maneuver. The pattern of exhalation-swallow-exhalation may change in normal aging[18,19] and in disease (Clinical Corner 2-1).[20] The duration of swallow apnea in normal subjects varies from 0.75 to 1.25 seconds depending on the subject's age and bolus size.[21] In general, the larger the bolus size, the longer the duration of swallow apnea.[19] During swallow apnea the true vocal folds move medially but do not fully approximate.[15] It is possible that the cessation of respiration during swallowing is not physiologically tied to vocal fold movement because patients with laryngectomy show similar periods of swallow apnea compared with normal subjects.[22]

Pharyngeal Stage

The pharyngeal stage begins when the bolus arrives at the level of the valleculae and ends when the PES closes.[23]

When the bolus enters the pharynx, the hyoid bone continues its superior and anterior excursion toward the edge of the mandible, tilting the larynx under the retracting tongue base to protect the bolus from entering the upper airway. The false vocal folds offer further protection in conjunction with the closure of the laryngeal aditus by the aryepiglottic folds. As a result of contraction of the thyroepiglottic ligament and posterior tongue contraction, the epiglottic cartilage descends from its erect position over the laryngeal aditus. Thus many mechanisms are active in preventing the bolus from entering the upper airway. These include (1) cessation of active respiration, (2) approximation of the true and false vocal folds, (3) closure of the laryngeal aditus, (4) deflection of bolus material by the tongue base

over a rising larynx, and (5) division of the bolus through the valleculae that direct the bolus around the superior aspect of the airway entrance.

As the bolus enters the pharynx, the superior, middle, and inferior constrictor muscles are activated sequentially to narrow and shorten the pharynx, contributing to peristalsis-like movements in the posterior pharyngeal wall that aid in bolus propulsion into the esophagus. The duration of pharyngeal muscle contraction is unaffected by bolus size.[24]

The forward excursion of the hyoid bone is important in applying traction forces on the PES to achieve maximum opening.[25] Before the bolus arrives in the pharynx, muscles in the region of the PES that had been closed before swallow are relaxed by parasympathetic signals carried by CN IX to the brainstem. After relaxation, the PES is pulled open during hyolaryngeal movements. As the bolus continues its descent toward the region of the PES, it remains divided as it passes lateral to the larynx into the piriform recesses of the hypopharynx, where the bolus is rejoined as it enters the esophagus. Preference for bolus flow through the pharynx has been found in healthy normal patients. Seta et al.[26] studied the preference of bolus flow in 167 normal patients. Although all patients had bolus flow in both halves of the pharynx, 58% showed no difference, 35% had left dominance, and 7% showed right dominance.[26] In addition to PES relaxation and mechanical traction, the PES is distended by the driving force of the bolus. The neurologic and biomechanical processes required for distention and closing of the PES are summarized in Figure 2-6.

As the tail of the bolus passes the region of the PES, primary esophageal peristalsis begins as the PES closes. The airway reopens and the hyoid bone returns to its resting

---

CLINICAL CORNER 2-1: HEIMLICH MANEUVER

While dining one evening a couple noticed someone at an adjoining table suddenly jump up and complain loudly that something was sticking in his throat. He seemed quite uncomfortable and was starting to sweat. Because of the commotion the waiter rushed over and began the Heimlich maneuver by pressing his hands around the diner's waist, forcefully pushing on his diaphragm with rapid thrusts. Unfortunately, this did not relieve his customer's symptoms and he continued to complain that something was stuck.

Critical Thinking
1. Why didn't the Heimlich maneuver relieve the customer's symptoms?
2. What might have been the problem?

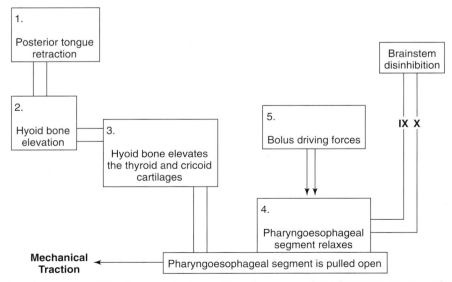

FIGURE 2-6 Schematic representation of the three mechanisms of the pharyngoesophageal segment opening. They include mechanical traction (1, 2, and 3), brainstem disinhibition (relaxation) (4), and bolus driving forces (5).

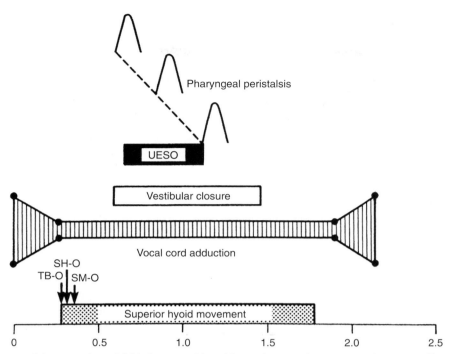

FIGURE 2-7   The relation of the time of vocal fold closure and hyoid bone elevation during a 5-mL barium swallow. Bolus transit through the pharynx and across the upper esophageal sphincter (UES) begins and ends while the vocal folds are at maximal adduction. SH-O, Onset of superior hyoid movement; SM-O, onset of submental myoelectrical activity; TB-O, onset of tongue base movement; UESO, UES opening. (From Shaker R, Dodds WJ, Dantas RO et al: Coordination of deglutitive glottic closure with oropharyngeal swallowing, *Gastroenterology* 98:1478, 1990.)

position. These activities signal the end of the pharyngeal phase of swallow. The timing of oropharyngeal swallowing events from the beginning of vocal fold closure to the reopening of the vocal folds at the end of the swallowing sequence is depicted in Figure 2-7. (For more detail on the activity of the PES during swallowing, see Chapter 5.) The structural and biomechanical aspects of the oral and pharyngeal phases of swallowing seen in the lateral and anteroposterior planes can be appreciated in a narrated version of a videofluoroscopic examination of swallowing (Video 2-3). Video 2-4 provides a narrated version of the normal swallow as seen by endoscopy.

Esophageal Stage

Before the bolus enters the esophagus, the esophageal lumen remains closed within the chest cavity under negative pressure. Pressures generated in the closed upper esophageal sphincter vary from 30 to 110 mm Hg depending on patient age and the type of manometric catheter used to gather the data.[27] Esophageal swallowing tasks require an ordered pattern of function that depends on coordinated activities in three distinct zones: the proximal, striated muscle zone; the body; and the specialized smooth muscle of the distal zone. Bolus movement through these zones is

characterized by an orderly, ringlike progression of contractions until the bolus enters the LES and the stomach. Liquid boluses, depending on **viscosity**, often precede this wave of contractions. The cervical portion of the esophagus works in conjunction with the hypopharynx, allowing the PES to fully relax and distend to accommodate bolus size. As the bolus enters the esophagus, a primary contraction wave (primary peristalsis) is triggered in the proximal, striated portion by vagal (CN X) efferent activity. This activity may be inhibited by multiple swallow attempts if the pharynx fails to clear its contents.[28] The motor activity in the cervical esophagus is rapid and gradually slows as it approaches the mid (level of the aortic arch) and distal esophageal regions.[29] Typically, the contraction force in the cervical esophagus is the strongest and is accompanied in time by a drop in pressure (relaxation) in the LES to allow the bolus to enter the stomach. Esophageal smooth muscle contraction (distal two thirds) has a sequential behavior by which proximal activity successively inhibits the next most distal portion of the esophagus.[30] The bolus propagation pressures generated in the esophagus are typically measured by manometric techniques. A visual representation of primary peristalsis is presented in Figure 2-8. The radiographic representation of esophageal peristalsis is presented in Video 2-5. The patient is standing while swallowing a

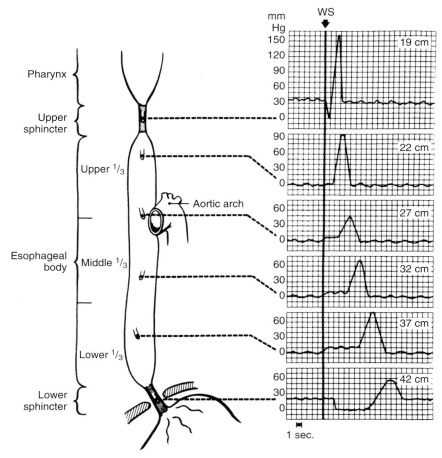

FIGURE 2-8 A manometric tracing of primary esophageal peristalsis. Pressure catheters are placed at various levels of the esophagus (19 cm from the incisors to 42 cm). Their representative measures of pressure are seen as peaks of activity on the right of the figure. Before the first pressure wave, a drop in pressure is seen from approximately 40 mm Hg (closed sphincter) to 0. This drop in pressure represents the opening and relaxation of the upper esophageal sphincter. The first primary esophageal contraction is the highest and therefore the strongest. As the bolus reaches the level of the aortic arch, the pattern of contraction is reduced because of the bending of the esophagus around the arch and the transition from striated to smooth muscle. Note that as the primary peristaltic wave begins, there is a corresponding drop in the pressure of the lower esophageal sphincter from approximately 25 mm Hg to 0 as it relaxes to await the oncoming bolus. A positive wave in the lower esophageal sphincter after this drop in pressure can be seen as a consequence of the sphincter closing.

liquid and a semisolid bolus. The ringlike contraction waves of the esophageal lumen can be appreciated, as can the bolus entering the stomach through the LES. The primary peristaltic wave on the liquid bolus is followed by a secondary wave. It is apparent that the semisolid bolus flows at a slower pace.

Primary peristalsis is followed by secondary peristalsis. The secondary peristaltic wave follows the primary wave and is propagated by the bolus distending the esophagus. Its propagation may begin at any point in the esophageal body and often assists in primary transport of solid food boluses because the primary wave may fail to push the bolus to the level of the LES. Primary and secondary peristalsis are accompanied by longitudinal muscle contraction, resulting in shortening of the esophagus by its proximal attachments to the hypopharynx and distal attachments to

the stomach (see Chapter 5 for a discussion of Zenker's **diverticulum** and esophageal shortening).

Tertiary contractions of the esophagus are random contractions that are not peristaltic (orderly) in nature and are inefficient in assisting in bolus transport. In general, they occur independent of swallowing activity but have been reported to occur more frequently in older adults.[31] Tertiary contractions may be the result of air trapped in the esophagus, or they may result from irritation of the esophageal lumen such as from gastroesophageal reflux.

BOLUS AND DELIVERY VARIATION

Altering volume, texture, taste, and delivery method may affect the biomechanics of the normal swallow. Dietary modifications are frequently used in the treatment of patients with dysphagia (see Chapters 9, 10, and 15 to assist in compensating for their deficits). The prescribed modifications in volume, texture (viscosity), and taste to facilitate normal swallowing are based on studies on the effects of these parameters on normal swallowing. Results from such studies are not uniform because of subject variability, measurement tools used (e.g., intramuscular and surface electromyography, ultrasound, manometry, videofluoroscopy), subject instructions (cue versus no cue),[32-34] type of bolus used and number of swallows tested,[35,36] and definitions of when specific biomechanical events begin and end. After reviewing 16 studies that investigated the temporal measurements of the normal swallow, Molfenter and Steele[35] concluded that while timing variations were apparent, they were the most stable for PES opening and the time between laryngeal closure and PES opening.[35] There are few published outcome data on the precise effects of volume, texture, and taste modification in patients with dysphagia, although these parameters are routinely modified in clinical care. Lee et al.[37] prospectively enrolled a mixed group of 82 patients suspected of oropharyngeal dysphagia. The group was divided almost equally into a group that did not aspirate on thin or thick fluids and a group that aspirated only on thin fluids. Both groups were given 5 mL of a thin and thickened liquid. **Kinematic** analysis revealed that the thick bolus arrived earlier in the valleculae in the thin-aspirator group, resulting in longer laryngeal elevation times that delayed the opening of the PES. They concluded that changes in bolus viscosity in dysphagic patients do not affect biomechanics.

Volume and Biomechanics

Studies have shown that the normal amount of a liquid taken per swallow attempt may range from 10 to 25 mL depending on the test instructions, gender, type of cup, and body size.[38,39] Most studies that examine the effects of volume on swallowing biomechanics have studied bolus volumes that range from 1 to 20 mL. These studies have focused on the effects of volume on the movement of the hyoid bone. Movement parameters can include maximal displacement and the duration of movement, documenting total time and velocity. Some investigators have found minimal effects of hyoid displacement between small and larger boluses,[40,41] whereas others have documented larger total displacement with an incremental increase in bolus volume more prominent in men.[42,43] One study found that larger volumes had a greater effect on superior, rather than anterior hyoid, movement.[44] Other studies have not focused specifically on hyoid mechanics but rather on the biomechanical and pressure changes associated with oral and pharyngeal transit, duration of swallow apnea, and PES mechanics.

Lingual swallowing pressures with varying bolus volumes were unaffected as bolus size was increased,[45] suggesting that increased effort in oral-stage transit is not needed as the size of a liquid bolus increases. However, the tongue changed its contour to contain larger boluses before swallow onset.[36] Ekberg and Nylander[30] found no change in the speed of pharyngeal transit between small and large boluses.

A direct relation appears to exist between bolus size and the length of time the PES stays open and the onset time of relaxation. Cook et al.[46] studied 21 normal volunteers using concurrent videofluoroscopy, surface electromyography, and manometry with four different bolus sizes ranging from 2 to 20 mL. In general, as the bolus size increased the PES stayed open longer, and the onset of relaxation was closer to the onset of the anterior movement of the hyoid bone. These results suggest a possible relation between the sensory aspects of the oral stage of swallow (bolus volume) and the mechanics of the PES. These results provide further evidence of the interdependence of the stages of swallowing.

Viscosity

Studies of the effects of viscosity, taste, and bolus delivery on swallowing have focused on the changes in biomechanical effort that may be needed as these variables are changed. Measurement of swallowing effort is accomplished best with manometric techniques, allowing the investigator to document changes in swallow-generated pressures.

In general, researchers agree that swallow-generated pressures are more sensitive to changes in viscosity than are changes in volumes of the same consistency. As the consistency of the bolus becomes thicker, greater tongue pressures are needed to transport it from the oral cavity.[45] Studies have shown no differences in this effect between healthy, younger men and women.[47] The increase in generated tongue force in 62 healthy adults was highest at the point where the anterior tongue made contact with the hard palate.[48]

Pelletier and Dhanaraj[49] studied the effects of sweet, salty, sour, and bitter on swallowing pressures in 10 healthy, young subjects. Subjects were also asked to judge the palatability of each test substance from "extremely like" to "dislike." Although palatability judgments did not affect swallowing pressures, higher pressures (compared with water) were generated with the moderate-sucrose, high-salt, and high–citric acid test samples. In 8 normal subjects using intramuscular electomyographic measurements, Palmer et al. concluded that a sour bolus provided increased activation of the suprahyoid musculature compared to a water bolus.[50] They concluded that the use of a sour bolus was justified as a treatment intervention, although the time of effect within a meal requires further investigation. Krival and Bates studied the swallowing pressures of 20 young women with three bolus types: carbonated, carbonation with taste, and water. Compared to water, the other two conditions showed a significant increase in swallow-related pressures.[51]

Straw drinking is a typical method to deliver a liquid bolus (Video 2-6). The patient takes multiple sips by straw. There are brief periods between each swallow when the airway opens briefly. Successful straw drinking requires adequate lip strength and intraoral pressures to draw the fluid into the oral cavity from the cup. In general, the airway must remain closed during sequential swallow attempts; therefore the biomechanical requirements may differ from single or multiple swallows from a cup. Daniels and Foundas[52] identified three distinct airway protection patterns during sequential straw drinking in 15 healthy young men, suggesting variation in how the upper airway is protected during sequential swallows using a straw with variations in the length of time the laryngeal vestibule remained closed (Clinical Corner 2-2). Younger and older normal subjects show hypopharyngeal accumulation on sequential straw swallows prior to bolus flow into the esophagus.[53]

Saitoh et al.[54] studied the effects of mastication on the normal swallow in 15 healthy, younger subjects. Boluses that required mastication usually were characterized by vallecular accumulation prior to the initiation of the swallow response because of weaker tongue-to-palate contact during mastication. Two-phase foods such as a liquid mixed with a solid may not be as easy to control in the valleculae and could put dysphagic patients at greater risk for aspiration.[52] Because viscosity often is manipulated as a treatment intervention, it is important to recognize that some ingested materials entering the oral stage requiring mastication may have their **rheologic** properties altered from the preswallow to the swallow-ready state. Hwang et al.[55] studied 20 normal subjects swallowing a cookie, banana, tofu, and cooked rice. As mastication cycles increased, mass increased and viscosity decreased only on the banana, tofu, and rice. The

importance of this study is to remind clinicians that if they wish to recommend a certain food item because of its viscous, adhesive, or cohesive properties, they may need to remember that deformation of that item may provide a different rheologic profile than that associated with premasticatory measurements.

SWALLOW AND NORMAL AGING

In persons older than 65 years, some demonstrable changes in swallowing performance are attributable to age alone. These changes may interact to decompensate swallowing. Some of these changes may appear as early as age 45 years.[56] These changes may be attributable to peripheral alterations in sensory perception, such as smell and taste, and decreased muscle strength secondary to changes in mass and contractility. Loss of muscle strength (force) and speed in older persons results in increased, but normal, swallow durations compared with younger cohorts.[57] Increased swallow durations were also found in healthy older adults who had more **periventricular white matter** lesions compared with healthy older adults without them.[58] Other structures involved in swallowing that may show changes in mass and contractility include the tongue, lips, jaw, velum, and lungs. Loss of elasticity in lung tissue coupled with reduced respiratory capacity and control may indirectly affect swallow because of the known interactions between breathing and swallowing. Brodsky et al.[59] found differences in respiratory patterns before and after swallows in older, healthy subjects compared with younger subjects. They speculated that this might be the result of a reduction in pharyngeal contraction pressures. Although these changes may not directly precipitate dysphagia, they may exacerbate conditions that are primary causative factors (e.g., neurologic disease). It is safe to assume that some aspects of swallowing are decompensated by normal aging and that the degree of compensation may enhance these effects in the diseased state. Robbins et al.[54] found that the ability of older persons to sustain **isometric** tasks involving the tongue may be different than in younger cohorts. These findings suggest that normal swallowing biomechanics may change under conditions of stress, such as might be imposed by hospitalization. Separating the effects of normal aging on swallowing from those in which disease is considered the primary causative factor presents a difficult clinical challenge.

Oral Stage and Aging

Tongue **hypertrophy** from fatty deposits and an increase in connective tissue results in a reduction of tongue mobility and tongue force as measured manometrically.[60] Some investigators have not found a significant difference in tongue pressure generation between normal, healthy older

---

CLINICAL CORNER 2-2: STRAW USE

A 75-year-old patient with respiratory disease was evaluated for difficulties swallowing liquids. Physical evaluation revealed that he had generalized weakness in the lips and tongue. He could take his liquids from a cup without any coughing episodes, but he had some coughing while using a straw. The patient reported that he was more comfortable using a straw and preferred it to the cup. The speech pathologist cut the straw in half and the patient then took his liquids with the straw without any difficulty.

Critical Thinking
1. Why might this patient have more difficulty using a straw than a cup?
2. Why might shortening the length of the straw improve his swallowing performance?

adults and younger cohorts,[47,61] although the time to reach maximum swallow pressures during swallowing was slower in older adults.[61] Significant differences are observed when comparing younger and older cohorts on their ability to generate maximum tongue pressures on nonswallowing tasks.[61,62] Youmans et al.[63] found that older women generated more pressure on swallows than men, and that both genders had a similar reduction of reserve strength, women greater than men. The difference between maximum isotonic pressures and the maximum pressure needed to complete a normal swallow seen in older persons, but not in younger cohorts, was discussed by Logemann et al.[62] They noted that the difference between these two measures in older persons represents a lack of pressure reserve and speculated that the difference may be important only when older persons need to rely on a pressure reserve, such as during illness. Fei et al.[64] compared 40 healthy younger subjects younger than the age of 40 to 38 healthy persons older than 60. They confirmed that older persons did generate lower maximum isometric pressures, and that these differences affected swallow-generated pressures by bolus type that were not seen in the younger cohort. Using maximum pressure generation as a covariate when comparing the two groups, they concluded that the effect of age alone on water and saliva swallows did not account for the differences.[62]

Tanaka et al.[65] compared the frequency of swallows in a fixed time frame between healthy and semi-bedridden older and younger adults.[65] There were significant differences in swallow frequency between older and younger adults and between healthy and semi-bedridden older adults. Semi-bedridden older adults had significantly fewer swallows than age-matched older adults without disability. Because dysphagia is a more frequent occurrence in older adults, some investigators have postulated that swallow frequency measurements may be a useful tool to predict dysphagia and risk for aspiration (see Chapters 7 and 8).

Sensory changes related to aging include decrements in smell and taste,[66,67] although it is not clear whether these changes are attributable to primary loss of sensory receptors, poor oral hygiene, poor health, medications that reduce salivary flow, impaired nutritional status, or a combination of these factors.[68] Alterations in the ability to discriminate between materials with varying viscosity have been reported, although whether this is the result of primary sensory changes or a loss in the cortical representation of viscosity discrimination is not clear.[69]

Alterations in dentition necessitating the use of dentures may affect oral-stage mechanics. Ill-fitting dentures affect oral-stage preparation and may also interfere with access to the sensory receptors on the hard palate. For bolus materials that require mastication, older persons require additional time because of decreased jaw biting force.[70]

Pharyngeal Stage and Aging

Cinefluorography has shown that a decrease in the connective tissue in the suprahyoid musculature that supports laryngeal excursion may result in inadequate anterior laryngeal movement that secondarily reduces the opening of the PES.[71] Radiographic studies of healthy older persons show that pharyngeal constriction is normal compared with younger cohorts.[72] The restriction of PES opening is also evident on manometric studies, as evidenced by higher hypopharyngeal and intrabolus pressures in addition to increased pharyngeal contraction pressures.[58] In videofluoroscopic recordings of normal older and younger men, the older men showed significantly reduced anterior hyoid bone movement, resulting in less distention of the PES.[73] Failure of the PES to adequately distend results in shorter PES relaxation times and may explain increased higher pharyngeal contraction pressures as a compensation for shorter opening times.[74] High intrabolus pressures may be consistent with a restriction of flow through the PES and in selected older patients may explain reports of cervical dysphagia (see Chapter 5). Resting pressures within the PES are lower in older cohorts and may affect the competency of that barrier of swallowed contents that may move from the esophagus to the posterior pharynx.[75]

Videofluoroscopic swallowing studies comparing older and younger male cohorts revealed more instances of airway penetration after age 50 years.[76] Even though these threats to airway protection were evident, no subject demonstrated evidence of aspiration as a consequence of material entering the upper airway.

Studies have shown that the duration of the airway closure time in older persons is longer compared with younger cohorts.[56,77] This difference may be related to documented slower oral- and pharyngeal-stage transit times in older cohorts, resulting in a physiologic compensation to maintain airway closure and swallow safety. Changes in sensitivity in the protective reflexes in the upper airway may occur with aging. When calibrated puffs of air were delivered to the supraglottic larynx of older and younger subjects, laryngeal reflex (closure) responses were not as evident in the older subjects until the puffs of air achieved higher pressure levels.[78] Aviv et al.[78] suggest that this weaker response may indicate that the sensory mechanisms involved in upper airway protection may decompensate with normal aging.

Esophagus and Aging

In general, radiographic studies and manometrics document that esophageal motor activity decreases with age, but aging alone does not always explain dysphagic complaints. Reduction in the amplitude of esophageal contractions caused by smooth muscle thickening has been reported,[71]

CLINICAL CORNER 2-3: AGING ESOPHAGUS

An 82-year-old man went to his primary care physician and reported that it had become more difficult to swallow solid foods over the past few months. Six months previously he started taking an antidepressant because he was not adjusting well to his wife's recent death. He denied choking episodes, so his doctor ordered a barium esophagram. The radiologist noted that with solid boluses there was a mild delay of bolus flow at the level of the aortic arch and no evidence of a stricture.

Critical Thinking
1. Did the patient's physician believe the swallowing problem represented new disease or normal aging?
2. Speculate on why the patient did not have a swallowing problem 1 year ago.

as well as delay in esophageal emptying and an increase in nonperistaltic contractions resulting in increased esophageal dilation and stasis[79] (review Clinical Corner 2-3).

NEUROLOGIC CONTROLS OF SWALLOWING

Neuroregulation of swallowing involves the activation of multiple levels of afferent and efferent pathways at different levels of the nervous system, including the cranial nerves, brainstem, cerebellum, subcortex, **limbic cortex**, and **neocortex**. Some aspects of swallowing appear to operate at a purely reflexive level, but it is more likely that swallowing does not represent a truly reflexive, brainstem-mediated response because food items are rarely swallowed the same way each time regardless of similarity in bolus type and size. As such, swallowing is believed to represent a more patterned type of neurologic response that can be influenced by control centers above the level of the brainstem. The peripheral muscles of swallowing contract sequentially but can be altered to accommodate the feeding activity. Therefore swallowing relies on both peripheral and central neurologic control systems that are activated differentially depending on the feeding circumstance. For instance, a person normally does not volitionally "think" about starting a swallowing response when eating but can "think" about swallowing when trying to swallow a pill. Although the mechanism is not totally understood, the act of swallowing potentially involves nervous system connections at multiple levels.

Peripheral and Medullary Controls

Pharyngeal swallow is initiated by sensory impulses transmitted as a result of stimulation of receptors on the fauces, tonsils, soft palate, base of the tongue, posterior pharyngeal

TABLE 2-5 Afferent Controls Involved in Swallowing

Sensory Function	Innervation (Cranial Nerve)
General sensation, anterior two thirds of the tongue	Lingual nerve, trigeminal (V)
Taste, anterior two thirds of the tongue	Chorda tympani, facial (VII)
Taste and general sensation, posterior third of the tongue	Glossopharyngeal (IX)
Mucosa of valleculae	Internal branch of superior laryngeal nerve (vagus; X)
Primary afferent	—
Secondary afferent	Glossopharyngeal (IX)
Tonsils, pharynx, soft palate	Pharyngeal branch of vagus (X)
Pharynx, larynx, viscera	Glossopharyngeal (IX) Vagus (X)

TABLE 2-6 Efferent Controls Involved in Swallowing

Efferent/Stage	Innervation (Cranial Nerve)
Oral	
Masticatory, buccinators, floor of mouth	Trigeminal (V)
Lip sphincter	Facial (VII)
Tongue	Hypoglossal (XII)
Pharyngeal	—
Constrictors and stylopharyngeus	Glossopharyngeal (IX)
Palate, pharynx, larynx	Vagus (X)
Tongue	Hypoglossal (XII)
Esophageal	
Esophagus	Vagus (X)

wall, and anterior surface of the epiglottis.[80] These sensory impulses reach the NTS of the medulla primarily through the seventh, ninth, and tenth CNs. The efferent function is mediated through the ninth, tenth, eleventh, and twelfth CNs by the nucleus ambiguus (NA) (Tables 2-5 and 2-6; Figure 2-9). The highly integrated activities of swallowing depend on a combination of voluntary and involuntary control of the position of the lips, teeth, jaw, cheeks, and tongue—all mediated by multiple cranial nerves. Through innervation by the fifth CN, the masseter and pterygoid muscles provide the control of leverage, stabilization, and centering of the movable parts of the buccal cavity. Mastication depends primarily on CN V, whereas the muscles of the lips and cheeks depend on motor functions of CN VII. The extrinsic muscles of the tongue depend on the motor function of the CNs V and XII, except for the palatoglossus (elevator of the tongue root), which is innervated by CNs

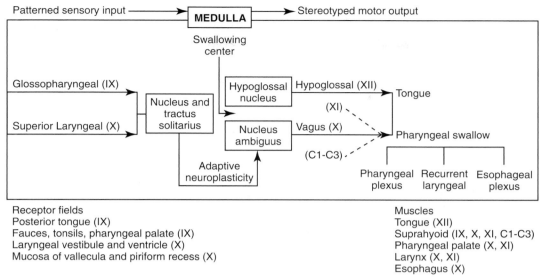

Patterned sensory input ⟶ **MEDULLA** ⟶ Stereotyped motor output

FIGURE 2-9 Conceptualization of the components of pharyngeal swallow as sensory-cued, stereotyped behaviors.

X and XI. All the intrinsic tongue muscles are innervated by CN XII. All the muscles of the soft palate are innervated primarily by CN X except the tensor veli palatini, which is innervated by CN V. The stylopharyngeus, a longitudinal muscle, widens the pharynx and is innervated by CN IX, whereas the palatopharyngeus is innervated primarily by CNs X and XII. The maxillary and mandibular sensory divisions of CN V are primarily involved in providing sensation pertaining to the lips, palate, teeth, inner mouth, and proprioceptive aspects of the muscles of mastication. The gag reflex and nasal regurgitation depend on the function (or dysfunction) of the glossopharyngeal and vagus nerves. Some controversy exists over the origin of the PES (cricopharyngeal) resting tone, which may not rely solely on the cervical sympathetic nervous system but may depend more heavily on vagal input for both contraction and relaxation.[81]

The literature refers to a swallowing center composed of key nuclei involved in afferent and efferent swallow control functions with interneuronal connections to respiratory centers in the medulla at the level of the **obex** of the fourth ventricle. This swallowing center has been defined as the dorsal NTS and ventral NA and the adjacent reticular formation.[82] In an excellent review of brainstem nuclei that are activated for swallow, Lang[83] identified medullary control centers based on swallowing stage; oral stage activity is mediated by the trigeminal nucleus and reticular formation, the NTS receives sensory neurons for pharyngeal and esophageal function, and the NA and dorsal motor nuclei provide the motor input for the pharynx and esophagus. Based on current evidence, it is more likely that major contributions from neural activity in supramedullary structures, such as pons, mesencephalon, and limbic and

cerebral cortices, also are involved in modulation of oral and pharyngeal swallowing and voluntary and involuntary behaviors.

The brainstem coordinates efferent impulse flow by way of the trigeminal, vagus, and hypoglossal cranial nerves to the muscles of the oropharynx, by way of CN X to the muscles of the hypopharynx, by way of CNs V and XII to the extrinsic muscles of the larynx, and by way of CN X to the intrinsic muscles of the larynx and esophagus. The cervical esophagus may receive two vagal efferent supplies from nerves within the neck. One comes from the recurrent laryngeal nerve (RLN) and another from the pharyngoesophageal nerve that rises proximal to the **nodose ganglion** or from an esophageal branch of the SLN. Such double innervation of the cervical esophagus in human beings has not been proved but might provide a margin of safety to prevent esophageal distention and reflux.

Sequentially timed discharges from the medulla result in movement of a bolus through successive levels of the esophageal musculature. Esophageal smooth muscle contractions have a sequential behavior by which proximal activity successively inhibits the next most distal portion of the esophagus.[84] Esophageal distention is signaled on visceral afferent nerves passing in the upper five or six thoracic sympathetic roots, presumably to the thalamus and inferior postcentral gyrus, where they may cause symptoms described as pressure, burning, gas, or aching. When such symptoms are described as pain, the referral patterns are based on sensory impulses from tissues innervated by somatic nerves that cross the corresponding spinal levels.

Motor fibers originating in the NA innervate the pharyngeal, laryngeal, and upper esophageal striated muscles. By way of the dorsal vagal nucleus, the NA also innervates the heart, lungs, and gastrointestinal tract smooth muscle.[85] Rootlets emerging from the medulla form the peripheral vagus, which exits the skull through the jugular foramen. Above the nodose ganglion, the vagus nerve sends branches to the pharyngeal plexus, which supplies the mucosa and musculature of the pharynx, larynx, and PES (Figure 2-10).[85]

The highly important branch of the vagus—the SLN—is sensory to the laryngeal mucosa and motor to the cricothyroid muscle. The vagus terminates as the RLN that loops around the aorta and returns to the larynx and hypopharynx. The RLN supplies muscles intrinsic to the larynx and is

believed not to supply the cricopharyngeus, which apparently derives its innervations from the pharyngeal plexus.[86]

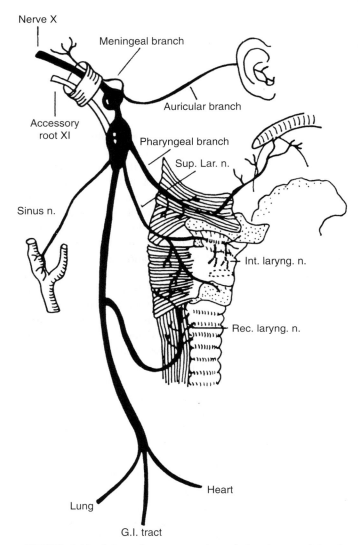

Nerve X

Meningeal branch

Auricular branch

Accessory root XI

Pharyngeal branch

Sup. Lar. n.

Sinus n.

Int. laryng. n.

Rec. laryng. n.

Heart

Lung

G.I. tract

FIGURE 2-10 Schematic representation of the three peripheral branches of cranial nerve X: the pharyngeal branch to the region of the velum and pharynx; the internal and recurrent branches to the larynx; and the autonomic branch to the heart, lungs, and gastrointestinal (GI) tract. *Sup. lar.,* Superior laryngeal nerve; *Int. laryng. n.,* internal laryngeal nerve; *Rec. laryng. n.,* recurrent laryngeal nerve.

CLINICAL CASE EXAMPLE 2-1

An 86-year-old man recently had heart surgery. After surgery he had a stroke affecting the premotor cortex of the left hemisphere. The man has a past history of depression treated with an antidepressant. He also had a history of Bell's palsy that affected CN VII in the upper and lower half of the left side of his face. He presented to the clinician with dysphagia. On examination the patient reported difficulty chewing and stated that food did not taste good. He noted considerable choking and a feeling that food was sticking in his throat. Physical examination of CN function revealed weakened right facial musculature from the stroke and weakened left facial musculature from the previous Bell's palsy. He was unable to make a tight lip seal because of bilateral CN VII nerve weakness. His tongue deviated to the right on protrusion, and range of motion was reduced (CN XII). Inspection of the oral cavity revealed moderate **xerostomia**. His voice was hoarse and breathy, although the velum rose evenly during testing of the gag reflex. His swallowing study showed poor bolus preparation, limited laryngeal elevation, pharyngeal stasis on pudding textures, and aspiration of thin liquids at the moment of swallow. It was concluded that the patient's poor bolus preparation could have been caused by multiple factors: tongue weakness, poor motor control from the involvement of a cortical motor area known to be important to bolus preparation, lack of taste appreciation from xerostomia (medication side effect), and probable involvement of the chorda tympani branch of CN VII (on the left). It was further concluded that his pharyngeal symptoms were attributable to poor laryngeal elevation caused by tongue weakness. This resulted in reduced opening of the PES, thus making it difficult for pudding to enter the esophagus, which caused the feeling that food was sticking in his throat. Liquids were aspirated because the vocal folds could not close fast enough because of the involvement of the recurrent branch of CN X that may have been damaged during the heart surgery, combined with the failure of the larynx to forcefully elevate and tilt forward because the tongue was weak. The pharyngeal branch of CNs IX and X was unaffected as evidenced by an intact gag reflex.

The neural control systems that subserve pharyngeal swallow are initiated by the action of CN afferents, but isolated central activation is not possible even though voluntary components exist. It appears that afferent impulses competent to initiate swallowing must conform to highly codified stimulus patterns that enter the NTS of the brainstem by way of its fasciculus and are relayed into the reticular formation, where connections exist to motor

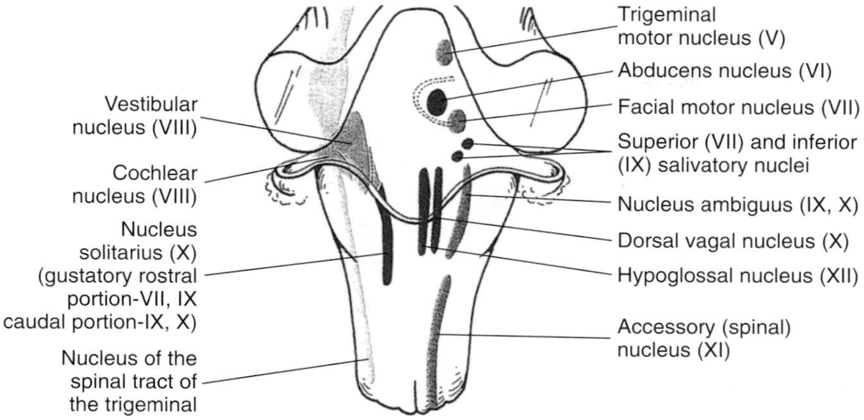

Trigeminal motor nucleus (V)

Abducens nucleus (VI)

Facial motor nucleus (VII)

Superior (VII) and inferior (IX) salivatory nuclei

Nucleus ambiguus (IX, X)

Dorsal vagal nucleus (X)

Hypoglossal nucleus (XII)

Accessory (spinal) nucleus (XI)

Vestibular nucleus (VIII)

Cochlear nucleus (VIII)

Nucleus solitarius (X) (gustatory rostral portion-VII, IX caudal portion-IX, X)

Nucleus of the spinal tract of the trigeminal

FIGURE 2-11   A view of the relations of the key brainstem nuclei involved in swallowing. Most nuclei are within close proximity in the dorsal and ventral parts of the medulla.

neurons lying in the nuclei of the fifth, seventh, and twelfth CNs and the NA.

Other brainstem motor neurons of interest in the neuroregulation of swallowing include the salivatory nuclei on either side of the genu of CNs VII and IX that provide saliva to the oral cavity and the dorsal motor nucleus of the vagus that innervates the esophageal smooth muscle (Figure 2-11).

The neuroregulatory brainstem mechanisms for pharyngeal swallow exist within the medullary reticular formation 1.5 mm from the midline on either side of the obex of the fourth ventricle. On each side of the midline is a site that communicates with the opposite side through cross-connections running behind the obex. As a result, bilateral symmetry of pharyngeal swallow is achieved. Each half of the medullary reticular formation exerts ipsilateral inhibition and excitation on appropriate motoneurons, with the exception of the inferior constrictor muscles, whose excitation is strictly contralateral.

Pharyngeal swallow involves a sequence of excitation and inhibition produced by several motor neuronal pools on each side of the brainstem.[82] Experimental unilateral destruction of the medulla eliminates swallowing in the ipsilateral musculature, except for the crossed pharyngeal constrictor muscle pathway. However, the responsiveness of the contralateral side to afferent input for the side of the lesion is still normal. For example, destruction of the left lateral medulla does not prevent right-sided swallowing if the left SLN is stimulated. This has immediate clinical relevance, especially in the case of unilateral destructive lesions to the brainstem.

The peripheral neural organization of swallowing has been largely elucidated by recording the electrical activity of involved muscles, beginning with onset of contraction in the mylohyoid and including concurrent activity in muscles innervated by CN V and those of the posterior

tongue, superior constrictor, palatopharyngeus, palatoglossus, stylohyoid, and geniohyoid. These initiators constitute what has been called the leading complex.[85] Because the pharyngeal constrictor muscles form a continuous sheet of striated muscle, an overlapping "firing sequence" is observed beginning with the superior pharyngeal constrictor (the principal muscle), the middle pharyngeal constrictor, and the inferior pharyngeal constrictor, with distinct rostral (thyropharyngeus) and caudal (cricopharyngeus) components. The superior constrictor is active at the same time as the leading complex activity. A reconstruction of firing patterns leads to the conclusion that inhibition probably surrounds or brackets (in a time sense) the excitation of swallowing.[87]

The convergent supranuclear afferent systems (rostral to the brainstem) include the maxillary branch of CN V and CNs IX and X. These lead to the descending or spinal trigeminal system and the fasciculus and nucleus solitarii. The magnocellular part of the NTS receives input from the sensorimotor cortex and the ventromedial thalamus.[88] Some fibers of CNs IX and X project to the lateral cuneate nucleus (lateral portion of posterior spinal column), serving as a relay to the ventroposteromedial nucleus of the thalamus and limbic cortical system.

There are intrinsic and extrinsic neurologic controls for the esophageal components of swallowing. The extrinsic portion includes fibers that innervate the striated and smooth muscle portions of the esophagus. The striated (proximal third) portion of the esophagus is innervated by the recurrent branch of the vagus by the NA in the brainstem. Sympathetic and parasympathetic fibers leave the dorsal vagal nucleus in the brainstem, course through the NA, and innervate the smooth (distal two thirds) muscle of the esophagus. The intrinsic portion of esophageal nervous innervation is supplied by a neural network that lies between the circular and longitudinal esophageal musculature, referred to as the mesenteric plexus.

Supranuclear Swallowing Controls

Normal oral feeding appears to involve brainstem reflex initiation by way of several types of peripheral excitation as well as a central facilitation of its limbic and cortical sensorimotor pathways. The importance of peripheral afferent stimulation cannot be underestimated because a bolus appears to be required to sustain repetitive swallowing activity. It is difficult to conceive of the act of swallowing as either purely reflexive (brainstem mediated) or purely voluntary (supranuclear mediated) because the repetitive nature of motor activity and potential differences in sensory inputs undoubtedly need to be modulated by higher cortical structures. It is conceivable that supranuclear connections to the brainstem swallowing center are necessary to continue, modify, and monitor swallowing activity when necessary as well as respond appropriately to different sensory stimuli. Conceivably, supranuclear systems are organized so that repetitive and overlearned efferent response networks (such as chewing) are maintained by a series of feedback loops that connect jaw activity to frontal motor areas. These networks interact with interneurons that communicate with lower brainstem centers.[89] Other cortical centers appear to be reserved for modifications in swallowing activity depending on either the volitional nature of the task or changes in afferent information that may require alterations in motor performance. Kennedy and Kent[90] theorize that swallowing takes place at three different levels of nervous system organization: (1) a peripheral level that is linked to afferent bolus characteristics, (2) a subcortical level that organizes and executes learned patterns of efferent activity, and (3) a descending cortical portion that responds to any needed changes in motor activity based on perceived changes in the need to modify feeding behavior. Examples of volitional behaviors might include the need to eat faster, the need to expectorate an unwanted bolus, or perhaps the need to talk and masticate simultaneously. Investigations of these multiple pathways and centers have been conducted in human beings and animals with various laboratory techniques, including functional magnetic resonance imaging, electrical stimulation, ablation of suspected control centers, positron emission tomography, and transcranial magnetic stimulation. A complete understanding of the interrelations among centers during varying volitional and nonvolitional swallowing tasks remains speculative.

Regions of the cerebral cortex identified as active participants during swallowing are the anterior **insular cortex** with connections to the primary and **supplementary motor cortices**,[91] **orbitofrontal operculum**,[92] and the medial and superior portion of the **anterior cingulate gyrus**.[93] Interestingly, some of these areas appear to be active only for particular bolus types, such as water or a thicker liquid.[93] In animals, activation of the primary sensorimotor cortices during swallow show both inhibitory and excitatory effects that depend on the perceived strength of the stimulus.[94] Using functional magnetic resonance imaging, Shibamoto et al.[91] found that a swallow attempt with the combination of water and a capsule activated limbic and neocortical structures as well as the cerebellum. Other studies have shown activation of multiple cortical and subcortical sites, including the basal ganglia.[95,96] From preliminary data on a small number of subjects the right cortical hemisphere appears to be more active during volitional swallows, whereas the left is more active during reflexive activity.[97]

TAKE HOME NOTES

1. Swallowing is accomplished by a complex interaction of striated and smooth muscles whose sensory and motor components are carried by multiple cranial nerves.
2. The cranial nerves involved in swallowing send sensory information to the NTS. Motor components are organized in the NA. Together the NTS and NA compose the "swallowing center" located in the medulla of the brainstem.
3. Higher cortical control centers are capable of influencing the brainstem swallowing center.
4. The preparation and movement of a bolus during swallowing can be theoretically conceived as a series of valves that must open and close in a coordinated manner. This activity creates zones of high pressure around the bolus and zones of negative pressure below the level of the bolus. These pressure mismatches, together with gravity, create bolus flow.
5. Respiration ceases during swallowing. Protection of the airway to achieve a safe swallow is multifaceted. It is accomplished by primary airway closure at the level of the true and false vocal folds, laryngeal elevation, tongue base retraction, and epiglottic tilt.
6. The process of aging alone does not create dysphagia but may contribute to it, especially during disease-related decompensation.

REFERENCES

1. Leopold NA, Kagel MA: Dysphagia—ingestion or deglutition? A proposed paradigm. *Dysphagia* 12:202, 1997.
2. Stephan JR, Taves DH, Smith RC, et al: Bolus location at the initiation of the pharyngeal stage of swallowing in healthy older adults. *Dysphagia* 20:266, 2005.
3. Kendall KA: Oropharyngeal swallowing variability. *Laryngoscope* 112:547, 2002.
4. Mishellany A, Woda A, Peyron MA: The challenge of mastication: preparing a bolus suitable for deglutition. *Dysphagia* 21:87, 2006.
5. Hiiemae KM, Palmer JB: Food transport and bolus formation during complete feeding sequences on foods of different initial consistency. *Dysphagia* 14:31, 1999.
6. Kapila YV, Dodds WJ, Helm JF, et al: Relationship between swallow rate and salivary flow. *Dig Dis Sci* 29:528, 1984.

7. Steele CM, Miller AJ: Sensory input pathways and mechanisms in swallowing: a review. *Dysphagia* 25:323, 2010.

8. Ponderoux P, Logemann JA, Kahrilas PJ: Pharyngeal swallowing elicited by fluid infusion: role of volition and vallecular containment. *Am J Physiol* 270:G347, 1996.

9. Widdicombe JG: Airway receptors. *Resp Physiol* 125:3, 2001.

10. Engelen L, Fontijn-Tekamp A, van der Bilt A: The influence of product and oral characteristics on swallowing. *Arch Oral Biol* 50:739, 2005.

11. Wilson EM, Green JR: Coordinative organization of lingual propulsion during the normal adult swallow. *Dysphagia* 21:226, 2006.

12. Pearson WG, Langmore SE, Zumwalt AC: Evaluating the structural properties of suprahyoid muscles and their potential for moving the hyoid. *Dysphagia* 26:345, 2011.

13. Logemann JA, Kahrilas PJ, Cheng J, et al: Closure mechanisms of the laryngeal vestibule during swallowing. *Am J Physiol* 262(2 Pt 1):G388, 1992.

14. Cook IJ, Dodds WJ, Dantas RO, et al: Timing of videofluoroscopic, manometric events, and bolus transit during the oral and pharyngeal phases of swallowing. *Dysphagia* 4:8, 1989.

15. Martin-Harris B, Brodsky MB, Price CC, et al: Temporal coordination of pharyngeal and laryngeal dynamics with breathing during swallowing: single liquid swallows. *J Appl Physiol* 94:1235, 2003.

16. Palmer JB, Hiiemae KM: Eating and breathing: interactions between respiration and feeding on solid food. *Dysphagia* 18:169, 2003.

17. Cichero JAY, Murdoch BE: What happens after the swallow? Introducing the glottal release sound. *J Med Speech Pathol* 11:31, 2003.

18. Shaker R, Li Q, Ren J, et al: Coordination of deglutition and phases of respiration: effect of aging and tachypnea, bolus volume, and chronic obstructive pulmonary disease. *Am J Physiol* 263(5 Pt 1):G750, 1992.

19. Hiss SG, Treole K, Stuart A: Effects of age, gender, bolus volume, and trial on swallowing apnea duration and swallow/respiratory phase relationships of normal adults. *Dysphagia* 16:128, 2001.

20. Leslie P, Drinnan M, Ford G, et al: Swallow respiration patterns in dysphagic patients following acute stroke. *Dysphagia* 17:202, 2002.

21. Klahn MS, Perlman AL: Temporal and durational patterns associating respiration and swallowing. *Dysphagia* 14:131, 1999.

22. Hiss SG, Strauss M, Treole K, et al: Swallowing apnea as a function of airway closure. *Dysphagia* 18:293, 2003.

23. Kendall KA, McKenzie S, Leonard R, et al: Timing events in normal swallowing: a videofluoroscopic study. *Dysphagia* 15:74, 2000.

24. Ekberg O, Olsson R, Sundgren-Borgstrom P: Relation of bolus size and pharyngeal swallow. *Dysphagia* 3:69, 1988.

25. Ishida R, Palmer JB, Hiiemae KM: Hyoid motion during swallowing: factors affecting forward and upward displacement. *Dysphagia* 17:262, 2002.

26. Seta H, Hashimoto K, Inada H, et al: Laterality of swallowing in healthy subjects by anterior-posterior projection using videofluoroscopy. *Dysphagia* 21:191, 2006.

27. Castel JA, Castell DO: Modern solid state computerized manometry of the pharyngoesophageal segment. *Dysphagia* 8:270, 1993.

28. Bardan E, Xie P, Aslam M, et al: Disruption of primary and secondary esophageal peristalsis by afferent stimulation. *Am J Physiol Gastrointest Liver Physiol* 279:G255, 2000.

29. Castell DO: Esophageal manometric studies: a perspective of their physiological and clinical relevance. *J Clin Gastroenterol* 2:91, 1980.

30. Ekberg O, Nylander G: Cineradiography of the pharyngeal stage of deglutition in 150 patients without dysphagia. *Br J Radiol* 55:253, 1982.

31. Ren J, Shaker R, Kusano M, et al: Effect of aging on the secondary esophageal peristalsis: presbyesophagus revisited. *Am J Physiol* 268:G379, 1995.

32. Daniels SK, Schroeder MF, Degeorge PC, et al: Effects of verbal cue on bolus flow during swallowing. *Am J Speech Lang Pathol* 16:140, 2007.

33. Bennett JW, von Lieshout PHHM, Pelletier C, et al: Sip-sizing behaviors during natural drinking conditions compared to instructional experimental conditions. *Dysphagia* 24:152, 2009.

34. O'Kane L, Groher ME, Silva K, et al: Surface electromyography and normal swallowing activity. *Ann Otol Rhinol Laryngol* 11:398, 2010.

35. Molfenter SM, Steele CM: Temporal variability in the deglutition literature. *Dysphagia* 27:162, 2012.

36. Lawless HT, Bender S, Oman C, et al: Gender, age, vessel size, cup vs. straw sipping, and sequence effects on sip volume. *Dysphagia* 18:196, 2003.

37. Lee SI, Yoo JY, Kim M, et al: Changes of timing variables in swallowing of boluses with different viscosities in patients with dysphagia. *Arch Phys Med Rehabil* 94:120, 2013.

38. Adnerhill I, Ekberg O, Groher ME: Determining normal bolus size for thin liquids. *Dysphagia* 4:1, 1989.

39. Lawless HT, Bender S, Oman C, et al: Gender, age, vessel size, cup vs. straw sipping, and sequence effects on sip volume. *Dysphagia* 18:196, 2003.

40. Wintzen AR, Badrising UA, Ross RAC, et al: Influence of bolus volume on hyoid movements in normal individuals and patients with Parkinson's disease. *Can J Neurol Sci* 21:57, 1994.

41. Ekberg O, Olsson R, Sundgren-Borgström P: Relation of bolus size and pharyngeal swallow. *Dysphagia* 3:69, 1988.

42. Leonard RJ, Kendall KA, McKenzie S, et al: Structural displacements in normal swallowing: a videofluoroscopic study. *Dysphagia* 15:146, 2000.

43. Chi-Fishman G, Sonies BC: Effects of systematic bolus velocity and volume changes on hyoid movement kinematics. *Dysphagia* 17:278, 2007.

44. Jacob K, Kahrilas PJ, Logemann JA, et al: Upper esophageal sphincter opening and modulation during swallowing. *Gastroenterology* 97:1469, 1989.

45. Miller JL, Watkin KL: The influence of bolus volume and viscosity on anterior lingual force during the oral stage of swallowing. *Dysphagia* 11:117, 1996.

46. Cook IJ, Dodds WJ, Dantas RO, et al: Timing of videofluoroscopic, manometric events, and bolus transit during the oral and pharyngeal phases of swallowing. *Dysphagia* 4:8, 1989.

47. Youmans SR, Stierwalt JAG: Measures of tongue function related to normal swallowing. *Dysphagia* 21:102, 2006.

48. Gingrich LL, Stierwalt JAG, Hageman CF, et al: Lingual propulsive pressures across consistencies generated by the anteromedian and posteromedian tongue by healthy adults. *J Speech Lang Hear Res* 55:960, 2012.

49. Pelletier CA, Dhanaraj GE: The effect of taste and palatability on lingual swallowing pressure. *Dysphagia* 21:121, 2006.

50. Palmer PM, McCulloch TM, Jaffe D, et al: Effects of a sour bolus on the intramuscular electromyographic (EMG) activity of muscles in the submental region. *Dysphagia* 20:210, 2005.

51. Krival K, Bates C: Effects of club soda and ginger brew on linguapalatal pressures in healthy swallowing. *Dysphagia* 27:228, 2012.

52. Daniels SK, Foundas AL: Swallowing physiology of sequential straw drinking. *Dysphagia* 16:176, 2001.

53. Daniels SK, Corey DM, Hadskey LD, et al: Mechanism of sequential swallowing during straw drinking in healthy young and older adults. *J Speech Lang Hear Res* 47:33, 2004.

54. Saitoh E, Shibaba S, Matsuo K, et al: Chewing and food consistency: effects on bolus transport and swallow initiation. *Dysphagia* 22:107, 2007.

55. Hwang J, Kim DK, Bae JH, et al: The effect of rheological properties of foods on bolus characteristics after mastication. *Ann Rehab Med* 36:776, 2012.

56. Robbins JA, Hamilton J, Lof G, et al: Oropharyngeal swallowing in normal adults of different ages. *Gastroenterology* 103:823, 1992.

57. Robbins J: Normal swallowing and aging. *Semin Neurol* 16:309, 1996.

58. Levine R, Robbins JA, Maser A: Periventricular white matter changes and oropharyngeal swallowing in normal individuals. *Dysphagia* 7:142, 1992.

59. Brodsky MB, McFarland DH, Michel Y, et al: Significance of non-respiratory airflow during swallowing. *Dysphagia* 27:178, 2012.

60. Shaker R, Lang IM: Aging and deglutitive motor function: effect of aging on the deglutitive oral, pharyngeal, and esophageal motor function. *Dysphagia* 9:221, 1994.

61. Nicosia M, Hind JA, Roecker EB, et al: Age effects on the temporal evolution of isometric swallowing pressure. *J Gerontol A Biol Sci Med Sci* 55:634, 2000.

62. Logemann JA, Pauloski BR, Rademaker AW, et al: Temporal and biomechanical characteristics of oropharyngeal swallow in younger and older men. *J Speech Lang Hear Res* 43:126, 2000.

63. Youmans SR, Youmans GL, Stierwalt JAG: Differences in tongue strength across age and gender: is there a diminished reserve? *Dysphagia* 24:57, 2009.

64. Fei T, Polacco RC, Hori SE, et al: Age-related differences in tongue-palate pressures for strength and swallowing tasks. *Dysphagia* 28:575, 2013.

65. Tanaka N, Nohara K, Kotani Y, et al: Swallowing frequency in elderly people during daily life. *J Oral Rehabil* 40:744, 2013.

66. Murphy C, Shubert CR, Cruickshanks KJ, et al: Prevalence of olfactory impairment in older adults. *JAMA* 288:2307, 2002.

67. Schiffman SS: Taste and smell losses in normal aging and disease. *JAMA* 278:1357, 1997.

68. Schiffman SS, Graham BG: Taste and smell perception affect appetite and immunity in the elderly. *Eur J Clin Nutr* 54:S54, 2000.

69. Smith CH, Logemann JA, Burghardt WR, et al: Oral and oropharyngeal perceptions of fluid viscosity across the age span. *Dysphagia* 21:209, 2006.

70. Peyron MA, Blanc O, Lund JP, et al: Influence of age on the adaptability of human mastication. *J Neurophysiol* 92:773, 2004.

71. Jones B, Donner MW: *Normal and abnormal swallowing: imaging in diagnosis and therapy*, New York, 1991, Springer-Verlag.

72. McKee GJ, Johnston BT, McBride GB, et al: Does age or sex affect pharyngeal swallowing? *Clin Otolaryngol* 23:100, 1998.

73. Logemann JA, Pauloski BR, Rademaker AW, et al: Temporal and biomechanical characteristics of oropharyngeal swallow in younger and older men. *J Speech Lang Hear Res* 43:1264, 2000.

74. Van Herwaarden MA, Katz PO, Gideon M, et al: Are manometric parameters of the upper esophageal sphincter and pharynx affected by age and gender? *Dysphagia* 18:211, 2003.

75. Shaker R, Ren J, Podvrsan B, et al: Effect of aging and bolus variables on pharyngeal and upper esophageal sphincter motor function. *Am J Physiol* 264:427, 1993.

76. Daggett A, Logemann JA, Rademaker AW, et al: Laryngeal penetration during deglutition in normal subjects of various ages. *Dysphagia* 21:270, 2006.

77. Selley WG, Flack FC, Ellis RE, et al: Respiratory patterns associated with swallowing. Part 1. The normal adult pattern and changes with aging. *Age Aging* 18:168, 1989.

78. Aviv JE, Martin JH, Jones ME, et al: Age-related changes in pharyngeal and supraglottic sensation. *Ann Otol Rhinol Laryngol* 10:749, 1994.

79. Zboralske FF, Amberg JR, Soergel KH: Presbyesophagus: cineradiographic manifestations. *Radiology* 82:463, 1964.

80. Jean A: Brainstem organization of the swallowing network. *Brain Behav Evol* 25:109, 1984.

81. Mu L, Sanders I: Sensory nerve supply of the human oro- and laryngopharynx: a preliminary study. *Anat Rec* 258:406, 2000.

82. Jean A: Brain stem control of swallowing: neuronal network and cellular mechanisms. *Physiol Rev* 81:929, 2001.

83. Lang I: Brain stem control of the phases of swallowing. *Dysphagia* 24:333, 2009.

84. Ekberg O, Nylander G: Cineradiography of the pharyngeal stage of deglutition in 150 individuals without dysphagia. *Br J Radiol* 55:253, 1982.

85. Rontal M, Rontal E: Lesions of the vagus nerve: diagnosis, treatment, and rehabilitation. *Laryngoscope* 87:72, 1977.

86. Mu L, Sanders I: Muscle fiber-type distribution patterns in the human cricopharyngeus muscle. *Dysphagia* 17:87, 2002.

87. Doty RW, Bosma JF: Electromyographic analysis of reflex deglutition. *J Neurophysiol* 19:44, 1956.

88. Bass N: The neurology of swallowing. In Groher ME, editor: *Dysphagia: diagnosis and management*, ed 3, Boston, 1997, Butterworth-Heinemann.

89. Martin RE, Sessle BJ: The role of the cerebral cortex in swallowing. *Dysphagia* 8:195, 1993.

90. Kennedy JG, Kent RD: Physiologic substrates of normal deglutition. *Dysphagia* 3:24, 1988.

91. Daniels SK, Foundas AL: The role of the insular cortex in dysphagia. *Dysphagia* 12:146, 1997.

92. Martin RE, Kemppainen P, Masuda Y, et al: Features of cortically evoked swallowing in the awake primate. *J Neurophysiol* 82:1529, 1999.

93. Shibamoto I, Tanaka T, Fujishima I, et al: Cortical activation during solid bolus swallowing. *J Med Dent Sci* 54:25, 2007.

94. Power M, Fraser C, Hobson A, et al: Changes in pharyngeal corticobulbar excitability and swallowing behavior after oral stimulation. *Am J Physiol Gastrointest Liver Physiol* 286:G45, 2004.

95. Hamdy S, Rothwell JC, Brooks DJ, et al: Identification of the cerebral loci processing human swallowing with H2(15)O PET activation. *J Neurophysiol* 81:1917, 1999.

96. Suzuki M, Asada J, Ito K, et al: Activation of cerebellum and basal ganglia on volitional swallowing detected by functional magnetic resonance imaging. *Dysphagia* 18:71, 2003.

97. Kern MK, Jaradeh S, Arndorfer RC, et al: Cerebral cortical representation of reflexive and volitional swallowing in humans. *Am J Physiol* 280:G354, 2001.

CHAPTER 3

Adult Neurologic Disorders

Michael A. Crary

To view additional case videos and content, please visit the evolve website.

CHAPTER OUTLINE

OBJECTIVES

1. Explain why is it important to possess a basic understanding of the nervous system to clinically manage swallowing disorders resulting from neurologic disease.
2. Name some of the sensorimotor characteristics associated with impairments at different levels of the nervous system.
3. Identify some of the dysphagia characteristics that might be seen in diseases affecting various levels of the nervous system.
4. Describe some of the dysphagia-related problems that might be seen in patients with neurologic disease.
5. Describe some aspects of change in dysphagia over time in neurologic diseases.
6. Identify some of the more common treatment issues, decisions, options, and practices in different forms of neurogenic dysphagia.

PRELIMINARY CONSIDERATIONS: SWALLOWING SYMPTOMS AND NEUROLOGIC DEFICITS

Swallowing disorders are symptoms of underlying disease processes. One implication of this perspective is that swallowing disorders in patients with neurologic disorders should manifest the characteristics of damage to different areas of the nervous system. This premise has long been accepted in the arena of motor speech disorders (**dysarthria**).[1] For example, spastic dysarthria results from damage to the upper motor neuron system governing speech production. Upper motor neuron damage results in specific patterns of neuromotor impairment, including spasticity, slowed movement, exaggerated reflexes, and reduced range of movement. The characteristics of spastic dysarthria are believed to be the direct result of spasticity in the corticobulbar system governing speech production. Patients with spastic dysarthria demonstrate a slow rate of speech, limited movement of the speech articulators, equalized stress patterns, and other characteristics reflecting the underlying neuromotor characteristics of spastic weakness.

A similar framework helps clinical specialists evaluate and plan treatment for patients with swallowing disorders resulting from neurologic deficit. Patients with damage to upper motor neuron systems characteristically demonstrate spastic weakness with resultant slowness and reduced range of movement. This may translate to reduced speed of swallowing (i.e., a delay in initiating one or more components of the swallow) or reduced range of movement in the swallowing mechanism (i.e., reduced transport of the bolus contributing to postswallow residue). To understand better the potential clinical applications of such a framework, clinical specialists must be familiar with neuroanatomy, neurologic functions and dysfunctions of various nervous system components, and sensorimotor components of swallowing at different stages of the swallow. Chapter 2 describes the basic anatomy and neuroanatomy of swallowing functions. A summary of some common neurologic functions associated with various levels within the central nervous system follows.

Brief Overview of Functional Neuroanatomy Relative to Swallowing Functions

Adequate swallowing depends heavily on adequate movement of structures within the upper aerodigestive tract. Motor and sensory systems work together to produce movement, including movement associated with swallowing. However, in clinical practice motor and sensory functions frequently are described separately as they may relate to impaired swallowing physiology. To facilitate a clinical perspective, a top-down approach to the nervous system is followed in which sensory and motor components are described at each level. Figure 3-1 is a simplified schematic depicting each "level" of the nervous system. Table 3-1 summarizes neurobehavioral and sensorimotor functions associated with each level.

CORTICAL FUNCTIONS

Functional control of sensorimotor behaviors in the human cortex frequently is described in reference to various areas

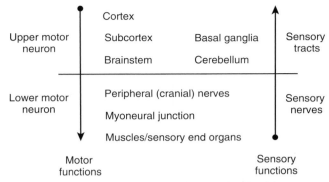

FIGURE 3-1 Simplified schematic of various levels of the nervous system.

TABLE 3-1 Basic Sensorimotor Functions Associated with Different Levels of the Nervous System

Level	Motor	Sensory
Cortical	Intent	Recognition
	Initiation	Awareness
	Programming	Motor tuning
	Execution	
Subcortical (basal ganglia)	Initiation	Motor tuning
	Refinement	Awareness
	Inhibition	Sensory conduit
Brainstem	Junction box:	Reflexes
	upper motor neuron/ lower motor neuron	Sensory conduit
	Motor/sensory "centers":	
	Swallow	
	Respiration	
	Heart	
Cerebellum	Refinement	Refinement
	Inhibition	
Peripheral nerves	Lower motor neuron	Sensory conduit
	Drive movement	
Muscles and sensory receptors	Effect movement	Sensation reception

or regions. The frontal lobe cortex is deemed responsible for multiple aspects of motor control, ranging from intent and initiation of movement to coordinating a movement in time and space to executing the movement in an organized and timely fashion. In general, parietal lobe regions are responsible for recognizing and interpreting sensory functions. These functions might include identifying the presence of a sensory stimulus or the interpretation of a sensory stimulus in reference to an appropriate motor response. Sensorimotor impairments resulting from cortical damage may vary in response to the location of neurologic deficit, extent of the deficit (larger areas of damage are believed to result in more severe or widespread behavioral impairments), and whether the neurologic damage is unilateral or bilateral.

Other important functions housed within the cortex are those of human communication and cognition. Damage to primarily the left side of the brain may result in a number of difficulties in the ability to communicate. Focal attention is frequently afforded to the area of the inferior frontal lobe and superior temporal lobe, although damage to these areas often is accompanied by damage to adjacent motor control areas of the frontal lobe and/or sensory control areas of the parietal lobe. Cognitive deficits associated with cortical dysfunction may present in various forms with different levels of severity and different clinical courses depending on the location of damage and the nature of the underlying disease process.

Arriving to and leaving from the cortex are the major sensory and motor tracts within the central nervous system. Damage to the sensory tracts arriving in the primary sensory strip of the anterior parietal lobe results in loss of recognition of sensory stimuli in the corresponding body area. Damage to the motor tracts leaving the primary motor strip in the posterior frontal lobe (upper motor neurons) results in paresis or paralysis of the corresponding body area. Sensory or motor deficits are similar regardless of the location of the damage along the tracts. For example, cortical level damage to the upper motor neuron system results in the same type of motor weakness as subcortical or brainstem upper motor neuron damage.

Cortical Functions and Swallowing Impairment

If motor functions of the cortex range from intent to execution, then swallowing deficits resulting from cortical damage may range from no observable swallow activity to poorly coordinated execution of the act of swallowing. In considering these possibilities, frequent cortical pathologic conditions such as stroke, dementia, and traumatic brain injury (TBI) should be reviewed.

Before reviewing dysphagia characteristics in various cortical pathologies, a worthwhile question to ask is "Where is swallowing function represented in the human cortex?" Given the complexity of motor control involved in oropharyngeal swallowing, it is logical to implicate the frontal cortex, specifically areas involved in various components of motor control. In fact, results of both animal and human studies using lesion or cortical stimulation techniques implicate the importance of the lateral frontal cortex, the inferior frontal lobule, and the insula in various motor acts associated with feeding and swallowing. Recent studies using **functional magnetic resonance imaging (fMRI)** implicate a wide range of cortical, subcortical, and

brainstem structures involved in swallowing performed by healthy volunteers.[2-4] Not surprisingly, the primary motor and sensory cortical areas consistently participated in swallowing function. In a comparison of ischemic stroke patients with dysphagia and stroke patients without dysphagia, the internal capsule emerged as the only brain region significantly associated with dysphagia. However, other areas of the sensorimotor cortex and the basal ganglia also were frequently associated with the presence of dysphagia in stroke patients.[5]

Although findings from many studies implicate a dysphagia based in poor motor control resulting from damage to the anterolateral and precentral frontal cortex, no consensus exists concerning the specific characteristics of these dysphagias. Still, hemispheric damage to frontal areas underpinning motor control resulting in direct movement deficits should raise significant clinical concern for the presence of dysphagia.

What about cortical or hemisphere lesions that impair sensory function? These sensory areas of the hemisphere may be important in understanding swallowing functions and impairments. In fact, some studies report that many stroke patients with dysphagia have damage to the parietal lobe with associated sensory deficits.[6] Primary sensory areas of the cortex have extensive interconnections with the motor areas of the cortex. Sensory function is deemed important in the control of voluntary movement. Beyond direct sensory loss, we should consider conditions in which the patient cannot interpret sensory information, for example, **neglect**. Patients with neglect may not respond to a stimulus in the swallowing tract (food or liquid bolus), not because of direct sensory loss, but because of a cortical deficit in processing and interpreting sensory information. In at least one study, hemispatial neglect was related to clinician recommended nonoral intake of food and liquid, but not severity of dysphagia, in patients evaluated 3 days after hospital admission for stroke.[7] Unfortunately, these investigators did not interpret the association between neglect and nonoral intake. As a result, the presence of neglect may be related to feeding limitations rather than swallowing deficits leading to nonoral intake.

More recently, increased systematic attention has been afforded sensory functions in swallowing and swallowing impairment.[8-10] Continued emerging information and clinical observations suggest that impaired sensory functions may have a direct influence on swallowing functions. A better understanding of the role of sensory systems on swallowing function and impairment may lead to improved sensory-based interventions for dysphagia (see Clinical Corner 3-1).

Issues of Unilateral versus Bilateral Hemispheric Lesions

The issues previously raised regarding hemispheric contribution to swallowing control also raise the question of

CLINICAL CORNER 3-1: SENSORY DEFICITS AND SWALLOWING

Sensory deficits may be observed in many neurologic (and nonneurologic) diseases and disorders. They may range from a direct loss of sensory input (e.g., numbness, blindness) up to and including the inability to interpret an intact sensory signal (e.g., agnosia, cortical blindness). Depending on the nature of the sensory deficit, patients may have reduced (and at times insufficient) oral intake of food and liquid. However, this deficit level of oral intake of food and liquid may not represent a dysphagia (here meaning specific difficulty swallowing food). Rather, certain sensory deficits may contribute to feeding limitations that reduce oral intake of food and liquid. Clinical specialists in the area of dysphagia need to be able to differentiate various sensory deficits and interpret their impact on feeding versus swallowing impairments.

Critical Thinking

1. What types of sensory problems might occur within the swallowing mechanism—specifically the oral and pharyngeal components of the mechanism? Consider various diseases and disorders that might contribute to these sensory deficits. Be sure to consider direct sensory loss versus deficit interpretation of sensory input.

2. How would you evaluate sensory functions within the swallow mechanism from direct sensory loss up to poor interpretation of sensory information?

3. What practical impact might sensory deficits have on the oral intake of food and liquid? Consider specific clinical examples.

whether such control is unilateral or bilateral. A traditional perspective is that patients with bilateral lesions often demonstrate the most severe and persistent dysphagia characteristics.[11] Still, patients with unilateral hemisphere lesions may demonstrate dysphagia to varying degrees. Research using the technique of transcranial magnetic stimulation has suggested an interesting point of view on the hemispheric representation of swallowing function. Transcranial magnetic stimulation involves sending a magnetic current across the cranium over discrete hemisphere regions. These magnetic currents stimulate motor activity that is measured in various muscles by electromyography. This interesting work on the hemispheric control of swallowing function can be summarized as follows:

1. Swallowing motor functions are bilaterally represented in the hemispheres.

2. If the dominant hemisphere is impaired, a contralateral "backup" area may be available to facilitate recovery.

3. A form of **cortical plasticity** may occur over time, increasing the utility of the intact, nondominant hemisphere to control swallowing motor functions.

4. Bilateral strokes would result in the most tenacious dysphagias.[12-15]

In some respects, this perspective is consistent with traditional clinical observations; bilateral strokes produce the most severe dysphagia, and many patients with unilateral strokes often recover the ability to swallow after a period of dysphagia.

SWALLOWING DEFICITS IN HEMISPHERIC STROKE SYNDROMES

Several issues must be addressed when considering dysphagia secondary to hemispheric strokes. These issues may be simplified into two general considerations: location and extent of damage and functional consequences of the damage. These considerations are not mutually exclusive. Location and extent of the damage may be important in understanding sensory and motor impairments and in understanding the severity and potential for recovery based on unilateral versus bilateral lesions. In clinical practice, information on lesion characteristics often is not available at the time of the dysphagia evaluation. Therefore a strong reliance on the clinical examination of functional impairment after stroke may provide the best "road map" to understanding and perhaps predicting dysphagia characteristics. Table 3-1 provides a basic orientation to some of the functional impairments that may be clinically observed after impairment to various levels of the nervous system. At the hemisphere level, intent to swallow may be an important consideration. If the patient indicates such intent, a subsequent consideration would be motor initiation of the swallow. Patients with damage to premotor areas (e.g., supplemental motor cortex) may have generalized difficulty with motor initiation. The clinical picture may be that of a patient who holds a bolus in the mouth for an abnormally long period with associated movements that indicate the intent to swallow but without initiating a swallow (see Practice Note 3-1).

Patients with sensory deficits may demonstrate a variety of dysphagia characteristics, including retention of a portion of a bolus in the mouth, oropharynx, or hypopharynx with no attempt to clear the residue. These patients also may be more susceptible to aspiration of material into the upper airway as a result of the sensory deficit. Another category of sensory deficit may be seen in the patient with neglect. Such patients may not recognize material presented to one side of the swallowing tract. These patients may hold material in the mouth with no apparent intent to swallow, but in fact they are unaware of the material in the mouth.

Finally, patients with hemispheric stroke may have significant communication deficits or cognitive deficits that reduce their ability to relate to the clinical examiner the nature of the dysphagia complaints. Patients who are asleep, lethargic, have waxing and waning alertness, or difficulty

PRACTICE NOTE 3-1

The difference between intent to swallow and poor initiation of the swallow may be difficult to ascertain clinically. Some patients may hold food or liquid material in the mouth but not make any overt attempt to swallow. When this situation is encountered, one strategy is to observe differences in swallows when the patient self-feeds versus when the clinician provides the material to be swallowed.

Several years ago we encountered a young woman who had a severe stroke. Details of the stroke were sparse other than it was large and involved the frontal areas of the brain. She was nonverbal but did produce some vocalizations and demonstrated a very hypokinetic appearance. She was receiving all nutrition and hydration by gastrostomy tube. During the fluoroscopic swallowing study a clinician placed materials in the patient's mouth by spoon. No overt reaction was noted to the placement of liquid or pudding material in the mouth. A colleague who was observing the examination suggested having the patient self-feed. We did not believe this was viable because of the paucity of spontaneous movement demonstrated by this patient, but we placed a spoon in the patient's hand and assisted her through the movements of filling the spoon with a liquid and then placing it in her mouth. The difference in swallow was dramatic. The woman swallowed the liquid material almost immediately. She demonstrated little residue and no airway compromise. This pattern was repeated for all materials presented in this manner. This simple change in feeding strategy was subsequently used in her daily rehabilitation program and she eventually returned to total oral feeding.

Refer to Video 3-1, *A* and *B*, on the companion Evolve site for an example of fluoroscopic swallowing differences in a single patient. This patient had a large right hemispheric middle cerebral artery stroke. In her initial fluoroscopic swallowing examination the clinician "fed" the patient barium contrast materials. A week later, the fluoroscopic examination was repeated because the reported results did not match the clinical profile. In this second examination we asked the patient to self-feed. The differences were dramatic.

participating in the swallowing evaluation because of cognitive deficits present significant challenges to a valid evaluation of swallowing abilities (see Practice Note 3-2). Also, the inability to describe swallowing difficulties may delay or hinder clinical evaluation and implementation of rehabilitation strategies. Figure 3-2 depicts general hemisphere areas that may be associated with various sensorimotor functions associated with swallowing. The left hemisphere is shown for descriptive purposes only. Box 3-1 presents various swallowing characteristics that may be associated with sensorimotor deficits after hemispheric stroke.

A variety of swallowing deficits have been reported after hemispheric stroke. In general, hemispheric lesions (including both cortical and subcortical damage) contribute to many swallowing deficits (Box 3-2), including (1) poor initiation of saliva swallows (sometimes termed the *dry swallow*), (2) delay in initiation of the pharyngeal component of the swallow, (3) incoordination of the oral components of swallowing, (4) increased pharyngeal transit time and reduced pharyngeal constriction and clearing, (5) aspiration, (6) dysfunction of the pharyngoesophageal segment (cricopharyngeal muscle), and (7) poor relaxation of the lower esophageal sphincter. These collective observations indicate that hemispheric stroke can impair swallowing functions from the mouth to the stomach. Furthermore, a wide spectrum of swallowing deficits has been noted, ranging from impaired initiation of the swallow to poor transport of the bolus to aspiration into the airway. To date no report has emerged comparing specific sensorimotor stroke sequelae with specific swallowing impairments. However, the preceding list suggests that the array of potential swallowing deficits after

PRACTICE NOTE 3-2

Acute stroke patients may present a variety of clinical signs and certainly are at risk for a variety of morbidities. One issue that seems obvious but may not be apparent to all health care providers is the level of alertness presented by the patient. Some stroke patients may be generally lethargic, whereas others may demonstrate a waxing and waning level of alertness.

A few years ago, I was working on the inpatient service in our hospital when I received a request for a consultation from a neurologist whom I knew well. The consult was to "evaluate and treat" dysphagia in a patient who had survived a recent stroke. On entering the patient's room I found her asleep. I tried to gently awaken her by speaking close to her ear, then by speaking louder, then by washing her face and hands with a cloth rinsed in cold water. Nothing worked. I entered a note in the chart that the patient could not be aroused and that the service should reconsult when her status improved. The next day I received another consultation request from the same neurologist. I visited the patient at a different time during the day with the same result. In fact, I went back at different times on the same day with the same result. I called the neurologist and arranged to be with him when he next saw this patient. Together we agreed that this patient could not realistically participate in a swallowing examination and we would wait and watch. In another few days she "woke up" and we evaluated her swallow and began small amounts of oral intake.

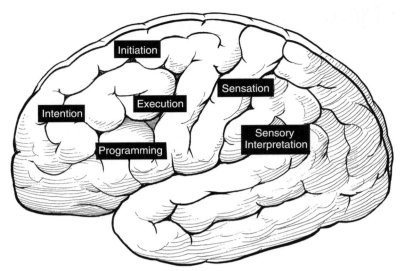

FIGURE 3-2 Various hemisphere areas that may be associated with sensorimotor functions supporting swallowing function.

BOX 3-1 GENERAL SENSORIMOTOR CONSIDERATIONS FOR VARIOUS SWALLOWING DEFICITS IN HEMISPHERE STROKE

- Volitional motor control
  - Initiation difficulties
- Paresis, paralysis
  - Transport difficulties
- Sensory recognition
  - Residue
  - Aspiration
- Communication deficits
  - Inability to describe difficulties

BOX 3-2 SWALLOWING DEFICITS IN PATIENTS AFTER HEMISPHERE STROKE

- Reduced ability to initiate a saliva swallow
- Delayed triggering of pharyngeal swallow
- Incoordination of oral movements in swallow
- Increased pharyngeal transit time
- Reduced pharyngeal constriction
- Aspiration
- Pharyngoesophageal segment dysfunction
- Impaired lower esophageal sphincter relaxation

---

stroke is extensive and may relate to the spectrum of post-stroke sensorimotor impairments (see Practice Note 3-3).

Dysphagia is highly prevalent in acute stroke, with estimates that well over 50% of all patients are affected. Early identification of dysphagia in acute stroke is a critical feature of clinical management as dysphagia is related to numerous health complications. Fortunately, the majority of acute stroke patients recover functional swallowing ability within the first 1 to 6 months after stroke, whereas swallowing problems develop in a small percentage of patients during the postacute period.[16-18] These observations emphasize the importance of accurate identification and management of swallowing deficits in acute stroke patients. Furthermore, it is important to understand factors that might predict persistent swallowing problems beyond the acute recovery period. The importance of this perspective is highlighted by the observation that acute and chronic swallowing problems in stroke patients are associated with many complications, including increased length of hospitalization, dehydration, malnutrition, aspiration, chest infections and, in some cases, death.[18-21] Furthermore, dysphagia during acute stroke is associated with poor long-term outcome, including death and an increased rate of institutionalization.[22]

Treatment Considerations

Perhaps the most obvious statement about dysphagia in stroke is that it changes over time. From that perspective, dysphagia intervention strategies should also change over time. Table 3-2 presents clinical considerations and decisions that may affect treatment planning over time. Early in the course of a stroke, focus should be given to basic decisions such as the safety of oral feeding versus the need for nonoral feeding routes, the presence of comorbid conditions such as pneumonia (or other infections), malnutrition, dehydration, and the overall medical condition of the patient.

The acute stroke patient is at greatest risk for dysphagia and morbidities associated with dysphagia. The presence, or more accurately, the risk of dysphagia in acute stroke is best identified with screening programs (see previous discussion and Clinical Corner 3-2). In general, any patient who "fails" an early dysphagia screen should be thoroughly assessed during the early acute stroke period to confirm the presence and detail the characteristics of any dysphagia.

PRACTICE NOTE 3-3

Recently I saw two patients within a short time frame who had similar histories and clinical presentations. Both patients were stroke survivors and at least 6 months past the stroke event. Both were deemed medically stable. Both depended on nonoral percutaneous endoscopic gastrostomy (PEG) feedings. And both had difficulty managing their oral secretions; they drooled and carried a towel to "mop up the problem." Finally, neither patient had functional speaking ability, but both could vocalize and phonate simple vowels. These patients were referred for evaluation and treatment of pharyngeal dysphagia.

On the surface, this clinical presentation may make sense. However, the basic problem for both patients was not pharyngeal dysphagia, but rather oral **apraxia**. Admittedly, oral apraxia was quite severe in both patients. Both presented with a persistent open-mouth posture but in the absence of overt weakness within the facial or oral musculature. Both could close the mouth in response to intraoral sensory stimuli and both spontaneously swallowed, though infrequently. A key feature of the clinical examination in both cases was the absence of overt cranial nerve deficits. Also, each patient had the ability to close the mouth, but this was context dependent (e.g., they did not close the mouth on command, but when liquid was placed in the posterior mouth they did close and a spontaneous swallow was observed). As part of the clinical swallow examination, liquid was placed in the oropharyngeal area with a straw as a pipette. As this liquid trickled into the hypopharynx, we occasionally observed a swallow. Under endoscopic inspection we delivered additional liquid to the oropharynx in this fashion. I also learned that both patients protected their airway and that no residue remained after these volume-dependent swallows.

Based on these clinical and endoscopic findings I did not enroll these patients in therapy for pharyngeal dysphagia. The dysphagia was primarily the result of a severe oral apraxia that limited oral motor control for voluntary tasks, including swallowing.

I did make simple recommendations that I hoped would improve oral functions for feeding and oral control for swallowing. Because I observed intermittent spontaneous swallows when liquid was placed in the posterior part of the mouth, I recommended this technique in an attempt to stimulate improved oral swallow initiation. I suggested to the local therapist that if the frequency of spontaneous swallowing improved, she should vary the type and amount of material used in this fashion and gradually place the material more forward within the mouth. Later I heard from one of the local therapists that her patient had increased the frequency of spontaneous swallowing and was taking more oral intake. Sometimes success comes in small steps.

Refer to Video 3-2, *A* and *B*, on the Evolve site for endoscopic and fluoroscopic examples of a single patient who demonstrated significant oral apraxia in the presence of preserved pharyngeal swallowing function.

CLINICAL CORNER 3-2: DYSPHAGIA SCREENING IN ACUTE STROKE

Identification of dysphagia in acute stroke is attempted by screening protocols (see Chapter 7). Successful dysphagia screening programs have been associated with reduced rates of poststroke pneumonia. However, screening programs are attempted differently across hospitals and no consensus exists on the most appropriate or beneficial screening protocol. Most screening protocols incorporate some form of limited clinical examination. Some incorporate a "test swallow" of one or more materials, whereas others do not ask the patient to swallow.

Critical Thinking
1. Why does early identification contribute to reduced pneumonia in stroke survivors? What other stroke and dysphagia complications might screening impact?
2. Discuss what might be the "ideal" screening program for dysphagia in acute stroke. Who should screen patients? Which patients should be screened? What is the "optimal" form for the screening tool?

During the acute phase of stroke, patients are likely to demonstrate significant weakness contributing to reduced stamina and perhaps reduced mental status, including alertness and attention. These factors significantly limit any meaningful clinical (or other) evaluation of swallowing ability. Thus a conservative strategy is to observe the patient's status and postpone any in-depth assessment or intervention until the patient is more alert and has better endurance. *Acute stroke patients also are at risk for respiratory abnormalities.* Respiratory abnormalities include basic weakness in expiratory muscles that might reduce cough effectiveness,[23] increased episodes of **oxygen desaturation**,[24,25] deviations in the respiratory rate,[26] and alterations in the coordination between respiration and swallowing.[27,28] Collectively, these respiratory deviations noted in acute stroke patients suggest an increased risk of aspiration of swallowed materials and pooled secretions and potential limitations in clearing aspirated secretions as a result of reduced cough efficiency. Given these potential risks, respiratory functions in the acute stroke patient should be evaluated as part of the comprehensive swallowing examination.

Pneumonia is noted in approximately 10% of acute stroke patients, with a higher prevalence if patients in the

TABLE 3-2 Treatment Considerations and Decisions for Dysphasia after Stroke*

Considerations	Decisions
Acute (0-1 Month)	
Most comorbid conditions	How to avoid or minimize complications
Resolving dysphagia	Need and readiness for therapy
Nutrition/hydration	How to maintain or improve nutrition and hydration
Improving (1-6 Months)	
Patient more stable with better endurance	Need and readiness for therapy
Comorbid conditions often under medical control	Type of therapy
Feeding routes established for most	
Malnutrition may still be a factor	
Chronic (After 6 Months)	
Feeding routes more established	Therapy or no therapy (prognosis?)
Patients eating orally may have impaired swallow	Type of therapy
Compensations that interfere with swallow	
Impact of prior therapy	

*Changing issues with time after onset.

intensive care unit are included.[29] Pneumonia is a significant morbidity because it is related to both an increased number of hospital readmissions[30] and short-term and long-term mortality.[31] Causes of pneumonia in the poststroke patient are multifactorial; however, dysphagia, especially dysphagia accompanied by aspiration, is significantly related to the presence of pneumonia.[18] In fact, dysphagia screening leading to early identification and treatment of swallowing deficits in acute stroke patients has been associated with a reduction in pneumonia rates.[32-34]

The presence of dysphagia after stroke may contribute to pneumonia in various ways. Although the focus is often on aspiration of orally ingested food and liquid, aspiration of pooled pharyngeal secretions also may contribute to chest infection. Aspiration of secretions may be especially problematic in the acute stroke population because oral bacteria colonization is prominent in these patients.[35] Patients dependent on tube feeding, specifically nasogastric tube feeding, may have a higher degree of bacterial colonization than patients who feed orally.[36] In fact, at least one clinical research team has reported that stroke patients who were dependent on nonoral feeding (e.g., nothing by mouth) demonstrated higher rates of respiratory infections than did stroke survivors who were feeding orally.[37-39] One implication of these findings is that reduced frequency of swallowing contributes to an increased risk of aspirating pharyngeal secretions in the presence of higher rates of bacterial colonization within the swallowing mechanism.[40] This premise is supported by treatment studies demonstrating that swallowing therapy[41] and strategies to improve oral hygiene[42,43] reduce the incidence of pneumonia in stroke patients. Thus the dysphagia clinician should consider more than aspiration of food and liquid when providing swallowing interventions to patients after acute stroke.

Nutrition and hydration deficits are prevalent among stroke patients on admission and may worsen during hospitalization. On admission, the prevalence of nutritional deficits has been estimated at approximately 16%; this figure increases to 22% to 26% through discharge from acute care.[44-46] Moreover, at least one study has identified an initial association between dysphagia and dehydration in acute stroke.[40] In this study 53% of acute stroke patients demonstrated some degree of dehydration based on laboratory values (blood urea nitrogen/**creatinine** >15:1). Patients with dysphagia demonstrated greater dehydration compared to those without dysphagia. Furthermore, the degree of dehydration as measured by the laboratory value increased selectively among dysphagia patients during acute care. Though preliminary, these results place a strong focus on the hydration status of acute stroke patients, especially those identified with dysphagia.

Nutritional decline continues beyond acute care. The prevalence of nutritional deficits in stroke patients at admission to rehabilitation approximates 50%.[47] At approximately 1 month after stroke, nutritional status begins to improve and continues to improve up to 4 months after stroke. In the acute stroke patient, nutritional deficits are not overtly linked to dysphagia.[45,48] However, later during the rehabilitation period and thereafter, swallowing and feeding difficulties may contribute to the maintenance or increase in poor nutritional status.[49] Still, some suggest that poor nutrition during the acute phase of stroke contributes to poor longer term functional outcomes.[50] Nutritional evaluation and intervention are outside the scope of practice for most dysphagia clinicians. However, all dysphagia clinicians should be aware of the potential impact of swallowing and feeding abilities on nutritional status and participate in multidisciplinary health care teams that include nutritional specialists.

As the patient's condition improves and more active rehabilitation is initiated (usually well within the first month after stroke), dysphagia treatment strategies also may change. One consideration is spontaneous resolution of dysphagia as the patient recovers from the effects of acute stroke. Although many stroke patients have some degree of recovery in swallowing ability, estimates of persisting dysphagia range from 11% to 50% at 6 months after stroke.[16,51] During this period of improvement the patient with persistent dysphagia is likely to be engaged in active swallowing rehabilitation. By this time a decision about oral or nonoral feeding has already been established and comorbid conditions are often under medical control. Of importance to active dysphagia rehabilitation are various patient issues and the nature of the swallowing deficit. If the patient is able to participate in active rehabilitation and is motivated, direct and intense swallowing therapy is expected to produce significant benefit. Benefits from swallowing therapy extend beyond improved swallowing abilities to include reduced pneumonia rates and improved nutritional status.[37,52-54] Decisions about therapy techniques selection depend in large part on the specific dysphagia characteristics demonstrated by individual patients (see Chapters 9-11).

Chronic dysphagia is reported in some stroke survivors, although no study has documented the prevalence of dysphagia in stroke patients beyond 6 months after stroke. Typically, if the swallowing deficit persists beyond 6 months, it is considered chronic. Available reports indicate that stroke patients with chronic dysphagia can benefit from intense therapy.[55-57] Such therapies are typically active and directed at changing specific physiologic features of the swallowing deficit.[58]

In summary, dysphagia is highly prevalent after stroke and may be related to pneumonia (and other infections), nutrition and hydration deficits, and other health complications. Dysphagia does resolve to varying degrees in the poststroke period, but the few estimates available suggest that up to 50% of stroke patients demonstrate some degree of persistent dysphagia. Dysphagia therapy has been shown to improve swallowing ability, reduce pneumonia rates, and improve nutritional status in stroke patients. Even stroke survivors with chronic dysphagia can experience functional benefit from intensive swallowing therapy.

SWALLOWING DEFICITS IN DEMENTIA

Another form of cortical impairment that can affect swallowing ability is the category of progressive diseases known as dementia. Several types of dementias have been described; the most frequent is Alzheimer's disease. Other forms of dementia include dementia caused by cerebrovascular disease, Lewy body dementia, frontotemporal dementia, alcoholic dementia, and metabolic and nutritional dementia.[59] The hallmark of all dementias is a progressive deterioration in cognitive abilities, including memory, judgment, abstract reasoning, and personality changes. Other cortical disturbances such as apraxia or aphasia might be noted.

BOX 3-3 SWALLOWING DEFICITS SEEN IN PATIENTS WITH COGNITIVE DECLINE (DEMENTIA)

- Unexplained weight loss*
- Oral-stage dysfunction*
- Pharyngeal-stage dysfunction
- Combined oral and pharyngeal dysfunction
  - Minor aspiration
  - Major aspiration
- Feeding limitations

*More commonly observed characteristics.

Swallowing deficits are well documented in advanced dementia.[60-63] A recent systematic review[64] reported that across all forms of dementia the prevalence of swallowing difficulties ranged from 13% to 57%. Persistent weight loss may be the first indication that patients with dementia have a significant swallowing problem; however, weight loss may not be directly related to feeding or swallowing difficulties.[62,65] As a result, such individuals are at significant risk for nutritional deficits that may further compromise their health status. Pneumonia is a common cause of death in patients with dementia.[63] Although dysphagia, including aspiration, is associated with pneumonia in this population,[65] it is not the only contributing factor and may not be the critical contributing factor.[62,63,66]

General characteristics of swallowing deficits in dementia are listed in Box 3-3. Prominent on this list is the presence of oral-stage dysfunction. Certain oral aspects of swallowing are under volitional motor control. From this perspective, generalized cognitive impairments in dementia may contribute to deficits in volitional motor control and hence oral aspects of dysphagia. Oral aspects of dysphagia in patients with dementia may be characterized by lack of initiation of the swallow in which the patient holds food in the mouth, incoordinated oral control of food and liquid, and/or delayed initiation of the oral component of the swallow. Each of these dysphagia characteristics contributes to prolonged mealtimes, which may put patients with dementia at nutritional risk from reduced food intake.

Although the majority of dysphagia information in dementia is derived from studies of patients in advanced stages of the disease, patients with mild-stage dementia also demonstrate feeding and swallowing deficits.[67,68] One interesting approach to identification of dysphagia early in patients with Alzheimer's disease was described by Sato et al.[69] These investigators evaluated a variety of oral and feeding activities during daily life (e.g., lip and tongue movement, ability to rinse and gargle orally, storing food in the mouth, appetite, etc.) and reported that oral rinsing ability was the single factor most significantly associated with dysphagia. At one level this observation is logical as

PRACTICE NOTE 3-4

Successful oral care and swallowing for the patient with advanced Alzheimer's disease is very much in the hands of the caregiver. I learned this firsthand by caring for my mother, who had Alzheimer's disease. As speech-language pathologists, we are often in a position to offer insight into the process of these two activities by combining our knowledge of swallowing with our knowledge of dementia. The following anecdotal examples illustrate this point.

First, how may the sensory input of taste trigger an oral behavior? Good oral hygiene is critical, but what do you do when it is no longer feasible to use regular toothpaste, because it is often mismanaged and swallowed? Toddler toothpaste (designed to be safe if swallowed) is an option and a popular flavor is bubble gum. There were occasions when my mother accomplished the desired swish and spit after the predictable brushing action. However, months later, when giving her liquid Tylenol (also in bubble gum flavor) she remembered to successfully swish and spit.

Second, and this may be very case specific, we encountered the dilemma of trying to cue chewing and swallowing during a meal. Although the process was slow and laborious, it seemed sensible that this should be done slowly with verbal and tactile cues with each step and a pause between each bite to check for residual food in the oral cavity. However, I stunned the nursing assistant by trying to follow a successful swallow with another bite without pausing. For a time this was a successful strategy. Why did I try this? One of the four "A's" of Alzheimer's disease is apraxia. I recalled that it is at the point of transition that motor planning seems to break down. Therefore if we minimized the pause between successful swallows, an almost "automatic" second swallow of food followed.

AUTHOR'S NOTE: This practice note was provided by my former student and good friend, Dr. Nancy J. Haak, who cared for her mother with Alzheimer's dementia in her home. In multiple conversations with Nancy, I learned much about the practical management of dysphagia in patients with dementia and felt it appropriate to share at least one example in this text.—MAC

BOX 3-4   EXAMPLES OF SWALLOWING AND FEEDING DEVIATIONS IN MILD-STAGE DEMENTIA

Swallowing Deviations
- Slow oral movement
- Slow or delayed pharyngeal response
- Overall slow swallowing duration

Feeding Deviations: Patients May Require the Following to Maintain Oral Intake
- Increased self-feeding cues (specifically related to food preparation or utensil use)
- Direct assistance with utensil use for food preparation or convenience
- Imitation of feeding behavior from the meal partner

mealtimes and hence increase the risk of involuntary weight loss and associated declining nutritional status. In addition, slowing of the pharyngeal response in swallowing may reduce airway protection, resulting in an increase of coughing and choking behaviors during mealtimes.

In addition to overall slowness in the swallowing process, individuals with dementia frequently demonstrate self-feeding difficulties. Self-feeding difficulties may relate to numerous factors, including cognitive impairment, motor deficits such as weakness or apraxia, loss of appetite, and food avoidance. Consequences of self-feeding difficulties can include weight loss and associated nutritional decline as well as dependency for feeding. Dependency for feeding can contribute to dysphagia-related health problems, including pneumonia.[70-72] Self-feeding difficulties may be noticed in the mild stages of the disease and become more pronounced as the disease progresses.[73,74] For patients with self-feeding difficulties, clinicians or caregivers may need to offer increased verbal or environmental cues or provide direct assistance. Refer to Video 3-3 on the companion Evolve website for this text for an example of feeding difficulties in a single patient with primary progressive aphasia (PPA). PPA is a form of dementia in which language and communication abilities deteriorate initially followed by deterioration of other functions. This patient appeared to have a specific form of apraxia that influenced her use of eating utensils.

At the beginning of this chapter the premise was offered that different neurologic deficits contribute to different clinical presentations of swallowing deficits. At least one study has evaluated differences in feeding and swallowing abilities in patients with Alzheimer's disease compared with patients with frontotemporal dementia.[75] As the name implies, frontotemporal dementia is often characterized by frontal lobe signs, including loss of insight, disinhibition, impulsivity, poor self-care, stereotypic behavior, and more. Conversely, Alzheimer's disease is characterized by progressive memory deficits that may affect many tasks of daily life because of forgetfulness, disorientation, or

successful oral rinsing requires a degree of oral motor control, which may be impaired among patients with Alzheimer's disease who have swallowing difficulties (see Practice Note 3-4). Box 3-4 summarizes salient findings regarding feeding and swallowing abilities in mild-stage dementia. These impairments are similar to, though not as severe as, those reported in more advanced stages of the disease. Specifically, patients with dementia demonstrate an overall slowing of the swallowing process from the oral aspects of food manipulation through the response of the pharynx accepting the bolus. This slowing of the swallowing process can have direct consequences for longer impaired **executive functions**. Ikeda et al.[75] used caregiver questionnaires to evaluate eating behaviors in patients with frontotemporal dementia versus Alzheimer's disease. They evaluated five categories: swallowing problems, appetite change, food preferences, eating habits (including table manners and stereotype behaviors), and other oral behaviors. In general, swallowing problems occurred less frequently than other limitations and the frequency of dysphagia did not differ among the types of dementia. However, swallowing problems tended to occur earlier in the course of disease progression in the patients with Alzheimer's disease. Patients with frontotemporal dementia demonstrated more frequent changes in appetite. These patients were more likely to demonstrate increased appetite compared with reduced appetite in patients with Alzheimer's disease. In addition, patients with frontotemporal dementia demonstrated more food preferences than patients in the Alzheimer's group. Still, more than 20% of the patients with Alzheimer's disease demonstrated increased preference for sweets and other taste-related changes. As might be expected from the basic profile, patients with frontotemporal dementia demonstrated more deviations in eating behaviors. Patients in the Alzheimer's disease group did demonstrate longer meal durations, decline in table manners such as eating with hands, and a tendency to prefer eating at the same time each day. Finally, the category of "other oral behaviors" included observations such as overstuffing the mouth, eating nonedible objects, snatching any food item within reach, or vomiting, including self-induced vomiting. In general, patients with Alzheimer's disease scored low on these behaviors with the exception of over-filling the mouth when eating. This is an interesting study in many ways. First, it details caregivers' observations of eating and swallowing behaviors in different groups of patients with dementia. Second, it supports the basic premise that the characteristics of the underlying neurologic disease affect the clinical presentation of dysphagia. Finally, it provides at least an initial description of feeding and swallowing behaviors that may be used by dysphagia clinicians in evaluating swallowing and related behaviors in patients with dementia.

Treatment Considerations

Dementia is a progressive disease with no known cure. Dysphagia intervention for patients with any form of dementia should keep that focus and incorporate basic principles of quality of life, dignity, and comfort.[76,77] Dysphagia treatment options for patients with dementia may range from simple environmental adjustments to the use of nonoral feeding sources. Depending on specific problems in individual patients, some potential treatment avenues may include special food preparations, diet restriction, enhanced taste and flavor, changing the mealtime environment, increased mealtime supervision and cueing, or a variety of other behavioral or environmental changes to facilitate increased food and liquid intake. Direct behavioral therapy to change swallowing mechanics also may be indicated (see Chapter 10).

Feeding tubes are frequently recommended for patients with advanced dementia as a mechanism to maintain nutritional support and avoid dysphagia-related comorbid conditions. However, the available evidence on the benefit of feeding tubes for this population suggests that they do not reduce the risks of aspiration pneumonia, may not prevent further decline in nutritional status, may not prolong survival, and seem to have no impact on overall functional status.[64,78,79] In fact, the American Geriatrics Society has issued a position statement that feeding tubes are not recommended for older adults with advanced dementia.[80]

A recent survey of national databases (Minimum Data Set and Medicare Claims Files) indicated that most feeding tubes were placed in nursing home residents with dementia during acute hospitalization.[81] The most common reasons for these hospitalizations included pneumonia, dehydration, and dysphagia. The 1-year mortality rate was 64%, with median survival of 56 days after tube placement. Patients with feeding tubes also had a significantly higher rate of health care use after tube insertion. These observations are nearly opposite the results of a survey completed by speech-language pathologists working in the area of dysphagia.[82] In that survey, many respondents believed that percutaneous endoscopic gastrostomy (PEG) improved nutritional status and increased survival, and nearly 40% believed that PEG was the standard of care for patients with advanced dementia. However, the majority of respondents did not believe that tube feeding improved quality of life or functional status for these patients. A slightly more recent survey of speech-language pathologists indicated that misperceptions about tube feeding in advanced dementia were common but that clinicians with more experience demonstrated greater knowledge about tube feeding outcomes in this population.[83] These misperceptions and lack of knowledge are not confined to speech-language pathologists. Pelletier[84] evaluated dysphagia and feeding knowledge of certified nursing assistants working in nursing homes. Even though these professionals were actively participating in patient feeding activities, their knowledge of dysphagia and feeding was greatly limited. The results of this study and others suggest that focused education is vital in managing dysphagia and feeding limitations in patients with dementia. In fact, at least one study has demonstrated that educational programs for medical and allied health staff on end-of-life care and feeding management in patients with dementia resulted in a reduction in feeding tube placement in these patients.[85] An additional study indicated that trained feeding assistance focusing on patients' self-feeding ability, social stimulation during meals or snack periods, and increased availability of choices for foods and liquids increased the daily intake of food and liquid in 90% of nursing home residents. Both feeding assistance and the availability of between-meal snacks resulted in increased oral intake.[86] Collectively, the available information suggests that (1) feeding tubes do not produce significant benefit to most patients with dementia, (2) they do not promote quality of life or compassionate care, (3) alternatives are available, and (4) education on the problems and intervention strategies can benefit patients. See Chapter 11 for more information on the use of feeding tubes.

SWALLOWING DEFICITS IN TRAUMATIC BRAIN INJURY

Traumatic brain injury (TBI) typically results in diffuse neurologic deficits that affect several aspects of behavioral control. Various studies have indicated the prevalence of dysphagia in acute or subacute TBI ranges from 60% to more than 90%.[87-89] Oral-phase difficulties and pharyngeal-phase deficits are roughly evenly distributed within this population.[88] The primary factor related to the presence of dysphagia in these patients is the severity of neurotrauma assessed by clinical scales such as the **Glasgow Coma Scale** (GCS), the **Rancho Los Amigos Scale** (RLAS), or the **Functional Independence Measure (FIM)**.[87-89] At least one study has suggested that the level of functional oral intake at admission to subacute rehabilitation as measured by the Functional Oral Intake Scale (FOIS; see Chapter 7) is one predictive component of return to total oral feeding in patients with TBI.[89] Another study reported that a level IV on the RLAS was required to initiate oral feeding and that a level VI on this scale was needed for return to total oral feeding.[87] Mandaville et al.[90] reported that increased age, low RLA score, presence of a tracheostomy tube, and aphonia combined to predict which patients would be discharged from acute care with a feeding tube. Recovery of swallowing function in TBI is good; most patients regain some degree of functional swallowing within the first 3 to 6 months after injury.[89,91,92] The severity of the initial injury emerges as a strong predictor of both the presence of swallowing deficits and time to recovery of functional swallowing ability.

Pneumonia is frequently seen in patients with TBI, especially early in the posttraumatic course of treatment.[93,94] Hansen et al.[94] reported that 27% of patients admitted with a brain injury for early rehabilitation were being actively treated for pneumonia and that pneumonia developed in an additional 12% during rehabilitation. Clinical factors associated with the presence of pneumonia included severity of neurotrauma (GCS, RLAS), no oral intake on admission, and presence of tracheostomy tube or feeding tube. Woratyla et al.[93] added prolonged intubation time and field intubation versus in-hospital intubation as risk factors for pneumonia. Furthermore, Hui et al.[95] reported that for patients requiring mechanical ventilation, each additional day on the ventilator was associated with a 7% increase in the risk of pneumonia. Thus level of consciousness, tracheostomy tube, nonoral feeding, type of intubation, and number of days on mechanical ventilation all appear related to the development of early pneumonia in patients with TBI.

In addition to the effects of neurotrauma on swallowing ability in patients with TBI, swallowing may be affected by factors such as the need for tracheostomy and/or ventilator support, the presence of communicative and cognitive deficits, and the presence of physical deficits that may interfere with self-feeding ability. Tracheostomy tubes indicate some degree of compromise in the respiratory system, which is integral in the swallowing process. Also, these tubes may have a mechanical impact on swallowing physiology. However, at least one study has reported that the presence of tracheostomy tubes was not associated with increased rates of dysphagia or aspiration in trauma patients.[96] Patients with communicative or cognitive deficits present additional challenges to clinicians in the design of swallowing assessments or rehabilitation strategies because of patients' reduced understanding and interaction. Finally, physical deficits impose a degree of dependency for activities such as self-feeding.[97]

Treatment Considerations

In as much as the deficits observed in TBI are multifactorial, the potential treatment strategies and techniques are also multifactorial. Cherney and Halper[98] provide a brief but excellent review of the roles of interdisciplinary team members that may be required in the management of dysphagia in patients with TBI. Standard intervention approaches included diet modifications, postural adjustments, feeding adaptations, and behavioral maneuvers and compensations (see Chapter 10).[99] In cases of severe injury with widespread comorbid conditions, alternate feeding routes may be indicated, especially in the early postinjury course. The good news is that many patients with dysphagia after TBI do regain the ability to eat by mouth with appropriate clinical intervention.

SUBCORTICAL FUNCTIONS

The basal ganglia are a group of cell bodies in the subcortical brain hemispheres that influence the quality of movement. Basal ganglia functions regulate tone (resting tension level of muscles) and steadiness of movement among other functions. Impairment to basal ganglia functions may create excessive tone and/or extra, unintended movements. Excessive tone may create delays in the initiation of movement,

BOX 3-5 GENERAL DYSPHAGIA CONSIDERATIONS IN PATIENTS WITH BASAL GANGLIA DEFICITS

- Poor bolus control: involuntary movements
  - Oral
  - Oropharyngeal
- Residue from inefficient swallow
  - Oral
  - Oropharyngeal
  - Pharyngeal
- Difference among swallow types
  - Automatic versus intentional movements
- Severity dependent

slowed movements, or a reduced amount of movement. Extra, unintended movements disrupt the smooth, coordinated nature of voluntary movement attempts. Movement disruptions may be seen as tremor, regular **clonic movements**, slow sustained postural interruptions (**dystonias**), or other unintentional movements superimposed on the normal resting state of muscle groups or during intended movements. Box 3-5 lists general swallowing problems that may be associated with various characteristics of basal ganglia deficits.

SUBCORTICAL FUNCTIONS AND SWALLOWING IMPAIRMENT: PARKINSON'S DISEASE

Parkinson's disease (PD) is a slowly progressive disease of the basal ganglia. The key problem is impairment in the execution of voluntary movement. The classic features of PD include **resting tremor**, **bradykinesia**, and **rigidity**. The cause of this disease is essentially unknown, but the immediate cause for the motor changes is the depletion of the neurochemical dopamine, which results in impaired basal ganglia functioning during voluntary movements. These changes may also result from long-term use of certain medications or may be part of more encompassing degenerative diseases that can influence basal ganglia performance.[100-102]

Patients with PD may present with a variety of interrelated clinical signs. They may demonstrate slowness in cognitive tasks and in some cases a form of dementia. As the disease progresses, they may show a masklike face that appears expressionless. They often demonstrate a characteristic dysarthria, impaired writing (**micrographia**), changes in body posture and gait, and other potential changes associated with reduced movement ability or instability. The progression of PD varies among patients, and no cure currently exists for PD. Medical management consists primarily of medications, although recent efforts have described surgical approaches to management.

Swallowing deficits in patients with PD are common and reflect the underlying motor impairments, the extent of the disease progression, and potentially the effects of medications. Miller et al.[103] identified dysphagia in 84% of a sample of 137 adults with PD; 23% demonstrated severe dysphagia and could not complete a 150-mL water swallowing task. These prevalence data may be lower than the true clinical picture because patients, especially those in the earlier, milder stages of the disease, do not reliably report swallowing difficulties.[103,104] For example, Kalf et al.[105] reported an objective (clinician assessed) prevalence of dysphagia of 82% versus a subjective (patient report) prevalence of 35% in community-dwelling PD patients. In general, oropharyngeal swallowing deficits may result from poor bolus control caused by involuntary movements or from residue or misdirection of the bolus from an inefficient, possibly weakened swallow (see also Clinical Corner 3-3). In addition, an overall slowness characterizes swallowing deficits in patients with PD that may reflect the degree of underlying bradykinesia.[106] In addition to the motor component of PD, sensory deficits may contribute to dysphagia and related difficulties. Hammer, Murphy, and Abrams[107] reported abnormal airway somatosensory functions and increased oropharyngeal residue in PD patients compared with healthy controls. Moreover, these investigators described a positive correlation between sensory thresholds and swallow impairment. These sensory deficits may be based in peripheral sensory nerve changes in the pharynx associated with the disease[108] and may contribute to aspiration of saliva and perhaps other liquids in this population.[109] Furthermore, these sensory limitations may contribute to underreporting of dysphagia symptoms by patients with PD.[107] Box 3-6 lists some of the oropharyngeal swallowing-related deficits in patients with PD.

Drooling, in some contexts termed **sialorrhea**, is a common problem for patients with PD and may be related to the presence and severity of dysphagia.[110] Sialorrhea in PD may result from a combination of sensory impairment and reduced frequency of spontaneous swallowing resulting in salivary retention.[103,107,111] Results from preliminary studies have suggested that patients with **diurnal** sialorrhea are at increased risk for silent aspiration,[112] which may, in turn, increase their risk for respiratory infections and subsequent death.[113] These risks are higher in later stages of the disease and in patients with severe sialorrhea.

Swallowing deficits in PD extend beyond the oral and pharyngeal components of the swallowing mechanism. Gross et al.[114] describe impaired coordination between swallowing and respiration that may contribute to reduced airway protection during swallowing. Moreover, various esophageal abnormalities have been reported, including delayed transport through the esophagus, esophageal stasis, abnormal contractions, and lower esophageal

---

CLINICAL CORNER 3-3: PARKINSON'S DISEASE AND AUTOMATIC SWALLOWING

Years ago I saw a patient with PD for whom a feeding tube was being considered. I do not recall the stage of the disease, but he was nonambulatory outside his home, had some obvious degree of rigidity, and presented with a significant dysarthria (likely a 4 or 5 on the Hoehn and Yahr functional rating scale). I do remember that his wife was pleading with me and the radiologist to recommend that this patient could continue oral feeding, even if a feeding tube had to be placed for nutritional support. He had already had one episode of pneumonia, which prompted his referral for swallowing evaluation. Furthermore, the wife insisted that her husband could drink milkshakes at home with no difficulty.

Initially, the fluoroscopic swallow evaluation incorporated small volumes (5 mL or less) of thin liquid, thickened liquid, and pudding material provided to the patient by spoon. As expected, we noted poor oral control with material entering the pharynx before the airway was closed. We also noticed residue that increased in amount as the thickness of swallowed material increased. Given the wife's report of successful milkshake drinking at home, we provided the patient with a cup of nectar-thickened liquid and a straw. To our surprise, his swallow improved dramatically under this condition. We observed no aspiration and only a small amount of residue once the sequence of multiple swallows was completed. This patient continued to take oral nutrition supplements by mouth for total nutrition for a short period. Even after a feeding tube was placed, he was able to continue drinking milkshakes by straw.

Critical Thinking

1. How would you explain the difference in swallowing performance based on straw drinking versus small volumes taken by spoon provided by the examiner? Consider neurologic, swallow mechanics, and context variables in your discussion.

2. Do you think this distinction may be specific to patients with PD or might other patients respond in a similar manner?

3. When do you think it is appropriate to evaluate swallowing abilities in patients diagnosed with PD?

Refer to Video 3-4 on the Evolve website for an example of how different swallowing strategies and different bolus volumes may affect swallow function in a patient with PD. The initial swallow is a thick liquid presented by the clinician from a spoon. Subsequent swallows are taken sequentially by the patient with a straw.

BOX 3-6 OROPHARYNGEAL SWALLOWING DEFICITS IN PATIENTS WITH BASAL GANGLIA DEFICITS (PARKINSON'S DISEASE)

Oral Stage
- Lingual tremor
- Repetitive tongue pumping*
- Prolonged ramplike posture
- Piecemeal deglutition
- Velar tremor
- Buccal retention*

Pharyngeal Stage
- Vallecular retention*
- Piriform sinus retention
- Impaired laryngeal elevation*
- Airway (supraglottic) penetration
- Aspiration

Sensory Deficits (Elevated Threshold for Sensation)
- Pharyngoesophageal segment dysfunction

*More commonly observed characteristics

abnormalities.[104] Patients with PD have been reported to demonstrate problems farther along the digestive tract—**gastroparesis** and various defecatory dysfunctions.[115-117] Again, these irregularities may be related to the movement disorder or to the influence of some of the medications used to treat the disease. Still, dysphagia clinicians should at least discuss the entire spectrum of gastrointestinal functions in evaluating dysphagia in patients with PD.

It is important to remember that patients with PD must cope with a widespread assortment of daily problems resulting from the disease and, at times, from the treatments for the disease. These deficits extend beyond the swallowing mechanism and may affect related acts such as food shopping, preparation of meals, and self-feeding activities.[118] Thus dysphagia in patients with PD and associated daily activities may contribute to increased patient and caregiver burden.[119] In the absence of appropriate support systems, these dysphagia-related impairments could have a direct, and potentially negative, influence on the nutritional and health status of individual patients.

Treatment Considerations

Clinical research on the effectiveness of dysphagia therapy for patients with PD is limited. In fact, a systematic reviews by Baijens and Speyer[120] and van Hooren et al.[121] identified only 16 and 12 articles respectively describing rehabilitative, surgical, pharmacologic, or other therapies for swallow difficulties in PD. Not surprisingly, most articles reported some degree of positive benefit from their particular interventions. In fact, it is conceivable that a variety of interventions may improve some aspects of swallow function in patients with PD. For example, Felix et al.[122] reported improved swallowing of water and to a lesser extent biscuits after a 2-week period of performing the effortful swallow technique with adjunctive biofeedback. Athukorala et al.[123] also used adjunctive biofeedback but employed a novel application in which patients focused on a skill that required spatiotemporal coordination rather than just increased strength of swallowing. Timing aspects of swallowing improved immediately following therapy and were maintained for 2 weeks following therapy. El Sharkawi et al.[124] reported that some swallowing variables improved after 1 month of Lee Silverman Voice Treatment (LSVT). LSVT is a well-known therapy for speech and voice improvement in patients with PD. This study examined the **cross-system effect** of LSVT on swallowing performance. Finally, Pitts et al.[125] reported that 4 weeks of expiratory muscle strength training improved both voluntary cough and some swallowing parameters. Collectively, these studies represent a wide range of behavioral interventions both in terms of the focus and outcomes of therapy. However, each intervention may be appropriate and helpful to select individual patients with dysphagia attributable to PD. In addition, dysphagia clinicians are advised to remember that medical and surgical interventions may be appropriate for certain patients. From an evidence-based perspective, the available literature reflects small numbers

of patients with generally weaker study designs. As the clinical sciences mature, the expectation is that clinicians and patients will benefit from more rigorous knowledge on the effectiveness of various dysphagia interventions for patients with PD.

As with all dysphagias, treatment planning interacts with an understanding of the underlying mechanisms contributing to the dysphagia. In addition, because PD is a progressive disease, intervention strategies are expected to change over time. Finally, some evidence suggests that medications may have a positive effect on swallowing function in patients with PD[126]; however, this benefit may not extend to all patients or to some aspects of swallow function.[127,128] Because medications tend to work in time cycles, it may be important to time meals in relation to the maximum beneficial effect of medications. Finally, Table 3-3 summarizes intervention strategies recommended by Yorkston et al.[129] that may be appropriate for patients with PD. Although clinicians should not limit treatment options to those listed in the table, the recommendations do reflect the changing nature of dysphagia in PD over time and represent a range of potential interventions from patient counseling and education to modifying swallowing activity to adjusting diets. As such, this information may serve as a general guide to dysphagia clinicians with common sense suggestions at various severity levels of PD.

TABLE 3-3 Summary of Swallowing Interventions in Parkinson's Disease

	Normal Swallow	Early Swallowing Problems	Moderate Swallowing Disability	Severe Swallowing Disability
Presenting features	No observable changes	Reduction in pharyngeal peristalsis	Pharyngeal peristalsis worsens	Aspiration both during and after swallow
		Repetitive rocking motion of the tongue	Delay in swallowing reflex	
			Cricopharyngeal dysfunction	
			Laryngeal closure during swallowing may be inadequate	
Intervention	Monitor weight	Provide counseling to bring swallowing under voluntary control	Introduce aids and devices to promote independence	Teach chin-tuck swallowing
	Answer questions	Monitor weight	Increase sensory input	Switch to soft diet
		Coordinate eating with drug cycle	Teach double swallow	
			Recommend small, frequent, highly nutritious meals	

(From Yorkston KM, Miller RM, Strand EA: Management of speech and swallowing in degenerative diseases, Tucson, AZ, 1995, Communication Skills Builders.)

BRAINSTEM FUNCTIONS

The brainstem is much like a junction box. Here the major ascending sensory tracts receive input from the head and neck region by way of the cranial nerves. The head and neck musculature also receives motor innervation from the **upper motor neurons** of the corticobulbar system. These upper motor neurons synapse with the motor components of the individual cranial nerves, which function as **lower motor neurons**. Thus damage to the brainstem typically results in sensory deficits to the head and neck region in addition to motor deficits associated with both upper and lower motor neuron damage. The first of these is characterized by spastic weakness and associated movement impairments, whereas the second is characterized by flaccid weakness and associated movement impairments. The term *alternating hemiplegia* is often applied to this pattern of motor impairment to describe flaccid weakness on one side of the body (head) and spastic weakness on the contralateral side (body). In simple terms, the "level" of brainstem deficit is noted by the cranial nerve level of flaccid weakness. Thus, facial alternating hemiplegia indicates a flaccid weakness in the facial or seventh cranial nerve with spastic weakness in the contralateral upper or lower extremities (or both).

The brainstem also is believed to be home to a "swallowing center" located in the rostral brainstem.[130,131] This group of nuclei (often focusing on the nucleus tractus solitaries and nucleus ambiguus) is believed to facilitate coordination among the various components of the swallowing mechanism (oral, pharyngeal, esophageal) and coordinate swallowing functions with respiration. Individuals with damage to this area of the brainstem usually demonstrate a severe dysphagia in addition to the basic sensory and motor signs associated with brainstem deficits.

Brainstem Functions and Swallowing Impairment

Swallowing deficits subsequent to brainstem stroke provide a good example of the relation between neurologic deficits and dysphagia. In general, dysphagia in brainstem stroke involves two aspects: incoordination presumably related to disruption of the "swallowing center" and weakness resulting from damage to the corticobulbar system (sensory deficits also may be present). The collective effects of these deficits often are manifest clinically as incoordination among "stages" of swallowing and between swallowing and respiration, as well as weakness in one or more of the muscle groups innervated by the corticobulbar system (velum, pharynx, larynx, pharyngoesophageal segment). The resulting swallow has been described as the incomplete swallow.[55,132] Although incomplete swallow is not a specific term, it does offer an overt description of the impairment

---

> **BOX 3-7** PHARYNGEAL SWALLOWING DEFICITS IN PATIENTS AFTER BRAINSTEM STROKE
>
> - Absent or delayed pharyngeal response
> - Reduced hyolaryngeal excursion
> - Reduced oropharyngeal constriction
> - Reduced pharyngeal constriction
> - Reduced laryngeal closure
> - Reduced pharyngoesophageal segment opening
> - Brief swallow event
> - Generalized incoordination (including respiration)

in swallow physiology observed in these patients. Box 3-7 summarizes features of the incomplete swallow often seen in patients with dysphagia subsequent to brainstem stroke. Video 3-6, *A* and *B*, on the companion Evolve website show endoscopic and fluoroscopic examples of the swallow incoordination typically seen after brainstem impairment. In this specific case, the patient had a tumor in the medulla. The author saw him nearly 3 years after medical treatment. He presented with deficits to cranial nerves X and XII on the left and depended on a feeding tube. Two months before the evaluation he had a thyroplasty to medialize a paralyzed left vocal fold. Additional descriptions of pharyngeal incoordination (or pharynx and pharyngoesophageal segment) subsequent to brainstem deficits based on manometric evaluation are provided by Lan et al.[133] and Huckabee et al.[134]

Treatment Considerations

Similar to hemispheric stroke patients, patients with brainstem stroke recover some degree of swallow function over time.[135] Likewise, the clinical presentation of dysphagia and comorbid conditions varies considerably. Given these perspectives, treatment approaches to dysphagia in the patient who has survived a brainstem stroke are symptomatic and change over time.

A careful assessment of the components of dysphagia and related deficits is mandatory in this group of patients. For example, the patient requiring tracheostomy for respiratory support presents a different clinical profile than does the patient who does not require tracheostomy. The patient with minimal cranial nerve deficits may have better physiologic support for rehabilitative efforts than the patient with multiple cranial nerve deficits. And the nonambulatory patient presents different challenges than the patient who can walk assisted or unassisted.

In the acute poststroke phase, intervention tends to be more cautious with a prophylactic component. At this point the patient may be at greatest risk for pulmonary complications from inappropriate oral intake. Depending on the severity of neurologic impairment and the overall health status of the patient, treatment strategies at this stage may range from nothing (monitoring recovery) to passive sensorimotor activities (oral hygiene and movement exercises) to more active swallowing efforts involving compensatory maneuvers (postural adjustments, changes in the swallow behavior, etc.) or even intensive rehabilitation exercises.

Because recovery facilitates an overall improvement in the patient's health status, dysphagia intervention may be more direct and aggressive. At some point the need for continuation of tracheostomy tubes should be addressed. Direct and intensive swallowing rehabilitation has been effective in facilitating return to oral feeding in chronic patients.[55-57] Although limited, clinical research has suggested that therapy approaches focused on increasing strength and coordination of swallowing are likely to improve swallow function (see Chapter 10 for examples of therapy approaches). The key for the dysphagia specialist is interaction with medical and other rehabilitative specialists to understand the patient's larger health status picture and selection of treatment strategies consistent with the patient's global needs and still provide the potential for improved swallowing function.

The Role of the Cerebellum in Swallowing

The cerebellum is adjacent to the brainstem and is located posterior and slightly superior to most brainstem structures. The role of the cerebellum in the control of swallowing is poorly understood. This structure does appear to play a role in swallow activity; several functional imaging studies have demonstrated activation, often bilateral activation, in the cerebellum on volitional swallowing.[136-138] A recent review of literature from 1980 forward concluded that the cerebellum likely has some role in modulating swallowing and can contribute to dysphagia when damaged.[139] From a clinical perspective, cerebellar damage results in unsteadiness (**ataxia**), **intention tremor** (tremor that is exaggerated at the initiation of movement), and **hypotonia** (low muscular tone). When present in the swallowing mechanism, these movement deficits are expected to impair coordinated swallowing functions. Motor unsteadiness and weakness resulting from cerebellar damage may contribute to difficulty in controlling a bolus, directing that bolus in a timely fashion, and residue from reduced swallowing effort. However, given the location of the cerebellum, clinicians must be vigilant of brainstem (cranial neuropathy and central pattern generator) contributions to any dysphagia resulting from primary damage to the cerebellum (see Practice Note 3-5). Video 3-7 on the companion Evolve website presents an endoscopic swallowing examination of a patient with cerebellar deficit who demonstrates tremor that contributes to poor oral control of a liquid bolus with subsequent aspiration.

PRACTICE NOTE 3-5

Our dysphagia treatment team received a referral to assess a young woman who had been on a feeding tube for 5 years. Her history indicated that a viral infection had interfered with her blood clotting ability, which resulted in a large midcerebellar stroke. Though the stroke did not directly affect the brainstem and she demonstrated no cranial nerve deficits, she did have a severe and persistent dysphagia and respiratory difficulties. She required months of hospitalization and ventilation support for breathing. Subsequently, she completed years of physical and swallowing rehabilitation. When we saw her, we dubbed her "the girl with no swallow." A brief fluoroscopic video of her swallow pattern can be found on the Evolve website (Video 3-5). Her pattern was to drop the base of her tongue to allow material to "fall" into the hypopharynx. Once at the level of the piriform recesses (entrance to the esophagus) she immediately "reversed gears" and regurgitated the material into her mouth. This pattern was repeated until she was forced to breath and the material was expectorated. In essence, she had lost any form of a functional swallow. The good news is that after intensive swallowing rehabilitation she was able to regain her swallow function and returned to a relatively normal oral diet.

LOWER MOTOR NEURON AND MUSCLE DISEASE

Lower motor neurons proceed through the body and connect with muscles at the **myoneural junction**. Deficits to the peripheral nerves or the myoneural junction produce flaccid weakness. However, myoneural junction deficits demonstrate significant deterioration of motor function with use but recovery with extended rest.

The end points in the sensorimotor chain of events are the muscle and sensory end organs. Motor impairments at the muscle level are termed myopathies. These are characterized by a severe flaccid weakness within the affected muscle groups. Sensory loss may come in many forms, resulting from both neurologic and nonneurologic processes. Reduction or loss of tactile sensation is considered particularly important in swallowing problems because it may lead to unawareness of residual food along the swallowing mechanism or it may contribute directly to aspiration of food and liquid materials into the airway.

Lower Motor Neuron Functions and Swallowing Impairment

Amyotrophic lateral sclerosis (ALS) is one disease that reflects the relation between lower motor neuron impairment and dysphagia. ALS, sometimes referred to as *Lou*

Gehrig's disease or *motor neuron disease,* is a progressive degenerative disease of unknown cause. The clinical presentation is progressive weakness; approximately 30% of patients show the initial effects of this disease in the corticobulbar musculature.[140] When present, corticobulbar deficits contribute to a significant and progressive dysphagia.

Neurologic deficits in ALS are not confined to the lower motor neurons of the peripheral nervous system. Central nervous system structures also are involved. As a result, the motor deficits in ALS are mixed—incorporating both flaccid (lower motor neuron) and spastic (upper motor neuron) weakness. The mixture of flaccid and spastic weakness may be seen in the musculature of the swallowing mechanism, in the respiratory musculature, and throughout the remainder of the body. ALS is progressive and terminal, and although many patients survive for longer than 5 years, the majority do not.[140,141] Substantial variability in progression rates exists among individuals. Respiratory failure is a common cause of death. Available research suggests that the different subtypes of ALS do not progress differentially.[142]

In addition to dysphagia, individuals with ALS experience movement difficulties with the arms and legs, dysarthria, respiratory decline from chest muscle weakness and, in some cases (though rare), cognitive changes (including **emotional lability** and dementia). Obviously the impact of this disease on all aspects of daily functions is severe. These factors certainly are considered in planning any rehabilitative efforts, including swallowing rehabilitation.

Swallowing deficits are progressive and widespread. As might be expected, they reflect a weakness across the muscle groups used to prepare and transport a bolus. Early in the course of the disease, dysphagia may be characterized by oral limitations resulting from lingual weakness.[143,144] In fact, lingual weakness has been associated with survival time in ALS in at least one study[145] and combined with respiratory measures may be a good indicator of a patient's ability to take oral food and liquid.[146] In addition to poor oral transport of a bolus, patients with ALS, even those with no bulbar symptoms, demonstrate pharyngeal residue.[147] This observation may be related to early, undetected weakness in pharyngeal muscles. Solazzo et al.[148] identified reported manometric irregularities in the pharynx and upper esophageal sphincter in the absence of fluoroscopic abnormalities in 10 patients with ALS. These findings suggest that weakness is present in swallowing musculature prior to clinical or fluoroscopic recognition of dysphagia. However, pharyngoesophageal segment opening and laryngeal excursion may demonstrate relative maintenance even in advanced dysphagia.[147] As might be expected, respiratory aspects of swallowing are negatively affected in ALS. Nozaki et al.[149] reported that swallow apnea, or **hypopnea**, was increased in patients with ALS and that patients with severe respiratory limitations or presence of aspiration on

fluoroscopic swallow examination presented the longest apnea durations. General considerations for dysphagia are listed in Box 3-8, and specific dysphagia characteristics are presented in Box 3-9. In general, these deficits reflect limitations in oral bolus control, reduced ability to transport the bolus with resulting residue, and reduced airway protection. Because lingual weakness is an early aspect of dysphagia in ALS, it is not surprising that speech production also is affected. In fact, speech and swallow functions in ALS tend to show a highly related course of deterioration.

Early in the disease course, no significant dysphagia may be reported. As weakness in the swallowing mechanism progresses, patients may have difficulty chewing solid food, loss of food or liquid from the lips, and food-specific difficulties. This may cause patients to begin to reject specific foods or to alter their diet or chewing or swallowing

---

BOX 3-8 GENERAL DYSPHAGIA CONSIDERATIONS IN PATIENTS WITH ALS AND ASSOCIATED SENSORIMOTOR DEFICITS

- Oral control of bolus
  - Perioral weakness
  - Lingual weakness
- Reduced transport
  - Velar leak
  - Reduced tongue pump
  - Reduced pharyngeal contraction
- Residue
- Airway protection
  - Bradykinesia
  - Residue
- Respiratory limitations
  - Increased swallow apnea

ALS, Amyotrophic lateral sclerosis.

BOX 3-9 OROPHARYNGEAL SWALLOWING DEFICITS SEEN IN PATIENTS WITH ALS

Oral Stage
- Leakage
- Mastication
- Bolus formation
- Bolus transport
- Residual pooling

Pharyngeal Stage
- Nasopharyngeal regurgitation
- Valleculae pooling
- Piriform sinus pooling
- Airway spillage
- Ineffective airway clearance
- Shortness of breath

ALS, Amyotrophic lateral sclerosis.

mechanics (see Practice Note 3-6). As the disease progresses further, patients need more extensive diet modifications and risk rapid weight loss, leading to nutritional decline. This situation, perhaps combined with the loss of a positive social environment surrounding mealtimes, may lead to the decision to use an alternate feeding source (see Chapter 11). Initially, patients may be able to continue some oral feeding, but at some point total reliance on alternate feeding sources may occur. Table 3-4 summarizes a variety of intervention strategies suggested by Yorkston et al.[129] across various stages of severity in ALS. Jenkins and colleagues[150] summarize the evidence for symptomatic treatments in ALS.

PRACTICE NOTE 3-6

A woman in her late 50s was referred for speech and swallow evaluation by her neurologist. Roughly 18 months before the evaluation she began to have speech difficulties. These were progressive, and roughly 5 months before the evaluation she noticed increased difficulty swallowing.

At the time of the clinical evaluation she was able to take all foods orally but she was avoiding "heavier" foods such as certain meats. She also engaged in swallow compensations, including cutting any masticated food into small pieces and using liquids to "wash" heavier food down when she ate them. She also reported difficulty controlling oral secretions, with resultant drooling day and night.

On clinical examination this woman demonstrated a mixed dysarthria. The tongue presented with bilateral **fasciculations** but other cranial nerves were grossly intact. Her score on the Mann Assessment of Swallowing Ability (MASA; see Chapter 7) was 166 of 200, indicating moderate dysphagia. Her score on the speech scale of the ALS Severity Scale was 6, indicating the need to repeat some messages, and her score on the swallowing subscale was 7, reflecting her diet changes.

Endoscopic and fluoroscopic swallowing examinations are presented in Video 3-8, A and B on the Evolve website. On endoscopic examination this patient demonstrates basic single and simple movement but impairment on rapid and sequential movements. Still, her swallow abilities seemed functional. On fluoroscopic examination, she demonstrated a pattern of slowness with possible weakness, but she again gave the impression of a functional swallow.

I saw her again 2 months later. At this point she demonstrated little clinical change, although her MASA score had lowered to 154 with noted changes in tongue function and increased coughing during meals. The patient was having obvious difficulty coping with the apparent diagnosis and indicated a desire for no further clinical follow-up. These wishes were respected and she has not returned for additional evaluation or clinical assistance or advice.

They conclude that few treatments alter the course of the disease, but that many symptomatic treatments can have a positive influence on a patient's quality of life. Noninvasive ventilation has been shown to support respiratory function, improve quality of life, and extend survival by approximately 7 months. Katzberg and Benatar[151] concluded that in the absence of strong evidence, the best available evidence suggested a survival advantage with improved nutrition of gastrostomy tube feedings for some patients with ALS. However, they caution that their findings are tentative. Furthermore, a pair of patient-oriented studies by Stavroulakis et al.[152,153] indicated that many patients preferred to delay feeding tube placement perhaps until swallowing difficulties reached a critical point, but that patient education both in the hospital and the community helped with the transition from oral to tube feeding. Finally, the role of exercise is still not clear for patients with ALS. Proponents of exercise suggest that especially in the early stages of the disease exercise benefits patients both physically and psychologically. Advocates indicate that exercise may slow muscle deterioration resulting from disuse.[154] However, a Cochrane review by Dal Bello-Haas and Florence[155] concluded that no evidence existed to claim benefit from exercise for patients with ALS. Likewise, no evidence existed that exercise was harmful to these patients. Based on the evidence (or lack thereof), the best clinical advice might be to evaluate the needs and motivation of each patient when considering an exercise approach to dysphagia in ALS.

Muscle Diseases and Swallowing Impairment

A variety of pathologic conditions may have a negative influence on muscles related to swallowing function. These diseases typically result in weakness in muscle groups that contribute to dysphagia. Examples of disease processes that might impair peripheral muscle function (in some cases including the peripheral nerve) include polyneuropathy, myasthenia gravis (MG), polymyositis, scleroderma, systemic lupus erythematosus, and dystrophy. Unless working as part of a specialized health care team, the typical dysphagia specialist does not encounter large numbers of patients with these disorders or diseases. However, it is important to recognize the potential impact of each condition on swallowing function and to be able to differentiate other causes of dysphagia from these clinical conditions. From that perspective, each of these muscle diseases with the potential to affect swallowing function is discussed briefly in relation to dysphagia characteristics.

Polyneuropathy

Literally meaning "pathology to many nerves," polyneuropathies may result from many sources. Systemic diseases such as diabetes can result in polyneuropathies, as can other

TABLE 3-4 Summary of Swallowing Interventions in ALS

	Early Swallowing Problems	Dietary Consistency Changes	Unable to Meet Needs Orally	Salivary Problems
Presenting features	Solid foods difficult to eat	Weight loss	Decline in calorie intake	Complaints of too much saliva
	Longer mealtimes	Chronic dehydration	Decline in fluid intake	Complaints of drooling
	Need for smaller bites	Loss of enjoyment	Food spillage from mouth	
			Respiratory fatigue	
Intervention	Use chin-tuck position	Change to soft diet	Insert PEG or insert nasogastric tube or insert intermittent orogastric tube	Maintain adequate hydration
	Maintain liquid intake	Maintain liquid intake		Use aspirator
	Try using a straw	Eat calorie-dense foods		Use medication
	Eliminate caffeine	Increase taste, temperature (colder), and texture sensations of liquids		Surgically relocate salivary ducts
	Use double swallow			
	Learn choking first aid			
	Avoid washing foods down with liquids			

ALS, Amyotrophic lateral sclerosis; PEG, percutaneous endoscopic gastrostomy.
(From Yorkston KM, Miller RM, Strand EA: Management of speech and swallowing in degenerative diseases, Tucson, AZ, 1995, Communication Skill Builders.)

processes that affect peripheral nerves. Perhaps most common to dysphagia, and often forgotten, is the peripheral nerve damage that can result from radiotherapy in the treatment of head and neck cancer. These patients have **fibrosis** in tissue as well as nerve deficits in the affected areas (see Chapter 4). Weakness in peripheral nerves innervating the swallowing musculature contributes directly to weakness in the muscles used for chewing and swallowing. Polyneuropathies also may result in sensory deficits with resulting effect on the ability to safely ingest food and liquid. Guillain-Barré syndrome is one example of a neurogenic polyneuropathy in adults. Nearly all patients with Guillain-Barré syndrome have some degree of dysphagia. According to Chen et al.,[156] the majority of patients present with moderate to severe pharyngeal dysphagia, but nearly half of the patients they studied also had oral-phase swallowing deficits. In fact, Orlikowski et al.[157] reported the reduced tongue strength was associated with dysphagia and respiratory limitations in patients with Guillain-Barré. Most patients recovered swallowing functions to varying degrees, but those with more severe dysphagia later in the disease tended to have persistent complaints.

Myasthenia Gravis

MG is a disease process in which the neurotransmitter substance between motor nerves and muscles is depleted with use. In this regard, initial movements (such as chewing) are often intact or at least at their strongest at the beginning of movement (such as a meal). With repeated use the muscles fatigue into a flaccid weakness. Thus any swallowing activity that requires sustained or repeated movement (i.e., most of them) results in fatigue and reduced function. Colton-Hudson et al.[158] described dysphagia characteristics in 20 adults with MG. These investigators reported oral and pharyngeal deficits in all patients, and approximately 30% demonstrated aspiration. In addition, Linke et al.[159] reported that esophageal transit often is compromised in MG. Thus patients with MG may present with dysphagia characteristics reflecting weakness along the entire course of the upper swallowing mechanism. Finally, Warnecke et al.[160] used a fiberoptic endoscopic examination of swallowing (FEES) (see Chapter 8) to evaluate the immediate effect of the Tensilon test. Injection of Tensilon into a symptomatic patient with MG reduced symptoms within a short time. These authors reported that the combination of the FEES examination and the Tensilon test represents a clinical tool useful in the early diagnosis of MG-related dysphagia. One additional factor merits consideration. Available literature contains multiple case reports in which dysphagia was the initial presenting symptom of what eventually was diagnosed as MG.[161-164]

Thus dysphagia clinicians should carefully examine any patients presenting with persisting dysphagia for the presence of any related neurologic signs.

Polymyositis, Scleroderma, and Systemic Lupus Erythematosus

Polymyositis, scleroderma, and systemic lupus erythematosus are inflammatory muscle diseases more generally classified as connective tissue diseases. A brief but informative summary of dysphagia in these diseases is provided by Sheehan.[165] Polymyositis (dermatomyositis) is an inflammation of striated muscle. It often is initially seen in proximal muscle groups, and when present in the head and neck musculature can contribute to oropharyngeal dysphagia. In these instances clinical characteristics may include nasopharyngeal regurgitation, residue in the pharynx, and airway compromise by food or liquid. Deficits of the cervical esophagus are also frequently reported.

Scleroderma (progressive systemic sclerosis) is an inflammation of smooth muscle tissue. In this respect dysphagia is often esophageal in nature, primarily resulting from dysfunction in the distal third of the esophagus. At some point in the disease process many patients with scleroderma experience solid food dysphagia as a result of esophageal dysfunction. However, oropharyngeal dysphagia also may be seen with this disease.

Systemic lupus erythematosus is a disease process that affects women more frequently than men. The clinical presentation may vary because the disease may involve many organ systems. The time course is also variable. Patients may demonstrate proximal muscle weakness (including head and neck musculature), cranial nerve abnormalities, or deficits in the central nervous system. Often the presentation is of acute deterioration with slow recovery between exacerbations. Many patients report esophageal-based dysphagias.

Other diseases in the category of connective tissue or **systemic rheumatic diseases** can contribute to dysphagia. The general presentation is fatigue, malaise, pain, reduced appetite, and often dysphagia. Dysphagia may present as oropharyngeal or esophageal or both. Often the determining factor is which muscle groups are involved.

Muscular Dystrophy

Muscular dystrophy is another muscle disease that can affect various muscle groups. One type of dystrophy that may directly contribute to dysphagia is oculopharyngeal muscular dystrophy (OPMD).[166,167] OPMD is a slowly progressive disorder characterized by dysphagia, dysarthria, **ptosis**, and face and trunk weakness. As the name implies, pharyngeal muscles are likely to be weakened and thus contribute to dysphagia. Depending on the stage of the disease, dysphagia may be mild or severe. Duchenne muscular dystrophy (DMD) is another variant of muscle

disorder affecting younger males. DMD is progressive with no known cure. The prevalence of dysphagia in DMD is not well estimated but rates between 18% and 30% have been cited.[168] The pattern of dysphagia in DMD often includes feeding difficulties, but pharyngeal abnormalities have been found more frequently than oral or esophageal difficulties.[169] Dysphagia symptoms are quite varied among individuals with DMD and may include prolonged meal times, difficulty swallowing hard food and thick liquids, and frequent coughing or expectoration during meals.[170]

Treatment Considerations

Many diseases that affect lower motor neurons and peripheral muscle groups are progressive and thus present special challenges to the patient and the clinician. As with other neurogenic dysphagias, swallowing interventions often are symptomatic, reacting to the specific set of clinical circumstances presented at any given time. Various strategies may be used; these range from behavioral compensations to diet modifications. The use of strengthening exercises or related strategies may be questionable in some situations. Exercise fatigues muscle groups. If the underlying disease creates weakness in muscles required for swallowing, attempts to over-exercise these same muscle groups may exaggerate the underlying weakness rather than ameliorate it. Available evidence neither supports nor contradicts the use of exercise in progressive neuromuscular disorders. Thus it is important to understand the impact of the underlying neurologic condition on sensorimotor capability of the individual patient.

Clinicians attempting to improve swallowing function also must remember that these patients are receiving ongoing medical care. They often take multiple medications that may be changed from time to time. It is important for the dysphagia specialist to maintain good communication with other members of the health care team to understand better the effects of various medications and make optimum decisions about changes in the dysphagia management plan. Remember, many of these diseases are progressive, necessitating changes in dysphagia management strategies over time. Hillel and Miller[171] provide an excellent perspective on the team approach to management of dysphagia and other bulbar symptoms in patients with ALS. Much of their sage clinical advice is applicable to management of dysphagia in patients with other progressive neuromuscular diseases.

IDIOPATHIC OR IATROGENIC DISORDERS OF SWALLOWING THAT RESEMBLE NEUROGENIC DYSPHAGIA

A variety of contributing factors may create a neurogenic dysphagia in the absence of overt neurologic disease. These

---

CLINICAL CORNER 3-4: IDIOPATHIC DYSPHAGIA?

A 75-year-old man was referred for evaluation of dysphonia and dysphagia after knee replacement surgery. His endoscopic swallow examination is presented in Video 3-9 on the Evolve website. Note the nonmoving left true vocal fold, weakness in the left hemipharynx, and pooled secretions.

Critical Thinking

1. What factors might contribute to both dysphonia and dysphagia in this specific patient?
2. Speculate about the relation between knee surgery and dysphonia and dysphagia in this patient.
3. What is the clinical significance of the hemipharyngeal weakness "on top" of the nonmoving left true vocal fold? How might this affect treatment planning for this patient?

---

factors include undetected vascular deficits (ministrokes), decompensation with advancing age, decompensation in complex medical conditions, medication-induced changes, initial symptoms of a progressive disease, and postsurgical changes.[172,173] When dysphagia appears to result from neurologic dysfunction in the absence of overt neurologic disease or damage, these factors should be considered. A good rule of thumb is to treat a suspected neurogenic dysphagia as the result of a neurologic process until proven otherwise (see Clinical Corner 3-4).

TAKE HOME NOTES

1. Dysphagia resulting from neurologic disorders reflects the underlying sensorimotor characteristics of the neurologic deficit.
2. Treatment of neurogenic dysphagias is often symptomatic but relies heavily on a strong understanding of the underlying neurologic process. In many cases behavioral treatment interacts significantly with medical treatment.
3. Many neurogenic dysphagias change over time, necessitating different intervention strategies. Change may occur both toward recovery or deterioration of function depending on the specific neurologic disease or disorder.
4. Medical treatments (including surgery) for various neurologic diseases and disorders also contribute to dysphagia.
5. In the absence of overt neurologic disease, dysphagia that appears to be neurogenic should be considered reflective of an underlying neurologic cause until proven otherwise.

CLINICAL CASE EXAMPLE 3-1

A 69-year-old man had a brainstem stroke 7 months before seeking rehabilitation for dysphagia. The patient takes no food or liquid by mouth and is receiving all nutrition by PEG. He expectorates saliva into a cup except at nighttime. Within the past month he has tasted food but not attempted to swallow. His anxiety level is high about the possibility of aspiration but he is highly motivated to initiate oral feeding. He has experienced no chest infections or other complications since discharge from acute rehabilitation. Clinical examination revealed a left facial weakness but he was able to make a strong lip seal. He demonstrated right-body weakness greater in the arm than the leg, and he was able to walk with a quad cane. Endoscopic evaluation revealed slight paresis of the left vocal fold and in the left hemipharynx. Fluoroscopic examination of swallowing function revealed incomplete swallow attempts with limited hyolaryngeal excursion, limited opening of the PES (a small amount of material entered the esophagus), postswallow residue for thicker materials, and a small amount of aspiration with thin liquid. He demonstrated a strong reactive cough to the aspiration and the ability to clear residue back into the mouth, where it was expectorated.

Interpretation

This patient would be considered in the chronic poststroke phase because more than 6 months have elapsed since his stroke. He has had no swallowing experience during that period, but the observation that he does not expectorate at night (and does not complain of a "soggy" pillow in the morning) possibly suggests that he is swallowing saliva while asleep. The fact that he has tasted food supports his motivation to undertake aggressive therapy. His anxiety about aspiration is understandable and may be a factor to consider once therapy begins. The fact that he has had no chest infections and no history of tracheostomy are positive indications for the respiratory system. Ambulatory status is considered a positive sign because active patients are believed to be less susceptible to respiratory infections than are bedridden patients. The alternating hemiplegia (left face, pharynx, and vocal fold versus right side of the body) is characteristic of brainstem stroke. The incomplete swallow is characterized by incoordination and limited excursion of movement of the hyolaryngeal complex with reduced PES opening. Material entering the esophagus is a positive finding, as is the strong reactive cough and the ability to clear residue.

This patient is a good candidate for direct, intensive swallowing therapy. An appropriate therapy program for this individual should address airway protection (either by choice of material to be swallowed or compensatory maneuver), hyolaryngeal excursion (increase upward and forward movement), and swallow coordination (in some cases slowing the speed of the swallow with prolonged maneuvers may accomplish this outcome). If successful, the functional outcome should be increased oral intake of food and liquid.

CLINICAL CASE EXAMPLE 3-2

A 72-year-old woman presented to the clinic with a diagnosis of primary progressive aphasia. The primary complaint was weight loss and unfinished meals. The patient lived independently and attended an adult day-care facility where she reportedly was observed to cough during lunch. Her brother had a history of esophageal disease and a concern was expressed by the family. The patient was ambulatory and presented no overt physical impairments. She was limited in her ability to communicatively interact. Her expressive communication was limited to head nods and a few vocalizations but no meaningful words were produced. She was able to respond appropriately to many basic commands and requests and participated interactively with a dysphagia examination. Oral mechanism examination was unremarkable with no overt signs of corticobulbar deficit. Videofluorographic examination of swallowing was completed. The only mild abnormality was the observation that the patient tilted her head upward as she initiated a swallow and that oral initiation and transit were prolonged. Subsequently, a feeding examination was completed in which the patient was provided a tray of food and liquid (regular-grade diet) and requested to eat. She surveyed the tray of food and promptly began to eat using her fingers. She was handed a fork and used this appropriately until she faced a situation in which she had to cut her food. She was handed a knife and proceeded to use it as a fork. Despite multiple cues she persisted to use the knife as a fork and could not be encouraged to use two tools (knife and fork) simultaneously.

Interpretation

This specific case contains features commonly associated with dementias (weight loss, reduced food intake, poor communicative interaction) in addition to a more rare and specific finding. Primary progressive aphasia is a form of dementia in which language skills are impaired early in the course of the dementia, rendering the initial symptoms to those of a progressive aphasia. The observations of utensil use by this patient suggest a form of apraxia that seemed specific to mealtime and self-feeding. Because at her age and in her situation these social functions were central to her life and her well-being, this form of apraxia had a significant functional impact on her life. The immediate therapy for this individual was environmental. The family was instructed to prepare meals that could be eaten with a single utensil (i.e., fork or spoon). The patient was quite successful with this strategy. Also, it is important to take into consideration the progressive, deteriorating nature of dementia. Although the mealtime adjustment of a single utensil was effective in the short term, as this disease progressed, this patient would require additional strategies to ensure adequate nutrition and hydration. In this respect, her treatment plan must contain periodic and regular monitoring of the success of any adaptation used to maintain oral food and liquid intake and the nutritional consequences of that intake (see Video 3-3 on the accompanying Evolve website).

REFERENCES

1. Duffy JR: *Motor speech disorders: substrates, differential diagnosis, and management*, ed 2, St Louis, 2005, Elsevier Mosby.
2. Humbert IA, Robins J: Normal swallowing and functional magnetic resonance imaging: a systematic review. *Dysphagia* 22:266, 2007.
3. Malandraki GA, Perlman AL, Karampinos DC, et al: Reduced somatosensory activations in swallowing with age. *Hum Brain Mapp* 32:730–743, 2011.
4. Malandraki GA, Sutton BP, Perlman AL, et al: Neural activation of swallowing and swallowing-related tasks in healthy young adults: an attempt to separate the components of deglutition. *Hum Brain Mapp* 30:3209–3226, 2009.
5. Gonzalez-Fernandez M, Kleinman JT, Ky P, et al: Supratentorial regions of acute ischemia associated with clinical important swallowing disorders: a pilot study. *Stroke* 39:3022, 2008.
6. Gordon C, Hewer RL, Wade DT: Dysphagia in acute stroke. *Br Med J (Clin Res Ed)* 295:411, 1987.
7. Schroeder MF, Daniels SK, McClain M, et al: Clinical and cognitive predictors of swallowing recovery in stroke. *J Rehabil Res Dev* 43:301, 2006.
8. Hays NP, Robers SB: The anorexia of aging in humans. *Physiol Behav* 30:257, 2006.
9. Perlman PW, Cohen MA, Setzen M, et al: The risk of aspiration of pureed food as determined by flexible endoscopic evaluation of swallowing with sensory testing. *Otolaryngol Head Neck Surg* 130:80, 2004.
10. Setzen M, Cohen MA, Mattucci KF, et al: Laryngopharyngeal sensory deficits as a predictor of aspiration. *Otolaryngol Head Neck Surg* 124:622, 2001.
11. Ickenstein GW, Kelly PJ, Furie KL, et al: Predictors of feeding gastrostomy removal in stroke patients with dysphagia. *J Stroke Cerebrovasc Dis* 12:169, 2003.
12. Michou E, Hamdy S: Cortical input in control of swallowing. *Curr Opin Otolaryngol Head Neck Surg* 17:166, 2009.
13. Hamdy S, Rothwell JC, Aziz Q, et al: Organization and reorganization of human swallowing motor cortex: implications for recovery after stroke. *Clin Sci (Lond)* 99:151, 2000.
14. Hamdy S, Aziz Q, Rothwell JC, et al: Recovery of swallowing after dysphagic stroke relates to functional reorganization in the intact motor cortex. *Gastroenterology* 115:1104, 1998.
15. Hamdy S, Aziz Q, Rothwell JC, et al: The cortical topography of human swallowing musculature in health and disease. *Nat Med* 2:1217, 1996.
16. Mann G, Hankey GL, Cameron D: Swallow function after stroke: prognosis and prognostic factors at 6 months. *Stroke* 30:744, 1999.
17. Smithard DG, O'Neill PA, England RE, et al: The natural history of dysphagia following stroke. *Dysphagia* 12:188, 1997.
18. Martino R, Foley N, Bhogal S, et al: Dysphagia after stroke: incidence, diagnosis, and pulmonary complications. *Stroke* 36:2756, 2005.
19. Crary MA, Humphrey JL, Carnaby-Mann G, et al: Dysphagia, nutrition, and hydration in ischemic stroke patients at admission and discharge from acute care. *Dysphagia* 28:69, 2013.
20. Foley NC, Martin RE, Salter KL, et al: A review of the relationship between dysphagia and malnutrition following stroke. *J Rehabil Med* 41:707, 2009.
21. Finestone HM, Greene-Finestone LS, Wilson ES, et al: Prolonged length of stay and reduced functional improvement rate in

malnourished stroke rehabilitation patients. *Arch Phys Med Rehabil* 77:340, 1996.

22. Smithard DG, Smeeton NC, Wolfe CD: Long-term outcome after stroke: does dysphagia matter? *Age Ageing* 36:90, 2007.

23. Harraf F, Ward K, Man W, et al: Transcranial magnetic stimulation study of expiratory muscle weakness in acute ischemic stroke. *Neurology* 71:2000, 2008.

24. Sulter G, Elting JW, Stewart R, et al: Continuous pulse oximetry in acute hemiparetic stroke. *J Neurol Sci* 179:65, 2000.

25. Ali K, Cheek E, Sills S, et al: Day-night differences in oxygen saturation and the frequency of desaturations in the first 24 hours in patients with acute stroke. *J Stroke Cerebrovasc Dis* 16:239, 2007.

26. Leslie P, Drinnan MJ, Ford GA, et al: Resting respiration in dysphagic patients following acute stroke. *Dysphagia* 17:208, 2000.

27. Leslie P, Drinnan MJ, Ford GA, et al: Swallow respiration patterns in dysphagic patients following acute stroke. *Dysphagia* 17:202, 2002.

28. Butler SG, Stuart A, Pressman H, et al: Preliminary investigation of swallowing apnea duration and swallow/respiratory phase relationships in individuals with cerebral vascular accident. *Dysphagia* 22:215, 2007.

29. Westendorp WF, Nederkoorn PJ, Vermeij JD, et al: Post-stroke infection: a systematic review and meta-analysis. *BMC Neurol* 11:110, 2001.

30. Bravata DM, Ho SY, Meehan TP, et al: Readmission and death after hospitalization for acute ischemic stroke. *Stroke* 38:1899, 2007.

31. Saposnik G, Hill MD, O'Donnell M, et al: Variables associated with 7-day, 30-day, and 1-year fatality after ischemic stroke. *Stroke* 39:2318, 2008.

32. Hinchey JA, Shephard T, Furie K, et al: Formal dysphagia screening protocols prevent pneumonia. *Stroke* 36:1972, 2005.

33. Lakshminarayan K, Tsai AW, Tong X, et al: Utility of dysphagia screening results in predicting poststroke pneumonia. *Stroke* 41:2849, 2010.

34. Yeh SJ, Huang KY, Want TG, et al: Dysphagia screening decreases pneumonia in acute stroke patients admitted to the stroke intensive care unit. *J Neurol Sci* 306:38, 2011.

35. Millns B, Gosney M, Jack CIA, et al: Acute stroke predisposes to oral gram-negative bacilli—a cause of aspiration pneumonia? *Gerontology* 49:173, 2003.

36. Leibovitz A, Dan M, Zinger J, et al: Pseudomonas aeruginosa and the oropharyngeal ecosystem of tube-fed patients. *Emerg Infect Dis* 9:956, 2003.

37. Langdon PC, Lee AH, Binns CW: High incidence of respiratory infections in "nil by mouth" tube-fed acute ischemic stroke patients. *Neuroepidemiology* 32:107, 2009.

38. Brogan E, Langdon C, Brookes K, et al: Can't swallow, can't transfer, can't toilet: factors predicting infection in the first week post stroke. *J Clin Neurosci* 22:92, 2015.

39. Brogan E, Langdon C, Brookes K, et al: Respiratory infections in acute stoke: nasogastric tubes and immobility are stronger predictors than dysphagia. *Dysphagia* 29:340, 2014.

40. Crary MA, Carnaby GD, Sia I, et al: Spontaneous swallowing frequency has potential to identify dysphagia in acute stroke. *Stroke* 44:3452, 2013.

41. Carnaby G, Hankey GJ, Pizzi J: Behavioural intervention for dysphagia in acute stroke: a randomized controlled trial. *Lancet Neurol* 5:31, 2006.

42. Kikiwada M, Iwamoto T, Takasaki M: Aspiration and infection in the elderly. *Drugs Aging* 22:115, 2005.

43. Sørensen RT, Rasmussen RS, Overgaard K, et al: Dysphagia screening and intensified oral hygiene reduce pneumonia after stroke. *J Neurosci Nurs* 45:139, 2013.

44. Axelsson K, Asplund K, Norberg A, et al: Nutritional status in patients with acute stroke. *Acta Med Scand* 224:217, 1988.

45. Davalos A, Ricart W, Gonzalez-Huix F, et al: Effect of malnutrition after acute stroke on clinical outcome. *Stroke* 27:1028, 1996.

46. Gariballa SE, Parker SG, Taub N, et al: Influence of nutritional status on clinical outcome after acute stroke. *Am J Clin Nutr* 68:275, 1998.

47. Finestone HM, Greene-Finestone LS, Wilson ES, et al: Malnutrition in stroke patients on the rehabilitation service and at follow-up: prevalence and predictors. *Arch Phys Med Rehabil* 76:310, 1995.

48. Crary MA, Carnaby-Mann GD, Miller L, et al: Dysphagia and nutritional status at the time of hospital admission for ischemic stroke. *J Stroke Cerebrovasc Dis* 15:164, 2006.

49. Poels BJ, Brinkman-Zijiker HG, Dijkstra PU, et al: Malnutrition, eating difficulties and feeding dependence in a stroke rehabilitation centre. *Disabil Rehabil* 28:637, 2006.

50. Yoo SH, Kim JS, Kwon SU, et al: Undernutrition as a predictor of poor clinical outcomes in acute ischemic stroke patients. *Arch Neurol* 65:39, 2008.

51. Smithard DG, O'Neill PA, Park C, et al: Complications and outcome following acute: does dysphagia matter? *Stroke* 27:1200, 1996.

52. Neumann S, Bartolome G, Buchholz D, et al: Swallowing therapy of neurologic patients: correlation of outcome with pretreatment variables and therapeutic methods. *Dysphagia* 10:1, 1995.

53. Elmståhl S, Bülow M, Ekberg O, et al: Treatment of dysphagia improves nutritional conditions in stroke patients. *Dysphagia* 14:61, 1999.

54. Foley N, Teasell R, Salter K, et al: Dysphagia treatment post stroke: a systematic review or randomized controlled trials. *Age Ageing* 37:258, 2008.

55. Crary MA: A direct intervention program for chronic neurogenic dysphagia secondary to brainstem stroke. *Dysphagia* 10:6, 1995.

56. Huckabee ML, Cannito MP: Outcomes of swallowing rehabilitation in chronic brainstem dysphagia: a retrospective evaluation. *Dysphagia* 14:93, 1999.

57. Crary MA, Carnaby-Mann GD, Groher ME, et al: Functional benefits of dysphagia using adjunctive sEMG biofeedback. *Dysphagia* 19:160, 2004.

58. Crary MA, Carnaby GD, LaGorio L, et al: Functional and physiological outcomes from an exercise-based dysphagia therapy: a pilot investigation of the McNeill Dysphagia Therapy Program. *Arch Phys Med Rehabil* 93:1173, 2012.

59. Focht A: Differential diagnosis of dementia. *Geriatrics* 64:20, 2009.

60. Easterling C, Robbins J: Dementia and dysphagia. *Geriatr Nurs* 29:275, 2008.

61. Langmore SE, Olney RK, Lomen-Hoerth C, et al: Dysphagia in patients with frontotemporal lobar dementia. *Arch Neurol* 64:58, 2007.

62. Kalia M: Dysphagia and aspiration pneumonia in patients with Alzheimer's disease. *Metabolism* 52:36, 2003.

63. Chouinard J: Dysphagia in Alzheimer disease: a review. *J Nutr Health Aging* 4:214, 2000.

64. Alagiakrishnan K, Bhanji RA, Kurian M: Evaluation and management of oropharyngeal dysphagia in different types of dementia: a systematic review. *Arch Gerontol Geriatr* 56:1, 2013.

65. Chouinard J, Lavigne E, Villeneuve C: Weight loss, dysphagia, and outcome in advanced dementia. *Dysphagia* 13:151, 1998.

66. Knol W, van Marum RJ, Jansen PA, et al: Antipsychotic drug use and the risk of pneumonia in elderly people. *J Am Geriatr Soc* 56:661, 2008.

67. Priefer BA, Robbins J: Eating changes in mild-stage Alzheimer's disease: a pilot study. *Dysphagia* 12:212, 1997.

68. Humbert IA, McLaren DG, Kosmatka K, et al: Early deficits in cortical control of swallowing in Alzheimer's disease. *J Alzheimers Dis* 19:1185, 2010.

69. Sato E, Hirano H, Watanabe Y, et al: Detecting signs of dysphagia in patients with Alzheimer's disease with oral feeding in daily life. *Geriatr Gerontol Int* 14:549, 2014.

70. Rothan-Tondeur M, Meaume S, Girard L, et al: Risk factors for nosocomial pneumonia in a geriatric hospital: a control-case one-center study. *J Am Geriatr Soc* 51:997, 2003.

71. Langmore SE, Skarupski KA, Park PS, et al: Predictors of aspiration pneumonia in nursing home residents. *Dysphagia* 17:298, 2002.

72. Wada H, Nakajoh K, Satoh-Nakagawa T, et al: Risk factors for aspiration pneumonia in Alzheimer's disease patients. *Gerontology* 47:271, 2001.

73. Bomfim FM, Chiari BM, Roque FP: Factors associated to suggestive signs of oropharyngeal dysphagia in institutionalized elderly women. *Codas* 25:154, 2013.

74. Park YH, Han HR, Oh BM, et al: Prevalence and associated factors of dysphagia in nursing home residents. *Geriatr Nurs* 34:212, 2013.

75. Ikeda M, Brown J, Holland AJ, et al: Changes in appetite, food preference, and eating habits in frontotemporal dementia and Alzheimer's disease. *J Neurol Neurosurg Psychiatry* 73:371, 2002.

76. Volicer L: Goals of care in advanced dementia: quality of life, dignity, and comfort. *J Nutr Health Aging* 1:481, 2007.

77. Amella EJ: Feeding and hydration issues for older adults with dementia. *Nurs Clin North Am* 39:607, 2004.

78. Finucane TE, Christmas C, Travis K: Tube feeding in patients with advanced dementia. *JAMA* 282:1365, 1999.

79. Cancy B, Sampson EL, Jones L: Enteral tube feeding in older people with advanced dementia: findings from a Cochrane systematic review. *Int J Palliat Nurs* 15:396, 2009.

80. American Geriatrics Society Ethics Committee and Clinical Practice and Models of Care Committee: American geriatrics society feeding tubes in advanced dementia position statement. *J Am Geriatr Soc* 62:1590, 2014.

81. Kuo S, Rhodes RL, Mitchell SL, et al: Natural history of feeding-tube use in nursing home residents with advanced dementia. *J Am Med Dir Assoc* 10:264, 2009.

82. Sharp HM, Shega JW: Feeding tube placement in patients with advanced dementia: the beliefs and practice patterns of speech-language pathologists. *Am J Speech Lang Pathol* 18:222, 2009.

83. Vitale CA, Berkman CS, Monteleoni C, et al: Tube feeding in patients with advanced dementia: knowledge and practice of speech-language pathologists. *J Pain Symptom Manage* 42:366, 2011.

84. Pelletier C: What do certified nurse assistants actually know about dysphagia and feeding nursing home residents? *Am J Speech Lang Pathol* 13:99, 2004.

85. Monteleoni C, Clark E: Using rapid-cycle quality improvement methodology to reduce feeding tubes in patients with advanced dementia: before and after study. *BMJ* 329:491, 2004.

86. Simmons SF, Schnelle JF: Individualized feeding assistance care for nursing home residents: staffing requirement to implement two interventions. *J Gerontol A Biol Sci Med Sci* 59:M966, 2004.

87. Mackay LE, Morgan AS, Bernstein BA: Swallowing disorders in severe brain injury: risk factors affecting return to oral intake. *Arch Phys Med Rehabil* 80:365, 1999.

88. Terré R, Mearin F: Prospective evaluation of oro-pharyngeal dysphagia after severe traumatic brain injury. *Brain Inj* 21:1411, 2007.

89. Hansen TS, Engberg AW, Larsen K: Functional oral intake and time to reach unrestricted dieting for patients with traumatic brain injury. *Arch Phys Med Rehabil* 89:1556, 2008.

90. Mandaville A, Ray A, Robertson H, et al: A retrospective review of swallow dysfunction in patients with severe traumatic brain injury. *Dysphagia* 29:310, 2014.

91. Ward EC, Green K, Morton AL: Patterns and predictors of swallowing resolution following adult traumatic brain injury. *J Head Trauma Rehabil* 22:184, 2007.

92. Terré R, Mearin F: Evolution of tracheal aspiration in severe traumatic brain injury-related oropharyngeal dysphagia: 1-year longitudinal follow-up study. *Neurogastroenterol Motil* 21:361, 2009.

93. Woratyla SP, Morgan AS, Mackay L, et al: Factors associated with early onset pneumonia in the severely brain-injured patient. *Conn Med* 59:643, 1995.

94. Hansen TS, Larsen K, Engberg AW: The association of functional oral intake and pneumonia in patients with severe traumatic brain injury. *Arch Phys Med Rehabil* 89:2114, 2008.

95. Hui X, Haider AH, Hashmi ZG, et al: Increased risk of pneumonia among ventilated patients with traumatic brain injury: every day counts! *J Surg Res* 184:483, 2013.

96. Sharma OP, Oswanski MR, Singer D, et al: Swallowing disorders in trauma patients: impact of tracheostomy. *Am Surg* 73:1117, 2007.

97. Duong TT, Englander J, Wright J, et al: Relationship between strength, balance, and swallowing deficits and outcomes after traumatic brain injury: a multicenter analysis. *Arch Phys Med Rehabil* 85:1291, 2004.

98. Cherney LR, Halper AS: Swallowing problems in adults with traumatic brain injury. *Semin Neurol* 16:349, 1996.

99. Schurr MJ, Ebner KA, Maser AL, et al: Formal swallowing evaluation and therapy after traumatic brain injury improves dysphagia outcomes. *J Trauma* 46:817, 1999.

100. Harris MK, Shneyder N, Borazanci A, et al: Movement disorders. *Med Clin North Am* 93:371, 2009.

101. Jankovic J: Parkinson's disease: clinical features and diagnosis. *J Neurol Neurosurg Psychiatry* 79:368, 2008.

102. Alverez MV, Evidente VG, Driver-Dunckley ED: Differentiating Parkinson's disease from other parkinsonian disorders. *Semin Neurol* 27:356, 2007.

103. Miller N, Allcock LM, Hildreth T, et al: Swallowing problems in Parkinson's disease: frequency and clinical correlates. *J Neurol Neurosurg Psychiatry* 80:1047, 2009.

104. Potulska A, Friedman A, Królicki L, et al: Swallowing disorders in Parkinson's disease. *Parkinsonism Relat Disord* 9:349, 2003.

105. Kalf JG, de Swart BJ, Bloem BR, et al: Prevalence of oropharyngeal dysphagia in Parkinson's disease: a meta-analysis. *Parkinsonism Relat Disord* 18:311, 2012.

106. Nagaya M, Kachi T, Yamada T, et al: Videofluorographic study of swallowing in Parkinson's disease. *Dysphagia* 13:95, 1998.

107. Hammer MJ, Murphy CA, Abrams TM: Airway somatosensory deficits and dysphagia in Parkinson's disease. *J Parkinsons Dis* 3:39, 2013.

108. Mu L, Sobotka S, Chen J, et al: Parkinson disease affects peripheral sensory nerves in the pharynx. *J Neuropathol Exp Neurol* 72:614, 2013.

109. Rodrigues B, Nóbrega AC, Sampaio M, et al: Silent saliva aspiration in Parkinson's disease. *Mov Disord* 26:138, 2011.

110. Nóbrega AC, Rogrigues B, Torres AC, et al: Is drooling secondary to a swallowing disorder in patients with Parkinson's disease? *Parkinsonism Relat Disord* 14:243, 2008.

111. Nicaretta DH, Rosso AL, Mattos JP, et al: Dysphagia and sialorrhea: the relationship to Parkinson's disease. *Arq Gastroenterol* 50:42, 2013.

112. Nóbrega AC, Rodrigues B, Melo A: Silent aspiration in Parkinson's disease patients with diurnal sialorrhea. *Clin Neurol Neurosurg* 110:117, 2008.

113. Nóbrega AC, Rodrigues B, Melo A: Is silent aspiration a risk factor for respiratory infection in Parkinson's disease patients? *Parkinsonism Relat Disord* 14:646, 2008.

114. Gross RD, Atwood CW, Ross SB, et al: The coordination of breathing and swallowing in Parkinson's disease. *Dysphagia* 23:136, 2008.

115. Pfeiffer RF: Gastrointestinal dysfunction in Parkinson's disease. *Lancet Neurol* 2:107, 2003.

116. Cloud LJ, Greene JG: Gastrointestinal features of Parkinson's disease. *Curr Neurol Neurosci Rep* 11:379, 2011.

117. Salat-Foix D, Suchowersky O: The management of gastrointestinal symptoms in Parkinson's disease. *Expert Rev Neurother* 12:239, 2012.

118. Andersson I, Sidenvall B: Case studies of food shopping, cooking and eating habits in older women with Parkinson's disease. *J Adv Nurs* 35:69, 2001.

119. Miller N, Noble E, Jones D, et al: Hard to swallow: dysphagia in Parkinson's disease. *Age Ageing* 35:614, 2006.

120. Baijens LW, Speyer R: Effects of therapy for dysphagia in Parkinson's disease: systematic review. *Dysphagia* 24:91, 2009.

121. Van Hooren MR, Baijens LW, Voskuilen S, et al: Treatment effects for dysphagia in Parkinson's disease: a systematic review. *Parkinsonism Relat Disord* 20:800, 2014.

122. Felix VN, Corréa SM, Soares RJ: A therapeutic maneuver for oropharyngeal dysphagia in patients with Parkinson's disease. *Clinics* 63:661, 2008.

123. Athukorala RP, Jones RD, Sella O, et al: Skill training for swallowing rehabilitation in patients with Parkinson's disease. *Arch Phys Med Rehabil* 95:1374, 2014.

124. El Sharkawi A, Ramig L, Logemann JA, et al: Swallowing and voice effects of Lee Silverman Voice Treatment (LSVT): a pilot study. *J Neurol Neurosurg Psychiatry* 72:31, 2002.

125. Pitts T, Bolser D, Rosenbek J, et al: Impact of expiratory muscle strength training on voluntary cough and swallow function in Parkinson disease. *Chest* 135:1301, 2009.

126. Monte FS, da Silva-Júnior FR, Braga-Neto P, et al: Swallowing abnormalities and dyskinesia in Parkinson's disease. *Mov Disord* 20:457, 2005.

127. Lim A, Leow L, Huckabee ML, et al: A pilot study of respiration and swallowing integration in Parkinson's disease: "on" and "off" levodopa. *Dysphagia* 23:76, 2008.

128. Melo A, Monteiro L: Swallowing improvement after levodopa treatment in idiopathic Parkinson's disease: lack of evidence. *Parkinsonism Relat Disord* 19:279, 2013.

129. Yorkston KM, Miller RM, Strand EA: *Management of speech and swallowing in degenerative diseases*, Tucson, AZ, 1995, Communication Skill Builders.

130. Miller AJ: *The neuroscientific principles of swallowing and dysphagia*, San Diego, 1999, Singular.

131. Lang IM: Brain stem control of the phases of swallowing. *Dysphagia* 24:333, 2009.

132. Crary MA, Baldwin BO: Surface electromyographic characteristics of swallowing in dysphagia secondary to brainstem stroke. *Dysphagia* 12:180, 1997.

133. Lan Y, Xu G, Dou Z, et al: The correlation between manometric and videofluoroscopic measurements of the swallowing function in brainstem stroke patients with dysphagia. *J Clin Gastroenterol* 49:24, 2015.

134. Huckabee ML, Lamvik K, Jones R: Pharyngeal mis-sequencing in dysphagia: characteristics, rehabilitative response, and etiological speculation. *J Neurol Sci* 343:153, 2014.

135. Chua KS, Kong KH: Functional outcome in brain stem stroke patients after rehabilitation. *Arch Phys Med Rehabil* 77:194, 1996.

136. Malandraki GA, Sutton BP, Perlman AL, et al: Neural activation of swallowing and swallowing-related tasks in healthy young adults: an attempt to separate the components of deglutition. *Hum Brain Mapp* 30:3209, 2009.

137. Harris ML, Julyan P, Kulkarni B, et al: Mapping metabolic brain activation during human volitional swallowing: a positron emission tomography using [18F]fluorodeoxyglucose. *J Cereb Blood Flow Metab* 25:520, 2005.

138. Suzuki M, Asada Y, Ito J, et al: Activation of cerebellum and basal ganglia on volitional swallowing detected by functional magnetic resonance imaging. *Dysphagia* 18:71, 2003.

139. Rangarathnam B, Kamarunas E, McCullough GH: Role of cerebellum in deglutition and deglutition disorders. *Cerebellum* 13:767, 2014.

140. Wijesekera LC, Leigh PN: Amyotrophic lateral sclerosis. *Orphanet J Rare Dis* 4:3, 2009.

141. Pupillo E, Messina P, Logroscino G, et al: The SLALOM Group. Long-term survival of amyotrophic lateral sclerosis: a population-based study. *Ann Neurol* 75:287, 2014.

142. Magnus T, Beck M, Giess R, et al: Disease progression in amyotrophic lateral sclerosis: predictors of survival. *Muscle Nerve* 25:709, 2002.

143. Kawai S, Tsukuda M, Mochimatsu I, et al: A study of the early stage of dysphagia in amyotrophic lateral sclerosis. *Dysphagia* 18:1, 2003.

144. Ruoppolo G, Schettino I, Frasca V, et al: Dysphagia in amyotrophic lateral sclerosis: prevalence and clinical findings. *Acta Neurol Scand* 128:397, 2013.

145. Weikamp JG, Schelhass HJ, Hendriks JC, et al: Prognostic value of decreased tongue strength on survival time in patients with amyotrophic lateral sclerosis. *J Neurol* 259:2360, 2012.

146. Easterling C, Antinoja J, Cashin S, et al: Changes in tongue pressure, pulmonary function, and salivary flow in patients with amyotrophic lateral sclerosis. *Dysphagia* 28:217, 2013.

147. Higo R, Tayama N, Nito T: Longitudinal analysis of progression of dysphagia in amyotrophic lateral sclerosis. *Auris Nasus Larynx* 31:247, 2004.

148. Solazzo A, Monaco L, Vecchio LD, et al: Earliest videofluoromanometric pharyngeal signs of dysphagia in ALS patients. *Dysphagia* 29:539, 2014.

149. Nozaki S, Sugishita S, Saito T, et al: Prolonged apnea/hypopnea during water swallowing in patients with amyotrophic lateral sclerosis. *Rinsho Shinkeigaku* 48:634, 2008.

150. Jenkins TM, Hollinger H, McDermott CJ: The evidence for symptomatic treatments in amyotrophic lateral sclerosis. *Curr Opin Neurol* 27:524, 2014.

151. Katzberg HD, Benatar M: Enteral tube feeding for amyotrophic lateral sclerosis/motor neuron disease. *Cochrane Database Syst Rev* (1):CD004030, 2011.

152. Stavroulakis T, Baird WO, Baxter SK, et al: Factors influencing decision-making in relation to timing of gastrostomy insertion in patients with motor neurone disease. *BMJ Support Palliat Care* 4:57, 2014.

153. Stavroulakis T, Baird WO, Baxter SK, et al: The impact of gastrostomy in motor neurone disease: challenges and benefits from a patient and carer perspective. *BMJ Support Palliat Care* 4:57, 2014.

154. de Almeida JP, Silvestre R, Pinto AC, et al: Exercise and amyotrophic lateral sclerosis. *Neurol Sci* 33:9, 2012.

155. Dal Bello-Haas V, Florence JM: Therapeutic exercise for people with amyotrophic lateral sclerosis or motor neuron disease. *Cochrane Database Syst Rev* (1):CD005229, 2013.

156. Chen MY, Donofrio PD, Frederick MG, et al: Videofluoroscopic evaluation of patients with Guillain-Barré syndrome. *Dysphagia* 11:11, 1996.

157. Orlikowski D, Terzi N, Blumen M, et al: Tongue weakness is associated with respiratory failure in patients with severe Guillain-Barré syndrome. *Acta Neurol Scand* 119:364, 2009.

158. Colton-Hudson A, Koopan WJ, et al: A prospective assessment of the characteristics of dysphagia in myasthenia gravis. *Dysphagia* 17:147, 2002.

159. Linke R, Witt TN, Tatsch K: Assessment of esophageal function in patients with myasthenia gravis. *J Neurol* 250:601, 2003.

160. Warnecke T, Teismann I, Zimmerman J, et al: Fiberoptic endoscopic evaluation of swallowing with simultaneous Tensilon application in diagnosis and therapy of myasthenia gravis. *J Neurol* 255:224, 2008.

161. Azeem N, Law RJ, Arora AS: 73-year-old man with recent-onset dysphagia. *Mayo Clin Proc* 89:845, 2014.

162. Breen E, Bleich L, Loeser C: Myasthenia gravis presenting with dysphagia in an elderly male: a case report. *Am J Med* 127:e7, 2014.

163. Klair JS, Rochlani YM, Meena NK: Myasthenia gravis masquerading as dysphagia: unveiled by magnesium infusion. *BMJ Case Rep* 2014, 2014.

164. Petit A, Constans T, Chavanne D, et al: Myasthenia gravis in the elderly: a rare case of undernutrition. *Aging Clin Exp Res* 24:398, 2012.

165. Sheehan NJ: Dysphagia and other manifestations of oesophageal involvement in the musculoskeletal diseases. *Rheumatology (Oxford)* 47:746, 2008.

166. Rüegg S, Lehky Hagen M, Hohl U, et al: Oculopharyngeal muscular dystrophy—an under-diagnosed disorder? *Swiss Med Wkly* 135:574, 2005.

167. Brais B, Rouleau GA, Bouchard JP, et al: Oculopharyngeal muscular dystrophy. *Semin Neurol* 19:59, 1999.

168. Aloysius A, Born P, Kinali M, et al: Swallowing difficulties in Duchenne muscular dystrophy: indications for feeding assessment and outcome of videofluoroscopic swallow studies. *Eur J Paediatr Neurol* 12:239, 2008.

169. Hanayama K, Liu M, Higuchi Y, et al: Dysphagia in patients with Duchenne muscular dystrophy evaluated with a questionnaire and videofluorography. *Disabil Rehabil* 30:517, 2008.

170. Archer SK, Garrod R, Hart N, et al: Dysphagia in Duchenne muscular dystrophy assessed by validated questionnaire. *Int J Lang Commun Disord* 48:240, 2013.

171. Hillel AD, Miller RM: Management of bulbar symptoms in amyotrophic lateral sclerosis. *Adv Exp Med Biol* 209:201, 1987.

172. Buchholz DW: Neurogenic dysphagia: what is the cause when the cause is not obvious? *Dysphagia* 9:242, 1994.

173. Buchholz DW: Oropharyngeal dysphagia due to iatrogenic neurological dysfunction. *Dysphagia* 10:248, 1995.

CHAPTER 4

Dysphagia and Head and Neck Cancer

Michael A. Crary

To view additional case videos and content, please visit the evolve website.

CHAPTER OUTLINE

OBJECTIVES

1. Define cancer and describe its potential impact on the individual patient.
2. Describe the various treatments for head and neck cancer and their side effects.
3. Describe factors that contribute to dysphagia in patients being treated for head and neck cancer.
4. Describe the dysphagia characteristics that might be associated with head and neck cancer treated with different modalities.
5. Elaborate on dysphagia-related complications seen in patients treated for head and neck cancer.
6. Describe unique features of dysphagia assessment for head/neck cancer patients.
7. Discuss the "when," "what," and "why" aspects of dysphagia intervention for patients being treated for head and neck cancer. What are the anticipated outcomes for the various dysphagia interventions?

CANCER AS A DISEASE

Cancer is currently the second leading cause of death in the United States. An estimated half of all men and one third of all women will have some form of cancer. Millions of people are either living with cancer or have had cancer. These facts clearly indicate that prevention, early detection, and treatment of cancer, as well as appropriate rehabilitation for the cancer survivor, are among today's primary health concerns.

What Is Cancer?

Cancer is the result of cell growth that is out of control. In simple terms, cells become abnormal and grow rapidly, forming extra, unwanted, and potentially destructive tissue. This proliferation of cell growth is called **hyperplasia**. The abnormality that causes cancer cells results from damaged DNA within cells. This damaged DNA may be inherited or it may result from exposure to an environmental cause such as smoking. In fact, the primary risk factors for head and neck cancer (with the exception of nasopharyngeal cancer) have been identified as tobacco (including smokeless tobacco) and heavy alcohol use. Other high-risk factors include human papillomavirus infection, poor oral hygiene, consumption of certain processed foods, radiation exposure, and mechanical irritation.[1] One potential problem caused by these abnormal cancer cells is that they can travel to various places in the body, begin to grow and proliferate, and replace normal body cells. This traveling of cells is referred to as **metastasis**. Metastasis may occur when cancer cells enter the bloodstream or the **lymph** system and travel to a different part of the body.

Cancer usually forms as a *tumor,* which technically means a swelling or enlargement, although not all cancers form tumors and not all tumors are cancerous. Some tumors are **benign** rather than **malignant**. Different types of cancers grow at different rates, create different problems, and respond to different treatments. One way to conceptualize cancer is as a group of diseases with different symptoms and signs. *Symptoms* are noticed by a patient and taken as an indication that something is not right in the body. *Signs* are also indicative of health problems but are more definitive of disease as observed by a physician or other health care professional. Symptoms and signs of cancer may change as the disease changes over time. The specific symptoms and signs depend on the location of the cancer; the size of the tumor; the direct effect on any surrounding organs, blood vessels, or nerves; and any metastasis of the cancer. Both general and specific symptoms have been associated as warning signs of cancer. These are summarized in Box 4-1.

Different problems may be encountered depending on the type and location of a cancer. The symptoms listed in Box 4-1 provide general categories of problems that may be encountered. Pain is perhaps the most feared of cancer-related problems. Pain does not result from all cancers, but when it does occur it may be the result of tumor growth or result from the treatments used to eradicate the cancer. Another common problem is fatigue. Like pain, fatigue may result either directly from the cancer or as a side effect of cancer treatment. Box 4-2 summarizes some of the

salient characteristics that may be associated with cancer-related fatigue.

Cancers may also contribute to significant weight loss and impaired immune function. These problems are not mutually exclusive because malnutrition also contributes to impaired immune function. Impaired immune function contributes to increased complications, poor wound healing, and opportunistic infections. Together, poor nutrition and impaired immune function may contribute to a suboptimal outcome for patients with cancer. An estimated 30% to 50% of patients with head and neck cancer demonstrate some degree of malnutrition.[2-4] Up to half of patients with head and neck cancer reveal some degree of weight loss when cancer is first diagnosed.[5,6] Average weight loss has been estimated between 5% and 10% of baseline body weight[6-8] and weight loss is often long term.[9] Weight loss may result from reduced ingestion or digestion of food or from impaired absorption or utilization of nutrients by the body in the presence of adequate food and liquid intake. This latter situation may be complicated by the need for increased caloric intake resulting from increased energy expenditure in some patients with cancer. Thus some patients have a biologic need for more caloric intake, but as a result of poor food and liquid intake, absorption, or utilization, they actually have a significantly reduced caloric reservoir. This can become a vicious cycle leading to **cachexia**. Weight loss may be accompanied by **anorexia,** nausea, constipation, and fatigue. Box 4-3 summarizes some of the more general

---

BOX 4-1 GENERAL AND SPECIFIC SIGNS ASSOCIATED WITH CANCER (NOT SPECIFIC TO HEAD AND NECK CANCER)

General Cancer Warning Signs
- Unexplained weight loss
- Fever
- Fatigue
- Pain
- Skin changes

Specific Cancer Warning Signs
- Change in bowel or bladder function
- Sores that do not heal
- White patches in mouth or white spots on tongue
- Unusual bleeding or discharge
- Thickening or a lump in any part of the body
- Indigestion or difficulty swallowing
- Recent change in a wart or mole or any new skin change
- Nagging cough or hoarseness

BOX 4-2 SALIENT CHARACTERISTICS OF CANCER-RELATED FATIGUE

- Feeling tired, weary, or exhausted even after sleep
- Lacking energy to do regular daily activities
- Trouble concentrating, thinking clearly, or remembering
- Negative feelings, irritability, impatience, lack of motivation
- Lack of interest in day-to-day activities
- Less attention to daily appearance
- Spending more time lying in bed or sleeping

BOX 4-3 GENERAL CONSEQUENCES OF MALNUTRITION

- Increased susceptibility to infection
- Reduced immune functions
- Respiratory failure
- Poor wound healing
- Skin breakdown
- Death

consequences of malnutrition in patients with head and neck cancer.

Early detection and timely treatment for cancers of the head and neck often are associated with improved outcomes. From that perspective, it is important to facilitate early recognition of the symptoms and signs of cancer and obtain appropriate medical diagnosis early in the course of the disease.

Diagnosis of Cancer

As noted, the initial indications of cancer are often symptoms identified by the patient (see Clinical Corner 4-1). These should not be ignored because early detection and prompt treatment lead to a better outcome. Depending on the type and location of cancer, various diagnostic tests may be used. These tests are used to identify the specifics of the cancer and help plan the best possible treatment. Patients with head and neck cancer require careful examination by a multidisciplinary team of health care providers. Such teams may vary but a common core membership might include a head and neck surgeon, radiation oncologist, medical oncologist, dentist, social workers, and rehabilitation specialists. The goal of the team evaluation is to characterize the cancer and develop the best comprehensive treatment approach (including rehabilitation when indicated). The team may use a variety of diagnostic procedures, including radiography, computed tomographic or magnetic resonance imaging, endoscopy (including both laryngoscopy and esophagoscopy), biopsy and **histopathologic** confirmation, and physical examination.

Staging

A common procedure involved in evaluating cancer is *staging*. In simple terms, staging is the process of determining how far the cancer has spread. This process is important in determining the best treatment options, estimating complications or comorbid conditions, and formulating a

prognosis. Although more than one system is available for cancer staging, the TNM system is used most often.[10] *T* (tumor) describes the size of the tumor and extension into any neighboring tissues. *N* (nodes) describes any spread of the cancer into nearby lymph nodes. *M* (metastasis) describes spread of the cancer to other organ systems within the body. A number or additional letter after each letter is assigned to provide more detail. In general, lower numbers mean smaller, more localized cancers. Higher numbers

---

CLINICAL CORNER 4-1: EARLY SIGNS OF HEAD AND NECK CANCER

Some cancers are identified early, which is believed to lead to earlier treatment and better outcomes. In my practice, I typically ask patients what the initial signs were that "something was wrong." The answers vary greatly. Some men report that they felt a small lump (size of a pea) in their neck when shaving. Others have told me that their dentist found a growth during routine dental examination. Still others have reported sore throat, persistent dysphonia, or swallowing difficulties. However, the most unusual report was from an elderly man who indicated that he had trouble keeping his dentures in place. This man has a diagnosis of nasopharyngeal carcinoma (NPC). When I looked into his mouth, the reason for the ill-fitting dentures was obvious (Figure 4-1, *A*). Subsequently on endoscopic examination the complete tumor was clearly seen (Figure 4-1, *B*). Despite the size and location of this growth, this man reported no difficulties with either nasal breathing or the sense of smell.

Remember that NPC often has no early signs and these tumors may grow large before any overt signs are noted by the patient.

Critical Thinking
1. What other head and neck cancer shares the dubious distinction of few or no early symptoms?
2. How might NPC affect swallowing function?

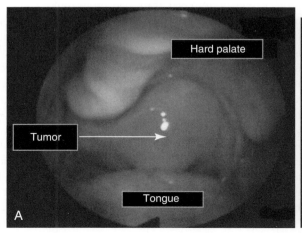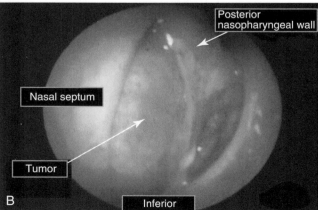

FIGURE 4-1   Photograph of a nasopharyngeal tumor protruding into oral cavity (*A*) and viewed with **transnasal** endoscopy (*B*).

mean larger, spreading cancers. Therefore a T1N0M0 tumor is small, has not invaded neighboring lymph nodes, and has not spread to other body organ systems. Conversely, a T4N2M1 tumor is large, has invaded neighboring lymph nodes, and has metastasized to other body organ systems. Box 4-4 lists TNM definitions for oropharyngeal cancer. Similar, but not identical, definitions are used for hypopharyngeal and laryngeal cancers. One difference is the inclusion of anatomic subsites for these latter areas.

After TNM description, cancers may be grouped together into stage classifications. In general, five stages are used (stage 0 through 4). Stage 4 has three subdivisions (A, B, and C). A lower stage classification indicates a smaller, nonmetastasized cancer. A higher stage classification indicates a more serious, widespread cancer. Box 4-5 shows the staging system based on TNM descriptions.

TREATMENTS FOR HEAD AND NECK CANCERS

Many cancers of the head and neck region can be cured if they are found early. Choice of treatment and outcome frequently depend on many factors, including location and stage of the cancer, the patient's age and general health status, the experience of the medical team treating the patient, and available facilities. Although curing the cancer is a primary goal, the patient's posttreatment function and quality of life are also important considerations in choosing the type of treatment because each treatment has potential side effects and sequelae. Another aspect to consider is whether the treatment is intended to be **palliative** or curative. Three primary options are frequently used in the treatment of head and neck cancers: surgery, radiation, and chemotherapy. These may be used in isolation or in various combinations depending on the type of cancer and the goals of treatment. Surgery and radiation therapy (RT) are considered the only curative therapies for cancer in the head and neck region. Chemotherapy is used in the **neoadjuvant** or **adjuvant** setting but is not considered a curative therapy.[11]

Surgery

Surgery refers to removal of the cancerous tumor and some of the surrounding healthy tissue, referred to as the *margin*. Surgery is intended to remove as much of the primary tumor as possible and leave no trace of cancer cells in the margin. However, this is not always possible, and surgery often is combined with RT and chemotherapy. In some cases, more than a single surgery may be required to remove the cancer or restore the anatomic or functional deficit caused by the primary surgery. For example, if the cancer has spread to the lymph nodes in the neck, the lymph nodes are removed. This is called a *lymph node dissection* or a *neck dissection*. In other situations reconstruction may be required. This involves moving tissue from another part of the body to fill a gap created by the cancer **resection.** A variety of procedures have been described to relocate tissue to the head and neck region. Generally referred to as *flaps,*

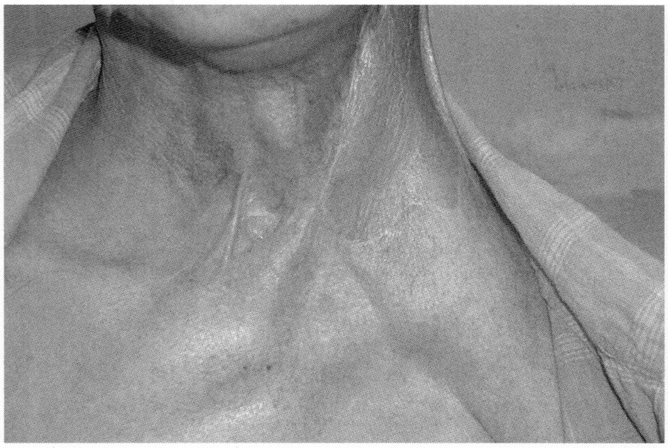

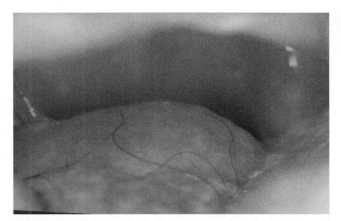

FIGURE 4-2 Photograph of a pectoralis major flap on the left side of the neck.

FIGURE 4-3 Photograph of a flap reconstruction of the tongue and floor of the mouth.

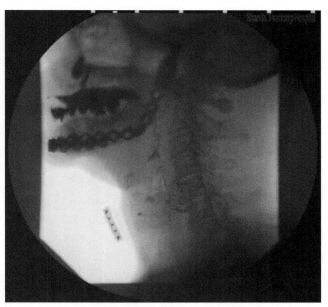

FIGURE 4-4 Example of mandibular reconstruction with an implant.

these are often named for the location from which the replacement tissue is taken. Therefore a pectoralis major flap is constructed from tissue obtained from the pectoralis major muscle. Other flaps might include a lateral thigh flap, a radial forearm flap, or similar procedures. Figure 4-2 depicts a pectoralis major flap on the left side. Figure 4-3 shows a flap reconstruction of the floor of the mouth and tongue. In some situations bone tissue may be relocated to reconstruct bony deficits in the mandible, or if a majority of the mandible is removed an implant may be used to replace the missing bone (Figure 4-4). If surgical reconstruction is not feasible, a **prosthodontist** may be consulted to construct artificial dental or facial parts to fill a space created by the initial surgery. If the primary tumor surgery creates a risk to breathing, a **tracheotomy** may be performed. If severe swallowing problems are anticipated, a **gastrostomy** may be performed. Either or both of these procedures may be performed at the time of the primary cancer surgery if the surgical team anticipates airway or swallowing problems as a direct result of the surgery.

Surgery is a primary treatment consideration for all small cancers. Contraindications to surgical removal of a small tumor are the possibility of significant deficits to function (speaking, chewing, swallowing) or cosmetic defects. Advanced cancers often require a combination of surgery and radiation or chemotherapy. Various surgical approaches may be used depending on the location and size of the cancerous tumor. Box 4-6 lists some of the more common surgeries associated with head and neck cancer treatment.

Surgery, like other cancer treatments, has a number of side effects that can be problematic for patients. Side effects typically depend on the location and type of surgery. Some of these are temporary and others are more permanent. All side effects affect the patient's quality of life. Box 4-7 lists some of the more frequent side effects from cancer surgery in the head and neck region. The length of time after surgery was performed is an indicator of the prominent side effects. For example, edema is pronounced in the acute postoperative period. Edema may be accompanied by pain. As the primary surgical site heals, scarring may reduce movement of anatomic structures spared and in the vicinity of the surgery. In addition, if cranial nerves are damaged during the primary surgery or as a result of postoperative scarring, the patient may sustain motor or sensory deficits from nerve damage.

Radiation Therapy

RT uses high-energy x-rays to kill cancer cells. Death of cancer cells leads to shrinkage of the tumor. RT may be

BOX 4-6 COMMON SURGERIES ASSOCIATED WITH HEAD AND NECK CANCER TREATMENT

Primary tumor surgery: removal of tumor and surrounding tissue

Mandibulectomy: removal of a piece of the jawbone

Mandibulotomy: splitting the mandible to gain access to a tumor

Maxillectomy: removing all or part of the hard palate

Mohs surgery: removal of a tumor in thin slices, evaluating each slice under a microscope for cancer cells until all cancer cells are gone

Laser surgery: using a narrow, intense beam of light to remove cancer

Laryngectomy: removal of the entire larynx

Partial laryngectomy: removal of part of the larynx: supraglottic, hemilaryngectomy, supracricoid, vocal cord

Laryngopharyngectomy: removal of larynx and pharynx

Tracheostomy: establishing a hole in the anterior neck (stoma) into the trachea to establish an airway

Gastrostomy: creating a fistula into the stomach by way of the abdominal wall; often used to place a feeding tube

Neck dissection: removal of lymph nodes and other tissue in the neck considered at risk for metastatic disease; radical neck dissection involves more tissue removal than modified neck dissection

Reconstructive surgery: any surgery that attempts to replace missing anatomy to improve function and/or appearance

BOX 4-7 POTENTIAL SIDE EFFECTS OF SURGERY TO TREAT HEAD AND NECK CANCER

- Swelling of the mouth or throat, resulting in difficulty breathing
- Impaired speech or voice
- Difficulty chewing and swallowing
- Facial disfigurement
- Numbness in the face, neck, or throat
- Reduced mobility in the neck and shoulder area
- Decreased function of the thyroid gland

used as the primary treatment for small tumors, after surgery to destroy residual small pockets of cancer cells, or before surgery to shrink tumors in the hope of more successful surgical removal with fewer residual deficits. Radiation may be administered in two ways: external-beam radiation and internal radiation. *External-beam radiation* involves aiming a high-energy radiation beam at the tumor and surrounding tissues. External-beam radiation may be applied on a conventional, once-daily schedule or on an altered fractionation schedule. The latter form of RT may increase acute toxicity, but late effects are similar between these two

techniques.[11] A newer form of external-beam radiation is known as *intensity-modulated radiation therapy (IMRT)*. This procedure allows more effective doses of radiation to be delivered to the tumor while hitting less healthy tissue around the tumor. This method is intended to result in fewer side effects. Other recent advances in RT include *radiosensitization* (using drugs to make cancer cells more sensitive to radiation) and *hyperfractionation* (giving radiation in small doses several times per day). In general, treatment strategies leading to a lower dose of RT or RT to more confined anatomic regions results in less-severe and more transient dysphagia.[12-16]

Internal radiation therapy, often referred to as **brachytherapy**, involves implanting small pellets or rods containing radioactive material into the cancer or near the cancer site. Patients remain hospitalized during this procedure while the implants remain in place.

Recently, proton therapy has been more frequently used in the treatment of some head/neck cancers.[17,18] Simply stated, proton therapy involves aiming a beam of protons at a tumor site. As protons pass through body tissue, they release energy. The point of peak energy release can be programmed, causing damage to the tumor with minimal damage to surrounding tissues.

Side effects from RT are common both during treatment (acute toxicity) and after treatment (late effects or late toxicity). Some of these effects are transient and others are persistent. In addition, certain side effects may be latent—that is, they may not appear for a substantial period (in some cases years) after the completion of RT. Many side effects of RT to the head and neck region contribute directly to dysphagia and resulting decline in nutritional status. If these occur during treatment, patients may experience interruptions in therapy. Box 4-8 lists several side effects that may occur from RT to the head and neck region.

Before the initiation of RT, all patients should undergo a complete dental examination. Damaged or decayed teeth may need to be removed because radiation can cause tooth decay. Also, patients who receive radiation to the anterior neck region are at risk for damage to the thyroid gland, contributing to **hypothyroidism**. This condition may worsen any feelings of fatigue already experienced by the patient. For these patients, thyroid gland function should be monitored on a regular basis.

Chemotherapy

Chemotherapy refers to the use of drugs to kill cancer cells. These agents are typically very powerful drugs that can cause several unpleasant side effects. Chemotherapy may be administered by mouth, intravenously, by injection into a muscle or under the skin, or by injection directly into the tumor. Chemotherapy may be used to palliate symptoms in patients with incurable disease or as an adjuvant to RT,

BOX 4-8 POTENTIAL SIDE EFFECTS OF RADIATION THERAPY TO TREAT HEAD AND NECK CANCER

- Redness and skin irritation in area treated
- Permanent change to salivary glands leading to persistent dry mouth or thickened saliva
- Bone pain
- Nausea and vomiting
- Fatigue
- Mouth sores and sore throat
- Dental problems
- Painful swallowing
- Loss of appetite
- Reduced or altered sense of taste (and sometimes smell)
- Earaches resulting from hardening of ear wax
- Hypothyroidism
- Fibrosis leading to reduced movement
- Peripheral neuropathy
- Bone, cartilage, soft tissue necrosis

BOX 4-9 POTENTIAL SIDE EFFECTS FROM CHEMOTHERAPY TO TREAT HEAD AND NECK CANCER

- Fatigue
- Nausea and vomiting
- Hair loss
- Dry mouth
- Loss of appetite
- Reduced sense of taste
- Weakened immune system
- Diarrhea or constipation
- Open sores in the mouth potentially leading to infection

surgery, or both. Chemotherapy may be used before (neoadjuvant) or after surgery (or RT). Chemotherapy has been used in combination with RT to treat certain laryngeal cancers in an attempt to preserve the larynx (i.e., avoid a total laryngectomy) and subsequent voice functions. As previously mentioned, certain drugs may be used in combination with RT as a form of radiosensitization. Although these approaches are promising, many combined therapies are still considered experimental. One negative aspect of combined therapies is the risk of increased severity or a wider range of side effects. For example, large clinical studies reported increased acute toxicity in patients receiving concomitant chemoradiation therapy (CRT).[19] However, at least one review has concluded that posttreatment swallowing dysfunctions noted in patients receiving concomitant CRT were similar to those seen in patients receiving only RT.[20] Box 4-9 lists several possible side effects from chemotherapy in the treatment of head and neck cancer.

Each patient should be evaluated for the presence of one or more of these possible side effects resulting from primary cancer treatments that may affect swallowing function.

DYSPHAGIA IN PATIENTS WITH HEAD AND NECK CANCER

Many—in fact, a majority—of patients treated for head and neck cancer have some degree of swallowing difficulty. Some dysphagia symptoms result directly from the cancer and thus may be present before medical treatment, whereas others are the result of various treatments for the cancer. In general, patients receiving RT (alone or in combination with surgery) are at greater risk for swallowing difficulties than are patients receiving surgical treatments without radiation.[21-25] Dysphagia subsequent to cancer treatments may be described as resulting from reduced swallowing efficiency, which may be complicated by anatomic changes within the swallow mechanism. Reduced swallow efficiency is characterized by reduced movement of structures within the swallowing mechanism, leading to prolonged duration of various aspects of the swallow and reduced opening of the pharyngoesophageal segment (PES).[26,27] The reduction of movement during swallowing contributes to postswallow residue along the swallowing mechanism and poor clearance of saliva.[20,28] Food and saliva residue may build up over time, increasing the risk of aspiration or necessitating frequent expectoration by the patient.

Dysphagia from Surgical Intervention

Surgery for head and neck cancer results in the loss, rearrangement, or reconstruction of structures that are important for swallowing function. A traditional rule for predicting dysphagia after surgery for head and neck cancer is the "50% rule."[29,30] This "rule," which seems to result from experiences with oral cancers, suggests that removal of less than 50% of a structure will not result in a significant and permanent swallowing problem. However, this rule has been challenged with the introduction of surgical reconstruction techniques as clinicians report good postoperative swallowing function after surgical flap reconstruction.[31,32] Thus individual patient characteristics should be carefully examined both before and after surgery to identify and manage any resulting swallowing impairments.[33] A general guideline is that the more tissue removed or relocated, the higher the probability for postsurgical dysphagia. Of course, this guideline requires modification when combined modalities are used (RT or chemotherapy in addition to surgery). The following text provides a brief overview of certain dysphagia characteristics that may result from surgery involving various aspects of the swallowing mechanism. Table 4-1 presents a summary of certain surgeries with the

TABLE 4-1 Common Swallowing Disorders Resulting from Various Surgeries to Treat Head and Neck Cancer

Resection	Physiologic Effect	Swallowing
Partial glossectomy	Removes <50% of tongue Anterior tissue removal difficulties	Difficulty holding and preparing a bolus for swallowing
Total glossectomy	Removal >50% of tongue Flap technique influences result	Difficulty moving materials from the oral cavity Reduced tongue driving force May show reduced pharyngeal clearance
Tonsil/base of tongue	Reduced anterior tongue range	Reduced tongue driving force Difficulty moving materials through the oropharynx
Palatal resection	Removal of >50% of soft palate Incomplete velar seal	Velar leak results in retrograde movement of materials into the nasopharynx
Anterior/lateral floor of mouth	Reduced anterior tongue range; unable to lateralize tongue Reduced ability to elevate hyoid or larynx Reduced opening of upper esophageal sphincter	Reduced control of oral bolus Reduced tongue driving force Difficulty moving material through the oropharynx Delayed triggering of pharyngeal swallow Reduced clearance of bolus from pharynx
Partial pharyngeal resection	Reduced pharyngeal wall constriction Reduced elevation of hyoid and larynx	Difficulty clearing materials from the pharynx Delay triggering swallow
Hemilaryngectomy	Unilateral resection Partial airway closure	Unilateral pharyngeal weakness Reduced airway protection
Supraglottic laryngectomy	Incomplete posterior tongue movement, restricted arytenoids motion, partial airway closure	Delay in bolus propulsion Difficulty with elevation of structures for swallow Reduced airway protection
Total laryngectomy	Removal of vibratory source Alternative source surgically developed	Issues with reduced negative pressure, bolus transit Anatomic or physiologic **stenosis** of PES possible

PES, Pharyngoesophageal segment.

associated physiologic impact and anticipated swallow deficit.

Surgery for Oral Cancers

Generally speaking, the oral cavity involves the anterior aspect of the tongue, floor of the mouth, submental structures, the mandible, and the maxilla. Oral surgeries often involve more than a single structure. For example, a **mandibulotomy** may be required to gain adequate surgical access to tumors in the floor of the mouth or other areas of the oral cavity. In general, surgeries for oral cancers may limit mastication, bolus formulation and containment, and bolus transport from the front to the back of the mouth. Surgeries restricted to the tongue often result in transient dysphagia with good functional outcome; however, this may depend on the extent of the tissue removed and the shape of the reconstructed tongue if flap reconstruction is completed.[34,35] When present, swallowing problems resulting from limited tongue resections involve bolus control and transport difficulties and may be transient.

With more extensive resections involving the tongue and floor of mouth with or without flap reconstruction, dysphagia may be expected for varying periods. Such dysphagia typically involves problems with mastication, bolus control, transport to the posterior oral cavity and, in some cases, airway protection as a result of loss of control of the bolus within the oral cavity.[36-38] In addition, pain may result from alterations to the temporomandibular joint. In cases of dramatic resection and reconstruction of the mandible, limitations in the PES may result from reduced upward pull from the hyolaryngeal complex that attaches to the mandible. Conversely, some patients with resection limited to oral structures will have functional pharyngeal aspects in swallowing and will do well if compensations can be used for oral deficits (see Practice Note 4-1). Video 4-1 on the Evolve website demonstrates functional pharyngeal aspects of swallowing in a patient with significant tongue reconstruction. Contrast liquid is delivered to the pharynx by a small straw connected to a syringe to compensate for limited oral control. Note the increase in residue resulting

PRACTICE NOTE 4-1

Many devices have been suggested to compensate for reduced oral transit in patients with limited tongue movement as a result of resection or paralysis. Glossectomy spoons have been described but are not always accepted by patients. We treated a patient who had floor of mouth and lingual resection and repair with a microvascular flap. As a result of these surgeries, the patient had reduced lingual movement, impaired ability to contain a liquid bolus in the mouth, and impaired ability to transit a pudding or thicker bolus posteriorly in the mouth. We were able to increase oral intake by placing a "cocktail straw" (small straw) on a syringe so that the patient could place liquid (thin and thick) in the posterior mouth where she could control delivery to the pharynx and swallow without complication. View Video 4-1 on the Evolve website for this text for an example of these types of deficits.

from thicker materials. Also note the patient's spontaneous compensations to adjust for limited tongue movement.

Surgery for Oropharyngeal Cancers

The oropharynx begins where the oral cavity stops, extending from the posterior hard palate to the hyoid bone inferiorly. This area includes the tongue base, faucial arches, tonsils and tonsillar fossa, **retromolar trigone**, soft palate, and the pharyngeal walls of the superior and lateral pharynx. General aspects of dysphagia resulting from surgery in the oropharynx include nasal regurgitation (sometimes called nasopharyngeal reflux), decreased bolus transit, aspiration, and PES dysfunction. Surgery in this area often involves multiple structures, thus increasing the extent of swallowing deficit.

Surgery limited to the tongue base may result in a reduced force applied by the tongue to move the bolus into the pharynx, which could result in postswallow residue in the area of the tongue base and valleculae. Surgery in this region also can result in reduced upward pull on the PES, contributing to reduced opening of this region and postswallow residue in the piriform recesses. In general, surgery limited to the tongue or to the tongue base has a favorable outcome regarding the ability to ingest food and liquid by mouth.[22,39,40] A related consideration is the use of reconstructive procedures in this region. Newer microvascular reconstruction techniques have shown promise for improved swallow function after surgery in the oropharynx[41,42]; however, at least one recent study has indicated that patients with tongue or floor-of-mouth cancers who received reconstruction surgery demonstrated more severe swallowing impairments in the acute phase of recovery than patients with primary closure.[43] This result could be related to numerous clinical variables, but the effect of reconstruction

surgery and possible concomitant treatments should be considered in postsurgical cases.

Patients undergoing surgery involving more than one structure in the oropharynx tend to have more severe and persistent dysphagia.[44] For example, if the tongue and palate are both resected, the patient may have difficulty propelling a bolus into the pharynx, poor bolus control, and nasal regurgitation. Patients who have extensive reconstruction with flaps may have swallowing difficulties related to both the ablative surgery and the flap reconstruction. Flaps used in reconstruction may contribute to swallowing problems related to altered sensation, poor movement, or bulk added to the oropharynx. Each of these factors should be clinically evaluated in patients with flap reconstruction in the swallowing mechanism.

Surgery for Hypopharyngeal Cancers

The pharynx is a tubelike structure extending from behind the nose to the entrance of the esophagus. The portion referred to as the hypopharynx is the section of the tube beginning at the hyoid bone and extending to below the cricoid cartilage of the larynx. The hypopharynx includes the piriform recesses, postcricoid area, and pharyngeal walls. The larynx rests within the hypopharynx but is not technically part of this structure. The most common site for hypopharyngeal cancer is the piriform recess. The hypopharynx has extensive lymph drainage into the cervical neck region, and metastasis to the cervical neck lymph nodes is frequent with hypopharyngeal cancer.[11] Thus neck dissection commonly is performed in combination with any surgery to the hypopharynx. Also, hypopharyngeal tumors often do not create overt symptoms early in the course of the disease. For this reason, hypopharyngeal tumors are often advanced and require extensive surgery that may involve both the larynx and the neck.[45] Such patients may have concurrent therapies, including extensive surgeries such as laryngopharyngectomy, along with a neck dissection. In some cases, only a partial removal of the larynx is required and vocal functions may be somewhat preserved. In advanced cancers in this region, reconstruction with a **gastric pull-up** or **jejunal transfer** may be used to retain as much swallowing function as possible. Given the location of hypopharyngeal cancers and the frequent spread of these cancers to adjacent structures (larynx, neck), dysphagia resulting from surgeries to treat these cancers is severe. However, newer surgical approaches using transoral laser microsurgery offer promise for good control of the cancer with lower rates of treatment-related morbidity.[46]

Surgery for Laryngeal Cancers

The larynx can be subdivided into three regions: the supraglottic region, glottic region, and subglottic region. Subglottic cancers are rare compared with cancers in the other regions, and when identified often involve the vocal folds

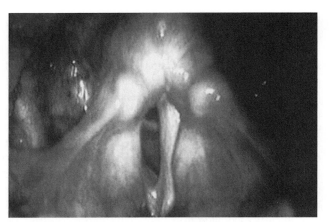

FIGURE 4-5 Photograph of a larynx after right true vocal cord removal by laser (laser cordectomy). The larynx is in the fully adducted (closed) position as indicated by approximation of the arytenoid cartilages. Note the large glottal opening resulting from the surgical procedure.

PRACTICE NOTE 4-2

Although patients with total laryngectomy are at minimal risk for aspiration during eating and drinking, some patients aspirate in an unusual way. A few years ago, I saw a patient who reported chronic coughing when he drank any liquids. We had been seeing him for minor adjustment with his tracheoesophageal speaking valve and wondered if he might be "leaking" around the valve. Clinically we did not see any visible signs of leaking around the valve, so we completed a fluoroscopic evaluation of swallowing. To our surprise, this patient had a long but narrow pharyngocutaneous fistula that opened in the anterior midline of the neck approximately 1 inch above the stoma. After a few sips of liquid barium he began coughing. The barium tracked along the fistula and dripped into his trachea through the stoma. A simple bandage reduced this unusual source of aspiration and the fistula was brought to the attention of our head and neck surgical team.

(glottic region). Supraglottic cancers have a higher rate of spread to the lymph system of the neck than isolated vocal fold tumors and thus may require neck dissection.[7] Supraglottic and glottic tumors both contribute to early overt changes in voice and swallowing and thus may be identified and treated early in the course of the disease. These small tumors may be successfully treated with limited surgeries, including laser surgery.[47-49] As the size of the tumor or metastasis to adjacent structures increases, the need for more extensive surgical resection is indicated; these may be considered as a partial laryngectomy or a total laryngectomy.

Partial laryngectomy procedures may include a cordectomy, in which only a true vocal fold is removed; a hemilaryngectomy, in which one half (right or left) of the larynx is removed; or a supraglottic or supracricoid laryngectomy, in which the structures above the glottis are removed. Figure 4-5 depicts the larynx of a patient after right cordectomy. Each partial laryngectomy procedure may contribute to a reduction in airway protection during swallowing by compromising either the glottis or the supraglottic mechanisms that contribute to airway closure. The extent of the surgery and the functional aspects of any reconstruction may be predictive of the presence and severity of any postoperative dysphagia. Recent reports suggest that partial laryngectomy, specifically supracricoid laryngectomy, has a good prognosis for return of functional swallowing, but airway protection is a persistent concern in the period after surgery.[50-53]

Patients with total laryngectomy typically do not present with risk of airway compromise because the airway and the swallowing tract are separated (see Practice Note 4-2). In these patients a new airway opening is established by way of a stoma in the anterior neck. By removing transnasal airflow and redirecting it to the neck stoma, these patients

also have a diminished sense of smell, which may further contribute to reduced food intake. The more common dysphagia problem faced by patients with total laryngectomy is stenosis in the **neopharynx** created after surgical removal of the larynx. The terms *anatomic stenosis* and *physiologic stenosis* may be applied as simple descriptors of whether this narrowing results from structural (anatomic) or muscle (physiologic) irregularities. Typically, this narrowing of the swallowing mechanism limits the ability of the patient to ingest solid foods, whereas liquids may be swallowed more easily. In cases of severe stenosis, patients may report difficulty swallowing both solids and liquids (see also Clinical Corner 4-2). Other problems faced by the patient after total laryngectomy may include tissue breakdown, leading to fistulas or surgical scarring. One variant of a postsurgical scar deficit in the neopharynx is the presence of a pseudoepiglottis, or pull-apart pouch. On lateral radiograph this "structure" may give the impression of an epiglottis in a patient who has none. Videos 4-2 and 4-3 on the Evolve website provide endoscopic and fluoroscopic studies of a pseudoepiglottis. Video 4-4 is a fluoroscopic study showing a stricture in the neopharynx of a patient after total laryngectomy. Video 4-5 is an endoscopic view of a patient who 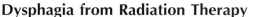 received a supraglottic laryngectomy.

Dysphagia from Radiation Therapy

RT in the treatment of head and neck cancer may be used in isolation or in combination with surgery and/or chemotherapy. RT may be used as the treatment of choice for small tumors to preserve tissue function (as in the larynx) or for advanced tumors that are not resectable. A general impression is that swallowing problems after RT either in isolation or in combination with surgery are worse than

CLINICAL CORNER 4-2:   STRICTURE IN THE PES

A 48-year-old man was treated with a concomitant chemotherapy–RT regimen for cancer at the base of his tongue. During his therapy a percutaneous endoscopic gastrostomy (PEG) tube was placed for primary nutrition and hydration. He attempted to maintain some oral intake, but this steadily declined and he eventually was limited to sips of water. At the time of our initial evaluation I reported the presence of an anatomic stenosis (stricture) beginning at the top region of the PES and continuing into the proximal esophagus. The entire length of this stenosis was estimated to be greater than 20 mm. The patient was referred to the gastroenterology service for dilatation. Several weeks after this procedure the patient returned for repeat fluoroscopic evaluation and reported increased oral intake but prolonged meal time. The report from the gastroenterology service indicated that the stricture was dilated to 48 Fr (approximately 16 mm). During the fluoroscopic study we again noted a severe stricture in the same area and the patient was unable to ingest more than a small sip of liquid without significant aspiration.

Critical Thinking

1. How do you reconcile the radiographic findings of a stricture with the gastroenterology report of a successful dilatation?
2. What next steps would you consider for this patient?

BOX 4-10 POTENTIAL COMPLICATIONS AND SIDE EFFECTS OF RADIATION THERAPY THAT MAY CONTRIBUTE DIRECTLY TO DYSPHAGIA

- Mucositis
- Xerostomia
- Sensory changes in taste and smell
- Fibrosis (including **trismus**)
- Neuropathy
- Changed anatomy (e.g., stricture)
- Odynophagia (painful swallowing)
- Loss of appetite
- Edema
- Infection (fungal, bacterial)
- Dental changes

those after surgery alone.[54,55] More recent use of IMRT appears to be associated with a reduction, but not elimination, of dysphagia posttreatment.[56-58] A recent review of strategies to reduce long-term dysphagia following CRT identified three promising approaches: (1) preventative exercise programs focused on oral and pharyngeal structures, (2) use of nasogastric (NG) tubes versus gastrostomy tube when supplemental nutrition or hydration is indicated, and (3) radiation dose restriction using IMRT.[15] More information on the first two of these approaches is provided later in this chapter.

RT contributes to a variety of mucosal and muscle tissue changes that can complicate any existing swallowing difficulties and create new problems. Box 4-10 lists several complications resulting from RT to the head and neck region that may contribute to dysphagia. One or more of these complications occur in almost every patient who receives RT for the treatment of head and neck cancer. These changes may occur to both mucosal tissue and muscle and nerve tissue. Recent work has assessed **symptom clusters** in patients treated with CRT for head and neck cancers. Results from one study identified two clusters: a head and neck cancer–specific cluster including dysphagia, mucositis, xerostomia, pain, taste deviations, fatigue, and skin changes; and a gastrointestinal cluster

including nausea, vomiting, and dehydration.[59] Another study[60] reported that although head and neck cancer patients treated with radiation demonstrated multiple symptoms, pain and swallowing difficulties were reported by the majority of patients. Furthermore, the pattern of reported symptoms can change over time both during and following RT. Clinical experience with this population suggests that in the early stages of treatment, pain and dryness as a result of mucositis and xerostomia and edema of structures in the swallowing mechanism directly contribute to reduced frequency and efficiency of swallowing ability. Swallowing difficulties that persist or develop after radiation treatment often are linked to fibrosis, muscle weakness from disuse atrophy, and peripheral nerve deficits. The time course of these tissue changes and resulting dysphagia are variable across patients and are related to many different factors. In general, an intense mucosal tissue response is noted within the first 3 to 4 weeks after the initiation of RT. Shortly thereafter the patient may be at greatest risk for development of new and severe dysphagia symptoms. If candidiasis (fungal infection) occurs, pain from mucositis may be increased and contribute further to dysphagia complaints. Finally, the effect of RT on dentition must be considered. Often, especially if the patient has poor dentition, a dentist will be consulted for corrective action before the initiation of RT. Even with this preventive action, the remaining teeth will be affected to some extent by RT. Figure 4-6 depicts various postradiation effects that can occur in the swallowing mechanism. Video 4-6 on the Evolve website is an endoscopic study revealing significant postradiation mucosal changes, including edema in the larynx, pharyngeal stenosis, and thickened secretions.

Dysphagia Characteristics after Radiation Therapy

General characteristics of dysphagia encountered by patients treated with RT for head and neck cancer are listed in Box 4-11. The listed percentages are from a single

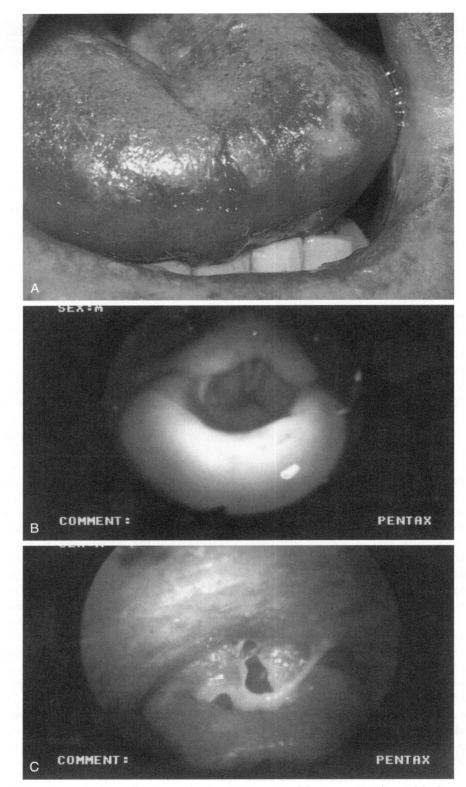

FIGURE 4-6 Postradiation changes to the swallowing mechanism. **A,** Mucositis of the tongue. **B,** Edema of the larynx, including epiglottis. **C,** Persistent and adhering mucus.

BOX 4-11 GENERAL CHARACTERISTICS OF DYSPHAGIA AND CONTRIBUTING FACTORS ASSOCIATED WITH RADIATION THERAPY FOR HEAD AND NECK CANCER*

- Bolus control deficits (63%)
- Small amounts per bolus and multiple swallow attempts
- Increased meal times
- Reduced frequency of swallowing
- Dry mouth (92%)
- Pain (58%)
- Altered taste (75%)

*Percentages are estimates.

PRACTICE NOTE 4-3

Sensory changes in patients treated with RT can have a profound effect on oral intake. On multiple occasions we have encountered patients who refuse to take any material beyond liquids by mouth. One reason is that more solid foods cause them to gag, often to the point of vomiting. Several years ago, in conjunction with an otolaryngologist we decided to "numb" the tongue of one patient with this complaint. We painted 4% lidocaine gel on the tongue dorsum and gave this patient the exact material on which he had gagged just minutes before. He was able to swallow this material without difficulty. The physician gave him a bottle of lidocaine to take home. On return to the clinic in 1 month, the patient had greatly increased the variety and amount of soft foods taken by mouth. Although this strategy has not always worked, we have since used it successfully for many patients. Whether gagging in these individuals was physiologic or psychological, altering the status quo sensory system by topical application of lidocaine seemed to help these patients improve oral intake.

published report and thus should be considered only as estimates.[61] This list contains both contributing factors (dry mouth, pain) and dysphagia characteristics (small amounts, multiple swallows). Only general characteristics are listed. In many but not all cases of dysphagia during or after RT, pain, dryness, and edema contribute to reduced frequency of swallowing, misdirection of a bolus leading to aspiration, inefficient swallow leading to postswallow residue, the need for multiple swallows, and prolonged mealtimes.

Pain from mucositis is a significant problem for patients early in the RT period and may last well beyond the initial treatment period. Oral mucositis also may result from chemotherapy and is enhanced in combined treatment protocols. The consequences of oral pain from mucositis extend beyond speech and swallowing functions and include potential interruption in the cancer treatment regimen[62] and economic consequences for the patient and family.[63] In general, oral mucositis is related to patient report of oral dysfunction and distress in patients receiving cancer therapy.[64]

Dry mouth, or xerostomia, is perhaps the most clinically significant and long-lasting difficulty faced by patients who undergo RT in the treatment of head and neck cancer. Patient surveys report associated xerostomia with significant negative emotional impact, in addition to difficulty talking and eating.[65] Interestingly, xerostomia may not be directly related to swallowing physiology. That is, the physiologic movement of a bolus through the swallowing mechanism is not significantly affected by xerostomia. Rather, xerostomia seems to have a negative effect on patients' perception of swallowing as a result of altered sensory processes.[66,67] However, xerostomia can be indirectly related to swallowing complaints as mastication of hard foods is negatively affected.[68] Head and neck cancer patients with xerostomia may avoid hard, masticated foods as they report difficulty chewing these materials, significant residue of masticated foods in the mouth, and a sensation of food sticking high in the throat.

Many patients describe reduced or altered senses of taste and smell that limit eating enjoyment.[69] Taste impairments may relate to reduction in the number of taste buds during RT, but in some instances taste buds return after cessation of RT and thus the sense of taste improves.[70] In fact, one study reported that the four basic tastes returned to baseline levels by 6 months after RT in patients who received either conventional or hyperfractionated RT for primary tumors of the oropharynx.[71] Note that these chemosensory impairments are not limited to diminished senses of taste and smell; some patients report abnormal and adverse tastes and smells that contribute to eating avoidance. Another perspective on taste aversions in patients with cancer is that they are learned through negative sensory experiences during RT and chemotherapy.[72] Thus primary sensory deficit or the learned negative reaction to it may contribute to reduced overall intake of food and liquid, resulting in threats to what may be an already compromised nutritional state (see Practice Note 4-3).

Poor dentition may further complicate any existing dysphagia by limiting the patient's ability to masticate solid foods. Reduced mouth opening from trismus also may limit the variety or amount of food or liquid that a patient may consume by mouth and may have negative implications for oral care. One group has operationally defined the degree of reduced mouth opening that may contribute to a functional cut-off point for trismus. By comparing vertical mouth opening with a mandibular function impairment questionnaire, this group identified a mouth opening of 35 mm or less as a functional cut-off for trismus in patients with head and neck cancer.[73] Trismus is not a trivial problem for head and neck cancer patients. Trismus affects more than one third of patients; often increases (further reduction in mouth opening) for months following RT; and is often associated with pain, swallowing difficulty, and xerostomia. Furthermore, trismus has been associated with reduced quality of life, negative effects on activities of daily living, and even depression in this population.[74,75]

ASSESSMENT STRATEGIES FOR DYSPHAGIA IN HEAD AND NECK CANCER

Chapters 7 and 8 provide detailed information on the clinical and imaging evaluation of dysphagia in adult patients. This section reviews certain assessment strategies of specific importance to the evaluation of swallow function in patients who are treated for head and neck cancer. Because of the diversity in clinical presentation of head and neck cancers (e.g., some cancers may contribute to pretreatment swallowing deficits, whereas others have minimal impact), the nature of their treatments, and the changing time course of the clinical signs and symptoms during and after treatment, patients who have been treated for head and neck cancer often present a unique clinical challenge to the dysphagia clinician. The basics of dysphagia assessment described in Chapters 7 and 8 are appropriate for these patients, but at least two additional factors should be considered: the timetable of evaluations and the assessment of impact factors.

Timing of Swallow Evaluations

Current summary reviews of dysphagia management in head and neck cancer patients strongly recommend a pretreatment evaluation of swallow function.[76,77] Many patients demonstrate some degree of swallow deviation before any medical treatment as a result of the cancer or other factors. Tumor stage (advanced tumors) and tumor site (laryngeal or hypopharyngeal) may be associated with pretreatment dysphagia in this population.[78] Interestingly, slightly more than half of these patients actually report swallow difficulty, and a majority demonstrate functional swallowing ability.[26] On the basis of these estimates, more than half of patients in whom head and neck cancer is diagnosed are not evaluated for swallow ability before cancer treatment. This approach may not provide the best patient care because neglected pretreatment deficits can have an impact on posttreatment dysphagia status and rehabilitation. In addition, a pretreatment evaluation provides the patient an additional opportunity to discuss potential difficulties that may occur during RT or posttreatment deficits that may occur after surgery or RT.[33]

Timing of the postsurgical evaluation of swallowing function should be determined between the speech-language pathologist (SLP) and the surgeon. In the early postsurgery period the patient may have significant edema that limits swallowing ability and the extent of any evaluation (recall that tracheostomy and gastrostomy tubes may be placed during the primary cancer surgery if the team suspects significant edema limiting breathing or swallow function postsurgery). Still, early evaluations may be helpful in determining the extent of dysphagia, identifying factors that contribute to any dysphagia, and establishing a time course for more intensive rehabilitation. In patients who demonstrate some functional swallow ability in the early postsurgery period, early evaluation may be critical to identify strategies that will facilitate safe "swallowing" with the potential to limit dysphagia-related complications during the hospital stay.

Patients treated with RT protocols should be evaluated before treatment as well as during treatment for acute toxicity side effects that will have a negative effect on swallow function. In fact, Denaro et al.[79] reviewed published literature through 2012 and concluded that dysphagia was underestimated during RT and that unidentified dysphagia contributed to increased morbidity, mortality, and decreased quality of life. Nearly one third of patients with dysphagia developed pneumonia with a mortality rate from 20% to 65%. Finally, these patients should have follow-up for the emergence of late-occurring effects of RT that may impair swallow function.[80] Late dysphagia from RT often includes lower cranial neuropathies and can contribute to serious complications, including hospitalization for pneumonia, related to the swallowing impairment.[81-83]

Swallow function and related oral morbidities may be evaluated with a variety of clinical tools and imaging studies when indicated (see Chapter 8) at multiple points before, during, and following cancer treatments. The Mann Assessment of Swallowing Ability (MASA) as described in Chapter 7 was initially validated for use with stroke and neurogenic dysphagia. The more recent MASA-C is a head and neck cancer–specific version of this standard clinical assessment tool for dysphagia that has been validated for use with patients who have head and neck cancer patients.[84] The Functional Oral Intake Scale (FOIS—see Chapter 7) is a validated tool to document the type and amount of oral diet intake by patients with dysphagia.[85] The Sydney Swallow Questionnaire (SSQ) is a patient-reported survey of swallowing difficulty with different food and liquid items. The original version of the SSQ was validated on a general population of adults with dysphagia complaints, but this tool has demonstrated **reliability** and **validity** in patients with head and neck cancer.[86] Finally, two patient survey tools were developed and validated at the MD Anderson Cancer Center in Houston. The MD Anderson Dysphagia Inventory (MDADI) is a reliable, valid questionnaire completed by patients with head and neck cancers to describe the effect of dysphagia on their quality of life.[87]

The MD Anderson Symptom Inventory–Head and Neck Module (MDASI-HN) is a patient-rated list of swallowing and related symptoms with established reliability and validity for application with patients with head and neck cancer. The MDASI-HN score represents the patient's symptom burden and impact of symptoms on daily life activities.[88]

Assessing Impact Factors

Impact factors are patient characteristics that directly or indirectly have a negative effect on swallowing functions. In patients with head and neck cancer, frequent impact factors include pain, xerostomia, taste and smell deviation, fibrosis, nutritional status, psychological status, and use of nonoral feeding methods.

Pain may be present after surgery or during or after RT. Alterations in swallowing related to painful swallowing (odynophagia) should be differentiated from dysphagia because the course of treatment differs. Pain is typically managed medically with a variety of analgesic medications. If pain medications—particularly narcotic-class medications—are used for a prolonged period, the dysphagia clinician must also consider gastroparesis in the profile of potential swallowing deficits.[89] As a minimal attempt to differentiate odynophagia from other forms of swallowing difficulty, clinicians should ask patients to identify, localize, and rate the severity of any pain within the swallowing mechanism. When pain is related to oral mucositis as a result of RT, oncologists and oncology nurses often use a standard rating scale to grade oral mucositis. Among these scales is the World Health Organization Grading Scale,[90] which relies heavily on the patient's ability to eat by mouth in determining the severity of oral mucositis (Table 4-2). Clinicians should become familiar with the rating scale used in their facilities and the functional interpretation of that scale as it may pertain to a patient's swallowing ability. In addition, clinicians should be aware that pain within the swallowing mechanism can result from fungal infections or peripheral nerve injury. A basic understanding of the source of pain within the swallow mechanism allows the dysphagia clinician to interact with the rest of the cancer rehabilitation team to best meet the patient's comprehensive needs. As pain diminishes with appropriate medical treatment, patients with reduced oral intake caused by odynophagia should increase both the amount and variety of foods and liquids taken by mouth.

Xerostomia is a common side effect of RT. As previously described, xerostomia may affect swallowing by altering the normal sensory function within the oral cavity and thus change the patient's perception of his or her swallowing ability. Xerostomia also has a direct and negative effect on mastication of more solid foods. Regardless of the specific effect of xerostomia on swallowing ability, it is a pervasive and long-lasting impairment in most patients treated with RT. The ability to rate the severity of xerostomia adds an objective dimension to the clinical evaluation of the patient with head and neck cancer. Researchers at the University of Michigan developed and validated a patient report scale for xerostomia that is widely used as a clinical scale.[91] The scale items from this xerostomia questionnaire are listed in Box 4-12. Patients rate each item from 0 to 10 (higher scores denote worse xerostomia). Clinicians should also discuss with the patient his or her perception of the effect of xerostomia on swallowing and other oral functions. Beyond the patient's report, clinicians should note the presence, type (thin and watery, thick, etc.), and amount of secretions on the tongue dorsum and in the anterior sublingual vault.

The senses of taste and smell are critical to the enjoyment of eating. Both RT and chemotherapy can have a negative effect on these senses. Taste is mediated by the tongue, with only five basic tastes identified (sweet, sour, bitter, salty, and **umami**). Many lingual tissue changes from RT or chemotherapy can diminish or alter the sense of taste. Flavor is mediated through olfaction. Often the sense of

---

TABLE 4-2 World Health Organization Scale for Grading Oral Mucositis

Grade	Clinical Findings
0	No symptoms
1	Sore mouth, no ulcers
2	Sore mouth with ulcers, but able to eat normally
3	Liquid diet only
4	Unable to eat or drink

BOX 4-12 UNIVERSITY OF MICHIGAN XEROSTOMIA QUESTIONNAIRE*

1. Rate your difficulty in talking because of dryness.
2. Rate your difficulty in chewing because of dryness.
3. Rate your difficulty in swallowing solid food because of dryness.
4. Rate the frequency of your sleeping problems because of dryness.
5. Rate your mouth or throat dryness when eating food.
6. Rate your mouth or throat dryness while not eating.
7. Rate the frequency of sipping liquids to aid swallowing food.
8. Rate the frequency of sipping liquids for oral comfort when not eating.

*Patients rate each item on a scale from 0 to 10. Higher scores indicate worse xerostomia.

smell is not impaired or perhaps is only temporarily diminished in the patient with head and neck cancer. Diminished senses of taste and smell can reduce a patient's enjoyment of eating and may negatively affect food choices and overall intake. Altered senses of taste and smell can have a direct, negative impact on oral intake because patients will avoid foods that are perceived as aversive. Although standard protocols exist for the systematic evaluation of taste and smell function, patient report is typically sufficient to document the presence of these sensory deficits and their effects on oral intake of food and liquid. If impaired senses of taste or smell are determined to be a primary factor affecting reduced oral intake, patients should be referred to an appropriate oral health professional for more extensive evaluation and potential treatment.

RT can damage skin and muscle along with devascularization and damage to peripheral nerves. Soft tissue of the skin and muscle can become fibrosed, which reduces movement in the swallowing mechanism and in the head and neck region in general. Dysphagia clinicians should attempt to differentiate the underlying cause of reduced movement primarily between muscle weakness and tissue fibrosis. Even passive movement will be restricted because of fibrosis. The patient with soft tissue fibrosis demonstrates hard, or "woody," presentation of a region that has been irradiated such as the anterior aspect of the neck. Simply grasping both sides of the larynx and trying to move this structure from side to side gives some indication of the degree of movement and hence fibrosis. Subsequently, the clinician can attempt to feel laryngeal movement during a volitional swallow. The combination of reduced passive and volitional movement suggests that fibrosis may be a limiting factor. If possible, endoscopic inspection of the larynx and pharynx helps determine whether the effects of fibrosis are limited to the superficial skin and muscles or if deeper structures are involved.

More details of this evaluation are provided in Chapter 8, but the key feature is to evaluate movement within the larynx, pharyngeal walls, and the base of the tongue.

Fibrosis may also alter other structures within the swallow mechanism. The upper esophageal sphincter (also termed pharyngoesophageal segment [PES]) may become fibrotic and stenosed as a result of RT. Strictures in this segment reduce the sphincter opening and limit the amount of food the patient is able to swallow. This impairment should be considered in patients with head and neck cancer who report difficulty swallowing solid foods. Finally, a common and potentially debilitating form of fibrosis can lead to reduced mouth opening, or trismus. Trismus may result from reduced flexibility of the masseter and temporalis muscles, which are the primary muscles of jaw closure. If these muscles become fibrotic, they pose a substantial force against the muscles of jaw opening and limit the degree of vertical opening of the mouth. This situation can negatively affect mastication, swallowing, speech, and general oral care. As previously mentioned, a vertical mouth opening of less than 35 mm may be considered reduced and indicative of trismus. TheraBite (Atos Medical AB, West Allis, Wis.) is a therapeutic device for the treatment of trismus; a simple cardboard "ruler" is available from the manufacturer of this device for the systematic measurement of mouth opening. Measurement of mouth opening is recommended for all patients who have been treated for head and neck cancer, but especially those who have been treated with a RT protocol. Figure 4-7 depicts the TheraBite mouth opening ruler and its use. One clinical tool that may be used to assess the effect of trismus on activities of daily living is the Gothenburg Trismus Questionnaire.[92]

Malnutrition in cancer patients is multifactorial and can lead to poor quality of life, reduced survival, and

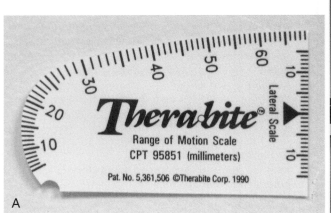
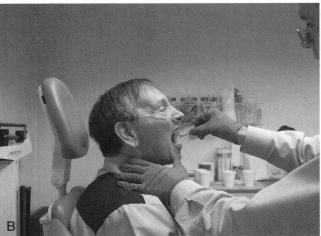

FIGURE 4-7 Measuring mouth opening. **A,** TheraBite mouth opening ruler. **B,** Use of the ruler in a patient to measure vertical mouth opening.

treatment-related morbidity.[93] As previously mentioned, between 30% and 50% of patients with head and neck cancer demonstrate a degree of malnutrition before, during, or after treatment. Reasons for malnutrition may include dysphagia, odynophagia, taste deviations, poor appetite (which in itself may be multifactorial), increased caloric needs, or other metabolic, physical, or psychological factors. Nutritional status may be evaluated by a variety of methods. Weight change is a general guideline for nutritional change, and unintentional weight loss is often used as a clinical sign of potential nutritional risk. The body mass index (BMI) is an extension of weight change reflected in a ratio between weight and height. BMI calculators are common and easily accessed on the Internet. Beyond these simple clinical tools, if significant nutritional deficit is suspected, the referring physician should always be notified and a consultation sought with a qualified nutritional specialist.

Psychological status may affect rehabilitation efforts. Cancer patients often cope with pain, fatigue, disfigurement, communication difficulties, dysphagia, and various gastric complaints, including nausea and vomiting. These conditions are chronic in many cases and may contribute to distress and depression. Psychological consultation is helpful in identifying potential factors and suggesting direction to minimize their impact on rehabilitative efforts.

Whether or not a patient continues to eat and drink orally during RT or CRT may be an important factor in long-term swallowing outcomes. Hutcheson et al.[94] have demonstrated that maintaining oral intake and adherence to swallowing exercises during RT or CRT were independently associated with better long-term diets in patients with head and neck cancer. However, if feeding tubes (nonoral feeding) are required for nutritional or medical reasons, the type of feeding tube and whether or not the patient maintains any oral intake may affect long-term swallowing outcomes. Although a recent review indicated that NG tubes may result in better swallowing outcomes, available data are inconclusive on the impact of NG versus gastric feeding tubes, with some studies claiming advantages for NG tubes and others claiming no difference. A related issue is the application of prophylactic versus reactive feeding tubes (either type). The intent of this practice appears to be to minimize medical treatment interruptions; however, swallow function following medical treatment may be more impaired if patients on prophylactic feedings cease or significantly limit oral intake of food and liquids.[95-98]

THERAPY STRATEGIES FOR DYSPHAGIA IN HEAD AND NECK CANCER

Chapters 9 and 10 provide more extensive detail on developing therapy plans for adult patients and a variety of therapeutic interventions. However, the patient who has been treated for head and neck cancer often represents a specific set of clinical challenges for dysphagia therapy resulting from both the cancer and its treatment. Most reports of therapy efforts in patients with head and neck cancer are based on small numbers of patients. For these reasons, much remains to be learned about the best therapy for such patients. Many patients, especially those with more advanced cancers, are treated with a combination of surgery and RT. In this situation, the effects of both treatments must be considered in therapy planning.

Timing of Swallowing Therapy

One important consideration for dysphagia therapy in patients treated for head and neck cancer is when to provide therapy. Many studies suggest that the sooner therapy is initiated after cancer treatment, the better the eventual outcome.[99-101] To the author's knowledge, no study suggests waiting for a prolonged period before initiating dysphagia therapy. Unfortunately, no consensus has emerged regarding the optimal time after cancer treatment to begin dysphagia therapy. As a general guideline, therapy should begin as soon as possible. It is advisable to consult with the head and neck surgeon regarding readiness of patients to initiate different therapeutic activities after surgery. Moreover, some patients who have only minor problems or those who substantially recover swallowing function after treatment develop new dysphagia symptoms or notice deterioration in swallowing function months or years after primary cancer treatment. Still, published clinical research does offer hope even for patients with chronic dysphagia after treatment of head and neck cancer.[102,103]

A different approach considers intervention strategies before or during cancer treatment that may prevent or reduce the severity of dysphagia after cancer treatment. This paradigm has been applied recently, primarily to patients being treated with RT with or without chemotherapy. Results from a single cancer treatment center indicate benefit to patient quality of life[104] and in certain aspects of swallow function[105] after RT (with or without chemotherapy) when patients completed swallowing-related exercises 2 weeks before cancer treatment. The exercises were commonly reported exercises (detailed in Chapter 10) and included tongue resistance, tongue hold, head lift, effortful swallow, and the Mendelsohn maneuver.

In at least one small, randomized clinical trial, active exercise-based therapy provided daily during RT treatment reduced the severity of dysphagia after cancer treatment with benefits lasting up to 6 months of follow-up.[106] Results of this study included preservation of muscle structure and functional maintenance of swallowing ability in patients who received intensive exercise-based therapy versus a sham therapy versus usual care involving no active intervention during cancer treatment. Exercises used in this study were simple and focused on tongue, larynx, pharynx, and jaw movement. They included tongue-resistance activities, effortful swallow, falsetto, and jaw stretch against mild resistance. Secondary findings from this study implicated preservation of salivary flow and smell sensation in the active exercise group. Both of these variables are considered contributory to dysphagia in this population. These initial findings are encouraging for patients and strongly suggest that engaging in active swallow exercises during (or before) RT may have widespread benefit for patients treated with this modality for head and neck cancer. Results of this study have been supported in other clinical studies despite differences in research designs and actual therapy methods employed.[107-109] Duarte et al.[109] completed a retrospective analysis of outcomes in patients completing swallowing exercises both before and during medical treatment (radiation or chemoradiation). One interesting aspect of their study was that they divided patients into two subgroups based on how compliant they were with the program of swallowing exercises. Compliant patients demonstrated superior outcomes (regular diet, fewer feeding tubes, and higher rate of diet maintenance or improvement) compared with noncompliant patients. This observation raises an important point regarding prophylactic dysphagia therapy in this population. Head and neck cancer patients are under enormous burden before, during, and even after medical treatments. The addition of dysphagia therapy during medical treatments, even though intended to reduce post-treatment swallowing limitations, adds to that burden. As a result of that burden, head and neck cancer patients may not adhere (e.g., be compliant) to swallow exercise regimens. Duarte et al.[109] reported that 67% of the patients were deemed compliant with the exercise program (defined as completing one full set of exercises per day). However, in a larger study reported by Shin et al.,[110] only 13% of patients were fully adherent with an additional 32% being partially adherent. The remaining 55% of patients were nonadherent, meaning they did not complete any swallowing exercises. Among reasons for nonadherence were "exercises too difficult," "kept forgetting," "pain," and even "too busy." Given the demonstrated benefit from adherence to these prophylactic exercises, strategies to improve patient adherence are important. A group in the Netherlands[111] developed a program called Head Matters that offered multimodal guided self-help exercises to patients treated for head and neck cancer. In a preliminary study Head Matters resulted in a 64% adherence rate with 58% of patients completing moderate to high levels of exercise. This approach may be a good initial step toward developing what Shin et al.[110] termed "supportive care strategies to optimize patient adherence" to prophylactic swallowing exercise programs.

Dysphagia characteristics may develop in patients receiving RT during the course of treatment. An **enteral** feeding tube may be used to maintain nutrition and hydration during and after treatment until oral food and liquid intake can be reestablished. In such situations, it is important to maintain contact with the patient during and after treatment to either initiate swallowing therapy or reevaluate for oral feeding possibilities. At the very least, patients should be given exercises focusing on both strength and flexibility of the swallowing mechanism to limit or eliminate weakness and restricted movement that may contribute to dysphagia after treatment. Although some patients do require long-term use of alternative feeding sources after treatment for head and neck cancer, many centers report only temporary use of these strategies (often between 2 and 4 months).[112] In these situations, the dysphagia specialist plays an important role in the patient's transition from nonoral to oral feeding.[113]

Given the variation in size and location of head and neck cancers and the resulting diversity in the medical and surgical treatments, no single approach to dysphagia therapy in this patient group is all-encompassing. In addition, the timing of dysphagia therapy after cancer treatment results in different clinical presentations within and across patients treated with the same medical and surgical strategies. Thus in an attempt to simplify what may be a complicated clinical issue, bolus transport and airway protection problems after head and neck cancer treatment are the focus of this section. In addition, an overview of interventions that may be indicated to address mucosal and muscle changes resulting from RT is provided.

Therapy for Bolus Transport Problems

In designing therapy for bolus transport problems, the first step is to identify the changes in the swallowing mechanism that are contributing to the transport problems. These changes may result from either surgical intervention or RT. The common attribute is reduced movement of the structures composing the swallowing mechanism. Surgical treatment may remove structures that are important to bolus movement. If structures have been removed, a maxillofacial prosthodontist is a valuable resource. In combination with a speech-language pathologist (SLP), this professional can fabricate palatal lifts, obturators, maxillary-shaping devices, or other intraoral prostheses that can contribute to improved swallowing function.[114] A palatal lift is helpful to lift the existing soft palate into a raised position, thus creating improved velopharyngeal closure. An obturator is a device that fills a gap created by surgical resection. If the soft palate is removed (or, for that matter, part of the hard palate), an obturator can be used to facilitate separation of the oral and nasal cavities. A maxillary-shaping device is a prosthesis that fits over the hard palate (much like an upper denture). This device may be thickened or shaped to facilitate maximal contact with a weakened or partially resected tongue. Increased lingual-palatal contact should facilitate improved oral bolus transport. However, at least one study has cast doubt on the overall benefit of these prostheses in patients who have been surgically treated for oropharyngeal cancer.[115] Yet Koyama et al.[116] reported oral swallowing benefit in three patients who received surgery for floor of mouth cancer using a combination of maxillary and mandibular reshaping prostheses. Video 4-7 on the Evolve website accompanying this text is an endoscopic study revealing a "gap" in the left aspect of the velopharyngeal sphincter. The SLP and the maxillofacial prosthodontist agreed that an obturator may provide benefit to both speech and swallowing functions in this patient. Video 4-8, *A* and *B,* show an endoscopic evaluation that (a) depicts a complete and symmetrical incompetence of the velopharynx and (b) a fluoroscopic evaluation showing sufficient soft palate tissue that may produce benefit from a palatal lift.

When structures are restricted in movement (from either surgery or radiation), changes in head posture, use of feeding devices, and dietary changes may be indicated. Range of motion (i.e., stretching) exercises also may be helpful in some instances. Patients who have limited tongue movement may benefit from elevating the chin to allow gravity to transport a bolus to the back of the mouth or even into the pharynx. In these cases, good airway protection is an important part of the clinical picture. The risk of aspiration is increased if the patient cannot protect the airway and propels a bolus into the pharynx by gravity. Another consideration is that elevating the chin may increase the pressure within the PES.[117] If patients have existing problems opening the PES, this technique may be contraindicated. Logic dictates that use of this postural technique requires a bolus that is amenable to movement by gravity. This may limit the oral diet to liquids or very soft and liquefied foods.

Feeding devices have been described that allow patients to place a more solid bolus in the posterior oral cavity.[118] These so-called glossectomy spoons have been used to place soft foods in the posterior mouth in patients who have lingual paralysis or otherwise restricted lingual movement. In cases of severe movement restriction, patients may use syringes or even soft catheters to place food into the posterior oral cavity, the pharynx, or in some cases directly into the upper esophagus (some patients can learn to pass an orogastric tube themselves).

Stretching exercises may be helpful, especially if performed before scarring or fibrosis is so severe that any movement is severely restricted. Positive results have been shown specifically in increasing mouth opening for patients with trismus. Two primary methods for stretching have been recommended. Active and passive stretching with physical therapy exercises has been suggested to be beneficial by some authors,[119] but this benefit has been questioned by other investigators.[120] Various devices also have been proposed to aid in passive stretching of the jaw in the

treatment of trismus. Traditionally, tongue blades were used by stacking the tongue blades, placing them between the incisor teeth (or gums in **edentulous** patients), and adding blades to increase the degree of stretch. Two commercially available devices include the Therabite and the Dynasplint Trismus System (Dynasplint Systems, Inc., Severna Park, Md.). All three systems have shown benefit in the treatment of trismus after irradiation in the treatment of head and neck cancer.[121,122] Among the three techniques, the Therabite device appears to have been studied most extensively in clinical research.[121] Improved mouth opening in patients with trismus has also been demonstrated in limited studies with microcurrent electrotherapy and use of the drug pentoxifylline, which is used to increase peripheral blood flow.[121]

Other maneuvers and compensations such as the effortful swallow or the Mendelsohn maneuver may also be useful in improving bolus transport in response to specific dysphagia characteristics (see Chapter 10 for a more complete review of various maneuvers and compensations and their effect on swallowing physiology and function). Finally, at least one study has implicated use of sour taste to improve pharyngeal transit of swallowed materials.[123] Although this was not an intervention study, the effect of sour taste on swallowing has received substantial attention (see Chapter 10).

Therapy for Airway Protection Problems

Airway protection deficits result from compromise of the laryngeal valve or from incoordination of the swallow event. Laryngeal changes may result either from surgical or radiation therapies that either impair the anatomy of the larynx or the movement of laryngeal structures. From this perspective, therapeutic endeavors to protect the airway will focus on improved laryngeal closure and improved coordination of the swallow focusing on airway protection.

In some instances, surgical correction of reduced glottal closure is indicated. Two frequently used techniques are medialization of a nonmoving vocal fold by a technique termed thyroplasty or injection of an acceptable biosubstance into a vocal fold. The determining factors in the selection of the specific technique may be the degree of glottal incompetence, the experience of the surgeon with the respective techniques, and factors regarding the patient's overall medical condition. Figure 4-8 shows the same larynx depicted in Figure 4-5 but after medialization by thyroplasty on the right side of the larynx. Note the improved glottal closure. Injection of biomaterials into one or both vocal folds has also been shown to be effective in improving glottal closure.[124-126] Although different techniques are available to surgeons to inject the vocal folds, recent techniques have focused on in-office procedures that allow

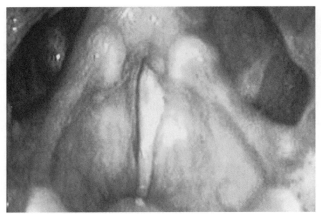

FIGURE 4-8 Photograph of the same larynx shown in Figure 4-5 after medialization of the right true vocal cord remnant by thyroplasty. Note the improved glottal closure by comparing the two photographs.

patients to avoid general anesthesia in the operating room. One such technique incorporates an injection through the thyrohyoid membrane and injecting the vocal fold with endoscopic visualization.[127]

Various behavioral therapy techniques have been shown to reduce aspiration during swallowing. These techniques may be appropriate in cases of altered laryngeal anatomy but should be considered when incoordination of the swallowing event contributes to aspiration of swallowed materials. These compensatory techniques include the chin-down position, the head-turn posture, the supraglottic swallow, and the super-supraglottic swallow. Each of these techniques is discussed in greater detail in Chapter 10. Video segments depicting these techniques are also described in Chapter 10. The chin-down position may be helpful when a patient demonstrates a delay in the pharyngeal component of the swallow. This head position narrows the oropharyngeal opening and causes the patient to swallow "uphill" over the tongue. The head-turn posture helps to both direct a bolus to one side (hopefully the more intact side) of the pharynx and to lower the intrasphincter pressure on the contralateral side of the PES. This postural adjustment during the swallow may help direct a bolus away from the airway and reduce the amount of postswallow residue that may be aspirated after the swallow event. Both supraglottic swallow maneuvers focus on closing the airway before the swallow occurs and coughing lightly to clear any residue in the larynx immediately after the swallow. The difference between these two maneuvers is that the "super" variation includes effort during the breath-hold phase in an attempt to ensure or increase the degree of laryngeal closure. One additional swallow maneuver, the Mendelsohn maneuver, may indirectly facilitate improved airway protection by improving swallowing coordination. Video 4-9 depicts changes in a patient's ability to

perform the Mendelsohn maneuver with progressing therapy over a 6-week span. Each video segment was obtained at 2-week intervals. The patient was a cancer survivor with a severe dysphagia and difficulty protecting his airway during swallowing. He was taught the maneuver during the initial fluoroscopic study (see Video 4-9, *A*) and with therapy he was able to learn the Mendelsohn maneuver and improved airway protection that led to increased oral intake. Note that even though this patient demonstrated increased skill with this maneuver, intermittent aspiration was still noted for some materials. This case raises a question as to what clinicians should expect as a result of any given technique or maneuver. A summary of this patient's history and progress in treatment follows.

Therapy for Mucosal and Muscle Changes Resulting from Radiation Therapy

When RT creates mucosal and muscle tissue changes that interfere with swallowing, it is in the patient's best interest for the therapy plan to incorporate activities directed at minimizing the effect of those tissue changes. Box 4-13 summarizes some of the more common interventions for both mucosal and muscle tissue changes created by RT in the treatment of head and neck cancer.

Xerostomia (dry mouth) can contribute to swallowing difficulties as a result of reduced watery saliva that mixes with food to assist in bolus transport. At least two studies have suggested that oral xerostomia after RT affects the sensory aspects more than the motor aspects.[66,67] Another function of saliva is to promote improved oral and dental health. Reduced salivary flow can contribute to impaired oral and dental health.[128,129]

CLINICAL CASE EXAMPLE 4-1   PNEUMONIA, ASPIRATION, AND SWALLOW REHABILITATION

A 66-year-old man had left neck dissection and RT for cancer of the left tonsillar fossa (T2N2A). The patient completed RT 4 months before his first visit to the outpatient dysphagia clinic. A left neck dissection was planned after RT; however, at the completion of RT he presented with pneumonia that was presumed to be related to aspiration and was hospitalized for treatment. A PEG tube was placed during that hospital stay. During that hospitalization a fluoroscopic swallowing evaluation revealed no aspiration. A left neck dissection was completed 2 months later (2 months before presentation to the dysphagia clinic). A repeat fluoro study did show aspiration 3 weeks after this surgery and the patient was recommended to take only thickened liquids. He presented to our outpatient dysphagia clinic 4 weeks later. Endoscopic assessment of swallowing functions identified no aspiration of thin liquids. Penetration of thick liquids was noted and these were effectively cleared with a cough. He showed moderate post-RT changes in the pharynx, including reduced movement of the pharyngeal wall during falsetto, adhering mucus in the pharynx, and postswallow residue that increased as the viscosity of the bolus increased. Subsequent fluoroscopic study indicated better swallowing performance (no aspiration, less residue) with thin liquids than with thicker materials. Swallow movements were deemed adequate to support functional swallowing but reduced in degree of movement (reduced hyolaryngeal excursion, reduced pharyngeal constriction, reduced PES opening). The recommendation at that time was to initiate oral intake of thin liquids and gradually increase viscosity as tolerated up to a soft food consistency. He was to be followed up by his local physician and SLP.

Ten months later this patient was again hospitalized with right lower lobe pneumonia. Fluoroscopic study at that time indicated aspiration with a recommendation for the patient to cease all oral intake of food or liquid. Two months later he again presented to the dysphagia clinic. Fluoroscopic study at that time indicated aspiration when attempting to swallow 10 mL of thick liquid but not with thin liquid or smaller volumes of thick liquid (5 mL). Both a supraglottic swallow and a Mendelsohn maneuver were taught and both were successful in reducing or eliminating aspiration during larger bolus swallows. At this point, intensive swallowing therapy was recommended with a focus on airway protection and increasing hyolaryngeal excursion, pharyngeal constriction, and PES opening during swallowing. The Mendelsohn maneuver with increasing effort was emphasized and a progression of materials beginning with thin liquid and progressing to thick liquids and pureed foods was introduced. Surface **electromyographic** (sEMG) biofeedback was used to teach the maneuver and monitor increased

swallowing effort. Postswallow airway clearance was monitored with cervical auscultation.

After 2 weeks of daily therapy sessions, the patient demonstrated increased base of tongue contact to the posterior pharyngeal wall, increased extent and duration of pharyngeal constriction, and increased hyolaryngeal excursion. He was able to take larger volumes of thin liquid without aspiration (cup drinking) and demonstrated less residue with swallows of thick liquid. After 2 additional weeks of daily therapy this patient was able to ingest thickened liquids without aspiration and minimal residue and able to ingest "moist puree" foods with only minimal residue and no signs of aspiration. At this point, he met with our team dietitian to discuss strategies for increasing to total oral feeding while reducing tube feedings. Subsequently, the PEG tube was removed and he returned to total oral intake of food and liquid. His diet was restricted to liquids and soft foods but he reported that this was indeed better for him than tube feedings.

This patient represents a case of moderate reduction of movement within the swallowing mechanism as a result of RT. His case was complicated by pneumonia after completion of RT and by the inconsistent findings of aspiration across swallow imaging studies. This inconsistency might result from variability within the patient over time or from variability in how these examinations were completed. One consistent finding was that he swallowed thin liquid better than thicker materials. This may result from less force applied to a bolus as a result of reduced movement of structures within the swallowing tract or perhaps from xerostomia, which would create more adherence between oral mucosa and thicker materials. The initial approach to increase oral intake for this patient was to start with material deemed safe based on a swallow imaging study and to allow him to progress at his own pace under supervision of his physician and local therapist. This was somewhat successful, but the level of intensity of his attempts and his compliance with a routine were unknown with this approach. The subsequent therapy program for this patient focused on attempting to increase movement of oropharyngeal structures during swallowing attempts while taking precaution to reduce the risk of aspiration of material into the airway. In this case, he improved even though it was more than a year after RT. Possibly because he was continuing to swallow during this period, some flexibility in the mechanism was retained or at least not further compromised. This case presents many interesting questions, not all of which can be answered directly. Still, this case does demonstrate that swallowing rehabilitation can be successful and safe even in patients with chronic conditions and those who are at risk for airway compromise.

Unfortunately, xerostomia can be long lasting or even permanent after RT. Various interventions have been introduced, but none has been completely effective across the wide array of patients with this disabling clinical problem.[129,130] For some patients, especially those with some preservation of salivary flow, chewing gum may increase salivary output. Flavored gum may be superior in this regard because saliva flows in response to taste (particularly sour and bitter). In this regard, some patients may benefit from gums or lozenges (sugar free!) that have the potential to increase salivary flow by mechanical and chemosensory stimulation. Synthetic saliva or other moisturizing agents are commercially available as a replacement or compensation for lost natural saliva. These agents come in various forms, including mouthwash, sprays, and gels. When saliva substitutes are used, it is important to instruct the patient to coat the entire oral mucosa and to place a small pool of the liquid under the anterior aspect of the tongue. Some patients will benefit from use of these materials and others reject them. In general, any obtained benefit typically is temporary; therefore if xerostomia is a factor in dysphagia, patients should be instructed to apply these agents before eating. Many patients report using a water spritzer bottle as needed for dry mouth. These patients also use liquids frequently during meals to help transport food through the swallowing mechanism and to remove post-swallow residue with this liquid wash. Of course, this strategy requires adequate airway protection to minimize or eliminate risk of aspiration.

Physicians may prescribe medication to increase salivary flow. These agents tend to require extended use and the cost may be prohibitive for some patients. These medications also increase fluid secretion from many glands in addition to salivary glands. Some patients report profuse sweating when taking these medications. In reality, many patients who have xerostomia experiment with different approaches to improving oral lubrication. Clinicians can help this process by providing a wide range of options and information. One consideration for patients with xerostomia is oral hygiene. Reduction of saliva can compromise oral and dental health. Clinicians should counsel patients to engage in a routine of frequent oral hygiene activities consistent with the condition of the oral cavity.

Xerostomia is a serious and long-lasting complication from RT. In general xerostomia is related to hyposalivation, but it is important to remember that xerostomia represents the patient's perception of dry mouth, which can be influenced by more than salivary flow. Xerostomia has a direct effect on mastication of solid, dry foods and appears to influence sensory aspects of swallowing. Multiple options have been investigated in the treatment of xerostomia in head and neck cancer patients, including topical and systematic medications, salivary substitutes, hyperbaric oxygen treatments, electrical stimulation, and acupuncture. An excellent review and **metaanalysis** of treatments for hyposalivation and xerostomia is presented by Lovelace et al.[131]

Oral pain from mucositis can be a significant problem resulting from acute toxicity in the patient treated with RT protocols (also with chemotherapy). In severe cases, this pain can be excruciating and cause the individual to reduce the frequency of swallowing or cease oral intake of food and liquid altogether. Few proven strategies are available to combat this situation. Simple techniques that do not require medical support include mechanical cleansing with saline solution and use of ice chips.[132] Foam "toothettes" are not recommended for mechanical cleansing because they tend to disintegrate on the dry mucosa. Instead, patients are encouraged to use a very soft toothbrush in light salt water and to brush the oral mucosa to remove any debris. Ice chips use both cold, which can provide temporary relief from oral pain in some cases, and water, which can help lubricate the oral mucosa. Some patients report using oral analgesic gels similar to those used for babies who are teething. For severe pain, physicians may prescribe analgesic patches of strong pain-suppressing medication. In milder cases, an over-the-counter liquid medication to suppress pain may be adequate.

A series of Cochrane reviews has been completed to evaluate the effectiveness of interventions for oral mucositis.[133] Conclusions from those reviews are that only weak, unreliable evidence was available to support the use of allopurinol mouthwash or other medical approaches, or more recently low-level laser applications. However, despite this absence of proven interventions in the treatment of oral mucositis, at least two positive views should be mentioned. Oral mucositis is a side effect of acute toxicity and thus is often a temporary condition. When it is well managed, the duration and impact of oral mucositis in the irradiated area can be contained to various degrees. Second, clinicians and researchers continue to investigate new and perhaps unusual methods to help patients with this disabling condition. Some novel approaches include the topical application of pure honey[134] and the use of low-level laser therapy.[135] Recently, the drug gabapentin has demonstrated promise as a prophylactic treatment for oral mucositis in this population.[136,137] Gabapentin (also known as neurontin) is a nonopiate medication that appears promising in control of pain associated with mucositis and thus may reduce potential side effects associated with opiate pain medications. Worthington et al.[138] summarize 10 interventions for oral mucositis related to cancer treatment that demonstrate some significant effect on preventing or reducing the severity of mucositis. Moreover, Campos et al.[139] provide a summary of oral mucositis in cancer treatment that includes the natural history along with a review of methods to prevent and treat this painful condition.

Changes in muscle tissue occur in the direction of restricted movement of structures resulting from fibrosis or

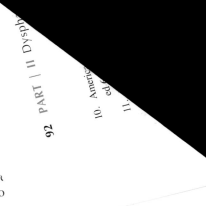

neuropathy in muscles that have been irradiated. Also, disuse atrophy leading to weakness should be considered in patients who are not taking food and liquid by mouth. No single therapy has been shown to be a panacea for all patients. Consultation with a physical therapist may be valuable to identify strategies to increase movement in fibrotic muscles, especially when fibrosis restricts functional head or neck movement. One general strategy is to stretch the restricted structure and thereby the fibrotic muscles. As previously described, repetitive stretching has improved movement, especially in the jaw. If movement is reduced from muscle weakness, exercise approaches to muscle rehabilitation should be investigated. This applies to the swallowing mechanism as well as the general head and neck region.

In severe cases of radiation changes in mucosa or muscle tissue, patients are not able to maintain any oral intake of food or liquid. In these cases, the physician providing the cancer treatment may opt for nonoral feeding strategies. Historical evidence supports the use of a PEG tube over an NG tube.[140] PEG feedings have been shown to be superior to NG feedings in regard to less mechanical failure, better nutritional outcomes, and fewer associated chest infections in this patient population. However, as mentioned previously, recent perceptions are that NG tubes may result in superior swallowing outcomes. In clinical practice, the specific application of the enteral feeding tube may determine the choice of a gastric versus nasal approach.[141] The decision to pursue nonoral feeding strategies is typically based on individual patient circumstances and is often done in consultation with a dietician and an SLP. As noted, it is important to monitor these patients over time to determine whether oral feeding may be reestablished or if swallowing therapy may be beneficial. In addition, it is important for these patients to follow a prophylactic exercise regimen to limit the potential atrophic effects of muscle disuse within the swallowing mechanism while the patient relies on a nonoral feeding source for nutrition and hydration.

TAKE HOME NOTES

1. Cancer within the swallowing mechanism and the treatments for cancer contribute to dysphagia and other life-altering changes. The primary treatments for cancer are surgery and RT. These may be used alone or in combination. Chemotherapy may be used in combination with one of these primary approaches.
2. Dysphagia characteristics resulting from treatments for head and neck cancer vary depending on the type and extent of the treatment. One common feature is reduced movement within the swallowing mechanism. This contributes to reduced swallowing efficiency, which may be observed in many ways. Knowledge of the nature and

extent of the cancer trea_
and developing therap_
dysphagia.
3. Patients who receive RT _
with surgery may have d_
movement of structures wi_
nism or from pain and dry_
structures. If present, these tr_
require direct intervention to_
lowing function.
4. In evaluating swallowing functi_ _ _e patient who has been treated for head and neck cancer, it is important to evaluate dysphagia-related conditions, including nutritional status, senses of taste and smell, endurance, and oral pain.
5. Therapy for dysphagia in patients with head and neck cancer often focuses on bolus transport issues and airway protection issues. A variety of surgical and behavioral therapy strategies are available to improve swallowing function. Recent research has suggested that the earlier therapy is initiated, the better the expected outcome. The most recent developments in dysphagia therapy focus on a prophylactic approach, which has been shown effective at reducing dysphagia and related morbidities in patients treated with chemoradiation.

REFERENCES

1. National Cancer Institute Factsheet: Head and neck cancer: Questions and answers: http://www.cancer.gov/cancertopics/factsheet/Sites-Types/head-and-neck. Accessed August 15, 2014.
2. van Bokhorst-de van der Schuer MA, van Leeuwen PA, Kuik DJ, et al: The impact of nutritional status on the prognoses of patients with advanced head and neck cancer. *Cancer* 86:519, 1999.
3. Silander E, Nyman J, Hammerlid E: An exploration of factors predicting malnutrition in patients with advanced head and neck cancer. *Laryngoscope* 123:2428, 2013.
4. Hébuterne X, Lemarié E, Michallet M, et al: Prevalence of malnutrition and current use of nutrition support in patients with cancer. *J Parenter Enteral Nutr* 38:196, 2014.
5. Fietkau R: Principles of feeding cancer patients via enteral or parenteral nutrition during radiotherapy. *Strahlenther Onkol* 174(Suppl 3):47, 1998.
6. Lees J: Incidence of weight loss in head and neck cancer patients on commencing radiotherapy at a regional oncology centre. *Eur J Cancer Care (Engl)* 8:133, 1999.
7. Johnston CA, Kean TJ, Prudo SM: Weight loss in patients receiving radical radiation therapy for head and neck cancer: a prospective study. *J Parenter Enteral Nutr* 6:399, 1982.
8. Ottosson S, Zackrisson B, Kjellén E, et al: Weight loss in patients with head and neck cancer during and after conventional and accelerated radiotherapy. *Acta Oncol* 52:711, 2013.
9. van der Berg B, Rütten H, Rasmussen-Conrad EL, et al: Nutritional status, food intake, and dysphagia in long-term survivors with head and neck cancer treated with chemoradiotherapy: a cross-sectional study. *Head Neck* 36:60, 2014.

n Joint Committee on Cancer: *AJCC cancer staging manual*, , New York, 2002, Springer.

Mendenhall WM, Riggs CE, Cassisi NJ: Treatment of head and neck cancers. In DeVita VT, Hellman S, Rosenberg SA, editors: *Cancer: principles and practice of oncology*, Philadelphia, 2005, Lippincott Williams & Wilkins.

12. Smith RV, Goldman Y, Beitler JJ, et al: Decreased short- and long-term swallowing problems with altered radiotherapy dosing used in an organ-sparing protocol for advanced pharyngeal carcinoma. *Arch Otolaryngol Head Neck Surg* 30:831, 2004.

13. Levendag PC, Teguh DN, Voet P, et al: Dysphagia disorders in patients with cancer of the oropharynx are significantly affected by the radiation therapy dose to the superior and middle constrictor muscle: a dose-effect relationship. *Radiother Oncol* 85:64, 2007.

14. Jensen K, Overgaard M, Grau C: Morbidity after ipsilateral radiotherapy for oropharyngeal cancer. *Radiother Oncol* 85:90, 2007.

15. Paleri V, Roe JW, Corry J, et al: Strategies to reduce long-term postchemoradiation dysphagia in patients with head and neck cancer: an evidence-based review. *Head Neck* 36:431, 2014.

16. Sanguineti G, Rao N, Gunn B, et al: Predictors of PEG dependence after IMRT + chemotherapy for oropharyngeal cancer. *Radiother Oncol* 107:300, 2013.

17. Frank SJ, Cox JD, Gillin M, et al: Multifield optimization intensity modulated proton therapy for head and neck tumors: a translation to practice. *Int J Radiat Oncol Biol Phys* 89:846, 2014.

18. Holliday EB, Frank SJ: Proton radiation therapy for head and neck cancer: a review of the clinical experience to date. *Int J Radiat Oncol Biol Phys* 89:292, 2014.

19. Adelstein DJ, Li Y, Adams GI, et al: An intergroup phase III comparison of standard radiation therapy and two schedules of concurrent chemoradiotherapy in patients with unresectable squamous cell head and neck cancer. *J Clin Oncol* 21:21, 2003.

20. Mittal BB, Pauloski BR, Harah DJ, et al: Swallowing dysfunction—preventive and rehabilitation strategies in patients with head-and-neck cancers treated with surgery, radiotherapy, and chemotherapy: a critical review. *Int J Radiation Oncology Biol Phys* 57:1219, 2003.

21. Logemann JA, Pauloski BR, Rademaker AW, et al: Swallowing disorders in the first year after radiation and chemoradiation. *Head Neck* 30:148, 2008.

22. Zuydam AC, Lowe D, Brown JS, et al: Predictors of speech and swallowing function following primary surgery for oral and oropharyngeal cancer. *Clin Otolaryngol* 30:428, 2005.

23. Pauloski BR, Rademaker AW, Logemann JA, et al: Speech and swallowing in irradiated and nonirradiated postsurgical oral cancer patients. *Otolaryngol Head Neck Surg* 118:616, 1998.

24. Shin YS, Koh YW, Kim SH, et al: Radiotherapy deteriorates postoperative functional outcome after partial glossectomy with free flap reconstruction. *J Oral Maxillofac Surg* 70:216, 2012.

25. Ryzek DF, Mantsopoulos K, Künzel J, et al: Early stage oropharyngeal carcinomas: comparing quality of life for different treatment modalities. *Biomed Res Int* 2014:421964, 2014.

26. Pauloski BR, Rademaker AW, Logemann J, et al: Pretreatment swallowing function in patients with head and neck cancer. *Head Neck* 22:474, 2000.

27. Kendall K, McKenzie S, Leonard R, et al: Timing of swallowing events after single-modality treatment of head and neck carcinomas with radiotherapy. *Head Neck* 20:720, 1998.

28. Kotz T, Abraham S, Beitler JJ, et al: Pharyngeal transport dysfunction consequent to an organ-sparing protocol. *Arch Otolaryngol Head Neck Surg* 125:410, 1999.

29. Conley JJ: Swallowing dysfunctions associated with radical surgery of the head and neck. *Arch Surg* 80:602, 1960.

30. Summers GW: Physiologic problems following ablative surgery of the head and neck. *Otolaryngol Clin North Am* 7:217, 1974.

31. Hsiao HT, Leu YS, Lin CC: Tongue reconstruction with free radial foreman flap after hemiglossectomy: a functional assessment. *J Reconstr Microsurg* 19:137, 2003.

32. Seikaly H, Rieger J, Wolfaardt J, et al: Functional outcomes after primary oropharyngeal cancer resection and reconstruction with the radial forearm flap. *Laryngoscopy* 113:897, 2003.

33. Crary MA, Carnaby-Mann GD: Rehabilitation after treatment for head and neck cancer. In DeVita VT, Hellman S, Rosenberg SA, editors: *Cancer: principles and practice of oncology*, ed 7, Philadelphia, 2005, Lippincott Williams & Wilkins.

34. Frazell EL, Lucas JC: Cancer of the tongue: report of the management of 1,554 patients. *Cancer* 15:1085, 1962.

35. Kimata YSM, Hishinuma S, Ebihara S, et al: Analysis of the relations between the shape of the reconstructed tongue and postoperative functions after subtotal or total glossectomy. *Laryngoscope* 113:905, 2003.

36. Hirano M, Kuriowa Y, Tanaka S: Dysphagia following various degrees of surgical resection for oral cancer. *Ann Otol Rhinol Laryngol* 101:138, 1992.

37. McConnell FMS, Logemann JA: Diagnosis and treatment of swallowing disorders. In Cummings CW, editor: *Otolaryngology, head and neck surgery (update II)*, St Louis, 1990, Mosby.

38. Khariwala SS, Vivek PP, Lorenz RR, et al: Swallowing outcomes after microvascular head and neck reconstruction: a prospective review of 191 cases. *Laryngoscopy* 117:1359, 2007.

39. Tei K, Maekawa K, Kitada H, et al: Recovery from postsurgical swallowing dysfunction in patients with oral cancer. *J Oral Maxillofac Surg* 65:1077, 2007.

40. Pauloski BR, Rademaker AW, Logemann J, et al: Surgical variables affecting swallowing in patients treated for oral/oropharyngeal cancer. *Head Neck* 26:625, 2004.

41. Reiger JM, Zalmanowitz JG, Sytsanko A, et al: Functional outcomes after surgical reconstruction of the base of tongue using the radial forearm flap in patients with oropharyngeal carcinoma. *Head Neck* 29:1024, 2007.

42. O'Connel DA, Rieger J, Harris JR, et al: Swallowing function in patients with base of tongue cancers treated with primary surgery and reconstructed with a modified radial forearm free flap. *Arch Otolaryngol Head Neck Surg* 134:857, 2008.

43. Blyth KM, McCabe P, Heard R, et al: Cancers of the tongue and floor of mouth: five year file audit within the acute phase. *Am J Speech-Language Pathol* 23:668, 2014.

44. Borggreven PA, Verdonck-de Leeuw I, Rinkel RN, et al: Swallowing after major surgery of the oral cavity or oropharynx: a prospective and longitudinal assessment of patients treated by microvascular soft tissue reconstruction. *Head Neck* 29:638, 2007.

45. Wycliffe ND, Grover RS, Kim PD, et al: Hypopharyngeal cancer. *Top Magn Reson Imaging* 18:243, 2007.

46. Martin A, Jackel MC, Christiansen H, et al: Organ preserving transoral laser microsurgery for cancer of the hypopharynx. *Laryngoscope* 118:398, 2008.

47. Preuss SF, Cramer K, Klussmann JP, et al: Transoral laser surgery for laryngeal cancer: outcome, complications and prognostic factors in 275 patients. *Eur J Surg Oncol* 35:235, 2009.

48. Hinni ML, Salassa JR, Grant DG, et al: Transoral laser microsurgery for advanced laryngeal cancer. *Arch Otolaryngol Head Neck Surg* 133:1198, 2007.

49. Hartl DM, de Mones E, Hans S, et al: Treatment of early-stage glottic cancer by transoral laser resection. *Ann Otol Rhinol Laryngol* 116:832, 2007.

50. Lewin JS, Hutcheson KA, Barringer DA, et al: Functional analysis of swallowing outcomes after supracricoid partial laryngectomy. *Head Neck* 30:559, 2008.

51. Pellini R, Pichi B, Ruscito P, et al: Supracricoid partial laryngectomies after radiation failure: a multi-institutional series. *Head Neck* 30:372, 2008.

52. León X, López M, García J, et al: Supracricoid laryngectomy as salvage surgery after failure of radiation therapy. *Eur Arch Otorhinolaryngol* 264:809, 2007.

53. Mannellia G, Meccarielloa G, Deganelloa A, et al: Subtotal supracricoid laryngectomy: changing in indications, surgical techniques, and use of new surgical devices. *Am J Otolaryngol* 35:719, 2014.

54. Pauloski BR, Rademaker AW, Logemann J, et al: Speech and swallowing in irradiated and nonirradiated postsurgical oral cancer patients. *Otolaryngol Head Neck Surg* 118:616, 1998.

55. Pauloski BR, Logemann J, Rademaker AW, et al: Speech and swallowing function after oral and oropharyngeal resections: one-year followup. *Head Neck* 16:313, 1994.

56. Roe JW, Carding PN, Dwivdei RC, et al: Swallowing outcomes following Intensity Modulated Radiation Therapy (IMRT) for head & neck cancer—a systematic review. *Oral Oncol* 46:727, 2010.

57. Lohia S, Rajapurkar M, Nguyen SA, et al: A comparison of outcomes intensity-modulated radiation therapy and 3-dimensional conformal radiation therapy in the treatment of oropharyngeal cancer. *JAMA Otolaryngol Head Neck Surg* 140:331, 2014.

58. Pauloski BR, Rademaker AW, Logemann JA, et al: Comparison of swallowing function after intensity-modulated radiation and conventional radiotherapy for head and neck cancer. *Head Neck* 2014. [Epub ahead of print].

59. Xiao C, Hanlon A, Zhang Q, et al: Symptom clusters in patients with head and neck cancer receiving concurrent chemoradiotherapy. *Oral Oncol* 49:360, 2013.

60. Haisfield-Wolfe ME, Brown C, Richardson M, et al: Variations in symptom severity patterns among oropharyngeal and laryngeal cancer outpatients during radiation therapy: a pilot study. *Cancer Nurs* 2014. [Epub ahead of print].

61. Epstein JB, Emerton S, Kolbinson DA, et al: Quality of life and oral function following radiotherapy for head and neck cancer. *Head Neck* 21:1, 1999.

62. Rosenthal DI: Consequences of mucositis-induced treatment breaks and dose reductions on head and neck cancer treatment options. *J Support Oncol* 5:23, 2007.

63. Murphy BA: Clinical and economic consequences of mucositis induced by chemotherapy and/or radiation therapy. *J Support Oncol* 5:13, 2007.

64. Cheng KK: Oral mucositis, dysfunction, and distress in patients undergoing cancer therapy. *J Clin Nurs* 16:2114, 2007.

65. Dirix P, Nuyts S, Vander Poorten V, et al: The influence of xerostomia after radiotherapy on quality of life: results of a questionnaire in head and neck cancer. *Support Care Cancer* 16:171, 2008.

66. Logemann J, Smith CH, Pauloski BR, et al: Effects of xerostomia on perception of performance of swallow function. *Head Neck* 23:317, 2001.

67. Logemann J, Pauloski BR, Rademaker AW, et al: Xerostomia: 12-month changes in saliva production and its relationship to the perception and performance of swallow function, oral intake, and diet after chemoradiation. *Head Neck* 25:432, 2003.

68. Hamlet S, Faull J, Klein B, et al: Mastication and swallowing in patients with postirradiation xerostomia. *Int J Radiat Oncol Biol Phys* 37:789, 1997.

69. Mirza N, Machtay M, Devine PA, et al: Gustatory impairment in patients undergoing head and neck irradiation. *Laryngoscope* 118:24, 2008.

70. Yamashita H, Nakagawa K, Tago M, et al: Taste dysfunction in patients receiving radiotherapy. *Head Neck* 28:508, 2006.

71. Sandow PL, Hejrat-Yazdi M, Heft MW: Taste loss and recovery following radiation therapy. *J Dent Res* 85:608, 2006.

72. Schiffman SS: Critical illness and changes in sensory perception. *Proc Nutr Soc* 66:331, 2007.

73. Dijkstra PU, Huisman PM, Roodenburg JL: Criteria for trismus in head and neck oncology. *Int J Oral Maxillofac Surg* 35:337, 2006.

74. Pauli N, Johnson J, Finizia C, et al: The incidence of trismus and long-term impact on health-related quality of life in patients with head and neck cancer. *Acta Oncol* 52:1137, 2013.

75. Johnson J, Johansson M, Rydén A, et al: The impact of trismus on health-related quality of life and mental health. *Head Neck* 2014. [Epub ahead of print].

76. Starmer HM: Dysphagia in head and neck cancer: prevention and treatment. *Curr Opin Otolaryngol Head Neck Surg* 22:195, 2014.

77. Kraaijenga SAC, van der Molen L, van den Brekel MWM, et al: Current assessment and treatment strategies of dysphagia in head and neck cancer patients: a systematic review of the 2012/13 literature. *Curr Opin Support Palliat Care* 8:152, 2014.

78. Starmer H, Gourin C, Lua LL, et al: Pretreatment swallowing assessment in head and neck cancer patients. *Laryngoscope* 121:1208, 2011.

79. Denaro N, Merlano MC, Russi EG: Dysphagia in head and neck cancer patients: pretreatment evaluation, predictive factors, and assessment during radiochemotherapy, recommendations. *Clin Exp Otorhinolaryngol* 6:117, 2013.

80. Zackrisson PMC, Strander H, Wennerberg J, et al: A systematic overview of radiation therapy effects in head and neck cancer. *Acta Oncol* 42:443, 2003.

81. Hutcheson KA, Lewin JS, Barringer DA, et al: Late dysphagia after radiotherapy-based treatment of head and neck cancer. *Cancer* 118:5793, 2012.

82. Hutcheson KA, Yuk MM, Holsinger FC, et al: Late radiation radiation-associated dysphagia (late-RAD) with lower cranial neuropathy in long-term oropharyngeal cancer survivors: video case reports. *Head Neck* 37:E56–62, 2015.

83. Awan MJ, Mohamed AS, Lewin JS, et al: Late radiation-associated dysphagia (late-RAD) with lower cranial neuropathy after oropharyngeal radiotherapy: a preliminary dosimetric comparison. *Oral Oncol* 50:746, 2014.

84. Carnaby GD, Crary MA: Development and validation of a cancer-specific swallowing assessment tool: MASA-C. *Support Care Cancer* 22:595, 2014.

85. Crary MA, Mann GD, Groher ME: Initial psychometric assessment of a functional oral intake scale for dysphagia in stroke patients. *Arch Phys Med Rehabil* 86:1516, 2005.

86. Dwivedi RC, St Rose S, Roe JW, et al: Validation of the Sydney Swallow Questionnaire (SSQ) in a cohort of head and neck cancer patients. *Oral Oncol* 46:e10, 2010.

87. Chen AY, Frankowski R, Bishop-Leone J, et al: The development and validation of a dysphagia-specific quality-of-life questionnaire for patients with head and neck cancer: the M.D. Anderson dysphagia inventory. *Arch Otolaryngol Head Neck Surg* 127:870, 2001.

88. Rosenthal DI, Mendoza TR, Chamgers MS, et al: Measuring head and neck cancer symptom burden: the development and validation of the M.D. Anderson symptom inventory, head and neck module. *Head Neck* 29:923, 2007.

89. Levin AA, Levine MS, Rubesin SE, et al: An 8-year review of barium studies in the diagnosis of gastroparesis. *Clin Radiol* 63:407, 2008.

90. World Health Organization: *Handbook for reporting results of cancer treatment*, Geneva, 1997, World Health Organization.

91. Meirovitz A, Murdoch-Kinch CA, Schipper M, et al: Grading xerostomia by physicians or by patients after intensity-modulated radiotherapy of head-and-neck cancer. *Int J Radiation Oncology Biol Phys* 66:445, 2006.

92. Johnson J, Carlsson S, Johansson M, et al: Development and validation of the Gothenburg Trismus Questionnaire (GTQ). *Oral Oncol* 48:730, 2012.

93. Farhangfar A, Makarewicz M, Ghosh S, et al: Nutrition impact symptoms in a population cohort of head and neck cancer patients: multivariate regression analysis of symptoms on oral intake, weight loss, and survival. *Oral Oncol* 50:877, 2014.

94. Hutcheson KA, Bhayani MK, Beadle BM, et al: Eat and exercise during radiotherapy or chemoradiotherapy for pharyngeal cancers: use it or lose it. *JAMA Otolaryngol Head Neck Surg* 139:1127, 2013.

95. Oozeer NB, Corsar K, Glore RJ, et al: The impact of enteral feeding route on patient-reported long term swallowing outcome after chemoradiation for head and neck cancer. *Oral Oncol* 47:980, 2011.

96. Prestwich RLD, Teo MTW, Gilbert A, et al: Long-term swallow function after chemoradiotherapy for oropharyngeal cancer: the influence of a prophylactic gastrostomy or reactive nasogastric tube. *Clinical Oncol* 26:103, 2014.

97. Lewis SL, Brody R, Touger-Decker R, et al: Feeding tube use in patients with head and neck cancer. *Head Neck* 36:1789, 2014.

98. Nugent B, Lewis S, O'Sullivan JM: Enteral feeding methods for nutritional management in patients with head and neck cancers being treated with radiotherapy and/or chemotherapy. *Cochrane Database Syst Rev* (1):CD007904, 2013.

99. Denk DM, Kaider A: Videoendoscopic biofeedback: a simple method to improve the efficacy of swallowing rehabilitation of patients after head and neck surgery. *Otorhinolaryngol* 59:100, 1997.

100. Denk DM, Swoboda H, Schima W, et al: Prognostic factors for swallowing rehabilitation following head and neck cancer surgery. *Acta Otolaryngol* 117:769, 1997.

101. Zuydam A, Rogers S, Brown J, et al: Swallowing rehabilitation after oro-pharyngeal resection for squamous cell carcinoma. *Br J Oral Maxillofac Surg* 38:513, 2000.

102. Crary MA, Mann GD, Groher ME, et al: Functional outcomes of dysphagia therapy with adjunctive sEMG biofeedback. *Dysphagia* 19:160, 2004.

103. Carnaby-Mann GD, Crary MA: Adjunctive neuromuscular electrical stimulation in the treatment of chronic pharyngeal dysphagia. *Ann Otol Rhino Laryngol* 117:279, 2008.

104. Kulbersh BD, Rosenthal EL, McGrew BM, et al: Pretreatment, preoperative swallowing exercises may improve dysphagia quality of life. *Laryngoscope* 116:883, 2006.

105. Carrol WR, Locher JL, Canon CL, et al: Pretreatment swallowing exercises improve swallow function after chemoradiation. *Laryngoscope* 118:39, 2008.

106. Carnaby-Mann GD, Crary MA, Schmalfuss I, et al: "Pharyngocise": randomized controlled trial of preventative exercises to maintain muscle structure and swallowing function during head-and-neck Chemoradiotherapy. *Int J Radiat Oncol Biol Phys* 83:210, 2012.

107. Van der Molen L, van Rossum MA, Burkhead LM, et al: A randomized preventative rehabilitation trial in advanced head and neck cancer patients treated with chemoradiotherapy: feasibility, compliance, and short-term effects. *Dysphagia* 26:155, 2011.

108. Kotz T, Federman AD, Kao J, et al: Prophylactic swallowing exercises in patients with head and neck cancer under chemoradiation: a randomized trial. *Arch Otolaryngol Head Neck Surg* 138:376, 2012.

109. Duarte VM, Chhetri DK, Liu YF, et al: Swallow preservation exercises during chemoradiation therapy maintains swallow function. *Otolaryngol Head Neck Surg* 149:878, 2013.

110. Shin EH, Basen-Engquist K, Baum G, et al: Adherence to preventive exercises and self-reported swallowing outcomes in post-radiation head and neck cancer patients. *Head Neck* 35:1707, 2013.

111. Cnossen IC, van Uden-Kraan CF, Rinkel R, et al: Multimodal guided self-help exercise program to prevent speech, swallowing, and shoulder problems among head and neck cancer patients: a feasibility study. *J Med Internet Res* 16:e74, 2014.

112. Al-Othman MO, Amdur RJ, Morris CG, et al: Does feeding tube placement predict for long-term swallowing disability after radiotherapy for head and neck cancer? *Head Neck* 25:741, 2003.

113. Crary MA, Groher ME: Reinstituting oral feeding in tube fed patients with dysphagia. *Nutr Clin Pract* 21:576, 2006.

114. Light J: A review of oral and oropharyngeal prostheses to facilitate speech and swallowing. *Am J Speech Lang Pathol* 4:15, 1995.

115. Pauloski BR, Logemann JA, Colangelo LA, et al: Effect of intraoral prostheses on swallowing function in postsurgical oral and oropharyngeal cancer patients. *Am J Speech Lang Pathol* 5:31, 1996.

116. Koyama Y, Ota Y, Sakaizumi K, et al: Swallowing appliance: intraoral reshaping prosthesis for dysphagia second to oral floor cancer: a pilot study. *Am J Phys Med Rehabil* 93:1008, 2014.

117. Castell JA, Castell DO, Shultz A, et al: Effect of head position on the dynamics of the upper esophageal sphincter and pharynx. *Dysphagia* 8:1, 1993.

118. Fleming SM: Treatment of mechanical swallowing disorders. In Groher M, editor: *Dysphagia: diagnosis and management*, ed 3, Boston, 1997, Butterworth-Heinemann.

119. Grandi G, Silva ML, Streit C, et al: A mobilization regimen to prevent mandibular hypomobility in irradiated patients: an analysis and comparison of two techniques. *Med Oral Pathol Oral Cir Bucal* 12:E105, 2007.

120. Dijkstra PU, Sterken MW, Pater R, et al: Exercise therapy for trismus in head and neck cancer. *Oral Oncol* 43:389, 2007.

121. Dijkstra PU, Kalk WW, Roodenburg JL: Trismus in head and neck oncology: a systematic review. *Oral Oncol* 40:879, 2004.

122. Shulman DH, Shipman B, Willis FB: Treating trismus with dynamic splinting: a cohort, case series. *Adv Ther* 25:9, 2008.

123. Pauloski BR, Logemann JA, Rademake AW, et al: Effects of enhanced bolus flavors on oropharyngeal swallow in patients treated for head and neck cancer. *Head Neck* 35:1124, 2013.

124. Umeno H, Chitose S, Sato K, et al: Efficacy of additional injection laryngoplasty after framework surgery. *Ann Otol Rhinol Laryngol* 117:5, 2008.

125. Dursun G, Boynukalin S, Bagis Ozgursoy O, et al: Long-term results of different treatment modalities for glottic insufficiency. *Am J Otolaryngol* 29:7, 2008.

126. Morgan JE, Zraick RI, Griffin AW, et al: Injection versus medialization laryngoplasty for the treatment of unilateral vocal fold paralysis. *Laryngoscope* 117:2068, 2007.

127. Amin MR: Thyrohyoid approach for vocal fold augmentation. *Ann Otol Rhinol Laryngol* 115:699, 2006.

128. Scully C: The role of saliva in oral health problems. *Practitioner* 245:841, 2001.

129. Cassolato SF, Turnbull RS: Xerostomia: clinical aspects and treatment. *Gerodontology* 20:64, 2003.

130. Fox PC: Salivary enhancement therapies. *Caries Res* 38:241, 2004.

131. Lovelace TL, Fox NF, Sood AJ, et al: Management of radiotherapy-induced salivary hypofunction and consequent xerostomia in patients with oral or head and neck cancer: meta-analysis and literature review. *Oral Surg Oral Med Oral Pathol Radiol* 117:595, 2014.

132. Symonds RP: Treatment-induced mucositis: an old problem with new remedies. *Br J Cancer* 77:1689, 1998.

133. Clarkson JE, Worthington HV, Furness S, et al: Interventions for treating oral mucositis for patients with cancer receiving treatment. *Cochrane Database Syst Rev* (8):CD001973, 2010.

134. Motallebnejad M, Akram S, Moghadamina A, et al: The effect of topical application of pure honey on radiation-induced mucositis: a randomized clinical trial. *J Contemp Dent Pract* 9:40, 2008.

135. Arora H, Pai KM, Maiya A, et al: Efficacy of He-Ne laser in the prevention and treatment of radiotherapy-induced oral mucositis in oral cancer patients. *Oral Surg Oral Med Oral Pathol Oral Radiol Endod* 105:180, 2008.

136. Bar AV, Weinstein G, Dutta PR, et al: Gabapentin for the treatment of pain related to radiation-induced mucositis in patients with head and neck tumors treated with intensity-modulated radiation therapy. *Head Neck* 32:173, 2010.

137. Starmer H, Yang W, Raval R, et al: Effect of gabapentin on swallowing during and after chemoradiation for oropharyngeal squamous cell cancer. *Dysphagia* 29:396, 2014.

138. Worthington HV, Clarkson JE, Bryan G, et al: Interventions for preventing oral mucositis for patients with cancer receiving treatment. *Cochrane Database Syst Rev* (4):CD000978, 2011.

139. Campos M, Campos C, Aarestrup FM, et al: Oral mucositis in cancer treatment: natural history, prevention, and treatment. *Molecular and Clinical Oncol* 2:337, 2014.

140. Magné N, Marcy PY, Foa C, et al: Comparison between nasogastric tube feeding and percutaneous fluoroscopic gastrostomy in advanced head and neck cancer patients. *Eur Arch Otorhinolaryngol* 258:89, 2001.

141. Koyfman SA, Adelstein DJ: Enteral feeding tubes in patients undergoing definitive chemoradiation therapy for head-and-neck cancers: a critical review. *Int J Radiat Oncol Biol Phys* 84:581, 2012.

CHAPTER 5

Esophageal Disorders

Michael E. Groher

To view additional case videos and content, please visit the evolve website.

CHAPTER OUTLINE

OBJECTIVES

1. Discuss the structural disorders of the esophagus that affect swallowing.
2. Discuss the motor disorders of the esophagus that affect swallowing.
3. Detail disorders of the pharyngeal esophageal segment.
4. Show how disorders of esophageal origin might affect other aspects of the swallowing chain.
5. Discuss possible treatment approaches for swallowing disorders of esophageal and pharyngoesophageal origin.

ROLE OF THE SPEECH-LANGUAGE PATHOLOGIST

It is not the role of the speech-language pathologist (SLP) to diagnose and treat dysphagia of esophageal origin. In most cases this is done by the gastroenterologist. However, because of the interdependency of the oral, pharyngeal, and esophageal stages of swallowing, it is important for the speech pathologist to be aware of how esophageal-based dysphagia might affect other compartments involved in swallowing. It also is important for the SLP to be aware of the types of swallowing problems that should be referred to the gastroenterologist and what types of treatments they might recommend. Sometimes treatments (e.g., medications) might affect other parts of the swallowing chain, and patients might need certain instructions about taking their medications reinforced by other health care providers. One example is patients who take medication to control their gastroesophageal reflux disease (GERD). On careful questioning, it is sometimes revealed that they take their medicine only when they perceive they might be eating a meal that would cause an increase in reflux events. In most cases patients should be taking their medication on a daily basis, so reinforcing this point or reviewing proper dietary restrictions may be needed to avoid an increase in reflux events. In these circumstances knowledge of other professional roles and methods of evaluation and treatment can be beneficial to improve patient compliance and answer any questions patients might have about their dysphagia.

It is becoming more common for the SLP to include a screening of the esophagus in patients who are able to stand during the modified barium swallow study. The screenings are useful because they might detect a disorder that helps explain the patient's oropharyngeal symptoms. It is the role of the radiologist—rather than the SLP—to document and comment on these abnormalities. If further tests are warranted, the SLP might include them in his or her progress note but with the approval of the radiologist.

STRUCTURAL DISORDERS

Esophageal dysphagia can be caused by a change in the ability of the esophagus to fully open during swallowing, resulting in a blockage of bolus passage. A change in the structure of the esophagus may be caused by a luminal stenosis or narrowing or by a luminal deformity such as another structure compressing it, thereby limiting its ability to open.

Esophageal Stenosis

Esophageal stenosis is conceptually the easiest mechanism of dysphagia to understand. When the lumen narrows, solid food may be too large to pass through it. Esophageal stenosis typically causes dysphagia for solid food. In addition, the type of solid material ingested often is important for symptom production. For instance, dysphagia of esophageal origin is more likely when solids are tough or fibrous. Softer, more easily chewed foods are much less likely to cause symptoms of esophageal dysphagia. An exception to this tough food–soft food dichotomy is that many patients also have particular trouble with soft, absorbent foods such as bread or pasta, which swell when mixed with saliva during mastication. Once bolus impaction occurs, the patient may have difficulty with liquids as well, obscuring the characteristic solids-only nature of esophageal stenosis. However, a careful history usually reveals that liquid dysphagia begins with ingestion of solids (see Differential Diagnosis later in this chapter).

Clinicians often rely too much on the patient's sensation of where food is sticking. The common wisdom that patients accurately localize symptoms to the site of obstruction is often inaccurate. In fact, approximately one third of patients with obstructing lesions of the distal esophagus point to the neck as the site of obstruction.[1] Conversely, one third of patients with dysphagia localized to the pharynx have an isolated abnormality of the esophagus (review Clinical Corner 5-1).[2]

It is surprising how well some patients fare despite dramatic stenosis. Based on radiographic observations in patients with Schatzki's rings, it is often stated that patients with luminal diameters of more than 18 to 20 mm are never symptomatic, whereas those with diameters less than 10 to 12 mm are always symptomatic.[3] When the radiologist examines the esophagus for suspected stenosis, a **radiopaque pill** that is 13 mm in diameter is used to detect a stenosis. Between these extremes (20 and 10 mm), symptoms vary both in frequency and severity depending on the presence of associated motor dysfunction and the choice

---

CLINICAL CORNER 5-1: FOOD STICKING

A 57-year-old man came to the clinic because of solid and liquid dysphagia. He felt that food was sticking in the back of his throat. He had a long history of GERD but could not afford his medication. His oral peripheral examination was normal, and a modified barium swallow with liquids and solids was performed. Because he was an outpatient and was able to stand, the bolus was followed by the radiologist from the mouth to the region of the stomach. The radiologist commented that it appeared that the bolus flow through the pharyngeal esophageal segment (PES) was normal but was delayed with solid food boluses in the midesophageal region. For this reason he recommended a full examination of the esophagus with the patient in the supine position to more fully investigate this impression.

Critical Thinking
1. Why is it necessary to study the esophagus with the patient in the supine or side-lying position?
2. How could GERD cause a swallowing problem?

---

and preparation of food. Stenosis is treated by opening or removing the narrowed segment, depending on the specific cause. This is usually accomplished with **Maloney (bougie) dilators** or with **balloon dilatation**.

Common intrinsic structural abnormalities that narrow the esophagus include mucosal rings, benign strictures, and malignant tumors.

Rings and Webs

The esophagus may be narrowed by a band of tissue composed of mucosa and submucosa. By tradition, this type of lesion is called a ring when located at the esophagogastric junction and a web when located elsewhere in the esophagus or hypopharynx.

Although classically described in patients with iron-deficiency anemia (sideropenic dysphagia), the majority of esophageal webs are not associated with iron deficiency. Webs of the PES or cervical esophagus are frequently asymmetric, most often impinging on the esophageal lumen from the anterior wall (Figure 5-1, *A*). A suspected web at the cervical level also can be seen in Video 5-1 on the Evolve website accompanying this text.

Schatzki's rings are the most common bandlike constriction of the esophagus. This lesion is typically symmetric and located at the esophagogastric junction (Figure 5-1, *B*). Asymptomatic Schatzki's rings are detected in approximately 10% of the population.[4] The ring is always noted in the presence of a **hiatal hernia**. However, most hiatal hernias are not associated with Schatzki's rings. The etiologic factors of Schatzki's rings are unknown. Because they are rarely seen in childhood and generally are first noticed in middle age, it is unlikely that a Schatzki's ring represents

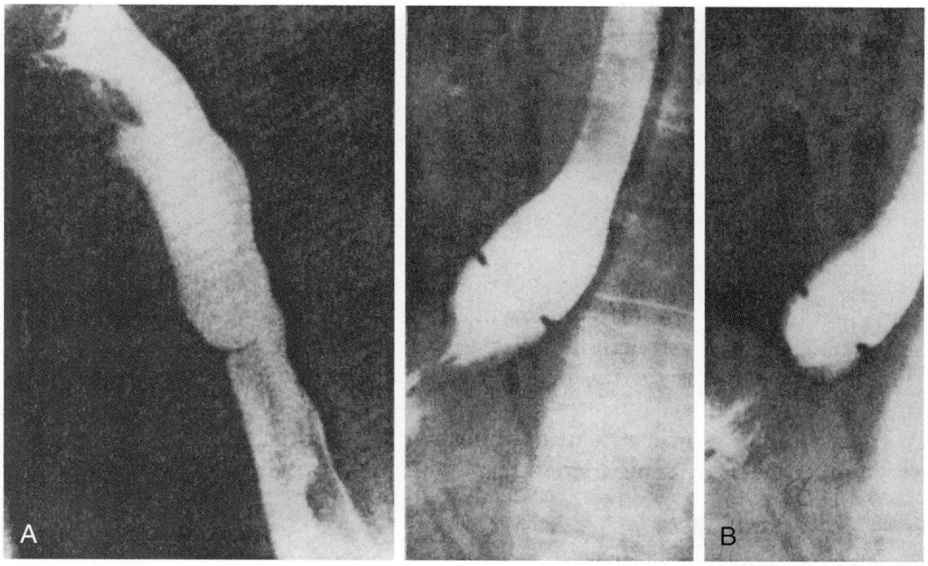

FIGURE 5-1   Thin, bandlike stenotic lesions are generally referred to as rings when located at or near the esophagogastric junction and webs when located elsewhere in the esophagus. **A,** A web is located at the pharyngeal esophageal segment. **B,** Schatzki's ring located at the esophagogastric junction. The webs are seen as darkened lines (slits) on the white barium column. (Courtesy Bronwyn Jones, MD.)

a congenital abnormality. A video image of a Schatzki's ring can be seen in Video 5-2 as a narrowing of the esophageal lumen in the distal esophagus during swallowing of a thicker bolus. Interestingly, the patient's presenting complaint was of solid food sticking in the back of his throat (see Chapter 7 for localization of symptoms, and review Critical Thinking Case 1).

Webs and rings typically produce dysphagia for solids only. Patients often report that symptoms are intermittent and less likely if they select their food wisely and chew carefully (see the section on Differential Diagnosis). Conversely, symptoms are more likely if the patient eats away from home or carries on a conversation while eating; in these situations the choice of food is more restricted and proper preparation of food before swallowing is more difficult. The patient often must end the episode by inducing regurgitation. Once the food is dislodged, the patient often can return to the meal without further difficulty.

The extent to which attention to the mechanics of cutting and chewing controls symptoms is limited. When the lumen is severely compromised, the patient may find it impossible to maintain the level of attention required to remain symptom free without avoiding solids entirely. The patient may describe symptoms without any apparent progression in frequency or severity that date back for many years. Progression, when it does occur, usually is slow.

Radiographically, rings and webs appear as thin (2 to 4 mm) bands that form shelflike constrictions anywhere along the esophagus. Although radiologists occasionally refer to thicker lesions as *webs* or *rings*, these are probably short strictures or abnormal muscular contractions.

Treatment of webs or rings involves dilatation or rupture of the ring by any one of a variety of esophageal dilator systems. The ring is thin, nonfibrotic, and easy to dilate. Complete, or nearly complete, symptomatic relief can be anticipated. Failure to respond is unusual. Dilatation may provide permanent relief, although a large proportion of patients need periodic redilatation at variable intervals.[5]

Benign Stricture

Strictures are rarely seen in children, although congenital strictures do occur. The majority of benign esophageal strictures are acquired in adulthood as a consequence of esophagitis. In a circular structure such as the esophagus, edema resulting from ongoing inflammation and fibrosis as part of the healing process occurs at the expense of luminal diameter.

As with webs and rings, dysphagia is generally for solids only. However, dysphagia is progressive, with episodes becoming more frequent and severe over a period of months or years. As luminal narrowing increases, the patient reports trouble swallowing food that previously caused no difficulty. Stenosis occasionally can become so severe that even thick liquids cause dysphagia. Even then, however, dysphagia is virtually always greater for solids than liquids.

Benign strictures are usually secondary to reflux-induced esophagitis, although most patients with GERD do not have esophagitis. Esophagitis refers to inflammation of the lining of the esophagus. Esophagitis may vary in severity from microscopic inflammation to mucosal edema to erosion, ulcerations, and stricture. Patients usually describe a history of heartburn or chest pain and may report the frequent use

---

BOX 5-1   DIFFERENTIAL DIAGNOSIS OF ESOPHAGITIS

1. Gastroesophageal reflux
2. Infections (*Candida*, viral)
3. Trauma (prolonged nasogastric intubation)
4. Acute chemical ingestion (lye, industrial acids)
5. Drug-induced esophagitis (tetracycline, iron, potassium, quinidine, nonsteroidal antiinflammatory drugs)
6. Radiation
7. Skin conditions (pemphigus, cicatricial pemphigoid, epidermolysis bullosa dystrophica, lichen planus, toxic epidermal necrolysis, Stevens-Johnson syndrome)
8. Others (Crohn's disease, Behçet's syndrome)

PRACTICE NOTE 5-1

One day my neighbor, aware of my background with swallowing disorders, came to tell me that her 18-year-old son suddenly could not swallow. Because sudden onset of a swallowing disorder is rare in younger persons, the only potential cause that came to mind was pill-induced esophagitis. When I asked whether he was taking medication, she reported that he had just started taking tetracycline for his acne and the day before he had forgotten to take his medication at home using the normal amount of water. Instead he took his dose in the classroom without water. Undoubtedly, the pill did not reach the stomach before it dissolved, which created an inflammatory reaction with subsequent stenosis. I speculated that he had temporary dysphagia from pill-induced esophagitis. His symptoms spontaneously resolved within 2 days.

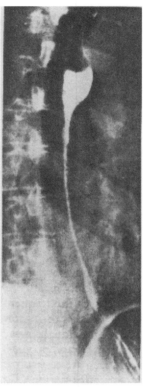

FIGURE 5-2   Long and symmetric benign stricture with a lumen that tapers gradually. The lumen follows the anticipated line of the normal esophagus. The barium within the narrowed lumen has a somewhat irregular appearance because of the erosions. (Courtesy Bronwyn Jones, MD.)

of antacids or other ulcer medications. In some patients the esophagus appears to be relatively insensitive to acid exposure. These individuals never experience significant reflux symptoms despite severe esophagitis and progression to stricture formation. Although most benign esophageal strictures are a result of reflux esophagitis, any source of esophagitis can cause stricture formation (Box 5-1).

Drug-induced or pill esophagitis can be seen in young or older adult patients (see Practice Note 5-1). Typically, commonly administered medications that are larger in size (tetracycline, potassium, quinidine) become lodged at the level of the aortic arch and dissolve, causing inflammation and stricture. Symptoms of chest pain, odynophagia, heartburn, and dysphagia may be present, usually more acutely in younger patients.[6]

Radiographically, a benign stricture is seen as a narrowed segment of esophageal lumen that may range from 1 cm to many centimeters long (Figure 5-2). The stricture usually is smooth and gradually tapering, with a symmetric

lumen that follows the anticipated path of the normal esophagus. Ongoing inflammation may produce an eroded appearance along its course. A lateral and anteroposterior (AP) video image of a midesophageal stricture caused by GERD can be seen in Video 5-3 on the Evolve website. In the AP view barium flow is interrupted, with barium building up above the stricture. The lateral view shows a long, tapered appearance of a stricture in the esophagus.

Proper management requires both treatment of the underlying inflammation and dilation of the stricture. Treatment of the cause of esophagitis requires accurate diagnosis. Although reflux is the most common cause of esophagitis, other possibilities must be considered, especially in patients with atypical histories, an unusual distribution of inflammation, or failure to respond to reflux treatment.

Dilatation often can be performed by using the same techniques available for a Schatzki's ring. However, the stricture may be relatively unyielding and require stiffer dilator systems. Effective dilatation usually improves symptoms, although edema from inflammation may result in less-complete symptomatic relief than with a Schatzki's ring and in relatively rapid restenosis. Frequent dilatations are more often required in benign strictures than with Schatzki's rings. Even when ongoing inflammation completely ceases, periodic dilatation may be necessary, especially during the first year after initial treatment, when maturation of the fibrotic reaction continues at the expense of luminal diameter.

Malignant Stricture

Although benign tumors may arise from the esophagus, the majority of clinically significant tumors of the esophagus are malignant. In the past, most esophageal malignancies were **squamous cell carcinomas**, although recent studies suggest a dramatic increase in **adenocarcinoma** of the distal esophagus. Most esophageal adenocarcinomas appear to arise from Barrett's esophagus, a premalignant condition in which columnar cells replace the usual squamous epithelium covering the lower end of the esophagus as a result of severe GERD.

As with other types of stenotic lesions, dysphagia initially occurs for solids only. However, it usually progresses rapidly, with dysphagia for soft foods and even liquids developing within a few months of the onset of symptoms.

Radiographically, esophageal malignancies appear as strictures of variable length. By the time of presentation, the cancerous tumor or area is usually many centimeters long and involves the entire circumference of the esophageal lumen, producing a stricture. The typical malignant stricture is characterized by its shelflike proximal margins and irregular channel, which may diverge substantially from the anticipated course of the esophageal lumen (Figure 5-3). However, not all esophageal cancers are obviously malignant on barium radiography, and occasional malignant-looking strictures may be benign.[6] For this reason, endoscopy with tissue sampling by biopsy with or without **cytologic brushing** is essential to differentiate benign and malignant strictures.

Curative treatment is primarily surgical, although apparent cures by radiotherapy have been reported. Unfortunately, by the time symptoms develop, the cancer is usually very advanced and incurable. The overall 5-year survival rate for esophageal cancer is only approximately 5%.[1] Even among those in whom resection for apparent cure is possible, the 5-year survival rate is only approximately 15%.[7] Recent studies suggested that the 5-year survival rate could be doubled with a combination of preoperative radiotherapy and chemotherapy.[8] Surprisingly, almost 25% of patients had no evidence of cancer by gross or histologic examination. Among these patients, survival was improved fourfold over rates reported for surgery alone and twofold over those with evidence of residual tumor at surgical resection.

For patients in whom curative resection is not possible, palliative resection often is still feasible and provides good symptomatic relief. In the past, a high perioperative

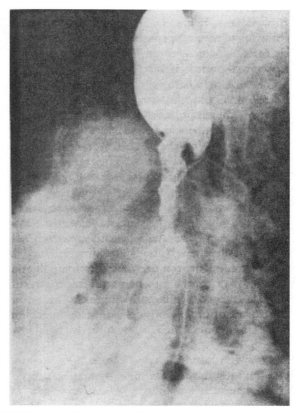

FIGURE 5-3   Malignant circumferential stricture. Characteristics distinguishing it from a benign stricture include the sharp, shelflike proximal margin and the more irregular configuration of the stenotic segment. Unlike some malignant strictures, this stricture follows the anticipated path of the esophageal lumen. Compare the appearance with the benign stricture shown in Figure 5-2. (Courtesy Bronwyn Jones, MD.)

mortality rate of approximately 29% combined with the infrequency of cure made surgery unattractive.[9] However, with better nutrition provided by preoperative and perioperative hyperalimentation the risk of palliative surgery has declined.[10]

Alternative approaches include dilatation, tumor ablation (thermal treatment to destroy tumor obstructing the esophagus) by laser or bipolar electrocautery, and **stent** placement. Each of these approaches is directed at opening the esophageal lumen to permit eating, in recognition that the major cause of early death in patients with esophageal cancer is malnutrition and aspiration pneumonia.

Dilatation generally provides limited and short-lived relief but is useful in preparing for other forms of therapy. The choice between other modalities depends on specific features of the tumor and local technical expertise and resources. Endoscopic laser therapy and bipolar electrocautery can be used to destroy tumor tissue that blocks the esophageal lumen; this may provide a number of months of relief, allowing continuing oral intake. Treatment can be repeated if obstruction recurs.

An esophageal stent is a tube with a large channel that can be placed through the strictured segment to maintain luminal patency. The stent permits ingestion of a modified diet, concentrating on soft, easily chewed foods and purees. The use of stents for palliation has decreased dramatically since the development of thermal methods of treatment. However, stents continue to be useful in certain situations, especially in the presence of a **tracheoesophageal fistula** that often complicates the natural history or treatment of esophageal cancer. In this situation, a properly placed stent can maintain the esophageal lumen while covering the opening to the airway. The recent introduction of expandable metal stents has made insertion easier and provides a larger internal luminal diameter, allowing patients to eat a less-restrictive diet.

Although endoscopic treatment with laser, bipolar electrocautery, or stent placement may be highly successful in reestablishing luminal patency, a substantial proportion of patients with esophageal cancer have poor appetites and are unable to gain weight. The early use of endoscopically placed or fluoroscopically guided gastrostomies should be considered in patients who do not eat once the lumen is reestablished or who are scheduled to undergo chemotherapy or radiotherapy, treatments that may produce or exacerbate anorexia (see Chapter 6 for a discussion of transhiatal esophagectomy).

Luminal Deformities

Extrinsic Compression

Some degree of luminal deformity caused by extrinsic compression by normal mediastinal structures (the aortic knob, the left mainstem bronchus, and the left atrium of the heart) is normally seen on barium studies and rarely, if ever, causes symptoms. More pronounced compression can occur with mediastinal conditions, such as aortic aneurysm, **cardiomegaly**, congenital abnormalities of the large mediastinal arteries (e.g., aberrant subclavian artery), enlarged mediastinal lymph nodes, and lung cancer. Video 5-4 on the Evolve website shows a patient with cardiomegaly and reduced bolus flow. The enlarged heart is seen as a large shadow (note heartbeat) in the middle of the video image. The elasticity of the contralateral esophageal wall usually tends to minimize symptoms until compression is far advanced. Dilatation is usually ineffective because the force of dilatation is absorbed by the elastic, uninvolved wall. Effective treatment, when necessary, requires shrinking or removing the mass producing the compression. Unfortunately, this is often not practical in patients in whom compression produces significant symptoms.

Esophageal Diverticulum

Compared with diverticula of the hypopharynx, esophageal diverticula are rare and usually asymptomatic, even when they are relatively large. When symptoms do occur, they include dysphagia for liquids and solids, regurgitation of previously swallowed food back into the mouth, or both. Regurgitation without dysphagia is not uncommon.

Most often, esophageal diverticula are a consequence of obstruction distal to the region of bolus collection. Increased pressure in the esophagus results in bulging at a point of relative weakness. Less commonly, diverticula can result from periesophageal inflammation, which causes traction on the esophageal wall (traction diverticulum). Although most traction diverticula occur in the midesophagus, most midesophageal diverticula, like their distal esophageal counterparts, are caused by **pulsion**. Video 5-5 shows a diverticulum that fills and causes a momentary obstruction to bolus flow.

Treatment of pulsion-type diverticula is necessary only if a diverticulum is symptomatic. Because they frequently give rise to motor or structural disorders, it is important to look for pulsion-type abnormalities as causes for the development of the diverticulum. It may be difficult to distinguish between the underlying obstructive disorder and the diverticulum as a cause of symptoms. It is appropriate to attempt to treat the underlying cause of increased pressure with dilatation in the case of structural obstruction or with drugs for dysmotility. In some patients symptoms initially believed to be a consequence of the diverticulum improve significantly or resolve entirely with such conservative therapy.

Surgical removal of the diverticulum is required if medical management fails. Surgery limited to diverticulectomy, however, is associated with a high incidence of early anastomotic leakage or late recurrence, probably because it fails to deal with the underlying cause of increased intraesophageal pressure and creates an area of relative esophageal wall weakness. Therefore diverticulectomy should be combined with treatment of the underlying disorder—motor (with a surgical **myotomy**) or structural (with dilatation).

ESOPHAGEAL MOTILITY DISORDERS

An orderly, progressive peristaltic wave is not uniformly present after every swallow, even in individuals without dysphagia. The dividing line between normal and pathologic degrees of dysmotility is poorly defined. The incidence of abnormal contractions changes with bolus type (it is increased with dry swallows), although not with age.

A variety of schemes have been proposed to classify esophageal dysmotility. In abnormalities of esophageal peristalsis, contraction amplitude may be too high or low, contraction duration prolonged, or the orderly progression of the contractile wave down the length of the esophagus uncoordinated. In abnormalities of lower esophageal sphincter (LES) function, the pressure may be too high or too low and relaxation may be incomplete. Finally, the esophageal body and LES can misbehave separately or together. The individual characteristics of commonly described motility disorders are not necessarily unique. In many ways the separation between entities is somewhat arbitrary.

Disorders of Peristalsis

Motor dysfunction of the body of the esophagus may cause symptoms of dysphagia, chest pain, or regurgitation. Dysphagia is usually for liquids as well as solids, although not necessarily in equal measure. Chest pain may mimic that of cardiac disease and cause considerable concern on the part of both patient and physician. Although pain initiated or exacerbated by swallowing strongly implicates the esophagus as the site of origin, a clear relation to eating is often absent. Similarly, the presence of other symptoms implicating the swallowing mechanism supports the possibility that the esophagus is the cause of chest pain. However, cardiac disease is sufficiently common, especially in older patients, to justify a cardiology evaluation.

Diffuse Esophageal Spasm

Esophageal spasm is a graphic term with an imprecise meaning. The diagnosis of esophageal spasm is used quite freely among physicians, including gastroenterologists. All too often esophageal spasm is diagnosed on the basis of minor degrees of dysmotility seen radiographically (Figure 5-4) or manometrically (Figure 5-5), or even on the basis of consistent symptoms in the absence of radiographic or manometric confirmation. Esophageal spasm constitutes the end of a spectrum of nonspecific esophageal dysmotility. At one end of the range are the abnormal contractions seen occasionally in normal individuals. At the other are repeated high-amplitude, prolonged, simultaneous, or multiphasic contractions or some combination of these in the absence of any normal peristaltic activity (Figures 5-5 and 5-6). Although few would argue against calling the latter spasm, little agreement exists on where less-severe abnormalities of esophageal peristalsis end and spasm begins.

An interesting feature of these criteria is the inclusion of high LES pressures and incomplete relaxation as an associated finding. LES dysfunction in **diffuse esophageal spasm** is well recognized, with failure of complete relaxation noted in one third of patients.[11] The presence of LES dysfunction in diffuse esophageal spasm and of spastic contractions in a variant of achalasia ("vigorous achalasia") obscures the distinction between the two (see Achalasia later in this chapter).

Nutcracker Esophagus

Brand et al.[12] described a group of patients with chest pain or dysphagia that occurred in association with manometric

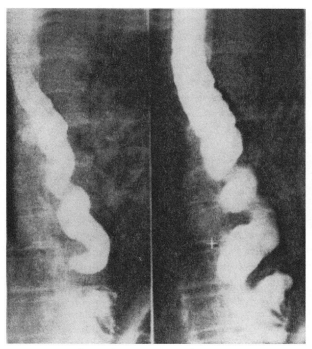

FIGURE 5-4 Radiographic appearance of esophageal dysmotility. A variety of patterns of abnormal peristalsis may be seen on barium radiography. In spot film, the silhouette of the barium column in the upper portion of the esophagus has a serrated appearance, whereas in the lower portion there is a corkscrew-like configuration. In addition, there is a hiatal hernia. (Courtesy Bronwyn Jones, MD.)

findings of high amplitude but with normally progressive peristaltic waves. This syndrome, often called the nutcracker esophagus, is considered by some authorities to be the most commonly detected disorder of esophageal motility.

A number of questions surround the manometric pattern of the nutcracker esophagus. First, the criterion for diagnosis has changed. Originally described as a mean pressure of more than 120 mm Hg, recent studies of healthy individuals indicate that this value is too low, especially for the older population. Castell[13] has suggested that to avoid overdiagnosis, the term *nutcracker esophagus* should be restricted to patients with mean pressures higher than 180 mm Hg.[13]

Second, the pressures measured during serial motility studies performed in the same individual may change substantially, resulting in the manometric interpretations changing from abnormal (i.e., nutcracker) to normal on different recordings in the same patient.[14] Interestingly, the pressures tend to be highest at the initial recording, suggesting that anxiety associated with the procedure may play a role in this manometric pattern.

Third, why nutcracker esophagus produces symptoms is not clear. Barium esophagrams demonstrate normal stripping function. Although increased pressure could conceivably

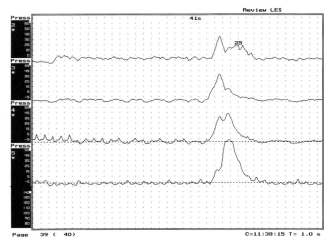

FIGURE 5-5 Manometric appearance of esophageal spasm. The manometric findings in esophageal dysmotility are characterized by various combinations of simultaneous, multiphasic, high-amplitude, and prolonged contractions. The more severe forms are designated diffuse esophageal spasm, although the boundaries between this diagnosis and lesser degrees of dysmotility are not well established. In addition, occasional abnormal contractions may be seen in normal individuals. In the manometric study shown, the four tracings are from pressure sensors spaced at 2-cm intervals in the distal esophagus (the distance of the distal sensor from the nares and timing of swallow are indicated by number and letter at the top). The initial upstroke in all leads is simultaneous. In addition, each demonstrates a secondary upstroke that also begins simultaneously. The amplitude and duration of contraction are within normal limits. The dashed lines represent intraesophageal resting pressure. (Vertical axis scale, 1 increment = 10 mm Hg; horizontal scale, 1 increment = 1 second.)

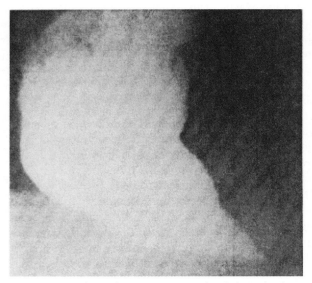

FIGURE 5-6 Radiographic appearance of achalasia. A barium esophagram with the patient in an upright position demonstrates the typical features of achalasia: a dilated esophagus and a smooth, tapering narrowing at the esophagogastric junction ("parrot-beaked deformity") holding up a column of barium mixed with retained food. In more extreme cases, the esophagus may take on a tortuous appearance (sigmoid esophagus). (Courtesy Bronwyn Jones, MD.)

cause discomfort, most patients with high-amplitude contractions during motility do not have pain at the time of the examination, and it is often difficult to appreciate differences between contraction amplitude and appearance during spontaneous episodes of pain that are witnessed manometrically.[15] Nutcracker esophagus may represent a marker of patients with intermittent diffuse esophageal spasm.

Nonspecific Motility Disorders

Disagreement about the criteria for esophageal spasm aside, a large number of patients referred to the esophageal function laboratory have abnormalities of esophageal motility in which the degree and type of motility abnormalities detected are not sufficient to be labeled esophageal spasm or nutcracker esophagus.[15] These lesser patterns of dysmotility are called nonspecific esophageal motor disorders. Their clinical significance remains unclear. On the one hand, it is difficult to ignore the potential significance of disordered peristalsis in patients with dysphagia. On the other hand, similar degrees of abnormality are so common in normal volunteers that their mere presence cannot be considered proof of causality.

Eosinophilic Esophagitis

Patients who complain of persistent solid food dysphagia, usually without pain or regurgitation and with a history of allergies such as hay fever, asthma, or allergic rhinitis, may have an abnormal build-up of **eosinophils** that interfere with the ability of the esophagus to move in a normal pattern.[16] This condition can be found in children (see Chapter 13) and in adults, more frequently in males than females. Diagnosis usually is confirmed by biopsy and often needs to be considered when other disorders that precipitate solid food dysphagia have been ruled out.

Treatment of Motility Disorders

The medical therapy for esophageal dysmotility is often of limited benefit. A variety of smooth muscle–relaxant drugs (nitrates, hydralazine, calcium channel blockers) have been used in an attempt to decrease esophageal contractile amplitude and repetitive contractions. Although some patients experience a dramatic response, many do not. Controlled clinical trials thus far have failed to demonstrate a convincing beneficial effect of these drugs on symptoms.[17] The symptomatic response to these drugs is quite variable and often incomplete. Potential side effects related to the **hypotensive** effects of the drugs severely limit their use.

The most common mistake in the treatment of esophageal dysmotility is to assume that the patient has a primary disorder of esophageal motility. Esophageal dysmotility is like anemia; it is a laboratory finding that requires further evaluation. As for anemia, there is a differential diagnosis of esophageal dysmotility. The most common cause of dysmotility is esophageal irritation, most commonly by GERD. Disordered esophageal peristalsis also may result from esophageal obstruction, ganglion degeneration (i.e., vigorous achalasia), autonomic neuropathies (e.g., caused by diabetes or alcohol abuse), or collagen vascular diseases (especially scleroderma and mixed connective tissue disease). Only patients with esophageal dysmotility in the absence of an underlying cause are considered to have a primary (or **idiopathic**) esophageal dysmotility.

Reflux-induced dysmotility is probably the most common cause of esophageal dysmotility and is more easily treated than idiopathic dysmotility. Because heartburn is not always present, reflux should be considered in any patient with symptoms of esophageal spasm. Ironically, the drugs used to treat idiopathic dysmotility may make reflux worse by further impairing LES pressure. Esophageal stenosis, another cause of esophageal dysmotility, may be missed occasionally by barium studies and endoscopy. Dilatation should be considered if there is any question of a structural obstruction.

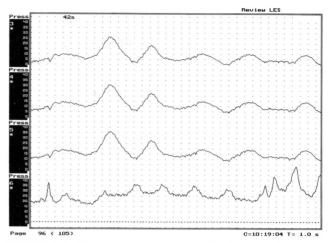

FIGURE 5-7 Manometric appearance of achalasia. The lower esophageal sphincter, examined in the bottom pressure channel, fails to relax to the level of the intragastric pressure *(dotted broken line)*. Additionally, the contraction in the other three pressure recordings are low and amplitudes are simultaneous. (Courtesy of William Ravich, MD.)

LOWER ESOPHAGEAL SPHINCTER ABNORMALITIES

Achalasia

Achalasia is a condition in which a nonrelaxing or incompletely relaxing LES prevents the passage of swallowed material into the stomach. Patients usually present with dysphagia for both liquids and solids. Regurgitation is common and characteristically results in regurgitation of recognizable food hours after it was eaten. Late regurgitation of undigested food is a feature seen in only a few cases of dysphagia, primarily achalasia and hypopharyngeal (Zenker's) or esophageal diverticulum. During barium swallow, with the patient in the upright position, the esophagus is generally dilatated and a column of barium of variable height is maintained above a tight esophagogastric junction (see Figure 5-6). The possibility that this appearance could represent a tight esophageal stricture is ruled out at endoscopy when the endoscope passes into the stomach with mild to moderate resistance.[15]

Although the impairment of LES response to swallow is key to the functional obstruction of the flow of food into the stomach, the motor abnormalities of achalasia include the complete loss of progressive peristalsis (Figure 5-7). In the more common variant of achalasia (classic achalasia), low-amplitude, aperistaltic contractions in the body of the esophagus are combined with a high or high-normal, nonrelaxing sphincter. The simultaneous low-amplitude increases in pressure with swallow are often attributed to pharyngeal pressure, transmitted into the dilated esophagus, rather than to true esophageal contractile activity.[15]

A variant of achalasia, called vigorous achalasia, has been recognized. In this condition, the typical LES findings of achalasia are associated with higher amplitude, prolonged, multiphasic contractions, indicating that intrinsic esophageal motor response to swallowing, however deranged, is still present.

The manometric features of achalasia include an LES with a high or high-normal resting pressure that fails to relax appropriately with swallow. In addition, a complete loss of progressive peristalsis occurs. Occasional patients with identical manometric findings as a result of tumor infiltration of the esophagogastric junction have been described; their condition is labeled secondary achalasia or pseudoachalasia.[18] Pseudoachalasia also has been described in a few nonmalignant conditions. Features that should raise suspicion of secondary achalasia include older age of onset, shorter duration of symptoms, modest dilation of the esophagus, and rapid and profound weight loss.

Compared with other primary esophageal motor disorders, identification and treatment of achalasia usually is successful. Although achalasia involves motor abnormalities of both the esophageal body and LES, the LES dysfunction is largely responsible for obstruction with resultant symptoms. Most patients are sufficiently affected by their symptoms at presentation to warrant therapy. The major absolute indication for treatment is nighttime regurgitation, which puts the patient at risk for aspiration during sleep. Treatment also is warranted if the obstruction is severe, nutrition is impaired, or the esophagus progressively dilates over time.

A number of treatment choices are available for achalasia, including smooth muscle–relaxant drugs, balloon dilatation, botulinum injections, and surgery. The treatment goal of all these choices is to decrease LES pressure, thereby diminishing the resistance to the flow of food and liquid. None has a clinically significant effect on abnormal motor function in the esophageal body.

Calcium channel blockers and long-acting nitrites do lower LES pressure significantly and have been used for achalasia, although complete relief of symptoms may not be achieved. Patients then may undergo either dilatation or surgery. Typically, if a trial of dilatation fails, a surgical myotomy is performed.

The endoscopic injection of a potent neurotoxin (botulinum toxin [Botox]) directly into the sphincter segment has been successful in treating achalasia. A placebo-controlled study has demonstrated a symptomatic response similar to that with dilatation.[19] This approach is technically simple and the risks appear to be confined to those associated with endoscopy alone. The effect of a successful injection lasts on average for 1 to 4 years. Those who respond initially often respond to repeated injection.

Isolated Abnormalities of the Lower Esophageal Sphincter

LES dysfunction is not limited to patients with achalasia. As previously mentioned, incomplete relaxation of the LES occurs in perhaps one third of patients with other evidence of severe esophageal dysmotility. In addition, occasional patients referred for esophageal manometry have isolated abnormalities of LES function, either hypertensive LES pressure or incomplete relaxation in response to swallow. Few of these patients have any radiographically detectable impairment of function. They may represent a preclinical stage in the evolution of achalasia, abnormalities related to esophageal spasm during periods of otherwise normal peristaltic activity, or a secondary reaction to intragastric phenomenon in which the LES reaction is directed at preventing GERD. In most patients the explanation and clinical significance of isolated abnormalities of LES function cannot be determined.

Motor Weakness

Intermittent impairment of contraction amplitude or peristalsis is relatively common. Radiologists frequently mislabel weakness as spasm when they see the escape of barium above the peristaltic wave.[15] This distinction is important because medication directed toward esophageal spasm, which generally decreases contractile amplitude, would be inappropriate if the problem actually is weakness. In practice, the esophagus can empty by gravity, and many patients with esophageal paresis are asymptomatic. Although some medications can increase esophageal contractility, their effect in patients with severe paresis usually is limited.

Severe esophageal weakness is relatively rare. It is most characteristically found in patients with collagen vascular disease, such as scleroderma and mixed connective tissue disease. The esophagus is the second most common organ involved in scleroderma.[20] Esophageal involvement varies from mild to nonspecific to the complete absence of a contractile response to swallow. The loss of esophageal motility can be appreciated on barium swallow studies. The patient in Video 5-6 initially had the diagnosis of rheumatoid arthritis and later reported solid food dysphagia. Eventually a diagnosis of overlap syndrome that included scleroderma was made. Many of these patients have low LES pressure on manometry. The resulting severe GERD with poor esophageal clearance makes them particularly susceptible to esophageal inflammation and strictures.

Patients with diabetes may have motor weakness in the esophagus secondary to autonomic neuropathy. In addition, gastroparesis with abnormal emptying of the stomach may contribute to esophageal-related dysphagic complaints.[21,22]

GASTROESOPHAGEAL REFLUX DISEASE

Gastroesophageal reflux is the normal movement of gastric contents into the esophagus. Because of constantly changing pressure relations between the stomach and esophagus during normal activity, this movement of contents is considered normal (physiologic reflux) and usually is not accompanied by dysphagia or heartburn. The relaxation of the LES is brief and the stomach contents that enter the distal esophagus typically are immediately cleared back into the stomach. Therefore all events of reflux are not pathologic. Gastroesophageal reflux is a common physiologic event. Many apparently normal individuals describe heartburn on a regular basis. A study of healthy hospital employees indicates that approximately 33%, 14%, and 7% reported they had heartburn on a monthly, weekly, and daily basis, respectively.[23] Therefore it appears that reflux is a feature of normal life and does not necessarily reflect a pathologic condition.

However, when gastric contents (usually acid, pepsin, and bile) entering the esophagus are not immediately cleared or when the transient relaxations are frequent, typical symptoms—such as heartburn, regurgitation, odynophagia, and dysphagia—may develop. Gastroesophageal reflux is not necessarily related to the levels of acid or pepsin but to the barriers that allow it to be pathologic. When symptoms become overt, it is referred to as gastroesophageal reflux *disease* (GERD). Despite its name, heartburn (or the sensation of burning in the chest) is generally of esophageal origin, although when severe it may be confused with cardiac disease. Heartburn is the archetypical symptom of GERD, although it may occasionally represent a nonspecific response to other types of esophageal dysmotility. Atypical symptoms, such as chest pain, recurrent sinusitis, chronic cough, hoarseness, asthma, laryngitis, **globus sensation**, and middle ear infections, also may be associated with GERD.[24] The negative effects on quality of life resulting from GERD are well known.[25] Detection and confirmation of typical and atypical GERD symptoms often can be done with a thorough history.[26] When the offending refluxate reaches the pharynx, it is called laryngopharyngeal reflux (LPR). Patients with LPR may represent a different diagnostic entity from those with classic GERD symptomatology (see Laryngopharyngeal Reflux later in this chapter).

Mechanisms of Reflux

Dysphagia associated with gastroesophageal reflux may be attributable to a variety of mechanisms. GERD, with or without esophagitis, is a common cause of esophageal dysmotility. Patients with GERD that does not result in esophagitis but who may have symptoms of heartburn and dysphagia are classified as patients with nonerosive reflux disease (NERD). The differential diagnosis between these two groups of patients is important because the management strategies (medication regimens) for controlling their symptoms may differ.[27] Although not definitely proven, it is conceivable that constant acid and pepsin irritation of the esophageal lumen results in edema that secondarily precipitates dysmotility with symptoms of heartburn and dysphagia, but not esophagitis. Patients with normal endoscopy and GERD symptomatology may have increase in the intercellular spaces as seen on tissue biopsy. A high mean value of the intercellular space may be a sensitive marker of acidic injury in those with suspected NERD.[28] A subgroup of patients with NERD are those with functional heartburn. These patients report heartburn symptoms but have normal 24-hour pH study findings, unlike some of those with NERD. Finally, chronic inflammation in the esophagus of any type can cause strictures and dysphagia.

A complete understanding of the pathophysiology of GERD has progressed substantially over the past decade but still remains incomplete. The major components of the "antireflux barrier" are the LES acting in combination with the anatomic configuration of the esophagogastric junction. In particular, the diaphragmatic crura act as a sphincter during inspiration through their contraction at the level of the esophagogastric junction, whereas the fibers of the LES are more active on expiration (Figure 5-8).

Together these structures maintain an equilibrium of pressure between the stomach and esophagus. Reflux was initially believed to be more likely when the tone in the LES was low; however, it is now known that abrupt periods of relaxation during nonswallow events with normal LES tone are the explanatory mechanism.[29] These abrupt periods of relaxation are called transient lower esophageal sphincter relaxations (tSLERs). Patients with symptomatic GERD

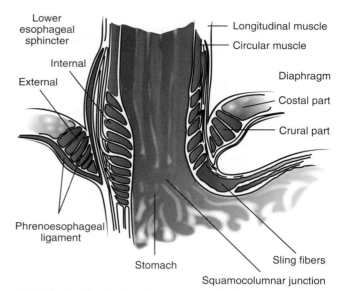

FIGURE 5-8 The distal esophagus pierces the diaphragmatic hiatus as it joins the stomach. On inspiration the crural diaphragmatic ligaments contract, pinching on the esophagus to maintain a pressure equilibrium between the stomach and esophagus. The longitudinal and circular fibers of the lower esophageal sphincter form the esophageal sphincter where the stomach and esophagus join. Together, this combination of muscular and ligamentous arrangement participates in the control of reflux.

tend to have more tSLERs than those without symptoms, although mucosal injury may depend more on the ability of the esophagus to clear refluxed contents and the mucosal defense system in the wall of the distal esophagus.[30] Some evidence suggests that the frequency of tSLERs may be related to high **postprandial** pressures accompanied by slow gastric emptying.[30] In addition, the LES protective barrier is compromised in patients with hiatal hernia, in which the stomach herniation pushes the LES into the chest cavity, effectively eliminating the protective mechanisms of the LES and crural diaphragm.

Measuring Reflux

Continuous (24-hour) pH monitoring allows the objective evaluation for reflux under near-physiologic conditions. In most studies of esophageal acidification, a pH of 4 or less is considered abnormal; however, even weakly acidic levels may cause symptoms in patients taking **proton pump inhibitors** to control stomach acid levels.[31] During the procedure, the patient performs the activities of normal daily living, including eating, working, and sleeping. A catheter is placed through the nose into the esophagus and is connected to a measurement device the patient wears at the waist. When the patient experiences heartburn symptoms, he or she depresses a button that records the time of the event. Continuous pH monitoring provides quantitative information on the presence and severity of acid reflux. The incidence and duration of reflux events can be calculated and analyzed for the entire recording period and for segments of particular interest. The severity of reflux detected by pH monitoring correlates fairly well with the probability of esophageal inflammation and Barrett's esophagus.[32] Continuous pH monitoring is currently considered the best single test for the diagnosis of GERD, with a sensitivity and specificity of approximately 90%.[33] Newer measurement techniques such as intraesophageal impedance monitoring combined with impedance-pH monitoring have been advocated as an important method in the identification of reflux events and esophageal transit disorders.[34] Kulinna-Cosentini et al.[35] compared the findings of pH studies in the identification of reflux in 37 patients using magnetic resonance imaging fluoroscopy. They concluded that when compared with 24-hour pH studies, the results were similar in 82% of the cases. Barium (imaging) studies, although important in evaluating patients with dysphagia, confirm the presence of reflux in only the minority of patients with symptomatic reflux disease.

Treatment of Gastroesophageal Reflux Disease

Treatment of GERD is directed at enhancing the strength of the antireflux barrier, improving esophageal clearance and gastric emptying, and decreasing the noxiousness of gastric contents. Antireflux therapy has three components: alteration in lifestyle, drugs, and surgery.

For many patients, reflux is provoked by dietary indiscretion and physical activity. Decreasing or eliminating foods that decrease LES pressure (e.g., fat, chocolate) or stimulate gastric acid production (e.g., coffee, tea) is important, especially in patients who ingest large amounts or note the association of symptoms with ingestion of these substances. In some patients with reflux, dietary modification is enough to control symptoms. Smoking and alcohol intake also impair esophageal function and should be eliminated. In addition, patients are instructed to elevate the head of the bed on 6-inch blocks and avoid lying down within 3 hours of eating. These measures allow gravity to assist in reflux prevention and enhance esophageal clearance.

Self-medication with antacids is common in patients with heartburn. Unfortunately, antacids alone are rarely sufficient to control esophagitis in patients with atypical symptoms. Antacids are primarily used for symptomatic relief of intermittent, infrequent heartburn. Most patients with severe symptoms or esophagitis require more potent acid-lowering agents. Prescribed most often are proton-pump inhibitors (PPIs) such as lansoprazole, rabeprazole, pantoprazole, or omeprazole. They are most effective in combination with lifestyle changes related to weight control and dietary modifications. Histamine antagonists, or H_2-blockers (e.g., cimetidine, ranitidine, nizatidine, famotidine), although less effective in curing esophagitis, are available in over-the-counter preparations. The control of typical and atypical manifestations in GERD is most effective with PPI therapy. Interestingly, control of symptoms in some patients does not always correlate with intraesophageal or intragastric acid suppression.[36] Because all patients in whom GERD is suspected respond uniformly to either H_2-blockers or PPI therapy, various algorithms that address success and failure, including dosage option and options other than medications, have been developed.[37]

Prokinetic drugs such as mosapride, tegaserod, urecholine, and metoclopramide have been used to improve gastric emptying to reduce intragastric pressure and events of reflux. Although these drugs have potential beneficial effects on upper gastrointestinal motor function, results have generally been disappointing when they are used as single agents. The use of metoclopramide has been further limited by the frequent occurrence of neuropsychiatric side effects, including agitation, insomnia, and lethargy. Prokinetic agents are occasionally used as adjunctive agents in combination with H_2-blockers and PPIs in patients with more severe disease.

Reflux can be controlled in the majority of patients with the judicious use of medication. Surgical intervention is generally reserved for occasional patients whose disease is **refractory** to medical management. A number of operations have been described; most involve reestablishing the intraabdominal location of the esophagogastric junction (hiatal hernia repair) in combination with wrapping a portion of the stomach around part or the whole circumference of the lower esophagus (**fundoplication**). **Laparoscopic** approaches to antireflux surgery have been developed and appear to be as effective as traditional surgical approaches with a more rapid recovery. Surgery is effective in controlling reflux in approximately 80% to 90% of patients in whom it is used.[15]

Newer nonsurgical, endoscopic approaches used to control GERD include suturing of the LES, electrical stimulation,[38] and radiofrequency ablation (Stretta procedure). Radiofrequency ablation attempts to place lesions in the wall of the stomach to reduce the frequency of tSLERs. Although no randomized trials have compared the Stretta procedure to other surgically based procedures, early data suggest a trend toward a reduction of PPI use and an increase in quality-of-life scores.[39] Specific subject selection for these procedures and efficacy data still need to be established.

LARYNGOPHARYNGEAL REFLUX

LPR occurs when stomach contents reach the laryngeal level, frequently resulting in odynophagia, hoarseness, sore throat, a globus sensation, and chronic throat clearing. Painful swallow and a feeling that something is sticking in the cervical region frequently give rise to reports of dysphagia. The mechanism by which refluxate reaches the level of the posterior larynx is unknown. Endoscopic evaluation of the upper airway shows mucosal abnormalities on the posterior pharyngeal wall, marked edema on the arytenoid cartilages, and generalized **erythema** in the laryngeal aditus. Patients with LPR differ from those with classic GERD in the following ways: (1) most events occur during the day without nighttime episodes, (2) higher doses of medication are needed for longer periods to achieve adequate control, and (3) esophageal motility and acid clearance mechanisms are normal. Patients with LPR and GERD are similar in the following ways: (1) results of 24-hour pH or radiographic studies may not always be positive, (2) the PES and LES often are normal, and (3) heartburn may be described.

DIFFERENTIAL DIAGNOSIS

Unlike disorders that affect oropharyngeal function, clues to the cause of esophageal disorders often can be determined with a thorough history. Because the disorders can be conveniently divided into structural and motor, and because of the importance of asking the question of whether solids, liquids, or both are important to the diagnosis, the use of a decision tree can be useful in guiding the clinician in the decision of what tests to order and what signs and symptoms to evaluate. Donner and Castell[40] suggest the use of a decision tree to guide differential diagnosis (Figure 5-9). The decision tree is normally used when the patient denies events of coughing and choking during meals

(highly correlated with oropharyngeal dysphagia) and most likely has more complaints about solid food than liquids.

DISORDERS OF THE PHARYNGEAL ESOPHAGEAL SEGMENT

The differential diagnosis of disorders from failed PES mechanics include disorders from poor traction (hyoid bone deficits); disorders of relaxation (neurogenic); disorders within the cricopharyngeal muscle, such as fibrosis, webs, **myositis**, and dystrophy; and disorders from failure of the cricopharyngeal muscle to relax or contract. Radiographic studies typically show a restriction of bolus flow through the region, particularly for solid food and often on multiple, consecutive attempts with fluids. When the diagnosis is confirmed as a PES abnormality, patients often initially report food sticking at the level of the cervical esophagus. However, most patients who describe solid food sticking at the level of the cervical esophagus often have disorders of esophageal origin (see Pharyngoesophageal Relations in this chapter).[41]

Cricopharyngeal Bar

The radiographic appearance of a "bar" at the level of the cricopharyngeal muscle (C6-C7) is believed to be the result of failure of the muscle to fully distend (Figure 5-10). In most cases manometric relaxation is found to be normal.[42] Failure of distention may range from mild to severe. In the severe forms, restriction of bolus flow may cause retrograde propulsion with spillage into the airway. Cricopharyngeal bars may be seen in 30% of older adults with no symptoms

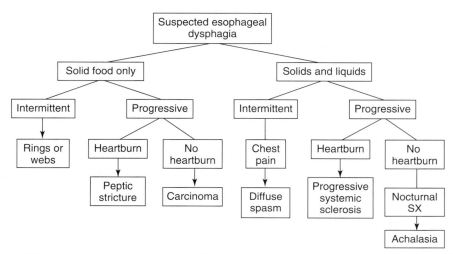

FIGURE 5-9   A differential diagnostic decision tree to be taken from patient report when suspicion for an esophageal-based disorder is high. Confirmation of the diagnosis is made with the appropriate laboratory tests. The decision tree may help in guiding the selection and order of testing. *SX,* Symptoms.

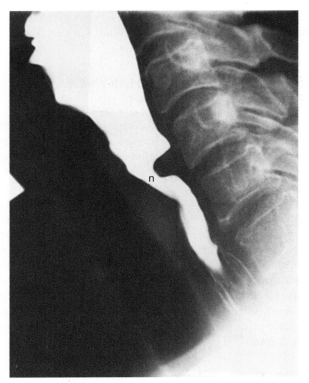

FIGURE 5-10 The cricopharyngeal muscle has pushed into the barium column, causing a narrowing (n) of the barium column. This creates the visual impression of a bar.

of dysphagia,[43] even though the intrusion of the muscle into the bolus pathway may be small or transitory. Some studies have suggested that the failure of the cricopharyngeal muscle to distend adequately is related to muscle hypertrophy rather than failed PES mechanics and is more common in older adults. These findings on autopsy suggest a change in muscle fiber composition with aging and the potential for decreased cricopharyngeal muscle performance.[44,45] One theory for the formation of cricopharyngeal bars is that they result from increased tone (higher PES pressures) in the cervical esophagus as a result of the failure of the LES to relax.[46] This suggests that patients with cricopharyngeal bars should have a complete evaluation of the esophagus, including manometric and radiographic swallowing studies. Treatment for symptomatic cricopharyngeal bars includes dilatation[47] and cricopharyngeal myotomy.[48]

The formation of so-called pharyngeal pouches (diverticula) may be related to the pathophysiology of cricopharyngeal bars, although they may not always coexist. Pharyngeal pouches are lateral protrusions on the pharyngeal wall seen at the level of the thyrohyoid membrane. When they are large, these pouches collect swallowed material, delay bolus flow, and may cause dysphagic symptoms. Pouches that empty after the swallow may result in piriform sinus accumulation with the possibility of postswallow aspiration.[49] Similar to cricopharyngeal bars, they may be the result of an unyielding PES with a subsequent increase in hypopharyngeal pressures that causes pouch formation above the level of the obstruction. Video 5-8 shows a patient with lateral pharyngeal pouches.

Zenker's Diverticulum

The name *Zenker's diverticulum* is reserved for a diverticulum that develops on the posterior pharyngeal wall in the region of the PES. Most often it represents a protrusion of the hypopharyngeal mucosa at the boundary of the transverse fibers of the cricopharyngeal muscle and the oblique fibers of the inferior constrictor muscle (Killian's dehiscence). These diverticula may be small and remain confined to the hypopharyngeal region. When larger, they may extend into the cervical esophagus. They often are associated with reduced flow through the PES and may cause postswallow aspiration. Figure 5-11, *C*, is representative of the radiographic appearance of a Zenker's diverticulum with tracheal aspiration. An example of a Zenker's diverticulum can also be seen in Video 5-9.

The origin of the development of a Zenker's diverticulum is controversial. Some have suggested that the pouch develops from high intrabolus pressure created by a resistance to flow through the PES, possibly either from failure of the cricopharyngeus muscle to relax or from premature closure.[42] Over time, the continued high pressures cause the hypopharyngeal mucosa to herniate through Killian's dehiscence, resulting in the formation of a diverticulum. Cook et al.[50] studied 14 patients with Zenker's diverticulum

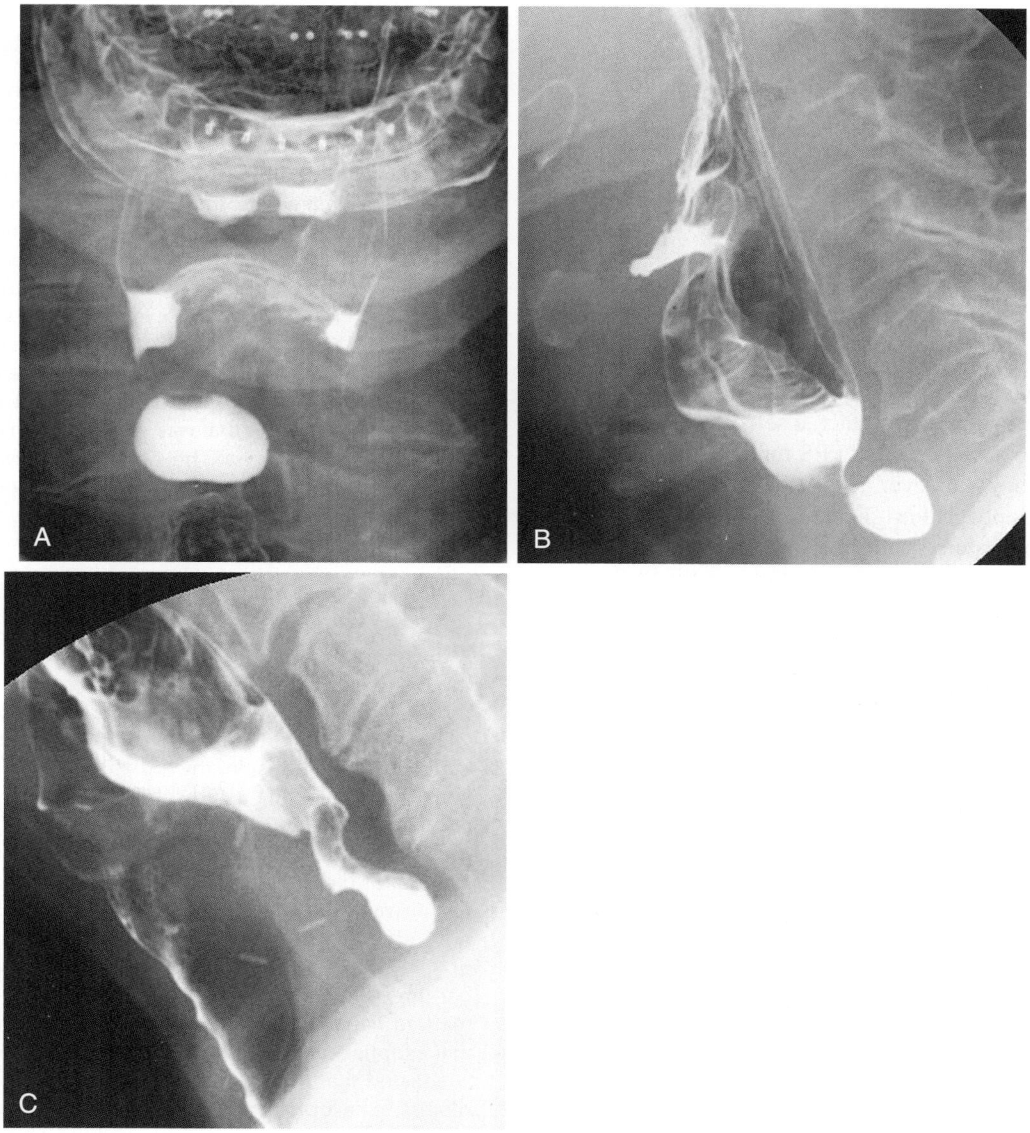

FIGURE 5-11 **A** and **B** show the frontal and lateral views, respectively, centered on the hypopharynx of a barium-filled diverticulum extending posteriorly near the junction with the cervical esophagus. **A,** The diverticulum is seen at the inferior portion of the image. Above the diverticulum the piriform and vallecular spaces also are filled with barium. **B,** In the lateral view the narrowing of the pharyngeal esophageal segment can be seen with the barium column in the piriform sinus above it. **C,** Another patient (lateral view) with a diverticulum seen inferiorly with a considerable collection of barium in the pharynx that has spilled into the trachea; this is seen as a line of barium on the left side of the image. (From Pickhardt PJ, Arluk GM: Atlas of gastrointestinal imaging: radiologic-endoscopic correlation, 2007, Saunders Elsevier.)

using videofluoroscopy and manometry. They concluded that the diverticulum was not responsible for the poor flow through the PES. They suggested that because mechanical traction and relaxation parameters were normal, the resistance to flow with subsequent development of a diverticulum must be from a lack of compliance (fibrosis or myopathy) within the cricopharyngeal muscle body, resulting in a higher than normal resting tone. Other investigators have found a relation between premature closure of the PES

caused by GERD, perhaps as a compensation for keeping any offending refluxate from entering the upper airway.[51] Sasaki et al.[52] have proposed the esophageal shortening theory and GERD as a possible explanation of the development of Zenker's diverticulum. During normal swallowing the esophagus shortens to propel the bolus to the stomach. In patients with chronic GERD, the inflammatory response to acid results in abnormal shortening capability of the esophageal longitudinal muscle. Therefore when the esophagus contracts abnormally, it pulls the hypopharyngeal musculature distally away from its caudal attachments, allowing the pouch to form. Zenker's diverticulum is treated either by surgical reduction to include cricopharyngeal myotomy[53] or by endoscopic stapling.[54]

PHARYNGOESOPHAGEAL RELATIONS

As detailed in Chapter 2, OK as is the stages of swallowing are interdependent. Primary disease in one stage may affect other stages. Examples of this concept may be common in patients who describe dysphagia localized to the neck but who may have a primary disorder of the esophagus as the cause of their symptoms. In fact, a select group of patients does appear to have abnormal PES function with dysphagic symptomatology; however, it is likely to be the result of a disorder of esophageal origin.

For instance, numerous investigators have found both manometric and radiologic abnormalities in the PES caused by achalasia.[46,55-57] One possible theory is that resistance to flow in the LES causes pressure changes in the esophagus above the level of obstruction perceived by the patient at the level of the PES. Interestingly, there is evidence that successful dilatation of the LES relieves the dysphagic symptoms localized to the neck in patients with achalasia.[58] There also is some evidence that patients with GERD may have dysphagia localized to the level of the PES, possibly as a response to esophageal acidification resulting in a esophageal-PES hypercontractility[59] or because chronic GERD may result in pharyngeal-based compensations that change the mechanics of the PES.[59,60] A change in pharyngeal biomechanics is subsequently perceived by the patient as dysphagia. The relation between GERD and PES symptoms has not been proven, and there is no evidence that controlling GERD reduces symptoms localized to the cervical esophagus. Nonetheless, patients who report cervical dysphagia without abnormal findings after modified barium swallow studies might be candidates for an evaluation of GERD, even in the absence of the traditional symptoms of heartburn and regurgitation.

TAKE HOME NOTES

1. The esophagus has two sphincters, the upper esophageal sphincter and the LES. The upper esophageal sphincter shares physiologic functions with the hypopharyngeal musculature. Physiologically this region is best described as the *pharyngeal esophageal segment (PES)*.
2. Structural disorders such as a stricture as a result of GERD affect the lumen of the esophagus, causing a reduction of bolus flow and dysphagia.
3. External compression of the esophagus, such as from an enlarged heart, could narrow the lumen of the esophagus with resultant dysphagia.

> **CLINICAL CASE EXAMPLE 5-2   SCHATZKI'S RING**
>
> A 64-year-old woman told her primary care physician that over the past 6 months she felt food was sticking in her throat. She was referred to the SLP for a modified barium swallow study. The evaluation of her oropharyngeal mechanism was normal, and she denied any history of esophageal-related disease. The modified barium swallow study was done with thin and thick barium while the patient was standing. The study showed normal flow through the region of the PES in the lateral view. In the frontal view, a restriction of flow was seen at the level of the LES as a mild indentation of the barium column (Video 5-10). A follow-up esophagram revealed a suspected Schatzki's ring that was confirmed on endoscopy by a gastroenterologist. The patient underwent dilatation and the cervical dysphagic symptoms resolved.

> **CLINICAL CASE EXAMPLE 5-3   CRICOPHARYNGEAL HYPERTROPHY**
>
> A 40-year-old man came to the clinic and stated that over the past year he felt that solid food was sticking in his throat. He reported that he had a significant history of GERD and was taking PPIs irregularly. He noted that he had lost 10 pounds in the past 3 months. A barium imaging swallowing study revealed a hypertrophic cricopharyngeal muscle that caused a reduction of solid food through the region of the PES. However, the solid food bolus did enter the esophagus and did not spill into the airway. Because the obstruction to solid food was not judged as severe and the patient had a past history of GERD that had not been reevaluated, a standard barium esophagram was ordered. This study revealed a marked narrowing in the region of the LES with abnormal esophageal motility and a dilated esophagus. It was suggested that the patient be referred to a gastroenterologist for esophageal endoscopy. Endoscopy revealed marked esophageal stenosis at the junction of the esophagus and stomach.
>
> In this case, the patient's report of solid food sticking in the neck was verified by the videofluorographic swallowing study. However, the history suggested that the patient had lost a significant amount of weight. The amount of weight loss seemed disproportionate to the degree of PES narrowing. In addition, the patient had a history of GERD that probably was not well controlled. Because of this, he was susceptible to primary esophageal disease, and tests confirmed this suspicion. The abnormality seen in the PES probably was a result of excessive pressure changes on the PES from a lack of esophageal motility. Alternate hypotheses for PES dysfunction include direct acid contact that resulted in cricopharyngeal hypertrophy, or an irritation of cranial nerve X that resulted in poor PES opening and closing mechanics. Treatment in this case would be aimed at dilatation of the LES stricture and medication to control the GERD.

4. Motor (motility) disorders affect the movement or peristalsis of the esophagus. Diffuse esophageal spasm and achalasia are examples of motor disorders.

5. Disorders of the PES may have numerous causes that result in either reduced relaxation or opening of the PES. These include oral and pharyngeal weakness that may cause disorders of traction (opening), neurologic disease (loss of relaxation), disorders within the PES musculature such as myositis and fibrosis, and disorders of esophageal motility that secondarily affect PES function.

6. Disorders specific to the region of the PES include cricopharyngeal bars, lateral pharyngeal pouches, and Zenker's diverticulum.

7. Patients who report solid food dysphagia with food sticking in the cervical region may be susceptible to disorders of the esophagus and not to disease affecting the hypopharyngeal or cervical region.

REFERENCES

1. Edwards DAW: Diagnostic procedures: history and symptoms of esophageal disease. In Vantrappen G, Hellemans J, editors: *Diseases of the esophagus*, New York, 1974, Springer-Verlag.

2. Jones B, Ravich WJ, Kramer SS, et al: Pharyngoesophageal interrelationships: observations and working concepts. *Gastrointest Radiol* 10:225, 1985.

3. Schatzki R: The lower esophageal ring: long term follow-up of symptomatic and asymptomatic rings. *Am J Roentgenol Radium Ther Nucl Med* 90:805, 1963.

4. Goyal RK, Bauer JL, Spiro HM: The nature and location of the lower esophageal ring. *N Engl J Med* 284:1175, 1971.

5. Groskreutz JL, Kim CH: Schatzki's ring: long-term results following dilatation. *Gastrointest Endosc* 36:479, 1990.

6. Ravich WJ, Kashima H, Donner MW: Drug-induced esophagitis simulating esophageal cancer. *Dysphagia* 1:13, 1986.

7. Earlam R, Cunha-Melo JR: Oesophageal squamous cell carcinoma: a critical review of surgery. *Br J Surg* 67:381, 1980.

8. Forastiere AA, Orringer MB, Perez-Tamayo C, et al: Preoperative chemoradiation followed by transhiatal esophagectomy for carcinoma of the esophagus. *J Clin Oncol* 11:1118, 1993.

9. Parker EF, Moertel CF: Is there a role for surgery in esophageal carcinoma? *Am J Dig Dis* 23:730, 1978.

10. Kinoshita Y, Endo M, Nakayama K, et al: Evaluation of ten-year survival after operation for upper- and midthoracic esophageal cancer. *Int Adv Surg Oncol* 1:173, 1978.

11. Dimarino AT, Cohen S: Characteristics of lower esophageal sphincter function in symptomatic diffuse esophageal spasm. *Gastroenterology* 66:1, 1974.

12. Brand Dl, Martin D, Pope CE: Esophageal manometrics in patients with anginal type chest pain. *Am J Dig Dis* 23:300, 1977.

13. Castell DO: The nutcracker esophagus and other primary esophageal motility disorders. In Castell DO, Richter JE, Dalton CB, editors: *Esophageal motility testing*, New York, 1987, Elsevier.

14. Dalton CB, Castell DO, Richter JE: The changing faces of the nutcracker esophagus. *Am J Gastroenterol* 83:623, 1988.

15. Ravich WJ: Esophageal dysphagia. In Groher ME, editor: *Dysphagia: diagnosis and management*, Boston, 1997, Butterworth-Heinemann.

16. Katzka DA: The skinny on eosinophilic esophagitis. *Gastroenterology* 145:1186, 2013.

17. Davis HA, Lewis MJ, Rhodes J, et al: Trial of nifedipine for prevention of esophageal spasm. *Digestion* 36:81, 1987.

18. Kahrilas PJ, Kishk SM, Helm JF, et al: Comparison of pseudoachalasia and achalasia. *Am J Med* 82:439, 1987.

19. Pasricha PJ, Ravich WJ, Hendrix TR, et al: Intrasphincteric botulinum toxin for the treatment of achalasia. *N Engl J Med* 332:774, 1995.

20. D'Angelo WA, Fries JF, Masi AT, et al: Pathologic observations in systemic sclerosis (scleroderma): a study of 58 autopsy cases and 58 matched controls. *Am J Med* 46:28, 1969.

21. Saltzman MB, McCallum RW: Diabetes and the stomach. *Yale J Biol Med* 56:179, 1983.

22. Enweluzo C, Aziz F: Gastroparesis: a review of current and emerging treatment options. *Clin Exp Gastroenterol* 6:161, 2013.

23. Castell DO, Johnston BT: Gastrointestinal reflux disease. Current strategies for patient management. *Arch Fam Med* 5:221, 1996.

24. Napierkowski J, Wong R: Extraesophageal manifestations of GERD. *Am J Med Sci* 326:279, 2003.

25. Liker H, Hungin P, Wiklund I: Managing gastroesophageal reflux disease in primary care: the patient perspective. *J Am Board Fam Pract* 18:393, 2005.

26. Manterola C, Munoz S, Grande L, et al: Initial validation of a questionnaire for detecting gastroesophageal reflux disease in epidemiological settings. *J Clin Epidemiol* 55:1041, 2002.

27. Dickman R, Bautista JM, Wong WM, et al: Comparison of esophageal acid exposure distribution along the esophagus among the different gastroesophageal reflux disease (GERD) groups. *Am J Gastroenterol* 101:2463, 2006.

28. Calabrese C, Fabbri A, Bortolotti M, et al: Dilated intercellular spaces as a marker of oesophageal damage: comparative results in gastro-oesophageal reflux disease with or without bile reflux. *Ailment Pharmacol Ther* 18:525, 2003.

29. Dent J: Patterns of lower esophageal sphincter function associated with gastroesophageal reflux. *Am J Med* 103:29S, 1997.

30. Richter JE, Castell DO: Drugs, foods and other substances in the cause and treatment of reflux esophagitis. *Med Clin North Am* 65:1223, 1981.

31. Mainie I, Tutuian R, Shay S, et al: Acid and non-acid reflux in patients with persistent symptoms despite acid suppressive therapy: a multicentre study using combined ambulatory impedance-pH monitoring. *Gut* 55:1398, 2006.

32. Iascone C, DeMeester TR, Little AG: Barrett's esophagus: functional assessment, proposed pathogenesis, and surgical therapy. *Arch Surg* 118:543, 1983.

33. Richter JE, Castell DO: Gastroesophageal reflux disease: pathogenesis, diagnosis, and therapy. In Castell DO, Johnson LF, editors: *Esophageal function in health and disease*, New York, 1983, Elsevier.

34. Conchillo JM, Smout AJ: Review article: Intraesophageal impedance monitoring for the assessment of bolus transit and gastro-oesophageal reflux. *Aliment Pharmacol Ther* 29:3, 2009.

35. Kulinna-Cosentini C, Schima W, Lenglinger J, et al: Is there a role for dynamic swallowing MRI in the assessment of gastroesophageal reflux disease and oesophageal motility disorders? *Eur Radiol* 22:364, 2012.

36. Milkes D, Gerson LB, Triadafilopoulos G: Complete elimination of reflux symptoms does not guarantee normalization of intraesophageal and intragastric pH in patients with gastroesophageal reflux disease (GERD). *Am J Gastroenterol* 99:991, 2004.

37. Tytgat GN, McColl J, Tack J, et al: New algorithm for the treatment of gastro-oesophageal reflux disease. *Aliment Pharmacol Ther* 27:249, 2008.

38. Rodriguez L, Rodriguez P, Gomez B, et al: Electrical stimulation therapy of the lower esophageal sphincter is successful in treating GERD: final results of open-label prospective trial. *Surg Endosc* 27:1083, 2013.

39. Reymunde A, Santiago N: Long term results of radiofrequency energy delivery for the treatment of GERD: sustained improvements in symptoms, quality of life, and drug use at 4 year follow-up. *Gastrointest Endosc* 65:361, 2007.

40. Donner MW, Castell DO: Evaluation of dysphagia: a careful history is crucial. *Dysphagia* 2:65, 1987.

41. Roeder BE, Murray JA, Dierkhising A: Patient localization of esophageal dysphagia. *Dig Dis Sci* 49:697, 2004.

42. Goyal RK: Disorders of the cricopharyngeus muscle. *Otolaryngol Clin North Am* 49:115, 1984.

43. Leonard R, Kendall K, McKenzie S: UES opening and cricopharyngeal bar in nondysphagic elderly and nonelderly adults. *Dysphagia* 19:182, 2004.

44. Torres WE, Clements JL, Austin GE, et al: Cricopharyngeal muscle hypertrophy: radiologic-anatomic correlation. *AJR Am J Roentgenol* 142:927, 1984.

45. Xu S, Tu L, Wang Q, et al: Is the anatomical protrusion on the posterior hypopharyngeal wall associated with cadavers of only the elderly? *Dysphagia* 21:163, 2006.

46. Zhang ZG, Diamant NE: Repetitive contractions of the upper esophageal body and sphincter in achalasia. *Dysphagia* 9:12, 1994.

47. Wang AY, Kadkade R, Kahrilas PJ, et al: Effectiveness of esophageal dilation for symptomatic cricopharyngeal bar. *Gastrointest Endosc* 61:148, 2005.

48. Bonavina L, Khan AN, DeMeester TR: Pharyngoesophageal dysfunctions: the role of cricopharyngeal myotomy. *Arch Surg* 120:541, 1985.

49. Jones B, Donner MW: *Normal and abnormal swallowing: imaging in diagnosis and therapy*, New York, 1990, Springer-Verlag.

50. Cook IJ, Gabb M, Panagopoulos V, et al: Pharyngeal (Zenker's) diverticulum is a disorder of upper esophageal sphincter opening. *Gastroenterology* 103:1229, 1992.

51. Brady AP, Stevenson GW, Somers S, et al: Premature contraction of the cricopharyngeus: a new sign of gastroesophageal reflux disease. *Abdom Imaging* 20:225, 1995.

52. Sasaki CT, Ross DA, Hundal J: Association between Zenker diverticulum and gastroesophageal reflux disease: development of a working hypothesis. *Am J Med* 115:1695, 2003.

53. Sen P, Lowe DA, Farnan T: Surgical interventions for pharyngeal pouch. *Cochrane Database Syst Rev* (3):CD004449, 2005.

54. Casso C, Lalam M, Ghosh S, et al: Endoscopic stapling diverticulotomy: an audit of difficulties, outcome, and patient satisfaction. *Otolaryngol Head Neck Surg* 134:288, 2006.

55. Jones B, Donner MW, Rubesin SE, et al: Pharyngeal findings in 21 patients with achalasia of the esophagus. *Dysphagia* 2:87, 1987.

56. DeVault KR: Incomplete upper esophageal sphincter relaxation: association with achalasia but not other esophageal motility disorders. *Dysphagia* 12:157, 1997.

57. Yoneyama F, Miyachi M, Nimura Y: Manometric findings of the upper esophageal sphincter in esophageal achalasia. *World J Surg* 22:1043, 1998.

58. Torrico S, Kern M, Aslam M, et al: Upper esophageal sphincter function during gastroesophageal reflux events revisited. *Am J Physiol Gastrointest Liver Physiol* 279:G262, 2000.

59. Sivit CJ, Curtis DJ, Crain M, et al: Pharyngeal swallow in gastroesophageal reflux disease. *Dysphagia* 2:151, 1988.

60. Mendell DA, Logemann JA: A retrospective analysis of the pharyngeal swallow in patients with a clinical diagnosis of GERD compared with normal controls. *Dysphagia* 17:220, 2002.

CHAPTER 6

Respiratory and Iatrogenic Disorders

Michael E. Groher

To view additional case videos and content, please visit the evolve website.

CHAPTER OUTLINE

OBJECTIVES

1. Detail how disorders of respiration might affect swallowing performance.
2. Discuss common medical and surgical complications that lead to or exacerbate dysphagia.
3. Review how artificial supports for respiration might interfere with swallowing.

BACKGROUND

As detailed in Chapter 2, the interactions between breathing and swallowing are well known. Swallow coordination and subsequent upper airway protection depend on the normal interaction between these two related phenomena. It follows that disorders of breathing, such as can occur after a stroke, might either be the cause of dysphagia or could exacerbate it.[1] Some patients enter the acute hospital setting with primary respiratory tract disease, such as congestive obstructive pulmonary disease with or without accompanying dysphagia. Others enter the acute care setting for medical reasons not related to their cardiopulmonary status but have cardiopulmonary complications, such as patients who undergo cardiac bypass surgery requiring **intubation**, support by respirator, or tracheotomy. Medical and surgical complications that result in dysphagic complications can be classified as iatrogenic. The side effects of radiation therapy on swallowing after treatment of cancer are classified as iatrogenic but are discussed in detail in Chapter 4.

ARTIFICIAL AIRWAYS

Patients with compromised respiratory status may require special interventions to support basic life functions. These supports include endotracheal or tracheostomy tubes that may or may not be connected to a mechanical respirator and oxygen delivered either by facial mask or through a nasal cannula. A potential side effect of oxygen use is xerostomia with its attendant negative effect on swallowing.

Endotracheal Tubes

Endotracheal tubes are long, plastic, flexible tubes that are inserted through the mouth, through the vocal folds, and

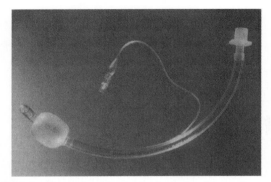

FIGURE 6-1 The endotracheal tube is designed to go through the mouth and below the level of the vocal folds into the trachea. This example shows the cuff on the end in the inflated position. The cuff is inflated by the small catheter in the middle of the photograph. (Photo courtesy Smiths Medical.)

into the trachea to aid the patient in respiratory distress. They are designed to be connected to a respirator to help the patient breathe. At the end of the tube is a cuff that is inflated to prevent oral secretions from entering the lungs by sealing the tracheal lumen and to keep air from escaping from the lungs past the tube (Figure 6-1). Keeping the desired respiratory volumes within the lungs is important to restore respiratory competence. Respirator settings are determined by the medical team and are implemented by the respiratory therapist. Placement of an endotracheal tube is considered a temporary measure (7 to 12 days) to establish respiratory competence. Longer periods of intubation may cause permanent laryngeal and lung injury because of local irritation to the mucosa. **Granulomas** and **hematomas** on the vocal folds and pharyngeal ulceration and edema may give rise to voice and swallowing complications. In some cases vocal fold paralysis or weakness may develop. Settings (inhalation and exhalation cycles) on the respirator are progressively adjusted to allow the patient to regain independent breathing. The endotracheal tube is removed as normal breathing patterns are achieved. Removal of the endotracheal tube does not guarantee that the patient will not experience further respiratory distress requiring reintubation. Multiple reintubations suggest that the patient's respiratory status is tenuous and may lead to a tracheotomy as a longer term approach to airway maintenance.

Bypassing the functions of the upper airway with an endotracheal tube precludes the patient from eating and swallowing because the presence of the tube means the vocal folds and oral cavity and pharynx are not available for swallowing activity. If successful extubation is achieved, the physician may request a swallowing evaluation before the patient starts oral feeding. Because the traditional method of breathing has been altered for some time, these patients may have difficulty speaking and swallowing immediately after the removal of the endotracheal tube.

Partik et al.[2] used videofluoroscopy to study 21 patients who were intubated for a mean of 24.6 days. They found that 86% of this group showed signs of aspiration after intubation. The majority of aspiration occurred before the swallow response, suggesting oral-stage weakness and subsequent poor laryngeal elevation. De Lariminat et al.[3] were interested in whether difficulty with postextubation swallowing was acute or chronic. Using swallow response times as the measurement of function, they found swallow delay on all bolus volumes on day 1, shorter but abnormal latencies on day 2, and normal response times by day 7. These results imply that interruptions in normal respiratory function may inhibit normal swallow response time but that, over time, they will recover without specific treatment. After systematically reviewing 14 articles that met inclusion criteria from a sample of 288, Skoretz et al.[4] found a wide variance in the reported prevalence of dysphagia following intubation (3% to 62%). Three studies reported prevalences of more than 50% in those who had prolonged intubation. These prevalence figures were not associated with any particular premorbid diagnosis.

Tracheotomy Tubes

Patients for whom weaning from endotracheal intubation is not possible may require the surgical placement of a tracheotomy tube. A vertical incision typically is made between the second and third tracheal rings so that the tube is below the level of the vocal folds to allow the medical team access to the lungs for suctioning. Other advantages over endotracheal intubation include the possibility for swallowing and speaking, less trauma to the vocal folds, and patient comfort. Tracheotomy tubes are available in various sizes, usually determined by the inner diameter of the lumen. Commonly used sizes are 8, 6, and 4 mm. The larger the tube size, generally the more difficult it is to get air around the tube up to the level of the vocal fold for phonation (Figure 6-2).

Decreasing the tube size from 8 to 6 mm is commonly done to reinvolve the upper airway for speech and swallowing and eventually for total decannulation. However, there are no prospective, empirical data studying the role of tracheotomy downsizing and its effect on speech and swallow (see Clinical Corner 6-2). Figure 6-3 shows a patient who underwent a tracheostomy with a close-up view of the tube in place. Complications of a tracheotomy tube include decreased sense of smell and taste because the direction of airflow is not through the nose and mouth, infection at the tracheotomy site, and increased secretions from the body's response to a foreign object. Tracheomalacia, or a breakdown of tissue on the posterior pharyngeal wall as a result of constant irritation, is rare. When severe, such tissue breakdown may create a tracheoesophageal fistula with resultant aspiration of food or secretions.

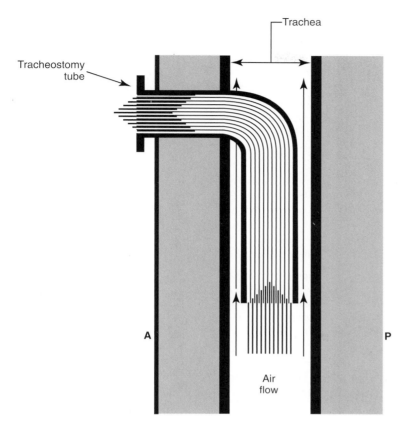

Trachea

Tracheostomy tube

A

P

Air flow

FIGURE 6-2 The tracheotomy tube is placed in the neck below the level of the vocal folds. The larger the diameter of the tube in the trachea, the more difficult it is to get air past the tube up to the vocal folds. Most of the pulmonary air for speaking would be directed through the tube. The smaller the tube lumen, the easier it is to get air up to the vocal folds. **A,** Anterior neck; **P,** posterior neck.

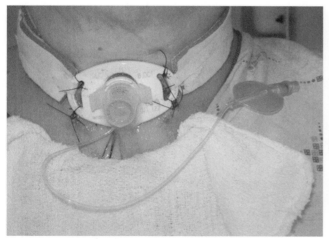

FIGURE 6-3 Close-up view of a tracheostomy tube. The tube is initially anchored by sutures and held in place around the neck by ties. The inner diameter of the tube can be read as 8 mm on the upper right section of the flange. The outer diameter is marked as 12.7 mm. The patient's secretions coughed from the lungs can be seen in and around the tube.

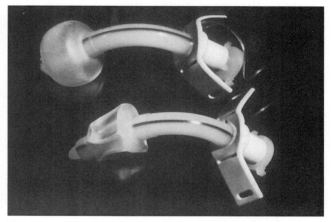

FIGURE 6-4 An example of a cuffed tracheotomy tube inflated (top) and deflated.

Tracheotomy tubes are either cuffed or noncuffed. The cuff is the portion on the end of the tube that can be inflated with air externally by using a syringe (Figure 6-4). When the cuff is inflated it theoretically seals off the entrance to the lungs in an effort to prevent aspiration of secretions or food. If the patient is also receiving ventilation from a respirator, the cuff ensures that the volume of air being delivered does not leak into the upper airway. The cuff may be advantageous in protecting the lungs, but its presence restricts voice and limits swallow by anchoring the larynx (Figure 6-5 and Clinical Corner 6-1). In a retrospective review of videofluoroscopic evaluations of patients swallowing with the cuff inflated and deflated, Ding and Logemann[5] found a higher prevalence

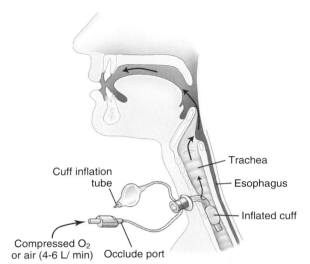

FIGURE 6-5 The inflated cuff protects the lung from secretions entering the airway above the level of inflation and keeps air from entering the upper airway. In addition, because the cuff is inflated, the laryngeal framework is anchored, potentially restricting laryngeal elevation during swallowing. (From Lewis S, Heitkemper M, Bucher L: http://www.us.elsevierhealth.com/product.jsp?isbn=9780323065 801 Medical-Surgical Nursing, ed 8, Mosby, St. Louis, 2011.)

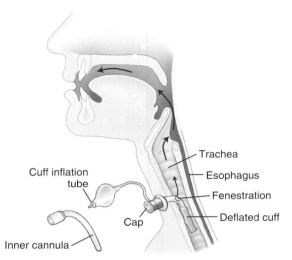

FIGURE 6-6 The fenestration in the top of the tracheotomy tube allows additional pulmonary air to flow to the vocal folds. (From Lewis S, Heitkemper M, Bucher L: http://www.us.elsevierhealth.com/ product.jsp?isbn=9780323065801 Medical-Surgical Nursing, ed 8, Mosby, St. Louis, 2011.)

CLINICAL CORNER 6-1: CARDIAC SURGERY

A 76-year-old man had cardiac bypass surgery and was doing well until the second postoperative day, when he had a respiratory arrest. An endotracheal tube was immediately placed and connected to a respirator. Eventually a cuffed tracheotomy tube had to be placed. The speech-language pathologist was consulted for a swallowing evaluation. As part of the evaluation he wanted to check the patient's voice.

Critical Thinking
1. Why is an evaluation of the patient's voice important?
2. To start the evaluation of voice, what should the speech-language pathologist ask the physician or nurse?

CLINICAL CORNER 6-2: DOWNSIZING TRACHEOSTOSTOMY

A 37-year-old woman had acute kidney and liver failure; eventually she required a tracheotomy and underwent multiple failed intubations. Her respiratory status was not stable, but the patient wanted to eat so the speech-language pathologist was consulted. She noted that with the no. 8 tracheotomy cuff down the patient was unable to phonate and suggested that if possible the medical staff consider either downsizing the tracheotomy tube or placing a no. 8 fenestrated tube. A no. 8 fenestrated tube was placed the next day and the speech-language pathologist went back for another evaluation. At this time, the patient was still unable to phonate.

Critical Thinking
1. What might explain why the patient still could not phonate?
2. Could the speech-language pathologist still check the patient's swallow even if she did not hear voicing?

---

of silent aspiration and changes in laryngeal biomechanics in the group with the cuff inflated.

Reexamination of Figure 6-3 shows the external catheter line to the internal cuff on the patient's chest. The balloon on the end of the catheter line is flat, indicating that the cuff on the end of the tracheotomy tube is deflated. When the balloon on the patient's chest is inflated, the cuff on the end of the tracheotomy tube can be assumed to be inflated.

In addition to the cuff versus no-cuff option, tracheotomy tubes may be fenestrated or nonfenestrated. A fenestration is a hole placed in the top of the tracheotomy tube to allow increased airflow to the upper airway, primarily for speaking (Figure 6-6).

SWALLOWING AND TRACHEOTOMY

Numerous studies from critical care medicine have noted a higher prevalence of aspiration events in patients with tracheotomy compared with those without tracheotomy.[6-8] Factors that may place patients with a tracheotomy at greater risk for aspiration include loss of subglottic air pressure,[9] poor laryngeal excursion related to the mechanical presence of the tube,[6] loss of upper airway sensitivity because of airway bypass, and loss of the normal laryngeal closure reflex during swallow.[10] Leder and Ross[11] used endoscopy to study 25 patients with multiple diagnoses prior to and after tracheotomy removal. Eighty-eight percent had a similar evaluation regardless of how long they had the tracheotomy or how old they were. These results appear to confirm that tracheotomy alone may not explain a higher prevalence of aspiration. Perhaps the fact that patients requiring tracheotomy are acutely ill and may not be able to coordinate a normal swallow because of muscle weakness or mental status fluctuations is a contributing factor to other studies that have found that those with tracheostomy tubes are at higher aspiration risk.

Laryngeal Excursion

Although many anecdotal descriptions exist of the tracheotomy tethering the larynx to the neck to reduce laryngeal excursion with subsequent aspiration, only one study has measured its effects on elevation. Terk et al.[12] studied seven patients with tracheotomy tubes without known dysphagia and concluded that elevation with the tracheotomy tube in place compared with when it was not in place showed no significant changes in laryngeal excursion measurements. However, factors of age, extent of respiratory illness, and prior medical history all must be considered before concluding that a tracheotomy tube does not affect laryngeal excursion.

Restoring Subglottic Pressure

Occlusion of the stoma at the tracheotomy site theoretically should help restore subglottic air pressure and improve swallow performance. Various methods of stoma occlusion have been studied, including digital occlusion, occlusion with a one-way valve such as a **Passy-Muir valve**, and occlusion from a cap placed at the stoma on the tracheotomy tube (see Practice Note 6-1).

Digital occlusion in eight patients with head and neck cancer showed mixed results.[13] In general, aspiration events were either reduced or eliminated. Some patients benefited with some bolus types, whereas others did not. All biomechanical measures, however, were normalized. The investigators concluded that the response to digital occlusion should be evaluated on a patient-by-patient basis. In a similar group of 16 postsurgical patients, Leder et al.[14] found no difference in

the prevalence of aspiration with or without finger occlusion. The use of one-way speaking valves and their effect on swallowing have been evaluated by numerous investigators with mixed findings.[15-18] Comparisons of studies are difficult because of subject selection variance, type of instrumentation to measure the effects on swallowing, swallowing outcome of interest, and length of time the valve was in place before the studies were conducted to assess swallowing status. All agree, however, that the placement of a valve improves speech and reduces upper airway secretions, restores olfaction, and improves patient ability to cough and clear secretions. In a mixed group of patients with chronic respiratory disease, Leder et al.[19] did not find any change in swallow-generated pharyngeal and cervical esophageal pressures with occlusion, either in those who aspirated or those who did not. Using endoscopy to study aspiration, Donzelli et al.[20] studied 37 patients—first with the tracheotomy in place and then with it removed with light digital occlusion over the tracheotomy site. Although some patients showed differences in aspiration and penetration patterns, for the majority there were no significant differences (review Practice Note 6-2).

CLINICAL CASE EXAMPLE 6-1

A 67-year-old man entered the hospital for knee replacement surgery. During the procedure he had a cardiac arrest and was resuscitated. After resuscitation he was intubated. Intubation includes insertion of an endotracheal tube and placement on a ventilator. A tracheotomy tube was inserted on the tenth postoperative day. The man's pulmonary status improved such that his physicians considered decannulation. He was being fed by nasogastric tube, and a modified barium swallow study was ordered to evaluate his ability to eat orally. Video 6-1 on the Evolve website shows the patient's modified barium swallow study, first with the tracheotomy tube unoccluded. On thin-liquid swallows there is obvious aspiration with cough that cleared some, but not all, of the aspirated contents. The chin-down position did facilitate airway protection. Thicker boluses showed penetration of the airway. After the study, the results were shared with the physician, who believed the feeding tube should remain in place. The physician was anxious to move toward decannulation and ordered that the patient's tube be capped as the first step. After tolerating the capped tube for 24 hours without difficulty, the patient was rescheduled for a modified barium swallow study before beginning oral feeding. Video 6-2 shows that with the tube capped (visible at the bottom of the image), the patient was able to protect his airway on all bolus types and volumes. A soft mechanical diet was ordered. After the patient successfully swallowed three meals, the tracheotomy tube was removed. The marked difference in swallowing safety demonstrated by this patient should not be generalized to all patients. Success or failure after tracheotomy occlusion should be put into the context of a patient's medical history and current medical status.

PRACTICE NOTE 6-1

Digital occlusion of a tracheotomy tube always is done with a gloved finger to prevent any contamination of the open airway. The examiner typically occludes the trachea at the moment of swallow. Digital occlusion is easiest with the thumb. Firm pressure is needed to achieve an adequate seal. Some patients can be taught self-occlusion and often benefit from a mirror to learn the process. Occlusion may assist in swallow performance and help the patient regain his or her speaking voice.

PRACTICE NOTE 6-2

Decannulation, or removal of a tracheotomy tube, although in the patient's best interest, may be one of the most disorganized and consequently lengthy processes in the medical center. Although some criteria for tube removal do exist—such as tolerances for breathing without supports and maintenance of adequate blood gases—rarely does one medical service or individual take responsibility for making the decision for removal. This is partly because of a lack of consensus on removal criteria and partly because of the physician's uncertainty that the patient will not incur any negative medical consequences and possibly require reintubation once the tube is removed.

POSTSURGICAL CAUSES OF DYSPHAGIA

Some surgical procedures, particularly those in the neck, predispose patients to postoperative dysphagia. Dysphagia results from (1) edema that restricts movement of swallowing structures such as the pharynx; (2) interference to the peripheral nerve supply to the muscles of swallowing, such as in **endarterectomy**, thyroidectomy, and cervical spinal fusion; (3) loss of central nervous system (brainstem) innervation, such as from posterior fossa or skull base surgery; or (4) replacement of swallowing structures that also may interfere with peripheral cranial nerves, such as in transhiatal esophagectomy. In surgical procedures that involve the neck region, it is difficult to identify the fibers of the pharyngeal plexus that innervate the pharyngeal constrictor muscles. This surgery may result in postoperative bilateral pharyngeal weakness that cannot be explained by isolated injury to the recurrent laryngeal nerve.[21] Using endoscopy, Leder et al.[22] found a 4.3% incidence of vocal fold immobility in those patients referred for dysphagia evaluation with multiple etiologic factors. Those with immobility were two and half more times likely to aspirate on thin liquids, and two times more likely to aspirate pureed foods. Using videofluoroscopy, Young et al.[23] noted that patients who demonstrated vocal fold paralysis that was central in origin had both oral and pharyngeal phase disorders, as opposed to those with paralysis of peripheral origin who demonstrated mostly pharyngeal abnormality.

Thyroidectomy

Surgical resection of all or part of the thyroid gland potentially can involve some disruption of motor and sensory branches of cranial nerve (CN) X. Unilateral vocal fold paralysis as a surgical complication compromises both voice and swallow. After follow-up of 39 patients for voice and swallow for 3 months after total thyroidectomy, Lombardi et al.[24] found persistent mild symptoms of voice and swallow abnormalities. In a series of 33 patients with thyroidectomy, Wasserman et al.[25] reported that 49% had preoperative swallowing difficulty, whereas 73% reported acute postoperative difficulty. They speculated that the prevalence of swallowing complaints was the result of injury to the extrinsic perithyroidal neural plexus innervating the pharyngeal and laryngeal structures. Using a questionnaire, Silva et al.[26] reported on 208 patients who underwent thyroidectomy. They found differences in reported symptoms of voice and swallowing disorders that depended on whether or not interoperative neuromonitoring was used during the procedure. In those without intraoperative monitoring, 26% had voice symptoms and 34% had dysphagia. In those with monitoring, 39% had voice symptoms and 27% were dysphagic. In a follow-up study of 60 patients, Pereira et al.[27] found that 15% of their patients had what they termed "nonspecific upper aerodigestive" complaints, including neck strangling, voice changes, and dysphagia. None of these studies provided objective, imaging swallowing data on the type or severity of the swallowing disorder.

Carotid Endarterectomy

Ekberg et al.[28] studied the swallowing ability of 12 patients before and after carotid endarterectomy. Findings for all swallowing studies were normal before surgery, but five patients had pharyngeal dysfunction and dysphagia after surgery. At 1 month after surgery, only two had swallowing complaints. These investigators speculated that the dysfunction was either attributable to peripheral nerve injury (vagus) or cerebrovascular damage during the procedure. Monini et al.[29] acknowledged the potential for cranial nerve involvement after carotid endarterectomy. Their follow-up of patients included serial examinations of voice and swallow for 60 days after surgery. Although most patients had only transient difficulty, 17.5% continued to have symptoms. Of those, only 9% required rehabilitation. In a related prospective study of 19 patients after endarterectomy, swallow endoscopies were done at 5 and 90 days after surgery. During the first evaluation, 15 of the 19 patients had dysphagia. Within 1 month, 10 patients returned to their regular diet, and an additional 6 did so by 90 days. The investigators suggested that the swallowing skills of patients after endarterectomy be closely monitored and rehabilitation strategies implemented if difficulties persisted.[30]

Cardiovascular Surgery

Patients who undergo procedures that reconstruct cardiac valves such as in coronary artery bypass grafts may suffer postoperative dysphagia. Because of the proximity of the tenth cranial nerve to the aorta, some patients may have temporary or prolonged vocal fold paralysis with accompanying dysphagia following their procedure. This may be complicated by postoperative complications requiring intubation or tracheotomy, or by general weakness following the procedure. In the absence of vocal fold involvement, patients who undergo major cardiovascular surgery may be at risk for dysphagia. In a large series of patients with multiple medical diagnoses precipitating their need for surgery, the incidence of postoperative dysphagia in this patient group was judged to be 4%.[31] Fifty-one percent of those requiring prolonged postsurgical intubation are dysphagic.[32] Silent aspiration is more prevalent in this patient group compared with other non–cardiac-related procedures.[33]

Cervical Spine Procedures and Conditions

Surgical stabilization of the cervical spine after trauma or surgery to eliminate pain and sensory or motor weakness from spinal nerve compression may secondarily result in oropharyngeal dysphagia. Surgical approaches to the cervical spine usually are through the anterior muscles of the neck. In some cases, a posterior approach or a combination of both may be used. Frequently, stabilization plates with screws are placed for long-term support of the cervical spine. Figure 6-7 shows a patient with an extensive posterior and anterior spine support at C2-C5 after a traumatic injury with accompanying anterior vertebral protrusions at C3-C4.

Abel et al.[34] provided demographic and outcome data for 73 patients with cervical spinal cord injury. Ten patients also sustained brain injury. Some patients required surgical intervention to stabilize the spine; others required intubation and tracheostomy. Oropharyngeal dysphagia was identified in 44% of patients. The authors concluded that surgical intervention was not related to dysphagia or the final outcomes but that the combination of tracheostomy and a rigid fixation device for postoperative stabilization **(halo)** predisposed patients to the most serious problems. Halo supports often put patients in a hyperextended position, which makes them more susceptible to tracheal aspiration.[35] Patients with dysphagia generally had longer hospitalizations and more medical complications.[34]

Surgical intervention into the cervical spine can cause injury to the pharyngeal plexus (CNs IX and X) with secondary pharyngeal weakness, direct injury to the esophagus causing local ischemia, edema in the prevertebral space resulting in loss of superior pharyngeal movement or, if the edema is extensive, the inability of the epiglottis to invert. Kepler et al.[36] used radiographic techniques to measure the amount of postsurgical edema at 2 and 6 weeks as it related to dysphagic complaints. After measuring the amount of postoperative edema in 43 patients they found no correlation between the amount of edema and dysphagia,

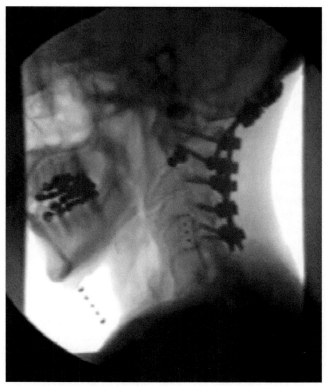

FIGURE 6-7 A metal appliance placed surgically in the posterior cervical spine for stabilization after an automobile accident is apparent. Patients with surgical procedures to the cervical spine may be at risk for postoperative dysphagia.

suggesting that other factors such as pharyngeal plexus injury may account for symptoms. It also is possible that retraction of the muscles and nerves in the neck to achieve exposure to the spine may result in peripheral nerve injury and vocal fold paralysis that contribute to dysphagia.[37] Patients with anterior cervical fusion (ACF) and swallowing disorders after surgery have received the most attention in the literature.

The incidence of dysphagic complications after ACF varies from 80%[38] to 6.5%.[39] The large variation is attributable to methods of detection (instrumental vs. patient report), definitions of dysphagia based on severity, and when the measurements were made. For instance, in a follow-up survey of patients at a mean duration of 3.3 years after surgery, 60% of the patients reported dysphagia, mostly with solids.[40] The evidence shows that dysphagia after ACF does improve with time. In a prospective study of 249 patients with ACF, Baraz et al.[41] documented the severity of dysphagic complaints by telephone at 1, 2, 6, and 12 months after surgery. The incidence steadily declined from 50.2% at 1 month to 12.5% at 6 months. Only patient gender (female) was related to an increased risk of dysphagia at 6 months. Other factors, such as age, type of procedure, level of surgery, and the type of stabilization hardware, were not related to the final outcome. After studying 135 patients with radiographic documentation of postoperative edema, Song et al.[42] concluded that there was a higher prevalence of dysphagia and dysphonia in those patients with higher cervical or multilevel procedures. Marquez-Lara et al.[43] and colleagues retrospectively analyzed a database of 1464 patients who had undergone ACF noting that 5.6% required reintubation from persistent airway compromise. This group tended to be older, had operated lesions involving three or more vertebra, and had a greater chance of developing aspiration pneumonia, presumably from dysphagic complications.

Buchholz et al.[44] used cineradiography to study patients who had ACF with cervical plates and dysphagic complaints (3 to 108 months later). The most common finding was a localized pharyngeal weakness at the site of the surgery with accompanying solid food dysphagia. They postulated that patients who initially had dysphagic complaints probably had some disruption in the pharyngeal constrictor muscles by way of the pharyngeal plexus and that a regeneration of those fibers was possible in those who totally recovered. Video 6-3 shows the same patient in Figure 6-7 on his fourth postoperative day. Note that the patient swallows thin liquids with some delay at the level of the piriform sinus, and what appears to be incoordination between pharyngeal contraction and pharyngeal esophageal segment (PES) relaxation is visible. As the bolus becomes increasingly thick, material collects at the vallecular level, causing the patient to report solid food sticking in the back of his throat. There is marked edema at the C3 level that restricts epiglottic inversion. The airway remains protected during all swallow attempts.

Osteophytes

Bony changes (osteophytes) in the vertebrae of the cervical spine may push on the posterior pharyngeal wall or esophagus, creating mechanical (obstructive) disorders of swallow (Figure 6-8). Often they are secondary to a syndrome known as *diffuse idiopathic skeletal hyperostosis*. Osteophytes are more common in older adults (20% to 30% of those who have them are in this age group) and most are asymptomatic.[45] In a series of 3318 patients referred for radiographic examination of suspected dysphagia, 1.7% had osteophytes that accounted for their symptoms.[46] Interestingly, 12 of the 55 patients with osteophytes had coexisting diseases, including histories of cancer surgery, thyroidectomy, and stroke. Osteophytes larger than 10 mm were associated with aspiration 75% of the time, whereas aspiration was found in 34% of those with osteophytes smaller than 10 mm. When they produce symptoms, osteophytes typically are at the C3 level, causing the epiglottis to not fully invert, or at the C6 level, resulting in disorders of flow through the PES and cervical esophagus. Osteophytes in both regions may result in aspiration. At the C3

level aspiration usually occurs during swallow, whereas at the C6 level it usually occurs after the swallow. In some cases osteophytes are associated with inflammation, edema, fibrosis, and pain with cricopharyngeal spasm, all of which can affect pharyngeal swallow mechanics.[47,48] Treatment options include neurosurgical intervention, postural changes such as the chin-down maneuver, and avoidance of solid food boluses. Zhang et al.[49] describe the successful surgical intervention in a 70-year-old with osteophytic changes that impeded cervical esophageal flow. Treatments are focused on the elimination of aspiration and subsequent pneumonia.

Postural Changes

Scoliosis, or changes in the alignment of the cervical spine, may interfere with the integrity of the pharyngeal swallow if the deformity is severe. Cervical **lordosis** or **kyphosis** has the potential to narrow the pharyngeal space with concomitant reduction of laryngeal elevation.[48] Congenital disorders such as **Klippel-Feil syndrome** and **Chiari-Arnold deformity** also may be at risk for cervical spine changes with accompanying risk for oropharyngeal dysphagia.[50]

Esophagectomy

Cancer of the esophagus most often necessitates the need for total esophagectomy. Typically, the esophagus is removed and replaced with tissue either from the stomach or **jejunum**. This tissue is connected to a remnant in the cervical esophagus and is referred to as the esophagopharyngeal **anastomosis**. For some patients, the anastomosis is made below this level in the thorax. In general, this procedure interferes with normal esophageal motility with presumed discoordination between the esophagus and pharynx, and may secondarily impair vagal innervation (recurrent laryngeal nerve) to the pharynx, although all pharyngeal-based symptoms cannot be accounted for on this basis alone.[48] Therefore patients who undergo esophagectomy may be at risk for oropharyngeal- and esophageal-based dysphagia. When dysphagia is present postoperatively in patients who have undergone esophagectomy, it is predictive of pneumonia and subsequent death.[48] Therefore early detection with fiberoptic endoscopy of swallow or videofluorographic swallowing studies and remediation before the initiation of oral feeding are important.[51,52] Atkins et al.[53] recommended serial evaluation of swallowing after esophagectomy to avoid the potential complications of aspiration. Using endoscopy, Leder et al.[51] found that immediately after surgery 21% of the 73 patients evaluated showed signs of vocal fold immobility and aspiration, implicating involvement of CN X. Patients with aspiration were not allowed to eat until examination results normalized. In a series of 26 consecutive patients who had

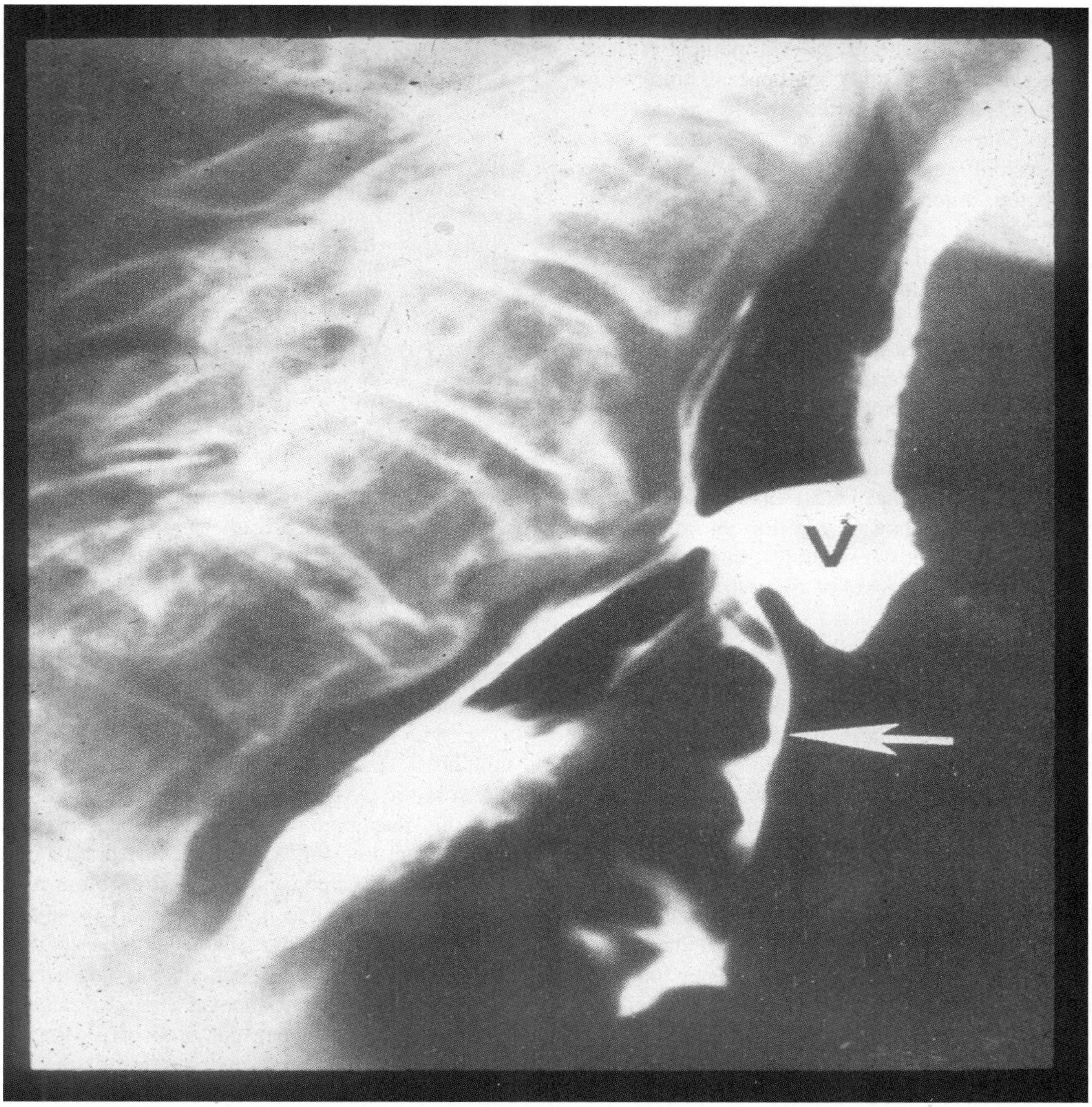

FIGURE 6-8 A large osteophyte at C3 is causing the bolus (in white) to collect in the vallecula (V) and eventually to spill into the airway (arrow). (Reprinted from Jonas B, Donner MW: *Normal and abnormal swallowing: imaging in diagnosis and therapy,* New York, 1991, Springer-Verlag.)

undergone esophagectomy, Lewin et al.[52] found that 81% of the patients showed signs of liquid aspiration at a mean postoperative period of 13 days; most instances of aspiration were the result of poor anterior laryngeal movement that resulted in residue in the piriform sinuses, with spillage into the airway. These authors speculated that tongue weakness secondary to involvement of the ansi hypoglossal innervation (C1-C3) to the tongue may be a complication of the surgery. This would explain why the hyoid bone did not move anteriorly. In their study, the chin-down maneuver eliminated the aspiration in 17 of the 21 patients.[52] Kato et al.[54] also found a limitation of hyoid movement with

resultant poor PES opening after esophagectomy regardless of the surgical reconstructive approach (retrosternal, posterior mediastinal, or intrathoracic). However, the poorest oropharyngeal biomechanics with subsequent aspiration were seen in patients who had the retrosternal reconstructive approach. Data on long-term outcomes in a significant number of those with esophagectomy and dysphagia are lacking. Martin et al.[55] found that in the 10 patients they studied, most had reduced or no swallowing difficulty in a range of 6 to 19 weeks after surgery. Heitmiller and Jones[56] studied 15 patients and found that their pharyngeal-based symptoms (aspiration/penetration, poor laryngeal elevation) had resolved at 1 month. Differences in these data can be attributed to the premorbid medical presentation, the surgical approach, and complications from aspiration or the surgery that would affect swallow recovery.

Patients in whom pulmonary complications develop after esophagectomy undergo swallowing studies to determine whether the source of their complication is related to aspiration. Typically, the first concern is that a leak has developed at the site of the anastomosis with resultant pulmonary complications. This situation is easily evaluated by radiographic studies. If a leak is not the source, then videofluoroscopic swallowing studies are conducted. A complication more common than an anastomotic leak after surgery is a stricture at the anastomotic site, often resulting in solid food dysphagia.[57] Such anastomotic strictures can be identified by standard radiographic studies. Video 6-4 shows a patient after a transhiatal esophagectomy. In the lateral view the patient shows aspiration during and after the swallow. The anteroposterior projection shows considerable bolus residue at the level of the anastomosis.

Skull Base/Posterior Fossa

Surgical procedures that involve the base of the skull and brainstem potentially can affect the peripheral cranial nerves important for swallowing (CNs V, VII, and IX through XII) or the central medullary controls for swallowing. Patients with dysphagia after posterior fossa surgery usually show bilateral pharyngeal impairment suggestive of brainstem, rather than peripheral nerve, injury.[37] Jennings et al.[58] detailed the swallowing disorders of 12 patients who had excision of skull-base tumors with varying involvement of the key cranial nerves for swallow. They found oral and pharyngeal involvement in all patients, including oral-stage delay, unilateral pharyngeal weakness, reduced hyoid excursion, and pharyngeal retention after the swallow. In addition, 75% aspirated, three of them silently. Compensatory swallowing strategies allowed seven of the patients to eat orally. At discharge, all patients were eating orally except the patient with involvement of CNs IX through XII. The prevalence and type of dysphagia following removal of tumor in the cerebellopontine angle was retrospectively studied in 181 consecutive patients by Starmer et al.[59] Following videofluoroscopic swallowing studies, 31% had evidence of oropharyngeal dysphagia with 91% involvement of the facial nerve versus 43% involvement in those without dysphagia. Sixty-five percent of those with dysphagia required special dietary manipulation, and 9% required tube feeding.

TRAUMATIC INJURIES

Trauma to the head and neck region has the potential to affect swallowing. Severe trauma (as to the spine) usually

requires respiratory supports and issues of intubation and tracheotomy tubes that already have been discussed. Trauma involving the cortical controls over swallowing was discussed in Chapter 3. Local trauma to bones involved in swallowing, such as laryngeal and mandibular fractures, may interfere with swallowing (see Practice Note 6-3). In laryngeal injury, the airway may be compromised, requiring tracheostomy, or the vocal folds may be injured, interfering with protection of the airway during swallow. Mandibular fractures of the jaw may need to be fixed (wired) in the closed position to promote healing. In some cases this may preclude oral ingestion or interfere with bolus preparation. Pineau and Ott[60] describe a case of isolated proximal esophageal injury from blunt trauma. The 52-year-old patient was in an automobile accident and had swelling in the left side of the neck, although a hematoma was ruled out. When the patient was unable to swallow solid foods the next day, an x-ray study revealed a stricture at the C6-C7 level. Pineau and Ott theorized that the trauma from the accident caused a disruption of the esophageal branches of the inferior thyroid artery that resulted in an ischemic stricture. The stricture was successfully dilated.

Patients with burn injuries also may be vulnerable to swallowing disorders as a result of respiratory complications and direct injury to the tissue and structures in the mouth and pharynx. Burn injuries frequently are a result of a traumatic event such as an explosion or automobile accident.

Dental Trauma

Oral surgery may result in a temporary loss of normal swallow function caused by pain. The removal of teeth may affect oral preparation. Teeth that are in poor repair also may affect oral preparation. Patients with ill-fitting dentures may sustain trauma to the mandibular or maxillary arches, creating inflammation, and in some cases permanent injury, to the mucosa, resulting in oral-stage preparation and delivery problems. Clinical examination of the dental arches reveals a reddened or whitish change in the mucosa at the point of denture contact where the patient feels the discomfort. Prolonged irritation can cause gingival hyperplasia, resulting in soft, sometimes flexible masses of tissue that appear markedly inflamed. Numerous studies have analyzed swallowing in older adults with and without their dentures in place.

Tamura et al.[61] found that dentures were important for older persons because they provided the posterior jaw stabilization necessary for a normal swallow. They also noted that older persons tend to have more xerostomia and that loss of saliva may affect patient perception of denture comfort. Furuya[62] and Yoshikawa et al.[63] found that the removal of dentures in older adults affected only the oral stage (delay) of swallowing and that more penetration of the airway occurred when the dentures were out. Hattori[64] did not find any differences in timing of oropharyngeal mechanics with dentures in or out but did find increased hyoid bone movement with the dentures removed. In none of these investigations were the patients at risk for pneumonia from events of aspiration.

Thermal Burn Trauma

Traumatic events that lead to thermal burn injuries can affect the structures and supporting tissue for swallow by direct contact, through inhalation of toxic gases with subsequent mucosal injury, and by the high incidence of respiratory complications requiring intubation and tracheostomy. Skin grafting procedures require intubation to achieve anesthesia with possible attendant injury to the upper airway. Grafts on the face may result in secondary fibrosis and restriction of facial and jaw musculature. Other respiratory complications that may compromise swallow include cough, hoarseness, stridor, **dyspnea**, increased mucus production, bronchospasm, necrosis, and ulceration. Video 6-5 on the Evolve website shows an endoscopic evaluation of the pharynx and larynx of a patient with an inhalation burn injury. There is generalized inflammation, particularly on the epiglottis, lateral pharyngeal walls, and in the interarytenoid space. Heavy mucus secretions are evident with ventricular fold edema. There is a visible ulceration on the right aryepiglottic fold. A feeding tube has been inserted through the PES.

Depletion of oxygen and carbon monoxide toxicity may result in diffuse brain injury that further complicates swallowing performance. Pain from burn injury is managed with sedatives and narcotics that compromise the levels of alertness needed for safe swallowing (see Medications later in this chapter). Severe burn injuries require immediate nutritional support by either enteral or **parenteral** routes. Hypermetabolic states are common, including increased oxygen consumption and cardiac demand, muscle wasting with a loss of lean body mass, and a compromised immune system. Because all these issues relate to swallowing and nutrition, stabilization of these medical problems often is a precursor to successful oral ingestion.

In a prospective review of 122 consecutively admitted patients to a burn unit, DuBose et al.[65] found that 18% had compromised swallowing. There were significant associations between the presence of oropharyngeal dysphagia and the number of days of mechanical ventilation, days to oral intake, age, length of hospitalization, and modified diet at discharge. The two highest predictors of dysphagia were age (odds ratio 2.18) and the presence of tracheotomy (odds ratio 26.9). After evaluating 438 consecutively admitted patients, Rumbach et al.[66] identified dysphagia in 11% of the cases. The speech pathologist was involved with these patients for a period of 1 month. A return to normal fluid consistencies was established by week 7 in 75% of the 49 dysphagics and to normal fluids and a regular diet in 85% at discharge. In a follow-up study of the physiologic characteristics of dysphagia using fiberoptic endoscopy in 19 burn patients, Rumbach et al.[67] noted a preponderance of pharyngeal-based deficits including, poor secretion management with loss of sensation, edema, and generalized weakness. Some had oral-stage deficits secondary to this weakness with accompanying lip contractures from their burns.

MEDICATIONS

Iatrogenic effects of medications may have negative effects on swallowing. In addition, they may negatively affect support systems needed for swallowing such as cardiac or respiratory function. Therefore it is important that the clinician review the medications a patient is taking because some may contribute directly to dysphagic conditions and others may exacerbate them. In general, side effects from medications that affect swallowing include those that interfere with cognition or motor performance, those that result in xerostomia, and those that affect gastrointestinal function. Side effects from medications that affect swallowing are not found in all patients and most likely will be found with higher doses. Combinations of drugs also may produce additive effects not found in single doses. Even though the clinical examination may suggest that a medication is responsible for dysphagia, it is not always possible to either reduce the dosage or discontinue the medication for medical reasons.

Drugs that depress the central nervous system also may depress the activity of striated muscle with subsequent negative effects on swallowing. Delay in swallow or an inability to sustain motor performance because of drowsiness or inattention may affect swallowing safety. Major classes of drugs that may affect motor performance and states of arousal include antipsychotics such as haloperidol or chlorpromazine, anticonvulsants such as carbamazepine

---

CLINICAL CORNER 6-3: MEDICATION COMPLICATION

An 83-year-old man was admitted to the psychiatry unit with acute onset of paranoia. His schizophrenia had been controlled successfully for many years with chlorpromazine (Thorazine). Chlorpromazine use had caused tardive dyskinesia that interfered with speech intelligibility but not with swallow. After dinner the patient became combative and a 5-mg dosage of haloperidol (Haldol) was ordered to control his behavior before bedtime. At breakfast he was noted to be coughing and choking on his regular diet and a request for consultation was sent to speech pathology.

Critical Thinking

1. Based on the patient's history, what potential causes might be considered in the differential diagnosis of his new problem with swallowing?
2. Based on your answer, what would be your next steps in managing his problem?

PRACTICE NOTE 6-4

An 81-year-old patient with a history of Parkinson's disease was admitted to the hospital with aspiration pneumonia that was believed to be attributable to increased oropharyngeal dysphagia. A progression of Parkinson's disease was suspected, and a nasogastric tube was inserted. A thorough medical history review revealed that the patient had recently seen his primary care physician because of increased pain in his right arm that had become progressively rigid. At that time he was given dantrolene sodium (Dantrium) to relax his arm and ideally relieve the pain. Because the patient had been eating fairly well before taking the Dantrium, I believed that the addition of the muscle relaxant was enough to remove any compensations he was making for his poor swallowing ability and probably led to his aspiration pneumonia. The Dantrium was discontinued while the man received treatment for his pneumonia, and he returned to successful oral feeding. Although the intent to relieve his arm pain was well meant, the side effects of the treatment outweighed the advantages.

---

and phenytoin, opioids such as morphine, and antianxiety preparations such as diazepam and clonazepam. Long-term use of antipsychotic drugs may result in tardive dyskinesia, a condition characterized by uncontrollable, repetitive, regular movements of the tongue and lips. When severe, tardive dyskinesia may interfere with the oral preparatory and oral initiation stages of swallowing (Clinical Corner 6-3).

Drugs such as dantrolene (Dantrium), which are intended to relax muscles that are spastic, may secondarily weaken the muscles for swallowing. Side effects from drugs used to lower cholesterol levels and steroids used to treat inflammatory disease may cause generalized myopathies and difficulty swallowing (Practice Note 6-4).

Many classes of drugs inhibit the flow of saliva through their anticholinergic effects on the nervous system. The resultant xerostomia may affect oral preparation and initiation, taste, and the patient's ability to neutralize stomach acid. Commonly used antidepressants with known xerostomic effects include amitriptyline, doxepin, and desipramine.

Medications that affect gastrointestinal function and that secondarily lead to or exacerbate dysphagic complications include those that change or alter appetite and those that lower esophageal sphincter (LES) pressures with the possibility of contributing to gastroesophageal reflux disease (GERD). Most medications used to treat cancer and other chronic diseases of the internal organs reduce appetite. Although these medications may not directly cause dysphagia, patients with dysphagia may have mechanical difficulty with swallowing and may not swallow enough because of lack of appetite. Insufficient caloric intake leads to protein-calorie malnutrition, loss of muscle mass, and further compromised muscle (swallowing) strength.

Medications used to treat respiratory disease, such as albuterol, beclomethasone, and theophylline, all reduce LES pressures, thereby increasing the risk of increased events of gastroesophageal reflux. The drug class of calcium channel blockers used to treat cardiac disease also may increase the patient's risk for GERD. For details on specific drug classes and drugs that affect patients with dysphagia, readers are referred to the work by Carl and Johnson.[68]

CHRONIC OBSTRUCTIVE PULMONARY DISEASE

As previously discussed, patients with respiratory-related disease may be at increased risk for dysphagia. One of the most prevalent disorders falls under the general category of chronic obstructive pulmonary disease (COPD). Subcategories of impairment include emphysema, chronic bronchitis, asthma, and cystic fibrosis. These diagnoses are characterized by airflow limitations, abnormalities in oxygen and carbon monoxide exchange, and lung hyperinflation characterized by failure to exhale sufficient amounts of carbon monoxide. Estimates of disease prevalence are difficult because of differences in measurement tools; however, the World Health Organization estimated that by 2020, COPD will be the third leading cause of death and the fifth leading cause of disability worldwide.[69] COPD is complicated by congestive heart failure in 20% to 30% of patients.[70]

Oropharyngeal swallowing performance has been studied in patients whose COPD is medically stable and in those with acute exacerbation. Mokhlesi et al.[71] used videofluoroscopy to compare the swallowing of 20 patients with stable COPD with 20 age-matched controls. No instances of aspiration were found in either group; however, those with COPD showed reduced hyoid bone excursion, earlier and longer airway closure durations, and earlier airway closure time relative to PES relaxation onset. The investigators noted that although no patient had evidence of airway protection problems, in instances of acute exacerbation these physiologic differences may become more pronounced, leading to swallow decompensation and the potential for airway protection disorders. Good-Fratturelli et al.[72] studied a group of 78 patients with COPD and other medical disorders such as stroke and myocardial infarction who were referred for suspected oropharyngeal dysphagia. Before evaluation, 95% were eating orally and 42% aspirated, primarily on thin and thickened liquids, often with ineffective or absent cough responses. Half of the 42% aspirated silently. Colodny[73] studied the swallowing and respiratory function of 15 patients with stable COPD. She found that only advancing age was the best predictor in those who aspirated. Interestingly, multisystem involvement did not predict aspiration in this cohort. Cvejic et al.[74] studied 16 stable COPD patients and 16 matched controls using various bolus volumes and a continuous drinking task using the Penetration-Aspiration (PA) scale as a measurement tool. Differences between groups were more pronounced on the continuous drinking task, with higher PA scores across most volumes for the COPD group. Episodes of penetration and aspiration were associated with an increase in respiratory rate and oxygen desaturation.

Coelho[75] studied 14 patients with COPD who were hospitalized for acute exacerbations. Thirteen had tracheotomies and five depended on ventilation support. On videofluorographic studies, 3 of the 14 aspirated, although all patients showed swallow delay in both oral and pharyngeal stages suggestive of generalized muscle weakness.[75] Shaker et al.[76] studied the respiration and deglutition cycle relations in those with acute COPD whose condition eventually stabilized. During an acute exacerbation more swallows were initiated during inspiration than in normal subjects, and there were some differences in the relation between deglutition apnea and total swallow durations compared with normal subjects. When their condition was stabilized, the patients returned to swallow initiation on the exhalatory cycle, and respiration-to-deglutition timing measures returned to normal. Nishino et al.[77] noted similar changes in inspiratory–expiratory cycle relations in patients with COPD compared with normal subjects. These changes occurred most often during periods of **hypercapnia**.

Of concern in patients with COPD and dysphagia is the issue of whether acute exacerbations are the result of aspiration or if they are unrelated. Or does an acute exacerbation of COPD increase the risk for aspiration? In one third of patients with COPD, the reason for an acute exacerbation is unknown.[78] Kobayashi et al.[79] studied the timing of the swallow reflex in patients with stable COPD and in patients who averaged 2.4 exacerbations within 1 year. All patients were eating orally at the time of the study. There was a significant difference between the two groups. Those with exacerbations showed swallow reflex delay that could be associated with the potential for swallowing dysfunction. These data do not show a cause-and-effect relation between oropharyngeal dysphagia and acute COPD exacerbations but suggest the two could be related. Tsuzuki et al.[80] reviewed the evidence that might establish a connection between dysphagia and COPD exacerbations and concluded that microaspiration could be the source. Such microaspiration might be the result of the loss of upper airway sensitivity. Using an air-pulse stimulator delivered by nasoendoscopy, Clayton et al.[81] studied laryngopharyngeal sensitivity in 20 patients with stable COPD compared with 11 controls. There was a significant difference in the elicitation of the laryngeal adductor reflex in the group with COPD, suggesting the potential for increased threat to the upper airway from sensory loss.

Other investigators have studied the changes of oxygen saturation levels during a meal. Presumably the work of eating may change saturation levels that secondarily may predispose the patient to aspiration. Brown et al.[82] found that not all patients with severe COPD experienced desaturation at mealtime. Only those whose baseline levels before the meal were below 90% desaturated. In 16 patients with severe COPD who had tracheotomies, Vitacca et al.[83] compared respiratory parameters during and after a 30-minute meal with and without ventilatory support. Respiratory rate, end-tidal carbon dioxide values, and an increase in dyspnea all were abnormally high when patients did not receive ventilatory assistance. This implies that in this specific group of patients that ventilatory support at mealtimes may be prudent to avoid the risk of aspiration.

Patients with COPD are at risk for aspiration from oropharyngeal sources as well as esophageal sources. It has been suggested that GERD may play a role in the exacerbation of COPD by three mechanisms: (1) direct infiltration of stomach contents into the lungs, (2) acid irritation to the esophageal vagal afferents with resultant bronchospasm and desaturation, and (3) primary disorders of the esophagus that secondarily affect PES physiology and subsequent airway protection.[84] Using videofluoroscopy, Stein et al.[85] studied 25 patients with severe COPD who were symptomatic for dysphagia. Disorders in flow through the PES were present in 21 of the patients. The authors suggested that the disorders in the PES for the older patients and those with more severe COPD may be related to compensatory activity of the PES resulting in its failure to adequately relax. This subgroup of patients was more likely to show signs of GERD. Using a questionnaire, Rascon-Aguilar et al.[86] found that 37% of 86 patients with COPD reported symptoms of reflux and that the rate of COPD exacerbations in those with such complaints was twice as high as in those with none.

This finding suggests that the presence of reflux-related symptoms may play a role in acute exacerbations in patients with COPD and that GERD control is important. Using 24-hour pH monitoring and measures of oxygen saturation, Casanova et al.[87] found pathologic reflux scores in 62% of patients with COPD. Of particular interest was that half of this group reported no GERD symptomatology. Kempainen et al.[88] found a similar prevalence of GERD in 41 (57%) patients with COPD, also noting that a high percentage reported no symptoms. In addition, 15% of the group with confirmed positive reflux studies had proximal esophageal reflux, suggesting there may be a threat to the airway. In addition to abnormal pH studies in 35% of 40 male patients, Gadel et al.[89] found disorders of motility at the LES in 65%, and at the PES in 53%. GERD in this sample was more prevalent in those who were older, heavy smokers, and had a low body mass index. Interestingly, in a large nonselected group of patients with well-documented GERD in the United States, higher body mass index was positively associated with GERD.[90]

Identification of those patients with stable COPD and GERD was the focus of a study by Bin-Miao and Yu-Lin.[91] Using the Reflux Diagnostic Questionnaire, 1486 patients with stable COPD were enrolled and divided into GERD-positive and GERD-negative groups. There was no difference between groups in age, body mass index, gender proportion, tobacco exposure and medication use. What differentiated the groups was expiratory volume in 1-second residual volumes and inspiratory capacity. These results suggest that pulmonary function testing may be of use in identifying those patients with COPD who may be at additional respiratory risk from GERD. Readers are encouraged to review the section on PES relations and GERD in Chapter 5 to fully appreciate the relationships among GERD, the esophagus, and the potential for pharyngeal swallowing dysfunction.

The mechanism for the increased prevalence of GERD in patients with COPD is speculative. One theory is that the number of transient LES relaxations is increased because of failure of the crural diaphragm or LES fibers as a result of short or irregular respiratory cycles. The crural diaphragm provides a barrier during inhalation, whereas the LES provides a barrier during exhalation. Therefore interruptions in respiratory competence may allow increased movement of stomach contents across the LES barrier. Because of the known relaxation of LES pressures caused by medications used to treat COPD,[68] the patient with COPD is at great risk for GERD and its potential negative consequences on swallowing.

TAKE HOME NOTES

1. Disorders of breathing often affect swallowing because of the close relation between breathing and swallowing.
2. Patients who require placement of a tracheotomy tube may be at risk for aspiration, particularly if they have multiple medical complications.
3. Swallowing disorders resulting from medical or surgical interventions may be referred to as iatrogenic.
4. Surgical procedures such as carotid endarterectomy, cardiac bypass, thyroidectomy, cervical spine fusion, esophagectomy, and skull base surgery may involve key cranial nerves needed for swallowing.
5. Traumatic injuries that result in fractures of swallowing structures, dental trauma, and thermal burn injuries all may increase the patient's risk of swallow safety.
6. The side effects from medications used to treat medical conditions may be the primary causative factor of dysphagia or may complicate preexisting dysphagia.
7. Patients with COPD are at risk for dysphagia, especially during periods of acute exacerbation, because of compromise to the respiratory system.

REFERENCES

1. Butler SG, Stuart A, Pressman H, et al: Preliminary investigation of swallowing apnea duration and swallow/respiratory phase relationships in individuals with cerebral vascular accident. *Dysphagia* 22:215, 2007.
2. Partik B, Pokieser P, Schima W, et al: Videofluoroscopy of swallowing in symptomatic patients who have undergone long-term intubation. *AJR Am J Roentgenol* 174:1409, 2000.
3. De Larminat V, Montravers P, Dureuil B, et al: Alteration in swallowing reflex after extubation in intensive care unit patients. *Crit Care Med* 23:486, 1995.
4. Skoretz SA, Flowers HL, Martino R: The incidence of dysphagia following endotracheal intubation; a systematic review. *Chest* 137:665, 2010.
5. Ding R, Logemann JA: Swallow physiology in patients with trach cuff inflated or deflated: a retrospective study. *Head Neck* 27:809, 2005.
6. Bonano PC: Swallowing dysfunction after tracheostomy. *Ann Surg* 174:29, 1971.
7. Nash M: Swallowing problems in the tracheotomized patient. *Otolaryngol Clin North Am* 21:701, 1988.
8. Elpern EH, Jacobs ER, Bone RC: Incidence of aspiration in tracheally intubated adults. *Heart Lung* 16:527, 1987.
9. Eibling D, Diez Gross R: Subglottic air pressure: a key component of swallowing efficiency. *Ann Otol Rhinol Laryngol* 105:253, 1996.
10. Sasaki CT, Susuki M, Horiuchi M, et al: The effect of tracheostomy on the laryngeal closure reflex. *Laryngoscope* 87:1428, 1977.

11. Leder SB, Ross DA: Confirmation of no causal relationship between tracheotomy and aspiration status: a direct replication study. *Dysphagia* 25:35, 2010.

12. Terk AR, Leder SB, Burrell MI: Hyoid bone and laryngeal movement dependent upon presence of a tracheotomy tube. *Dysphagia* 22:89, 2007.

13. Logemann JA, Pauloski BR, Coangelo L: Light digital occlusion of the tracheostomy tube: a pilot study of effects on aspiration and biomechanics of the swallow. *Head Neck* 20:52, 1998.

14. Leder SB, Ross DA, Burell MI: Tracheostomy tube occlusion status and aspiration in early postsurgical head and neck cancer patients. *Dysphagia* 13:167, 1998.

15. Dettelbach MA, Gross RD, Mahlmann J, et al: Effect of the Passy-Muir valve on aspiration in patients with tracheostomy. *Head Neck* 17:297, 1995.

16. Leder SB: Effect of one-way tracheotomy speaking valve on the incidence of aspiration in previously aspirating patients with tracheotomy. *Dysphagia* 14:73, 1999.

17. Elpern EH, Borkgren Okonek M, Bacon M, et al: Effect of the Passy-Muir tracheostomy speaking valve on pulmonary aspiration in adults. *Heart Lung* 29:287, 2000.

18. Suiter DM, McCulloch GH, Powell PW: Effects of cuff deflation and one-way tracheostomy speaking valve placement on swallow physiology. *Dysphagia* 18:284, 2003.

19. Leder SB, Joe JK, Hill SE, et al: Effect of tracheotomy tube occlusion on upper esophageal sphincter and pharyngeal pressures in aspirating and nonaspirating patients. *Dysphagia* 16:79, 2001.

20. Donzelli J, Brady S, Wesling M, et al: Effects of the removal of the tracheotomy tube on swallowing during the fiberoptic exam of the swallow (FEES). *Dysphagia* 20:283, 2005.

21. Buchholz DW: Oropharyngeal dysphagia due to iatrogenic neurologic dysfunction. *Dysphagia* 10:248, 1995.

22. Leder SB, Suiter DM, Duffey D, et al: Vocal fold immobility and aspiration status: a direct replication study. *Dysphagia* 27:265, 2012.

23. Young JY, Lee SJ, Lee SJ, et al: analysis of video fluoroscopic swallowing study in patients with vocal cord paralysis. *Dysphagia* 27:185, 2012.

24. Lombardi CP, Raffaelli M, D'Alatri L, et al: Voice and swallowing changes after thyroidectomy in patients without inferior laryngeal nerve injuries. *Surgery* 140:1026, 2006.

25. Wasserman JM, Sundaram K, Alfonso AE, et al: Determination of the function of the internal branch of the superior laryngeal nerve after thyroidectomy. *Head Neck* 30:21, 2008.

26. Silva ICM, Netto IPV, Guilherme J, et al: Prevalence of upper aerodigestive symptoms in patients who underwent thyroidectomy with and without the use of intraoperative laryngeal nerve monitoring. *Thyroid* 22:814, 2012.

27. Pereira JA, Girvent M, Sancho JJ, et al: Prevalence of long-term upper aerodigestive symptoms after uncomplicated bilateral thyroidectomy. *Surgery* 133:318, 2003.

28. Ekberg O, Bergqvist D, Takolander R, et al: Pharyngeal function after carotid endarterectomy. *Dysphagia* 10:62, 1989.

29. Monini S, Taurino M, Barbara M, et al: Laryngeal and cranial nerve involvement after carotid endarterectomy. *Acta Otolaryngol* 125:398, 2005.

30. Masiero S, Previato C, Addante S, et al: Dysphagia in post-carotid endarterectomy: a prospective study. *Ann Vasc Surg* 21:218, 2007.

31. Hogue CW, Lappas GD, Creswell LL, et al: Swallowing dysfunction after cardiac operations. *J Thoracic Cardiovasc Surg* 110:517, 1995.

32. Barker J, Martino R, Reichardt B, et al: Incidence and impact of dysphagia in patients receiving prolonged endotracheal intubation after cardiac surgery. *Can J Surg* 52:119, 2009.

33. Harrington OB, Duckworth JK, Starnes CL, et al: Silent aspiration after coronary bypass grafting. *Ann Thoracic Surg* 65:1998, 1599.

34. Abel R, Ruf S, Spahn B: Cervical spinal cord injury and deglutition disorders. *Dysphagia* 19:87, 2004.

35. Morishima N, Ohota K, Miura Y: The influences of Halo-vest fixation and cervical hyperextension on swallowing in healthy volunteers. *Spine* 30:E179, 2005.

36. Kepler CK, Rihn JA, Bennett JD, et al: Dysphagia and soft-tissue swelling after anterior cervical surgery: a radiographic analysis. *Spine* 12:639, 2012.

37. Buchholz D: Dysphagia due to iatrogenic neurological dysfunction. *Dysphagia* 10:248, 1995.

38. Welsh LW, Welsh JJ, Chinnici JC: Dysphagia due to cervical spine surgery. *Ann Otol Rhinol Laryngol* 96:112, 1987.

39. Martin RP, Nery MA, Diamant NE: Dysphagia following anterior cervical spine surgery. *Dysphagia* 12:2, 1987.

40. Winslow CP, Winslow TJ, Wax MK: Dysphonia and dysphagia following the anterior approach to the cervical spine. *Arch Otolaryngol Head Neck Surg* 127:51, 2001.

41. Baraz R, Lee MJ, Yoo JU: Incidence of dysphagia after cervical spine surgery: a prospective study. *Spine* 27:2453, 2002.

42. Song KJ, Choi BW, Kim HY, et al: Efficacy of postoperative radiograph for evaluating the prevertebral soft tissue swelling after anterior cervical discectomy and fusion. *Clin Ortho Surg* 4:77, 2012.

43. Marguez-Lara A, Nandyala SV, Fineberg SJ, et al: The incidence, outcomes and mortality of re-intubations following anterior cervical fusions. *Spine* 39:134, 2014.

44. Buchholz DW, Jones B, Ravich WJ: Dysphagia following anterior cervical fusion. *Dysphagia* 8:390, 1993.

45. Gamache FW, Voorhies RM: Hypertrophic cervical osteophytes causing dysphagia: a review. *J Neurosurg* 53:338, 1980.

46. Strasser G, Schima W, Schober E, et al: Cervical osteophytes imping-ing on the pharynx: importance of size and concurrent disorders for development of aspiration. *AJR Am J Roentgenol* 174:449, 2000.

47. Granville LJ, Musson N, Altman R, et al: Anterior cervical osteo-phytes as a cause of pharyngeal stage dysphagia. *J Am Geriatr Soc* 46:1003, 1998.

48. Atkins BZ, Shah AS, Hutcheson KA, et al: Reducing hospital mor-bidity and mortality following esophagectomy. *Ann Thorac Surg* 78:1170, 2004.

49. Zhang C, Ruan DK, He Q, et al: Progressive dysphagia and neck pain due to diffuse idiopathic skeletal hyperostosis of the cervical spine: a case report and literature. *Clin Interven Aging* 9:553, 2014.

50. Papadopoulou S, Exarchakos G, Beris A, et al: Dysphagia associated with cervical spine and postural disorders. *Dysphagia* 28:469, 2013.

51. Leder SB, Bayars S, Sasaki CT, et al: Fiberoptic endoscopic evalua-tion of swallowing in assessing aspiration after transhiatal esophagec-tomy. *J Am Coll Surg* 205:581, 2007.

52. Lewin JS, Hebert TM, Putnam JB, et al: Experience with the chin tuck maneuver in postesophagectomy aspirators. *Dysphagia* 16:216, 2001.

53. Atkins BZ, Fortes DL, Watkins KT: Analysis of respiratory complica-tions after minimally invasive esophagectomy: preliminary observa-tion of persistent aspiration risk. *Dysphagia* 22:49, 2007.

54. Kato H, Miyakaki T, Sakai M, et al: Videofluoroscopic evaluation in oropharyngeal swallowing after radical esophagectomy with lym-

phadenectomy for esophageal cancer. *Anticancer Res* 27:4249, 2007.

55. Martin RE, Letsos P, Taves DH, et al: Oropharyngeal dysphagia in esophageal cancer before and after transhiatal esophagectomy. *Dysphagia* 16:23, 2001.

56. Heitmiller RF, Jones B: Transient diminished airway protection following transhiatal esophagectomy. *Am J Surg* 162:422, 1991.

57. Rice TW: Anastomotic stricture complicating esophagectomy. *Thorac Surg Clin* 16:63, 2006.

58. Jennings SK, Siroky D, Jackson G: Swallowing problems after excision of tumors of the skull base: diagnosis and management in 12 patients. *Dysphagia* 7:40, 1992.

59. Starmer HM, Best SR, Agrawal Y, et al: Prevalence, characteristics, and management of swallowing disorders following cerebropontine angle surgery. *Otolaryngol Head Neck Surg* 146:419, 2011.

60. Pineau BC, Ott DJ: Isolated proximal injury from blunt trauma: endoscopic stricture dilatation. *Dysphagia* 18:263, 2003.

61. Tamura F, Mizukami M, Ayano R, et al: Analysis of feeding function and jaw stability in bedridden elderly. *Dysphagia* 17:235, 2002.

62. Furuya J: Effects of wearing complete dentures on swallowing in the elderly. *J Stomatol Soc Japan* 66:361, 1999 [in Japanese].

63. Yoshikawa M, Yoshida M, Nagasaki T, et al: Influence of aging and denture use on liquid swallowing in healthy dentulous and edentulous older people. *J Am Geriatr Soc* 54:449, 2006.

64. Hattori F: The relationship between wearing complete dentures and swallowing function in elderly individuals: a videofluoroscopic study. *J Stomatol Soc Japan* 71:102, 2004 [in Japanese].

65. DuBose CM, Groher ME, Mann GC, et al: *The prevalence of swallowing disorders following thermal burn injury*, Unpublished manuscript, University of Florida Health Science Center, 2006.

66. Rumbach AF, Ward EC, Cornwell PL, et al: Clinical progression and outcome of dysphagia following thermal burn injury: a prospective cohort study. *J Burn Care and Res* 33:336, 2012.

67. Rumbach AF, Ward EC, Cornwell P, et al: Physiological characteristics of dysphagia following thermal burn injury. *Dysphagia* 27:370, 2012.

68. Carl LL, Johnson PR: *Drugs and dysphagia: how medications can affect eating and swallowing*, Austin, TX, 2006, Pro-Ed.

69. Viegi G, Maio S, Pistelli F, et al: Epidemiology of chronic obstructive pulmonary disease: health effects of air pollution. *Respirology* 11:523, 2006.

70. LeJemtel TH, Padeletti M, Jelic S: Diagnostic and therapeutic challenges in patients with coexistent chronic obstructive pulmonary disease and chronic heart failure. *J Am Coll Cardiol* 49:171, 2007.

71. Mokhlesi B, Logemann JA, Rademaker A, et al: Oropharyngeal deglutition in stable COPD. *Chest* 121:361, 2002.

72. Good-Fratturelli MD, Curlee RF, Holle JL: Prevalence and nature of dysphagia in VA patients with COPD referred for videofluoroscopic swallow examination. *J Commun Disorders* 33:93, 2000.

73. Colodny N: Effects of age, gender, disease, and multisystem involvement on oxygen saturation levels in dysphagic persons. *Dysphagia* 16:48, 2001.

74. Cvejic L, Harding R, Churchward T, et al: Laryngeal penetration and aspiration in individuals with stable COPD. *Respirology* 16:269, 2011.

75. Coehlo CA: Preliminary findings on the nature of dysphagia in patients with chronic obstructive pulmonary disease. *Dysphagia* 2:28, 1987.

76. Shaker R, Li Q, Ren J, et al: Coordination of deglutition and phases of respiration: effect of aging, tachypnea, bolus volume, and chronic obstructive pulmonary disease. *Am J Physiol* 263:G750, 1992.

77. Nishino T, Hasegawa R, Ide T, et al: Hypercapnia enhances the development of coughing during continuous infusion of water into the pharynx. *Am J Respir Crit Care Med* 157:815, 1998.

78. Donaldson GC, Wedzicha JA: COPD exacerbations: epidemiology. *Thorax* 61:164, 2006.

79. Kobayashi S, Kubo H, Yanai M: Impairment of the swallowing reflex in exacerbations of COPD. *Thorax* 62:1017, 2007.

80. Tsuzuki A, Kagaya H, Takahashi H, et al: Dysphagia causes exacerbations in individuals with chronic obstructive pulmonary disease. *J Am Geriatr Soc* 60:2012, 1580.

81. Clayton NA, Carnaby-Mann G, Peters MJ, et al: The effect of chronic obstructive pulmonary disease on laryngopharyngeal sensitivity. *Ear Nose Throat J* 91:370, 2012.

82. Brown SE, Casciari RJ, Light RW: Arterial oxygen saturation during meals in patients with severe chronic obstructive pulmonary disease. *South Med J* 76:194, 1983.

83. Vitacca M, Callogari G, Sarua M, et al: Physiological effects of meals in difficult-to-wean tracheostomized patients with chronic obstructive pulmonary disease. *Intensive Care Med* 31:236, 2005.

84. Mokhlesi B: Clinical implications of gastroesophageal reflux disease and swallowing dysfunction in COPD. *Am J Respir Med* 2:117, 2003.

85. Stein M, Williams AJ, Grossman F, et al: Cricopharyngeal dysfunction in chronic obstructive pulmonary disease. *Chest* 97:347, 1990.

86. Rascon Aguilar IE, Pamer M, Wludyka P, et al: Role of gastroesophageal reflux symptoms in exacerbations of COPD. *Chest* 130:1096, 2006.

87. Casanova C, Baudet JS, Velasco MDV, et al: Increased gastroesophageal reflux disease in patients with severe COPD. *Eur Respir J* 23:841, 2004.

88. Kempainen RR, Savik K, Whelan TP, et al: High prevalence of proximal and distal gastroesophageal reflux disease in advanced COPD. *Chest* 131:2007, 1666.

89. Gadel AA, Mostafa M, Younis A, et al: Esophageal motility pattern and gastro-esophageal reflux in chronic obstructive pulmonary disease. *Hepatogastroenterology* 59:2498, 2012.

90. Corley DA, Kubo A: Body mass index and gastroesophageal reflux disease: a systematic review and meta-analysis. *Am J Gastroenterol* 101:2619, 2006.

91. Bin-Mia L, Yu-Lin F: Association of gastroesophageal reflux disease symptoms with stable chronic obstructive pulmonary disease. *Lung* 190:277, 2012.

Section 2
Evaluation of Swallowing

CHAPTER 7
Clinical Evaluation of Adults

Michael E. Groher

To view additional case videos and content, please visit the evolve website.

CHAPTER OUTLINE

OBJECTIVES

1. Describe the rationale for early detection of swallowing disorders.
2. Review the main components of the clinical evaluation of swallowing in adults.
3. Present the strengths and weaknesses of evaluation protocols.
4. Discuss noninvasive techniques for improving the diagnostic accuracy of the clinical examination.
5. Review screening and standardized tests for dysphagia.
6. Present potential adjunctive measures of swallowing performance.

RATIONALE

A comprehensive evaluation of a patient with known or suspected dysphagia involves a number of medical and allied health disciplines. Data collected for patients in an outpatient setting who reported dysphagia revealed that the diagnostic process involved an average of 3.5 disciplines per patient.[1] Therefore for most patients, the comprehensive evaluation of the patient with dysphagia should be considered a team evaluation. Relevant disciplines were discussed in Chapter 1. For the speech-language pathologist (SLP) the evaluation is intended to assess factors that relate to swallowing function, not to diagnose the underlying disease, although it may either obviate or clarify the need for further studies. In some cases the clinical examination of swallowing confirms a particular diagnosis because the swallowing characteristics are consistent with other aspects of the disease, such as the repetitive tongue pumping in the oral stage of Parkinson's disease.

The clinical evaluation of swallowing often is referred to as the bedside examination. Although the bedside examination encompasses the same procedures, clinical examination is the preferred terminology because the examination is performed in any setting and is not restricted to the bedside. However, modifications in the standard clinical evaluation of swallowing may need to be made at the bedside—often because of poor patient cooperation. The clinical evaluation of swallowing is to be distinguished from the *imaging evaluation* (see Chapter 8), which might include tests conducted outside the clinical environment, such as radiographic studies that require special space and equipment. Some patient settings, such as long-term care facilities, lack easy access to instrumental swallowing assessment environments. Patients must be transported to these settings. Therefore clinicians in these settings rely heavily on the clinical evaluation of swallowing to provide diagnostic and treatment information. Settings such as those in tertiary care hospitals can provide support for advanced swallowing studies. In this environment the clinician may not always rely totally on the clinical evaluation. Rather, it is viewed as complementary to the imaging evaluation. Interestingly, there are no **prospective data** that either support or refute the effect of each practice pattern on patient health outcomes.

The clinical evaluation of the patient with dysphagia has three main components: the medical history, the physical inspection of the swallowing musculature, and observations of swallowing competence with test swallows. Logemann et al.[2] list five reasons for performing a clinical (physical) evaluation for a swallowing disorder: (1) to define a potential cause (medical history), (2) to establish a working hypothesis that defines the disorder, (3) to establish a tentative treatment plan, (4) to develop a potential list of questions that may require further study, and (5) to establish the readiness of the patient to cooperate with any further testing. A lack of patient cooperation or performance may make it impossible to complete all elements of the physical evaluation. In this circumstance, the clinician must rely heavily on the medical history or, if the patient is eating, observations of his or her swallowing ability. Another valuable use of the clinical examination is its use as an outcome measure, either in a research protocol or in clinical practice. Changes in physical status after treatment intervention can be easily measured with a clinical examination with numeric values associated with each finding. Skilled examiners use baseline clinical evaluation data to track dysphagia severity over time in patients with progressive neurologic disease.

Practitioners might choose to use an abbreviated portion of the clinical examination of swallowing as a method to screen for or detect dysphagia. Once a high suspicion for dysphagia is established, the entire clinical examination is administered. Early detection of dysphagia is important because complications from dysphagia increase patient morbidity, lengthen hospitalization (health care cost), and may ultimately increase patient risk for death.[3] Most "screening" tools for dysphagia do not meet the strict criteria of a screening device. A valid screening tool for dysphagia should be able to detect dysphagia in a large group of patients who are not symptomatic for dysphagia, but who may, in fact, have dysphagia.[4] The advantage of a good screening tool is that it will rule out the presence of dysphagia and by implication allow the patient to take nutrition orally. If the screening tool suggests the patient might be at risk for dysphagia, the patient will undergo a complete dysphagia *assessment*. An assessment differs from screening because it encompasses an in-depth evaluation of a patient's swallowing skills with the intent of detailing the specific characteristics of the disorder. A valid screening tool for dysphagia also should be able to show improved health outcomes as a result of its administration.[5] To establish that improvement in health status is a consequence of effective screening, the screening device should be tested in a group with dysphagia who did not receive the screening and a similar group who did.[5] Current practice with dysphagia screening tools presupposes that the screening tool is administered because the patient already has a high suspicion for symptoms. After studying 254 older persons living independently, Serra-Prat et al.[6] concluded that routine screening of the presence of dysphagia would be very useful to avoid potential nutritional and respiratory complications in this age group. A good screening test has high sensitivity (detecting dysphagia when it is present) and a high negative **predictive value** (proportion of patients who have a negative finding that is verified to be correct). For instance, a patient who is classified as not at risk for dysphagia will be correctly classified most of the time. Ideally for patients with dysphagia the screening tool should be predictive of positive health outcomes, such as fewer cases of aspiration pneumonia, better nutritional status, or positive quality of life (QOL) scores as they relate to eating. The best tool will not only be able to identify frank aspiration, but also the risk for aspiration from the consequences of dysphagia.[7] Screening devices for dysphagia should be easily administered by any medical specialist in a short time. The clinical evaluation for swallowing as administered by the SLP is designed to provide a much broader perspective of the patient with dysphagia than a screening protocol would provide. The American Stroke Association has called for development of dysphagia screening devices. All patients, regardless of suspicion for dysphagia, should be screened for its presence. There are numerous screening tools available. In a **systematic review** of 35 identified screening protocols, Schepp et al.[8] concluded that only 4 had sufficient reliability and validity: the Barnes Jewish Hospital Stroke Dysphagia Screen, the Modified Mann Assessment of Swallowing Ability (MMASA), the Emergency Physician Swallowing Screening, and the Toronto Bedside Swallowing Screening Test (TOR-BSST). All have sensitivity measures and negative predictive values of more than 90%. The MMASA was standardized on 150 acute, poststroke patients.[9] It was designed to be given in 10 minutes by physicians in the emergency room. Test items and weighted scoring guidelines are presented in Table 7-1. The TOR-BSST also was validated on poststroke patients.[10] Validated with nurses, it uses three test items: water swallows, voice analysis before and after swallow, and tongue movement. Wilson and Howe[11] used a decision-analysis model and metaanalyses to study the cost effectiveness of screening for dysphagia, although their study analyses were geared more to full assessment rather than screening. They concluded that the most cost-effective method for reducing the cost of treating pneumonia related to dysphagia was the use of a single videofluoroscopic swallowing study, rather than the use of a clinical examination, or a clinical examination combined with a videofluoroscopic swallowing study.

Clinicians recognize that all clinical evaluations of patients with dysphagia are not the same, although clinician preference in selecting items for inclusion are items supported in the literature as discriminative.[12] Most clinicians combine data from the medical history, physical examination, and trial swallows.[12] The clinical examination for swallow suffers from lack of reliable methods of scoring and inconsistencies in agreement on observations, such as the definition of a wet-hoarse voice.[13] McCullough et al.[14] found that clinicians can reliably judge only 50% of items commonly administered in a clinical examination for swallow. The most reliable judgments were observation of the presence of tubes, oral motor data, and historical parameters. Inconsistency in recoding data carries the risk of diagnostic inaccuracy, which in turn affects the treatment plan. Clearly there is a need to standardize the clinical evaluation of swallowing (see Standardized Tests later in this chapter).

SYMPTOMS OF DYSPHAGIA

Symptoms usually are defined as any perceptible change in bodily function that the patient notices. This change eventually leads the patient to seek medical help when it causes pain or discomfort or negatively affects his or her lifestyle. Some people have adverse medical symptoms and ignore them until the severity of the problem significantly affects their physiologic or mental health. Others seek immediate medical attention. Both groups may have a diagnosis of a disorder that is similar in type and severity.

Patient Description

The physical examination of a patient with dysphagia may begin by asking the patient to describe the symptoms. Some common symptoms are detailed in Table 7-2. Because dysphagia often is secondary to neurologic disease that also may compromise communication skills, not all patients can provide a report of their symptoms. Others may give

unreliable or scant information because of cortical deficits. Anecdotal evidence suggests that many patients with dysphagia (particularly esophageal based) do not seek immediate medical attention. Rather, they make changes in their eating habits to accommodate their symptoms, such as chewing food more finely or eliminating troublesome items from their diet. Others know they have difficulty swallowing but cannot describe the specifics of their symptoms. Often it is difficult to remember how long the symptoms have been apparent; this may be from the inherent flexibility of the swallowing tract to accommodate changes in function. Only when these accommodations no longer provide relief or are too difficult to execute does the patient seek medical attention. Some patients may have symptoms of dysphagia but ignore them. For instance, one study of 56 older persons who did not report dysphagia found that a large majority had radiographic abnormalities during swallowing tests. Such abnormalities included poor esophageal motility and pharyngeal weakness.[15] Patients with Parkinson's disease often underreport their swallowing difficulty (see Chapter 1).

For those who are able to communicate symptoms of their dysphagia, a detailed description may be useful in helping establish a diagnosis. Detailed descriptions also may be used to help the examiner focus on the types of diagnostic tests that may be most useful in delineating the source of the complaint. The relation between the accuracy of a patient's complaint and the final diagnosis has not been investigated extensively. Whether the complaint is useful in guiding the diagnostic process also has not been experimentally verified. Nonetheless, asking the patient to describe the problem is a common point of departure in the dysphagia examination.

The literature suggests that asking patients to localize where they believe the problem exists is not always reliable and may not be useful in guiding the tests selected for patient examination, particularly when they report the problem is localized to the neck.[16] In one large study of patients who were found to have confirmed esophageal disease, most who pointed to the lower esophagus who had confirmed lower esophageal lesions were accurate. However, a significant number (30%) pointed to the upper neck and chest as the source of their discomfort.[17] Other investigators have found that a significant number of patients who described food sticking at the level of the pharynx did have abnormalities at this level; however, the primary source of that abnormality often was found to be in the esophagus.[18] This suggests that patients who report dysphagia localized to the neck and pharynx should not only have that specific region investigated, but also should have studies appropriate to the esophagus. After reading this chapter and Chapter 5, the reader should review Critical Thinking Cases #1 and #2 that presented with an initial complaint of solids sticking in the cervical region localized to the pharynx. In both

TABLE 7-1 Dysphagia Screen

Modified Mann Assessment of Swallowing Ability (Mini MASA)

INSTRUCTIONS: Circle the most appropriate *clinical findings* for each *indicator*. Calculate the total score by adding the points for each indicator. Do not add last item (i.e., water swallow).

Indicator	Clinical Findings (Points)				
Alertness	2	5	8		10
	no response to speech	difficult to rouse	fluctuates		alert
Cooperation	2	5	8		10
	no cooperation	reluctant	fluctuating cooperation		cooperative
Auditory comprehension	2	4	6	8	10
	no response to speech	occasional motor response if cued	follows simple conversation with repetition	follows ordinary conversation with little difficulty	WNL
Respiration	2	4	6	8	10
	chest infection suctioning vent dependent/ trach	coarse basal creps chest physio	fine basal creps	sputum upper airway other condition	chest clear
Dysphasia	1	2	3	4	5
	unable to assess	no functional speech sounds/single words	expresses self in limited manner short phrases/words	mild difficulty finding words or expressing ideas	NAD
Dysarthria	1	2	3	4	5
	unable to assess	speech unintelligible	speech intelligible but obviously defective	slow with occasional hesitation or slurring	NAD
Saliva	1	2	3	4	5
	gross drool	some drool consistently	drooling at times	frothy/ expectorated	NAD
Palate	2	4	6	8	10
	no spread or elevation	minimal mov't nasal regurg/ air escape	unilaterally weak	slight asymmetry mobile	NAD
Tongue movement	2	4	6	8	10
	no mov't	minimal mov't	incomplete mov't	mild impairment in range	full ROM
Tongue strength	2	5	8		10
	gross weakness	unilateral weakness	minimal weakness		NAD
Gag	1	2	3	4	5
	no gag	absent unilaterally	diminished unilaterally	diminished bilaterally	hypereflexive NAD
Cough voluntary	2	5	8	10	
	no attempt/ unable to assess	attempt inadequate	attempt bovine	NAD	
Optional: 3 oz water	2	5	8	10	
	violent cough/ expulsion/severe wet voice	moderately intense cough moderately wet voice	faint cough slightly wet voice	NAD	
TOTAL SCORE					

Score > or = 95 : Start oral diet and progress as tolerated. Monitor first oral intake and consult COMMUNICATIVE DISORDERS if patient has difficulty eating or drinking.
Score < or = 94 : Consult COMMUNICATIVE DISORDERS for a formal swallow evaluation.

Creps, creptitations: rales/rhonchi; mov't, movement; NAD, no abnormality detected; physio, respiratory physiotherapy; regurg, regurgitation; ROM, range of motion; WNL, within normal limits.
(From Antonios N, Carnaby-Mann G, Crary M. Behrouz R, Silliman S: Validation of a Physician Administered Bedside Screen for Dysphagia Associated With Acute Ischemic Stroke; The Modified-Mann Assessment of Swallowing Ability, Journal of Stroke and Cerebrovascular Diseases 19(1):49-57, 2010)

TABLE 7-2 Examples of Signs and Symptoms Associated with Dysphagia

Symptom	Sign
Difficulty chewing	Food spills from lips; excessive mastication time of soft food; poor dentition; tongue, jaw, or lip weakness
Difficulty initiating swallow	Mouth dryness (xerostomia); lip or tongue weakness
Drooling	Lip or tongue weakness; infrequent swallows
Nasal regurgitation	Bolus enters or exits the nasal cavity, as seen on radiographic swallowing study
Swallow delay	Radiographic study identifies transport beyond normal standard
Food sticking	Radiographic study identifies excessive residue in mouth, pharynx, or esophagus after completed swallow
Coughing and choking	Coughs on trial food attempts; material enters the airway on radiographic study
Coughing when not eating	Radiographic study shows aspiration of saliva or lung abnormality
Regurgitation	Undigested food in mouth; radiographic study shows food returning from esophagus to pharynx or mouth mucosal irritation on endoscopy; pH probe study positive for acid reflux
Weight loss	Unexplained weight loss; measurement of weight is below ideal standard

examples their primary problem that precipitated their complaint was esophageal, not pharyngeal in origin. Questioning patients about their disorder beyond localization often improves their accuracy. For instance, if the patient localizes the problem to the neck and reports coughing on fluids, the likelihood that the problem is pharyngeal based is high.[19] One study found that if patients who complained of food sticking in the region of the neck also reported respiratory symptoms (congestion, wheezing, cough), the sensitivity of dysphagia localized to the pharynx improved.[20] Another group of investigators found that subtypes of esophageal disorders (motility vs. obstructive) could be determined by patient report if the patient described a cluster of symptoms, such as heartburn with dysphagia, prior dilatation, pain, and weight loss, than if they reported heartburn alone.[21] In general, studies agree that the complaint (dysphagic symptoms) presented by the patient correlates better with the findings when the problem after diagnosis is judged to be severe. The fact that all studies do not agree on whether patient localization is accurate is largely attributable to inadequate numbers of subjects, the potential differences in final classification of the disease type, and the fact that some patients might have undergone other treatments and tests before being enrolled in the study.

Some clinicians find it useful to explore a patient's dysphagic symptoms by questionnaire. A sample questionnaire specific to patients with head and neck cancer that could be completed before their office visit is presented in Box 7-1. This method may help ensure that all relevant questions relating to the patient's symptoms are addressed by the examiner. It also gives the patient a chance to think carefully about the symptoms before responding. Other patient-specific questionnaires have been developed, including one specifically for stroke (the Burke Dysphagia Screening Test)[22] and one for patients with Parkinson's disease.[23]

Wallace et al.[24] sought to develop a symptom severity assessment tool. Their tool is a 17-point questionnaire designed to evaluate initial dysphagic symptom severity that could be used to judge outcomes after therapy. Questions range from the patient's difficulty in swallowing various textures to issues of swallow initiation, episodes of choking, and how the disorder interferes with the patient's QOL. Measurement of the effect of dysphagia on one's QOL can be important as a diagnostic and outcome measurement tool. McHorney et al.[25] developed a standardized measure of assessment of one's QOL as it relates specifically to swallowing disorders. Called the SWAL-QOL, the questionnaire contains 44 items that measure 10 areas of one's QOL particular to the effects of dysphagia. It may be accompanied by the use of SWAL-CARE, a questionnaire that contains 15 items assessing posttreatment care and overall patient satisfaction with that care.[25] Silbergleit et al.[26] developed a questionnaire consisting of 25 items, scored with a 7-point interval scale. Items surveyed included questions relating to one's physical, emotional, and functional problems as a result of their dysphagia. Eat-10 is a standardized, 10-question tool that focuses on a mix of questions that assesses QOL and swallowing symptoms.[27] It requires patients to self-report their symptoms on a 4-point scale ranging from no problem to a severe problem. Standardized QOL measurement scales specific to dysphagic populations such as those with head and neck cancer also have been developed.[28,29] For a critical review of measures that propose to measure the QOL as affected by dysphagia, the reader is directed toward the work of Timmerman et al.[30]

Regardless of which method is used—patient report to examiner questions or patient responses to a questionnaire—the patient's subjective complaint may not always fit the objective data gathered in the physical and instrumental evaluation. In another study, subjective complaints of

BOX 7-1 SAMPLE DYSPHAGIA QUESTIONNAIRE

1. Do you have difficulty chewing your food?	Yes	No
2. If so, which foods give you the most trouble? Underline any that apply.		
A. Solids (e.g., meats)		
B. Liquids (e.g., water)		
C. Semisolids (e.g., cottage cheese, applesauce, cereal)		
3. If you underlined a category in question 2, provide some examples:		
Specific solids:		
Specific liquids:		
Semisolids:		
4. Do you have difficulty lining up your teeth?	Yes	No
5. Does food go all over your mouth, and is it difficult getting it together to swallow it?	Yes	No
6. Do you have trouble opening and closing your jaw?	Yes	No
7. Is the sensation in your mouth decreased?	Yes	No
8. Do you choke when eating?	Yes	No
9. If you answered "yes" above, do you choke before you swallow, when you are chewing, or after you swallow?	Yes	No
10. Is it hard for you to:		
A. Lift your tongue?	Yes	No
B. Move it from side to side?	Yes	No
C. Move it from front to back?	Yes	No
11. Do you eat or drink more slowly now than before surgery?	Yes	No
12. Do you eat or drink one category more slowly than others?		
Solids:	Yes	No
Liquids:	Yes	No
Semisolids:	Yes	No
13. Does food catch in the:		
A. Left side of your throat?	Yes	No
B. Right side of your throat?	Yes	No
C. Left side of your mouth?	Yes	No
D. Right side of your mouth?	Yes	No
E. Behind your Adam's apple?	Yes	No
14. Do you need to pump your tongue many times to collect food to swallow?	Yes	No
15. Do you feel you have to swallow three or more times so all the food will go down?	Yes	No
16. Do you have trouble swallowing pills?	Yes	No
17. Do you cough up food?	Yes	No
18. If so, does the food come up:		
A. While chewing?	Yes	No
B. After the food is swallowed?	Yes	No
19. Do small amounts of food or liquids ever fall out of your mouth:		
A. Before you swallow?	Yes	No
B. After you swallow?	Yes	No
20. Do you have a gurgly voice after you eat?	Yes	No
21. Do you feel the need to clear your throat after swallowing or eating a meal?	Yes	No
22. Do you have trouble controlling drooling?	Yes	No
23. Does food or liquid leak out of your:		
A. Trachea?	Yes	No
B. Fistula?	Yes	No
24. Do you ever have to clean your mouth out after eating because food has become stuck?	Yes	No
25. Do you ever have to "wash down" your food with liquids?	Yes	No
26. Do you eat as much now as you did before your surgery?	Yes	No
27. Have you changed your diet in any way that is not mentioned above?	Yes	No
You are encouraged to add additional helpful information.		

NA, Not applicable.
(From Baker BM, Fraser AM, Baker CD: Long-term postoperative dysphagia in oral/pharyngeal surgery patients: subjects' perceptions vs. videofluoroscopic observations, *Dysphagia* 6:11, 1991.)

patients with head and neck cancer and oropharyngeal dysphagia were compared with the objective findings from the instrumental examination.[31] In general, many of the objective findings did not always support the patient's complaint. However, in some cases other findings that the patient did not consider important were documented. Jensen et al.[31] concluded that subjective complaints may be useful in guiding the examination but should be confirmed with objective data. There have been no comparisons between the standardized dysphagia questionnaire and the structured clinical interview as it relates to diagnostic approach or accuracy.

Asking pertinent questions in the initial interview is a clinical art and requires practice. Each question should build on another until there is clarity about the key elements of interest. Building a database from the patient's description of his or her problem provides useful information that may not be contained in a medical summary from another institution. Knowledge of what type of data may be most useful in planning the next step either in diagnosis or treatment is essential during the clinical interview. Clinical Case #2 provides an example of a clinical interview of a patient with recurrence of oral stage cancer who came to the outpatient clinic without any medical records. At selected intervals, you will be asked questions pertinent to the case history. Readers are advised to review Chapter 4 prior to reviewing this case.

Obstruction

One of the most common complaints from patients with dysphagia is that food or fluids "get stuck." Most frequently they report that the sticking sensation is in the throat or esophagus. Some patients do not use the word stuck but may use the word fullness. Especially when they localize the feeling of obstruction to the throat, patients often describe their complaint as "a lump in the throat" when eating. The medical term for this feeling is *globus*. Some physicians have used the term *globus hystericus* to describe this sensation, because it was once believed that the description of a lump in the throat was usually associated not with **organicity** but with symptoms of hysteria. Technically, globus hystericus is reserved for patients who complain of a lump in the throat that is relieved by swallowing or talking, not as a cause for dysphagia. The globus sensation is usually relieved by swallowing. However, use of the term *globus sensation* often is associated with the dysphagic person who reports that food is sticking at the level of the cervical esophagus. Although early investigators reported that they rarely found a cause for the globus sensation (i.e., patients were **hysterical**), recent reports suggest that with the appropriate battery of diagnostic tests, most who report the globus sensation have identifiable disease.[32] Moser et al.[33] found that when patients reported the globus sensation with chest pain or heartburn, they were likely to have an esophageal motility disorder.

Liquids Versus Solids

Patients may report a change in their dietary habits that is associated with perceived dysphagia. For instance, patients who describe the globus sensation often have more difficulty swallowing solids than liquids. Classically, those with solid food dysphagia are more likely to have disorders of esophageal origin, whereas those with dysphagia for liquids are more likely to have oropharyngeal dysphagia. This dichotomy, however, may be artificial because it is well known that those with oropharyngeal dysphagia can have dysphagia for liquids and solids, and some forms of esophageal dysphagia evoke complaints regarding liquids and solids.[16] When patients report choking on liquids or solids, it suggests a more pharyngeal-focused cause, whereas those who report dysphagia for liquids and solids without choking episodes may have a more esophageal-focused cause. Gastroenterologists who suspect the esophagus as the source of dysphagia may use a decision tree such as the one presented in Chapter 5 (see Figure 5-9) to assist in diagnosis. Such a decision tree has not been validated against a large number of patients with confirmed diagnoses; however, the concept is useful because the symptoms related to the diseases represented are well known. Patients are asked questions related to diet (solids vs. liquids), intermittent versus progressive symptoms, and the presence of heartburn. In general, patients with solid food dysphagia are at risk only for more obstructive types of dysphagia in the esophagus. Those who report problems with both liquids and solids more frequently have disorders of esophageal motility. A decision tree for suspected oropharyngeal dysphagia has not been developed, primarily because of overlapping (and therefore nonspecific) symptoms and signs that may be related to many disease entities. Therefore using a decision tree approach based on patient complaints would have little precision in helping establish a diagnosis for those with oropharyngeal dysphagia.

Gastroesophageal Reflux

Some patients report episodes of gastroesophageal reflux (heartburn) associated with their report of dysphagia. Some patients describe pain or fullness in the chest associated with their reflux. Others may have reflux and dysphagia but may be unaware that they have reflux because the overt symptoms of chest pain, or acid taste, are not present. Not all patients describe episodes of reflux unless questioned by the examiner because they may not relate their reflux symptoms to their dysphagia. This is particularly true when patients describe the globus sensation in the neck because they might not think that reflux in the esophagus could be related to a problem in the throat (see Chapter 5 for a full discussion of gastroesophageal reflux disease [GERD] and dysphagia).

Eating Habits

Reporting on changes in one's eating habits may signal the presence of dysphagia, its level of severity, and its psychosocial effect. Complaints that center on elimination of specific food items, such as avoidance of liquids or solids, or items that are sticky or crumbly, may help the examiner focus the evaluation. Excessive chewing of solid food to avoid a sticking sensation may be more consistent with esophageal disease versus the pharyngeal-focused complaint that liquids always seem to come back through the nose. Tiring with foods that require mastication may be consistent with neurologic impairment. Patients who report excessive time to finish a meal often have dysphagia that requires careful evaluation. Patients who report they no longer feel comfortable eating in a restaurant because they have to regurgitate or choke should be examined with care. Patients who have experienced marked weight loss or no longer enjoy the pleasures of eating probably have dysphagia that has reached a high severity level.

SIGNS OF DYSPHAGIA

Signs are objective measurements or observations of behaviors that people elicit during a physical examination. In a patient with dysphagia who is cooperative, this entails an examination of the cranial nerves relevant to swallowing and, if appropriate, interpretation of any laboratory findings. Examples of patient symptoms and corresponding signs are presented in Table 7-2. Some signs are seen on observation when the patient is eating a meal. Signs and symptoms may overlap. For instance, a patient may report (symptom) liquid going into the nose and food sticking. Both may be seen by the examiner (signs) on the videofluorographic swallowing study. In this circumstance the patient's symptoms have been confirmed.

The physical evaluation of a patient may reveal signs consistent with dysphagia, such as drooling from the lip; tongue weakness; poor dentition; or loss of strength or range of motion in the tongue, jaw, or velum. Poor strength or coordination may result in choking on liquids during test swallows or in lack of bolus flow. The patient's cognitive status may affect swallowing; signs of cognitive deficit may include failure to chew, talking while swallowing, or inattention to the feeding process. Patients who are hospitalized may have more overt medical signs such as the following: (1) feeding tubes already placed, (2) a tracheotomy tube, (3) respiratory congestion after eating, (4) need for excessive oral and pharyngeal suctioning, (5) eating refusals, (6) undernutrition and muscle wasting, (7) inability to maintain an upright feeding position, (8) an endotracheal tube, and (9) regurgitation of food.

CLINICAL CASE EXAMPLE 7-1

A 50-year-old woman comes to the clinic reporting a 6-year history of progressive weight loss. She tells the examiner it has become increasingly hard to swallow both solids and liquids. She denies heartburn. She reports that her dysphagia has interfered with her social life because it now takes an excessive time to finish her meal. The physical evaluation reveals a right facial weakness with atrophy of the left tongue. Her gag reflex is absent and her velum is weak on the left side. Her voice is weak and breathy. On test swallows of liquids and solids she coughs repeatedly.

By the patient's own report, her symptoms of weight loss and a change in social life because of increasing swallowing difficulty seem consistent with a diagnosis of dysphagia. On physical evaluation she has many signs consistent with dysphagia. This is manifest by the involvement of multiple cranial nerves that has resulted in misdirection of the food bolus into the airway, causing choking episodes that have made it embarrassing to eat in front of others. Her symptoms (complaints) are verified by the examination (signs).

MEDICAL HISTORY

The medical history can be assembled from prior or current medical records, from conversations with the medical staff if the patient is hospitalized, and verbally from the patient or family. Conversations with the patient often are needed to supply missing data or to elucidate or confirm data that are unclear. If the patient's mental status is not compromised, the physical examination often begins with the patient describing his or her dysphagic symptoms (see previous discussion). While the overall contribution of the medical history to the final dysphagia diagnosis is unknown, beginning examiners often do not appreciate its importance. This lack of recognition may be due to the possibility that multiple underlying causes may precipitate dysphagia, and that all of the potential etiologic factors are not always fully appreciated (see Practice Note 7-1). Some causative factors are rare, such as those with dysphagia secondary to **collagen-vascular disease**. A detailed history often provides clues that direct the clinician to the most definitive diagnostic tests. Each Critical Thinking Case provides the reader to integrate the importance of each element of the given history into a preliminary diagnosis and plan for evaluation.

Historical Variables

Figure 7-1 shows a sample medical history form. The form can be used to guide the examiner in gathering important historical elements that may affect the diagnosis and

PRACTICE NOTE 7-1

A 64-year-old man was referred to my outpatient swallowing disorders clinic and reported that he had been choking irregularly on liquids for 3 years. He told me that in each of the 3 years he had undergone a standard barium swallow examination and all results were normal. At this point I thought that perhaps his disorder had a pharyngeal focus and that the barium swallow only detailed his esophageal function. However, nothing in his history suggested he might have a reason for a pharyngeal pathologic condition until I asked if he had ever been hospitalized. There had been no record of a hospitalization in the medical file I had. He mentioned that 5 years earlier he fell down the basement stairs and was rendered unconscious. He was hospitalized and during his hospitalization had a tracheotomy for 2 months, even though he was discharged from the hospital after 3 weeks. I was unable to get any details about his tracheotomy tube tolerance, but I began to suspect that he might have sustained tracheal **malacia** with a subsequent tracheoesophageal fistula. I had a high suspicion for fistula because small ones frequently produce intermittent symptoms such as those the patient reported, and they may go undetected on standard barium swallow studies. A modified barium swallow study was ordered with particular attention to the anteroposterior projection. This projection provides the best opportunity to make the diagnosis. The radiologist confirmed a fistula, and the head and neck surgeons closed it.

treatment of a person with dysphagia. This information can be obtained from the patient, the caregiver, or the medical record. Some patients, such as those who have had a stroke and dysphagia, make the connection between their neurologic impairment and their complaint. Others, however, such as those who may have dysphagia after surgery unrelated to the swallowing mechanism, may not make the connection between their surgery and dysphagia. For instance, their dysphagia may be related more to the endotracheal tube placed in the airway during surgery for their knee. A thorough medical history pertinent to dysphagia sometimes reveals important data that either had been ignored by other specialists or may lead to a path of evaluation that had not been considered.

The medical history as presented in Figure 7-1 is divided into nine parts: congenital disease, psychiatric disease, surgical procedures, cancer-related procedures, metabolic disorders, respiratory impairment, esophageal disorders, prior evaluations of swallowing, and advance directive status.

Congenital Disease

Disorders from childhood, particularly those of neurogenic origin such as cerebral palsy, should be noted. These disorders may not have resulted in dysphagia in the past but may have more significance relative to the present complaint.

Neurologic Disease

Neurologic disorders are the most frequent cause of dysphagia. Stroke, head trauma, and progressive neurogenic diseases such as multiple sclerosis, amyotrophic lateral sclerosis, and Parkinson's disease often precipitate dysphagia. (For a full discussion of neurologic swallowing disorders in adults, see Chapter 3.) It is important to note any medical complications from the disease, particularly any side effects from medications to control the disease that may have adverse effects on swallowing. For instance, a patient who is taking a central nervous system depressant to control seizures may have a concomitant depression in motor function that affects swallowing.

Surgical Procedures

Any surgical procedure has the potential to create dysphagic symptoms, particularly if the patient underwent general anesthesia that required the placement of an endotracheal tube through the vocal folds. Damage to the vocal folds could interfere with airway protection, resulting in dysphagia. Any surgical procedure that involves the aerodigestive or respiratory tract should be noted. Patients who have undergone a surgical wrap (**fundoplication**) of the lower esophageal sphincter (LES) to control GERD may be dysphagic because the wrap is too tight. Patients who have undergone surgical relaxation (**myotomy**) of the PES or LES should have the circumstances of the outcome explored. Surgery to control cancer in the head, neck, or esophagus is of particular importance. Noting whether a patient's cancer was treated by chemotherapy or radiation therapy also may help explain common side effects from those therapies that may cause dysphagia (see Chapter 4). Other specific surgical procedures to note include cardiopulmonary surgery, thyroid surgery, surgery in the upper airway, and cervical spine surgery. The risk in these procedures of damaging cranial nerve (CN) X is higher than in other surgical procedures in these regions and therefore places the patient at greater risk for dysphagia (see Chapter 6 for a full discussion).

Systemic and Metabolic Disorders

Disturbance in the body's chemical balance that may result from toxins (as a result of medication intolerance) or infections may act on the central nervous system, resulting in symptoms of dysphagia. Disorders of metabolism may result in dehydration and undernutrition that compromise physical and mental performance. Physical weakness and mental confusion can be precursors to, or exacerbations of, the dysphagic condition. Asking the patient to comment on any recent weight loss or compare his or her current weight

Patient's name: _____

Date of birth: _____

Gender: _____

Medical record number: _____

Chief complaint: _____

_____

_____

Source of information:

——Patient

——Family

——Recent medical record

——Past history

——Other source

Congenital Family Illness:

　Neurologic disease:

　　——Stroke

　　——Progressive disease

　　——Traumatic injury

　　——Other CNS disorders

　　——Medications taken for:

　Psychiatric disease:

　　——Medications taken for:

　　——Movement disorder

　Surgical procedures:

　　——Spinal fusion

　　——Myotomy

　　——Alimentary tract

FIGURE 7-1 Sample medical history form. *CNS,* Central nervous system.

___ Fundoplication

___ Head/neck cancer

___ Thyroidectomy

___ Cardiac

Cancer-related:

___ Irradiation

___ Chemotherapy

Systemic/metabolic:

___ Nutrition/hydration status

___ Current and ideal weight

___ Laboratory values related to nutrition

___ Infections

___ Toxins

___ Diabetes

Respiratory impairment:

___ Chronic obstructive pulmonary disease

___ Prior history of aspiration pneumonia

___ Cardiopulmonary disease

Esophageal disease:

___ Reflux/regurgitation

___ Motility disorder

___ Dilatation

Prior test results:

___ Radiographic

___ Manometric

___ Scintigraphic

___ Endoscopic

Current Advance Directive Status:_____

FIGURE 7-1, cont'd

with previous weight may provide insight into the severity of the dysphagia. Diabetes is an example of a systemic, metabolic disorder that may affect swallowing, particularly esophageal peristalsis.

Respiratory Impairment

Because respiration and deglutition share common interactions, any compromise to the respiratory system may decompensate swallowing. Therefore it is important to ask patients if they have any respiratory disease such as chronic obstructive pulmonary disease (see Chapter 6) or asthma in their medical history. Patients who report being treated for suspected aspiration pneumonia already have shown signs of not being able to protect their airway adequately.

Esophageal Disease

Problems with esophageal motility or stenosis of the esophageal body can provide important clues in defining the dysphagic condition. Some patients may have a history of an enlarged heart that could be compressing the esophagus. Others may have a history of regurgitation or reflux that has required treatment such as dilatation. If patients have received specialized treatment or tests in the esophagus, the response to such treatment should be noted.

Previous Test Results

Results of any laboratory study, such as endoscopy of the upper airway, esophagus, or stomach, should be explored. The results of any radiographic results, such as a barium swallow, a modified barium swallow, or an ultrasound of the aerodigestive tract, also are of interest. Some patients with dysphagia and reflux may have undergone a scintigraphic evaluation in nuclear medicine to define the amount and extent of their reflux. Other patients may have undergone a 24-hour pH study to evaluate the presence and frequency of reflux.

Advance Directive

A patient may not have executed an advance directive stating his or her preference about tube feeding if dysphagia is severe. If an advance directive has been executed and is part of the medical record, it should be reviewed. If the patient has chosen not to have tube feeding under any circumstances, the need for further testing or treatments may be contraindicated (see Chapter 11).

PHYSICAL EXAMINATION

The physical examination specific to swallowing impairment typically includes observations of medical interventions that may affect swallowing, such as a tracheotomy tube, and an assessment of the patient's mental status and the cranial nerves involved in swallowing. If patients are eating, observations of their swallowing and feeding skills during test swallow attempts are made. A checklist of items of interest in the clinical evaluation of patients with dysphagia is presented in Box 7-2.

Investigators have sought to determine which elements in the clinical examination for swallow are more important in detecting and defining the disorder. Elements for which research evidence supports their importance, particularly in stroke patients, include dysphonia (harshness and breathiness), a wet-sounding voice, dysarthria, poor secretion management, cough on trial swallows, and decreased laryngeal elevation.[2,34,35] Some of these clinical markers were found to be more predictive of dysphagia and unsafe swallow if two or more of these features were found after clinical examination.[36] McCullough et al.[37] also found that a cluster of clinical findings was more predictive of aspiration than one sign alone. Their results suggested that dysphonia after trial swallows of 5 and 10 mL of thin and thickened liquids, unilateral jaw weakness, and failure on the 3-oz water test were most predictive of aspiration. Chang et al.[38] analyzed five parameters of vocal quality following a liquid swallow as a method to detect either penetration or aspiration of the airway. In a group of 44 patients suspected of dysphagia, there was no relationship between airway penetration or aspiration during videofluoroscopy and abnormal vocal quality postswallow. Similar findings were reported by Waito et al.[39] in 40 patients suspected of dysphagia following head and neck cancer. They concluded that a clear postswallow vocal quality did provide evidence that penetration or aspiration were not present; however, the chance for false-positive and false-negative results in prediction aspiration using voice alone was high. After systematically reviewing 37 articles related to physiologic events associated with swallow as they might relate to aspiration risk, Steele and Chichero[40] concluded that abnormal tongue strength, hyoid excursion, respiratory patterns, and pharyngeal residue were most likely to be associated to either airway penetration or aspiration. Of these four parameters, evidence was the strongest for abnormal respiratory patterns.[40] One investigation found that in acute stroke patients, the clinical examination of swallowing compared with videofluoroscopic examination underestimated the detection of dysphagia but overestimated the frequency of aspiration.[41] During trial swallows, the most important elements in predicting airway safety included failure on thin liquids, a wet voice after swallow, failure on thick liquids, a cough after swallow, and inability to self-feed.

Clinical Observations

A portion of the physical examination can be completed with basic observations of the patient's medical status. These observations are particularly important for patients

---

BOX 7-2 GUIDELINES FOR THE CLINICAL EVALUATION OF SWALLOWING

Clinical Observations

Feeding Method
- Nasogastric
- Gastrostomy
- Jejunostomy
- Intravenous

Respiratory Status
- SpO_2 level
- Tracheostomy
- Ventilator
- Rate

Mental Status
- Level of alertness
- Orientation
- Cooperation
- Sustained attention

Cognitive Screening
- Memory
- Language
- Perception

Cranial Nerve Assessment

CN V
- Jaw opening and closing
- Jaw lateralization
- Muscle strength, bite down

CN VII
- Facial muscles at rest
- Pucker, smile
- Raise eyebrow
- Lips closed against resistance

CN IX, X
- Gag reflex
- Velum
- Voice
- Cough
- Dry swallow

CN XII
- Tongue range of motion
- Tongue strength
- Fasciculations, atrophy

Oral Cavity Inspection
- Lesions, thrush
- Moisture
- Dentition

Test Swallows
- Thin liquid
- Thick liquid
- Pudding consistency
- Semisolid

Cervical Auscultation Results
- Normal sounds
- Abnormal sounds
- Swallow delay
- Respiratory changes

Mealtime Observations
- Posture
- Ambiance
- Self-feeding skills
- Utensil use
- Assistance needed
- Diet level
- Respiratory pattern changes

CN, Cranial nerve; *SpO₂*, oxygen saturation.

---

who are bedbound and undergoing medical or surgical treatment. Some assumptions can be made about swallowing performance based on observational data.

Feeding Tubes

Some patients may not be eating orally or may be taking part of their nutrition through a feeding tube. Nasogastric tubes, which are inserted through the nose and into the stomach, are easily visible (Figure 7-2). Feeding tubes come in various sizes. Larger tubes may be needed to pass medications without clogging. Smaller, more flexible ones (e.g., Dobhoff tubes, Sherwood Medical Supplies, Forest Hills, NY) are more comfortable for the patient. Evidence in healthy (normal) subjects indicates that the presence of a feeding tube through the nose may slow the sequence of the pharyngeal swallow regardless of tube size.[42] Feeding tubes placed in the stomach (gastrostomy) or jejunum (jejunostomy) may not be visible unless they are connected to a feeding pump or a bag hanging on a support stand (Figure 7-3). Other patients may be hydrated through intravenous feeding catheters placed in the arm and connected to a plastic bag containing specialized nutrients or medications.

Tracheotomy Tubes

The presence of a tracheotomy tube should be noted. Tracheotomy tubes are placed when the medical team requires access to the lungs to maintain pulmonary toilet. Often they are placed when the patient is in respiratory distress or when the upper airway is blocked after trauma or surgery. (Readers are advised to review the discussion of tracheotomy tubes in Chapter 6).

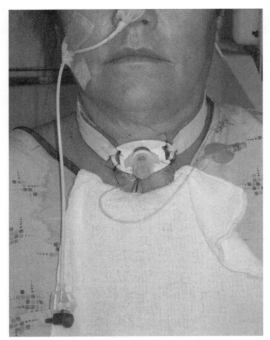

FIGURE 7-2 The patient has a small-bore feeding tube in place. The tube is taped away from her nostril to avoid nasal ulceration and taped to her cheek for comfort.

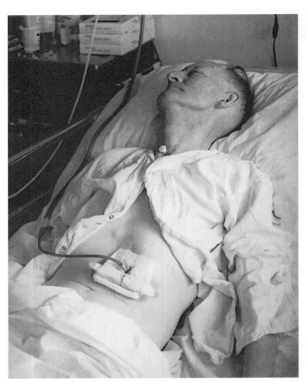

FIGURE 7-3 The patient has a gastrostomy tube in place. He is being fed specialized formula through the tube from a bag above his head.

Respiratory Pattern

Bedbound patients may be connected to a respirator to assist in the ventilation of the lungs and have a mask over the mouth or a cannula in the nose, both of which may supply oxygen. Most clinicians prefer for the medical team to achieve partial weaning of the patient from ventilator support before attempting oral feeding. Observations of the patient's ventilatory pattern can be made by watching the chest rise and fall. Rapid rates (more than 40 cycles/min) may make it difficult to close the airway for a sufficient time during the swallow. The respiration rate and oxygen saturation levels of some patients are measured by sensors attached to the skin. Oxygen saturation levels (percentage of hemoglobin attached to it) that drop to less than 90% may be an indicator for some patients that they are at risk for swallowing impairment. Respiratory rates and oxygen saturation levels can be monitored on a screen at the patient's bedside (Figure 7-4). For cooperative patients, a screening of vital and tidal respiratory capacities can be studied in the clinic or at the bedside with a portable respirometer. Declining respiratory capacities have been shown to be predictive of airway protection disorders in patients with amyotrophic lateral sclerosis.[43]

Mental Status

Observations of the bedbound patient may provide a preliminary indicator of mental status. For instance, patients who are alert often respond when the examiner enters the room,

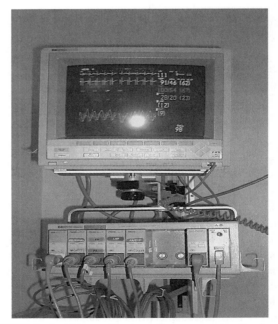

FIGURE 7-4 Bedside monitors track the oxygen saturation level (as a percentage), heart rate, and blood pressure on a single screen. The oxygen saturation level is monitored by a sensor that is attached to the hand or foot. On the lower right corner of this screen, the oxygen saturation (SpO_2) can be read as 98%.

PRACTICE NOTE 7-2

Patients with acute traumatic brain injury often are combative and are not able to cooperate with a formalized evaluation of their swallowing mechanism. A 24-year-old patient was in bed and restrained because he was combative with the nursing staff and at risk for pulling out his tracheotomy and feeding tubes. I needed to get him into a sitting position to attempt the physical examination. Positioning him required the restraints to be relaxed, but maintained. Once upright, it was clear he did not want to cooperate with the physical examination because of his poor cognitive status. However, he was attending to me and, although unintelligible, he was able to make a normal voice. He also showed signs of swallowing his own saliva. It seemed appropriate to try to see if I could get him to respond to a swallowing stimulus. I gave him a spoonful of crushed ice that he swallowed immediately without any cough or contents coming from the tracheotomy site. Sometimes, even with an uncooperative patient, information can be gathered about swallowing. Some patients do not have the cognitive skills to cooperate with a cranial nerve evaluation, but they do understand the learned behavior of taking a food item from a spoon.

CLINICAL CORNER 7-1: RIGHT BRAIN STROKE

A consultation was received for a 65-year-old patient who had a right brain stroke. He had left hemiplegia and left facial weakness. The patient was choking each time he drank liquids but did not seem particularly concerned. When attempting to eat solids he ate at a rapid rate and was asking when he could leave the hospital.

Critical Thinking
1. What could explain why this patient was not concerned about choking on liquids?
2. What other behavioral factors might need to be evaluated with this patient during his meal?

either visually by making eye contact or verbally with a greeting. These positive responses allow the examiner to assume that the patient may be able to cooperate with the remainder of the physical examination. Patients who are not readily alert to the examiner's presence or who are unable to sustain attention even after constant encouragement probably are not candidates for safe oral ingestion. The physical examination may be limited by the patient's inability to cooperate (see Practice Note 7-2). Patients who are uncooperative, either from lack of attention or extreme agitation, or who are difficult to arouse should be reexamined periodically during the day. In some cases, the side effects of medications may interfere with normal mental status; in other cases, medications may improve mental status. If the patient is able to cooperate, orientation, linguistic skills, perceptual ability, and memory should be assessed (review Clinical Corner 7-1). These learning modalities are important in giving the examiner an impression of the patient's ability to cooperate and learn during dysphagia treatment. For instance, patients who are confused and disoriented may need maximum assistance with eating, for feeding, and for reminders of how to perform therapeutic techniques needed for their care. The importance of a mental status examination that included questions about orientation and the ability to follow a single stage auditory command were studied by Leder, Suiter, and Warner.[44] In a retrospective review of 4070 patients suspected of dysphagia, those who were disoriented or who could not follow a single stage command were 69% more likely to be unsafe for any oral intake compared with those who could accurately complete both tasks.

Cranial Nerve Examination

Chapter 2 contains a review of the key cranial nerves involved in swallowing: V, VII, IX, X, XI, and XII. When smell and taste may be an issue, assessment of CN I is appropriate. The physical examination of the head and neck musculature for swallowing should focus on gathering information on the function of these cranial nerves. The examination begins by examining the muscles that can be seen easily and then proceeding into the oral cavity and oropharynx. The examination usually is focused on the motor aspects of relevant muscles, although gross, intraoral sensation may be of interest in patients who do not perceive a bolus once in the mouth. The examiner should look for any abnormality, including asymmetry, weakness, abnormal movements at rest, and abnormal movements during volitional efforts.

Facial Muscles

Observations of the facial muscles can be made with the patient at rest and during tasks such as lip pursing and smiling. Asking the patient to keep his or her lips closed against the examiner's attempt to pull them apart serves as a test for judging lip strength. The lower and upper facial muscles should be tested to differentiate between upper and lower motor neuron damage.

Muscles of Mastication

An assessment of the muscles of mastication begins by having the patient move the jaw up and down and laterally. Restrictions in mouth opening (**trismus**) should be noted. The strength of the masticator muscles can be appreciated by palpation as the patient bites down (Figure 7-5, and Clinical Corner 7-2).

Pathologic Reflexes

A number of brainstem-level primitive reflexes are associated with the chewing and swallowing mechanisms. Normally, these reflexes are inhibited in the adult by higher centers of the brain. Their presence in the adult patient suggests that these higher inhibitory centers are impaired.

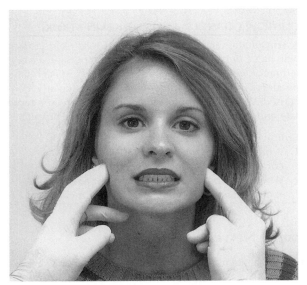

FIGURE 7-5 Asking the patient to bite down while palpating the response of the masseter muscles provides information about the integrity of the motor function of cranial nerve V.

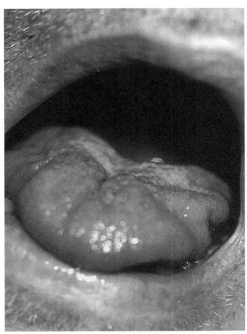

FIGURE 7-6 Lower motor neuron damage is assumed from the significant tongue atrophy (loss of tissue bulk) seen as deep grooves throughout the entire tongue surface.

CLINICAL CORNER 7-2: TRISMUS

A 58-year-old woman came as an outpatient with increased dysphagia and weight loss over the past 3 months. Five years ago she had completed a full course of radiation treatment for tonsillar cancer. The clinical evaluation revealed severe trismus, which made it very difficult to get a spoon in her mouth. She was treated with TheraBite (Atos Medical AB, West Allis, Wis.) for 3 weeks, resulting in improved jaw opening.

Critical Thinking
1. What is the probable source of her trismus?
2. What is TheraBite? How does it work?

These pathologic reflexes are seen most commonly in patients with bilateral hemispheric or frontal lobe damage.

The suck reflex may be elicited either by tapping the upper lip with a reflex hammer or by stroking the lips rapidly with a tongue blade. Movement of the lips in the direction of the stimulus is an abnormal response.

The bite reflex is often elicited in patients with severe neurologic lesions by touching the lips, teeth, or gums with a tongue blade and observing a strong closure of the jaw. This reflex can be particularly troublesome for the examiner because it may prevent a good oral examination. Attempts to force a jaw open usually result in a stronger bite. The examiner should avoid strong resistance that could result in fracture or dislocation of the mandible. In some patients, spontaneous mouth opening will occur as a stimulus object, such as a spoon or food, is seen approaching the mouth. Although the bite reflex can interfere with feeding

management, this mouth-opening reflex can be used to aid in the feeding plan.

Tongue Musculature

The examiner asks the patient to protrude the tongue and move it laterally. Rapid tongue movements may be assessed by asking the patient to repeat tongue-tip sounds such as "ta" rapidly. Ask the patient to move the tongue tip to the roof of the mouth, an activity important during bolus transfer. After reviewing the clinical examination of 3919 patients at risk for dysphagia, Leder et al.[45] found that reduced tongue range of motion was associated with aspiration independent of reduced labial closure and facial asymmetry. Protruding the tongue against a tongue blade gives the examiner a gross estimate of tongue strength. Objective measures of tongue strength can be accomplished with a cooperative patient as he or she pressures against a pressure transducer.[46] Inspect the tongue for atrophy, particularly along the lateral borders. Look for fasciculations if atrophy is seen (Figure 7-6, and Clinical Corner 7-3). Both are consistent with lower motor neuron involvement. If the patient has had tongue resection because of cancer, note how much has been spared. Sensation can be tested with a tongue blade in the region of the reconstruction by asking the patient if there is a difference between touch in the reconstructed region and the region that has not been reconstructed. Knowing the most sensitive area may be important in food placement during treatment.

CLINICAL CORNER 7-3: TONGUE ATROPHY

A 48-year-old told her dentist that she was choking on her saliva at night but not during the day. However, she did admit to choking on carbonated liquids. The dentist referred her to the speech pathologist for an evaluation of her swallowing. The physical evaluation was normal except for some atrophy on the left lateral border of her tongue.

Critical Thinking

1. What types of disorders might explain her tongue atrophy?
2. What referral should the speech pathologist make after this appointment?

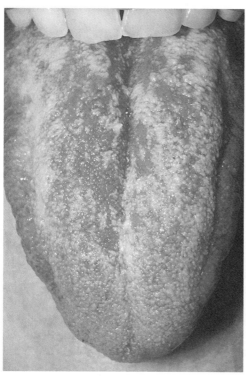

FIGURE 7-7 Whitish lesions on the tongue are consistent with thrush (oral candidiasis). (From Neville B, Damm DD, Allen CM et al: *Oral and maxillofacial pathology,* ed 2, Philadelphia, 2002, WB Saunders.)

Oral Cavity

With the patient's mouth open, the examiner inspects the oral cavity for any lesions. The milky-white appearance of candidiasis (thrush) indicates a fungal infection (Figure 7-7). If left untreated, thrush may cause odynophagia, which is frequently seen in those whose immune system has been decompensated by acute or chronic disease. Check to determine whether the amount of saliva is normal.

Patients with xerostomia often have little moisture throughout the oral cavity and report poor taste. The tongue may appeared reddened and secretions thick. Inspect the dentition. Teeth in poor repair or ill-fitting dentures may contribute to dysphagia.

Oropharynx

Observations of the velum at rest and during tasks of phonation should be made. The posterior dorsum of the tongue is stimulated on both sides with a tongue depressor to assess the gag reflex. If the patient has a gag response, it is important to note if the velum is elevated symmetrically and if the patient coughed. Some patients do not demonstrate a gag reflex until the tongue base is stimulated. Elicitation of the gag reflex accompanied by a cough provides information about the integrity of CNs IX (sensory) and X in the oropharynx (velum) and at the level of the larynx (vocal fold closure). The presence or absence of a gag reflex is not an indication that the patient has a normal swallowing response or is at risk for aspiration,[47] although for some examiners the absence of this reflex might suggest that the patient's swallow is compromised. The absence of a gag reflex as an isolated abnormal finding in the examination of the cranial nerves for swallowing may not be important (see Practice Note 7-3).

Pharynx

There are no tests of pharyngeal function that can be easily appreciated during the physical evaluation of the swallowing response. In some patients, the activity of the superior pharyngeal constrictor muscle can be observed after an active gag reflex as the posterior pharyngeal wall contracts or during the production of a falsetto voice. The activity of the pharyngeal constrictor muscles is best visualized by endoscopy during tasks such as producing a falsetto voice.

Larynx

Asking the patient to phonate or listening to his or her vocal quality in conversation provides useful information on the integrity of the airway protective mechanisms and on the coordination of articulatory structures during phonatory tasks. Speech is an extremely complex, overlearned behavior, and as such serves as a barometer from which the examiner can assess the status of the neuromuscular system that also serves swallowing. Patients should be asked to sustain a vowel, with the examiner noting duration, quality (hoarseness, breathiness, and harshness), pitch, and intensity. Articulation should be assessed for precision and speed. The use of oral diadochokinetic tasks (forced rapid alternating movements) using consonant-vowel combinations is recommended. Both hypernasal and hyponasal resonance qualities should be noted. Hypernasality suggests impaired palatopharyngeal function. Hyponasality implies filling of the nasopharynx or occlusion of nasal passages. For patients with unimpaired voice and speech, the clinician may reasonably conclude that the swallowing problem either resides in the late pharyngeal stage (cricopharyngeal function) or is related to esophageal and LES function. The remaining physical examination should confirm the integrity of the peripheral sensory-motor swallowing mechanism.

Asking the patient to produce a "dry" swallow while palpating the larynx at the level of the thyroid notch (Figure 7-8) helps the examiner assess the presence and extent of laryngeal elevation. Normal elevation ranges from 2 to 4 cm.

Test Swallows

In a cooperative, alert patient, who up to this point in the examination has not demonstrated significant neurologic impairment and has been able to swallow secretions without significant airway compromise, the examiner may want to grossly assess the swallow response with real food items. This part of the examination is useful because it provides the examiner information about swallowing dynamics. Before this portion of the examination, each cranial nerve should be evaluated in isolation. Some investigators have suggested that the risk–benefit ratio of this part of the evaluation is poor[2,48]; however, it is commonly performed in most settings. Test trials provide the opportunity to see the coordinated integration of all the swallowing muscles. Most examiners use an array of items ranging from thin to thickened liquids, to pudding and softer items, to items that require mastication. Initially it is advisable to use a substance that is relatively safe if it is partially aspirated and to be absolutely certain that the patient is able to cough to protect the airway in situations of suspected aspiration.[49] A spoonful of crushed ice is relatively safe and provides a

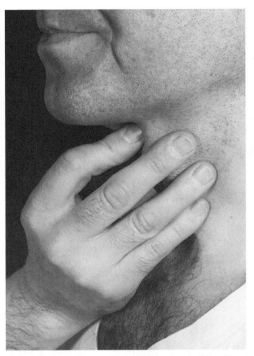

FIGURE 7-8 The examiner palpates at the level of the thyroid notch to feel for laryngeal excursion as a sign that a swallow response has been elicited.

good medium for eliciting the chewing reflex because of its texture and cold stimulation to the gums.

Once it has been determined that the patient adequately elevates the larynx and that there is an adequate protective cough, the examination can proceed to other substances with different textures and consistencies. Volumes usually range from 5 to 10 mL, starting first with a smaller bolus and, if successful, moving toward larger boluses. Traditionally, changing volumes precedes changing textures. If successful with 10-mL boluses, the examiner may wish to test the swallow with a 20-mL bolus. Groher et al.[50] found that the most discriminative items to use in test trials if the examiner is interested only in using cough as a sign of aspiration were thin liquids in 5-mL amounts and thickened liquids in 5- and 10-mL amounts. Methods of delivery, such as cup versus straw, may yield important differences in performance since the latter requires longer and more coordinated airway closure mechanics. Clinicians should observe chewing and bolus preparation. One clinical method of making a judgment of whether the swallow response is delayed is the use of cervical auscultation.[51,52] The examiner places a stethoscope on the neck at the level of the vocal folds and listens for the sounds associated with swallowing (Figure 7-9). Preswallow sounds can be heard before the swallow as the bolus size increases,[53] probably as a result of the tongue trying to contain a larger bolus.

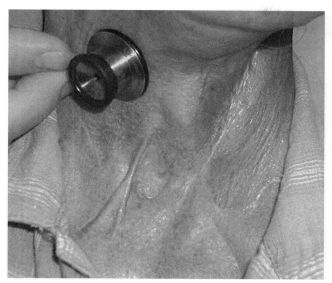

FIGURE 7-9 A stethoscope placed on the side of the neck can provide important acoustic information about the swallow response.

The three audible sounds associated with swallowing have both low- and high-frequency energy. The first two sounds are low-frequency energy, whereas the last sound (exhalatory burst) contains high-frequency energy. Microphones and accelerometers are capable of detecting the full frequency spectrum of these swallowing sounds; however, not all stethoscopes have this capability. Hamlet et al.[58] studied the frequency response characteristics of stethoscopes and identified two that had the capability of meeting these requirements: the Littman Cardiology II (3M, St. Paul, Minn.) and the Rappaport-Sprague pediatric size (Hewlett-Packard, Palo Alto, Calif.). There are two sides to a stethoscope—the flat, or diaphragm, side and the concave, or bell, side. Hamlet and colleagues found that the bell surface was best in detecting the sounds associated with swallowing.

Larger boluses produce more intense sound.[53] Before the swallow, the examiner should be cognizant of the respiratory rate. Comparisons should be made between the predeglutitory and postdeglutitory patterns. Marked change in the respiratory rate or an increase in respiratory congestion may be a sign of airway compromise. During swallow, respirations should cease (period of apnea). Within the short apneic period, two bursts of sound are markers of the presence of a swallow; these can be heard by cervical auscultation (see Practice Note 7-4). After listening to patients with normal swallows, the examiner can begin to appreciate what might constitute swallow delay in abnormal patterns, since the timing of the pattern from swallow onset to the first and second bursts of energy is consistent. Simultaneous videofluoroscopy and swallowing sound recordings have shown that the first burst of sound is associated with the bolus content that has entered the pharynx, whereas the second sound is associated with the bolus as it leaves the pharynx and enters the esophagus (Figure 7-10). After most swallows a short exhalation can be heard as a single, short burst of acoustic energy (release of subglottic air pressure). This exhalatory burst, or glottal release sign, is present in normal swallows and is affected by age and bolus volume.[54] Delay in detecting these sounds or failing to hear any of these sounds may serve as a potential marker of swallow abnormality.[54] In a series of patients with head and neck cancer, Uyama et al.[55] found that cervical auscultation could differentiate between normal and dysphagic swallows if the patient was asked to produce a voluntary exhalation after the swallow.[55] Changes in the frequency band from 0 to 500 Hz were more prominent in those with dysphagia compared with the changes in normal swallows. In 11 patients who showed signs of aspiration by endoscopy imaging, Shirazi et al.[56] found that the low frequency components detected after the swallow were reliable predictors of aspirators versus nonaspirators. Furthermore, a more specific analysis of the low-frequency power bands predicted silent aspiration in this small sample with 86% accuracy. Although interrater agreement on swallow abnormality with auscultation alone is only fair, agreement on abnormality versus no abnormality improves with group discussion, suggesting that individuals are capable of making decisions about safe swallow using acoustic data.[52] Borr et al.[57] also found only fair interrater reliability when rating seven parameters of acoustic recordings of swallows in normal (healthy) subjects, older adults, and subjects with known dysphagia. However, experienced clinicians were able to detect reliably events of aspiration or penetration, with 70% sensitivity and 94% specificity. Interestingly, the significant distinguishing factor between normal aging swallows and dysphagic swallows was that the patients with dysphagia swallowed twice instead of once on small bolus sizes. Borr et al.[57] concluded that cervical auscultation may be a viable tool to screen for airway compromise as part of a complete clinical evaluation.

An acoustic representation of an entire respiratory–swallowing sequence obtained with a microphone coupled to a computer with sound analysis capability is presented in Figure 7-11.

Feeding Evaluation

Patients who are unable to cooperate with a physical evaluation and who may be eating with suspected dysphagic complications can be partially evaluated through careful observation at the bedside. Bedside data should be gathered for three meals because the eating circumstance, including

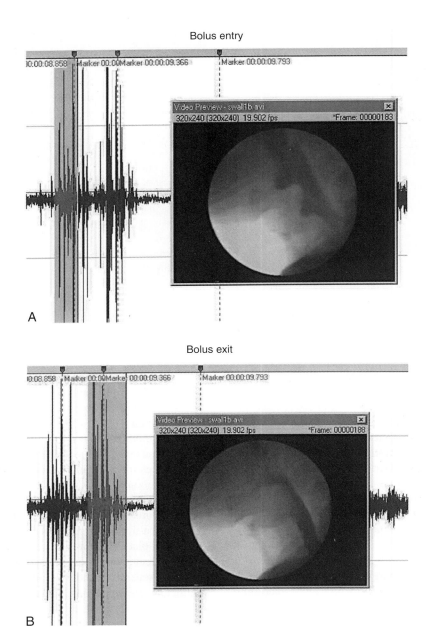

FIGURE 7-10 **A,** Simultaneous recording of the videofluoroscopic image of swallow and the corresponding acoustic pattern. The first swallow sound burst is associated with the bolus entry into the pharynx. **B,** The second sound burst should be associated with the bolus leaving the pharynx and entering the esophagus. (Courtesy T. Neil McKaig.)

differing food items, may vary from breakfast to lunch to dinner. When possible, the entire meal should be observed because patients often fatigue. Swallowing competence therefore may change as the meal progresses.

Environment

Patients with cortical brain damage and dysphagia may be highly distractible. If the distraction causes the patient to talk while eating or to not focus on the process of feeding, swallowing safety may be sacrificed. Typical distractions include the feeding assistant asking the patient for a verbal response while eating, listening to the radio, and viewing television. Other distractions include those that are patient centered. For instance, the patient's glasses not being positioned properly, resulting in distraction, or attention being focused on an ill-fitting denture that is causing discomfort.

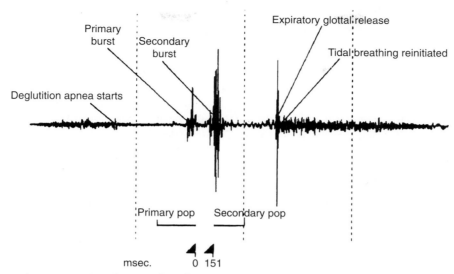

FIGURE 7-11 An acoustic representation of a normal swallow sequence. It is marked by the cessation of tidal airflow and two bursts of swallowing sounds within the apneic period *(between first two dotted lines)*, followed by a burst of exhalation and the resumption of tidal breathing *(final dotted line)*. (Courtesy T. Neil McKaig.)

Feeding

If the patient is self-feeding, is he or she able to open all containers, find the food on the tray, and use the utensils properly? Can the patient use the utensils to transport food to the mouth? Is the feeding rate appropriate? Are bite sizes appropriate? Are there differences in swallowing performance between taking liquids using a straw and taking them by cup? If the patient is to use special feeding utensils, are they provided? If dentures are needed, are they in place and properly fitted?

Posture

Because an upright posture is best for swallowing, it is important to note whether the patient is in that position and if he or she can maintain that position throughout the meal. If the patient is to use a special posture such as chin-down as a method of airway protection (see Chapter 10), the examiner should observe whether this posture can be achieved. Even patients who are fed by gastrostomy tube should have the head of the bed slightly elevated to avoid the possibility of reflux from the stomach.

Eating

The diet level (soft, pureed, mechanical soft, or regular) should be noted. Some patients receive a diet level that is not appropriately matched to their disorder.[59] If fluids are to be altered by thickening, is the consistency appropriate? If thickened fluids are allowed to sit too long before serving, they may become too thick for safe ingestion. Does the patient have more difficulty with liquids than semisolids or vice versa? When the patient places a chewable item in the mouth, is adequate chewing motion evident, or does the food sit without any apparent attempt by the patient to start a swallow? Does the patient have choking episodes, either before a swallow attempt, during the swallow, or after the swallow has been completed? The use of cervical auscultation or observations of laryngeal excursion may assist the examiner in this determination. The examiner should observe whether the eating process is more efficient at the beginning or end of the meal because fatigue may decompensate safe swallowing in some patients. An estimate of the amount eaten and the total time to finish the meal is an important marker of swallowing efficiency and may serve as useful functional outcome measures after swallowing treatment. Changes in respiratory status, taken from bedside monitors or from audible respiratory distress, such as wheezing or difficulty clearing secretions, should be part of the observational data pool.

Assistance

If prior recommendations have been made to improve the patient's feeding or eating performance, are these suggestions being followed by the patient? Or if the patient needs a feeding assistant who must provide reminders to accomplish safe feeding, are those reminders being provided?

TESTS TO DETECT ASPIRATION

In studies comparing the utility of the clinical evaluation compared with videofluoroscopy to detect aspiration, most have shown that only 60% to 70% of the patients who aspirate are correctly identified after the clinical examination.[19,34,60]

CLINICAL CASE EXAMPLE 7-2

An older adult woman came to the hospital to have her hip replaced. Her medical history was remarkable for childhood polio from which she recovered, **hypertension**, and coronary heart disease. After the hip surgery a nurse noted she was choking on liquids and a request for a consultation was sent to speech pathology.

The physical evaluation revealed that the patient was alert, oriented, and cooperative. She was able to sustain a cogent conversation while sitting upright in bed. She told the examiner that because she was choking on liquids, they no longer put them on her meal tray, which consisted of a soft mechanical diet. She was noted to have an intravenous feeding line in her right arm. An evaluation of her oral peripheral speech mechanism revealed generalized weakness of the tongue and lips, more severe on the right than left side. Examination of the muscles of mastication was normal. Her oral cavity was xerostomic and she was **edentulous**. The gag reflex was present but not brisk. She was able to produce a voluntary cough and swallow response. Normal laryngeal elevation was noted during her dry-swallow attempt. Her voice was markedly hoarse but not breathy. She did not show any signs of dysarthria. During test swallows of 5 mL of thin liquid, she coughed briskly, without delay, as the larynx was elevating. A commercial thickener was added to the thin liquid. During a test swallow with this consistency, the swallow was prompt without cough or delay. This was repeated with success on 10-mL and 20-mL boluses. The patient was then given a spoonful of pudding. This was swallowed without delay or cough. All swallow attempts were monitored with cervical auscultation so that a judgment of swallowing delay could be made.

In this case, the patient was able to express her difficulty swallowing thin liquids. Her difficulty was noted by the nurses, who reported that she coughed when swallowing thin liquids. Her problem was compensated by adding thickeners to the thin fluid. Failure to protect her airway on thin fluids could have been related to a temporary decompensation of her airway closure reflex related to the endotracheal tube from recent surgery. Airway closure problems frequently are most obvious with thinner fluids because of their speed of movement through the pharynx. This possibility was supported by the patient's severe hoarseness. An alternate explanation might be that she had generalized weakness in the bulbar musculature from her childhood polio that became more apparent at the laryngeal level after her surgery. That muscle weakness still was present was supported by diminished strength in the lip and tongue musculature. Her xerostomia was a side effect from medications to control her coronary artery disease. The patient started a diet of thickened liquids with a soft mechanical diet. The recommendation was made to discontinue her intravenous fluids because it was believed she could maintain her hydration with thickened liquids. The prognosis for returning to regular fluids was judged to be good because it was believed that the decompensation of her airway closure would be temporary. Continued monitoring of her respiratory status was recommended to ensure her safety on this dietary level. Because her complaint was explained and ultimately resolved by the clinical evaluation, no further testing was considered.

These findings have led to numerous investigations of tests to improve the accuracy of clinically based methods to detect tracheal aspiration. Another rationale to improve the accuracy of the ability of the clinical examination to detect aspiration is that many clinicians do not have easy access to instrumental examinations such as videofluoroscopy and its capability to visualize aspiration. The presumed consequence of failing to detect aspiration is that aspiration pneumonia with its attendant morbidity and mortality will develop in these patients. Interestingly, no data have prospectively studied in homogeneous groups the health risk of not detecting aspiration with a clinical examination. For instance, screening examinations for the detection of aspiration may identify those with severe aspiration and not detect those with minor aspiration and that minor aspiration may not be a threat to health outcomes[37] (review Clinical Corner 7-4).

Most studies of aspiration prediction have involved acute poststroke patients because they remain a population at risk for events of aspiration. Comparisons are made between the clinical examination's ability to detect

CLINICAL CORNER 7-4: DETECTING DYSPHAGIA

Investigators found that when patients with dysphagia were given 20 mL of a thickened liquid their eyes would tear ostensibly as a result of cough and congestion. They reported that their "eye-tearing test" had a sensitivity of 50% and a specificity of 40% at predicting aspiration.

Critical Thinking

1. How would you interpret the sensitivity data? Is this a good test to use to detect aspiration?
2. What is the consequence to the patient clinically given the 40% specificity of the test?

aspiration with confirmation by an instrumental examination such as endoscopy or videofluoroscopy.

Mann and Hankey[61] used regression analysis and studied 23 clinical features related to swallowing in 71 poststroke patients to identify significant independent predictors of aspiration. Significant predictors of aspiration included an impaired pharyngeal response, male gender, disabling stroke (**Barthel score** <60), incomplete oral clearance, palatal weakness or asymmetry, and age greater than 70 years. They argued that together these six variables could be used to detect aspiration risk, potentially providing a more efficient approach to a clinical evaluation. In a group of patients referred for a swallowing evaluation as a result of burn injury, Edelman et al.[62] found that the standardized clinical examination was highly predictive of aspiration subsequently verified by videofluoroscopy.[62] However, this may be because their patients had severe oropharyngeal dysphagia from their pathologic conditions, biasing the results toward the high prediction accuracy of aspiration from the clinical examination. Leder and Espinoza[63] compared six clinical features from the clinical examination with endoscopic detection of aspiration. In 49 poststroke patients they concluded that the clinical examination underestimated those who aspirated and overestimated those who did not aspirate on endoscopy. Bianchi et al.[64] sought to use objective pulmonary function testing to predict those patients who may be at risk for pulmonary complications secondary to aspiration. In a retrospective study of 55 patients with dysphagia with mixed diagnoses, 33% of those with pulmonary complications had significantly lower cough peak flow measures on pulmonary function tests than those without pulmonary complications.[64] In a series of 21 patients with spinal cord injury and tetraplegia who underwent a clinical evaluation and a videofluorographic imaging study, 38% were classified as dysphagic.[65] In only one subject was the diagnosis of dysphagia changed following the imaging study. Solid food dietary recommendations were altered in four patients, and liquid modifications in eight following the imaging studies. The authors concluded that in this patient group the clinical evaluation was a useful screening tool.[65]

Water Tests

Water tests presumably are to be used in patients who are alert enough to accept a bolus of water as a method to clinically detect aspiration or risk for aspiration. The assumption is that water is chosen as the bolus of choice because, if aspirated, it is relatively innocuous in the lungs.

The first water test was the 3-oz (85-mL) water test in which the patient attempts to swallow 3 oz of water at any rate he or she chooses.[66] The examiner then makes a clinical judgment of aspiration based on the patient's response. DiPippo et al.[66] reported a sensitivity of 76% and specificity of 59%, with incorrect identification of aspiration in 34% of cases. The high number of false-negative results (41%) suggests a high number of silent aspirators in this cohort because cough is the feature judged to help make the prediction of aspiration. Garon et al.[67] expressed concern that the 3-oz water test would become the standard test for detecting

aspiration. They studied patients with mixed neurogenic causes, comparing the 3-oz water test with videofluoroscopy. In their study only 35% of the patients were correctly predicted as aspirating. However, it is important to note that this subject sample was different from the original sample reported by DiPippo et al.[66] (mixed neurogenic vs. stable stroke). After studying 3000 patients with mixed ages and dysphagia diagnoses, Suiter and Leder[68] concluded that failure on the 3-oz test did not necessarily predict swallowing failure (71% were deemed safe for oral alimentation), and that passing the test suggested recommendations for oral alimentation could be made without further objective testing.

Sensitivity and specificity data similar to the 3-oz water test were found on the timed water test.[69] Patients are required to swallow 150 mL of water. Observations of cough, the number of swallows, the total time to finish the entire amount, and the amount of residue remaining if the patient could not finish are calculated. Accuracy of prediction is based on the speed of completing the swallow and amount of water swallowed.

Combinations of clinical evaluation procedures and water tests also have been studied. Mari et al.[70] combined a patient symptom checklist, a clinical examination, and the 3-oz water test as a method to detect aspiration compared with videofluoroscopy as the reference standard for aspiration documentation. The predictive value of the 3-oz water was 76% versus poor predictive values for the other two clinical measures. Sensitivity values were not as good as other studies because patients judged to have negative findings for aspiration showed silent aspiration on the videofluorographic study. Lim et al.[71] combined a 50-mL water test and oxygen saturation (SpO_2) data as a method of aspiration detection in acute poststroke patients with a 2% drop in saturation levels as the standard for abnormality and suspected aspiration during water swallows. The combination of the two tests showed 100% sensitivity and 70% specificity. Tohara et al.[72] designed a test battery that included a 3-oz water test, 4 g of pudding, and a standard plain x-ray film of the pharynx. They argued that some facilities may not have videofluoroscopy but probably did have the capability to obtain static images of the pharynx before and after swallow attempts. By summing the data from 63 patients on the three tests, they calculated 90% sensitivity in detecting aspiration and specificity of 56%. In an extensive systematic review of 11 studies that examined water tests and combinations of water testing, Bours et al.[73] found wide ranges of sensitivity and specificity in their use to detect dysphagia. Studies that combined water with oxygen saturation using cough and changes in voice postswallow as measurement endpoints appeared to be the best method to detect dysphagia in patients with neurologic disease. In a study that included suspected oropharyngeal disorders in 62 neurologic and nonneurologic patients, Schultheiss, Nusser-Muller-Busch, and Seidl[74] concluded that combining a test semisolid with a liquid bolus significantly increased the sensitivity and specificity levels of dysphagia detection by endoscopy to more than 80% with negative predictive values at similar levels.

Swallow Frequency

In a retrospective study of a mixed group of older adult patients, Murray et al.[75] used fiberoptic endoscopy to assess the presence of saliva aspiration as a predictor of aspiration-related pneumonia. As part of the study, they also counted swallow frequency during the examination. They concluded that saliva aspiration and reduced swallow frequency were related. The method of measuring swallow frequency was studied by Crary et al.[76] Comparing physiologic and acoustical measures of swallow occurrence, they found that acoustic measurement techniques can be a valid measure of swallow frequency and therefore may be an ideal non-invasive tool to measure swallow occurrence. Using acoustical analysis of swallows in acute stroke patients, they demonstrated that the measurement of swallow occurrence is a useful screening measuring to identify those at risk for dysphagia and its complications (see Chapter 3 for full discussion).[77]

Although water tests and combinations of tests using water may have some utility as screening devices for aspiration detection, all are hindered by design flaws that produce wide variability in results. Comparisons across studies are difficult because of differences in the diagnostic categories of subjects selected, differences in recruitment, time after onset of the patient's disease, variables measured and how measured, the reference test for confirmation of aspiration, and the clinical examination chosen.[78] These discrepancies make it difficult for the clinician to know if any one test is better than another to detect aspiration by a clinical examination.

Oxygen Saturation Tests

Numerous studies have examined whether a drop in oxygen saturation (SpO_2) levels using a pulse oximeter (Figure 7-12) could reliably detect events of aspiration. The rationale for this assumption is based on the fact that changes in respiratory status may signal a change in airway protection during swallowing events. Early investigators concluded that a drop in SpO_2 was associated with events of aspiration.[79,80] More recently, Smith et al.[81] found that a 2% drop in SpO_2 levels had an 86% sensitivity in predicting aspiration but poor predictive value. They argued for a combination of a standard clinical evaluation and SpO_2 monitoring to improve the predictive value. Using simultaneous measures of oxygen saturation and fiberoptic endoscopy, Colodny[82] studied 104 patients with dysphagia and 77 patients with no dysphagia. In neither group did reduced SpO_2 relate to events of aspiration; however, the trend

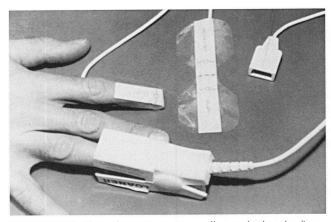

FIGURE 7-12 The pulse oximeter is usually attached to the finger in an adult and often is placed on the large toe in an infant. The device provides an estimate of the oxygenation in the blood as an indirect measure of respiratory status. Although oximetry is not as precise as an actual measurement of blood gases from a blood sample analyzed in the laboratory, it serves as a screening device for changes in respiratory status. (From Roberts J, Hedges J: *Clinical procedures in emergency medicine,* ed 4, Philadelphia, 2004, WB Saunders.)

indicated that a drop in saturation levels was most likely to be found in patients symptomatic for dysphagia. Those at particular risk for **oxygen desaturation** aspirated on solid food.

Modified Evans Blue Dye Test

The modified Evans blue dye (MEBD) test is another method used to detect aspiration at the bedside. The test is reserved for patients with tracheotomies who because of their illness may not be easily transportable to the radiographic suite for a videofluoroscopic swallowing study. The test protocol varies among institutions. The patient is given either a liquid or semisolid bolus that has been tinted with food coloring. The color is added so that any aspirated material is easily distinguished from other secretions. After the patient is given the test bolus, deep suctioning is performed through the tracheostomy site; suctioning is repeated in 15-minute intervals for an hour. The suction line is inspected for any coloration suggestive of aspiration (see Practice Note 7-5).

Thompson-Henry and Braddock[83] reported on the MEBD procedure in five patients. On follow-up videofluoroscopic and endoscopic procedures, all patients showed signs of aspiration, whereas no patient showed aspiration after the MEBD procedure. These authors concluded that the MEBD should be used with caution because of the high false-negative rate in this small sample. Brady et al.[84] used simultaneous videofluoroscopy and MEBD to study 20 patients. They divided their patients into two groups: those with only small amounts (trace) of aspiration and those with larger amounts of aspiration. Their results found 100%

PRACTICE NOTE 7-5

Protocols for the MEBD vary greatly among medical centers. Variation includes the type and amount of coloring used, the size of the test bolus, and the period after the test swallows in which the suctioning is attempted. Suctioning usually is done immediately after the test but may be done at hourly intervals for 3 hours up to 24 hours. Suctioning is continued with the intent that initially the patient may not have aspirated, but residual content in the mouth or pharynx may become aspirated at a later time. The test also is confounded by agreement of whether colored, aspirated material is present in the suction line. If a patient aspirates only a small amount, visualization through a clouded suction tube to make a decision on aspiration is not always reliable and is subject to considerable debate.

sensitivity in those with severe aspiration and 50% sensitivity in those with trace aspiration. It could be concluded from these data that MEBD is most useful in those with suspected severe aspiration. Although there is no experimental evidence to support it, even without the MEBD a standard clinical examination with inspection of trial swallows at the tracheostomy site might be as accurate in aspiration detection as the MEBD. O'Neill-Pirozzi et al.[85] also used simultaneous videofluoroscopy and MEBD with 50 patients. These investigators reported a sensitivity of 80% and a specificity of 62%. However, there was no association between aspiration on the MEBD and its severity as seen on videofluoroscopy, and the MEBD failed to detect some patients with severe aspiration. The differences across these studies are attributable to MEBD procedural differences, such as the bolus type and volume used, postswallow suction intervals, and potential differences in the severity of acute illness of the patients studied.

STANDARDIZED TESTS

Most clinicians design their own clinical swallowing evaluations based on the elements they have determined are most useful in detecting and defining the dysphagic condition. The majority of these tests are scored with a plus/minus (+/−) scoring system, present no data on the reliability of scoring, and do not compare their usefulness with other related measures (validity). Standardization implies that the test developer presents reliability and validity data on a large sample of patients with varying severity levels of the target disease. Evidence of the process of test development (theoretical rationale), comparisons to reference tests, the type of statistics used to support the reliability and validity, and a clear statement of how the test should be administered should be stated in the test manual.

The Mann Assessment of Swallowing Ability (MASA) is the first clinical test of swallowing with psychometric integrity.[86] It has reported reliability and validity data, positive and negative predictor values, and positive **likelihood ratios** on a population of 128 first-time, poststroke patients. The MASA allows the examiner to make judgments of dysphagia and aspiration severity with clinical diagnostic criteria (an ordinal risk rating) or by adding individual subtest scores and comparing them with the study sample for dysphagia and aspiration severity. Scoring guidelines are provided in 24 areas of assessment: alertness, cooperation, auditory comprehension, respiration, respiration rate after swallow, aphasia, apraxia, dysarthria, saliva management, lip seal, tongue movement, tongue strength, tongue coordination, oral preparation, gag reflex, palatal movement, bolus clearance, oral transit, cough reflex, voluntary cough, voice, tracheostomy, the pharyngeal phase, and the pharyngeal response. The MASA has not been evaluated for its predictive ability in the postacute phase of recovery or with patients with nonneurologic disorders such as head and neck cancer.

The McGill Ingestive Skills Assessment (MISA) is a standardized test developed to clinically assess patients' functional eating skills in a natural environment.[87] It assumes that the patient is already eating but has dysphagic symptoms or, if the patient is not eating, the examiner prepares varied food items for consumption and records the patient's attempt to eat. The MISA is to be used in conjunction with any extant data from the patient's medical history. Conceptually, the test is designed for clinicians working with older adults in skilled nursing facilities. Scores are assigned to patients in five areas of eating performance: positioning, self-feeding, liquid ingestion, solid ingestion, and texture management (manages a variety of foods). Within each area of swallowing performance there are subtests for a total of 43 test items. Each subtest is scored on a 3-point scale with clear instructions on what behaviors fit the numeric assignments. Each numeric category contains a detailed description of the desired performance that easily leads the examiner to the functional activities one would select in treatment. The MISA also has predictive data relating to health outcomes.[88] Seventy-three patients from skilled nursing facilities had follow-up for 563 days after administration of the MISA. Statistical analyses revealed that selective subtests such as solid ingestion, self-feeding, and texture management were predictive of time to death.

SUPPLEMENTAL TESTS

Occasionally the examiner who is assessing a patient with dysphagia may be interested in gathering data specific to the patient's complaint. Usually these tests are easily administered and scored. Ideally the tests will have

TABLE 7-3 Functional Oral Intake Scale

The Functional Oral Intake Scale is an **ordinal scale** that can be used to document the patient's functional eating status at the time of evaluation. It also is useful as a pretreatment and posttreatment outcome measurement tool.

Levels	Diet Level of Safe Oral Intake Meeting Nutritional and Hydration Needs
Tube dependent	1. Nothing by mouth (NPO) 2. Tube dependent with minimal attempts at food or liquid 3. Tube dependent with consistent intake of liquid or food
Total oral	4. Total oral diet of a single consistency 5. Total oral diet with multiple consistencies but requiring special preparation or compensations 6. Total oral diet with multiple consistencies without special preparation but with specific food limitations 7. Total oral diet with no restriction

CLINICAL CORNER 7-5: USING BIOFEEDBACK

A 58-year-old patient with myasthenia gravis reported increasing dysphagia with solid food. He underwent a modified barium swallow study with sEMG to measure the strength of his swallow. The patient had been taught to swallow hard to adequately clear his pharynx. By sEMG his swallow effort averaged 13 μV. During the study the examiner asked the patient to try to swallow with less force. The patient was still able to clear his pharynx with an average of 8 μV of effort.

Critical Thinking
1. How does the diagnosis of myasthenia gravis interfere with swallowing?
2. Why might it be important for this patient to swallow with less effort?

undergone the rigors of standardization. Data from these tests often serve as baseline measurement tools to assess outcome after intervention. Examples of supplementary testing include documentation of the patient's current dietary level, nutritional status, and documentation of the suspicion for GERD or laryngopharyngeal reflux (LPR).

A reliable and valid measure to document the patient's current dietary level is the Functional Oral Intake Scale (FOIS).[89] Originally validated on poststroke dysphagic patients, the FOIS is a 7-point ordinal scale that documents the patient's functional eating status ranging from total reliance on tube feeding to eating a diet with no restrictions or special preparation. Data are derived either from patient report or examiner observations. The FOIS is presented in Table 7-3.

A measure of nutritional status may be useful at the initial evaluation, particularly if the clinician does not have easy access to a dietitian. The Mini Nutritional Assessment (MNA) is a reliable and valid measure of nutritional status that can serve either as a screening device or, when used with additional test items, can provide a malnutrition indicator score.[90] The test items on the MNA are a mix of subjective examiner impressions, patient report, and objective measurements. The first five test items are used as a quick screening measure. Patients who score 11 points or less on this screening should be measured on 12 additional items. The only equipment the SLP needs to administer this test is the ability to measure midarm circumference, height, and weight.

Patients who present to the SLP with reports of food or liquid sticking at the level of the cervical esophagus should have a screening for GERD. Several reliable and valid methods for GERD screening have been developed, including the GERD score,[91] the Reflux Disease Questionnaire,[92] the Gastrointestinal Symptoms Rating Scale,[93] and the Reflux Questionnaire (ReQuest).[94] ReQuest has a short (5-minute) version, and a longer (20-minute) version in which the patient answers questions to relevant questions using a 7-point Likert scale.

Patients who present with the globus sensation, hoarseness, chronic cough, dysphagia or odynophagia, and chronic throat clearing should be screened for LPR. The easiest test to administer is the Reflux Symptom Index (RSI).[95] Patients are asked to answer questions about nine items that are sensitive to LPR detection. Each answer is scored on a 5-point scale. An RSI score greater than 10 suggests the presence of LPR. Follow-up fiberoptic endoscopic examinations should be used for symptom confirmation.

Although the use of surface electromyography (sEMG) has not been studied empirically as a method for clinical evaluation of swallow, it may be useful in the detection of swallow events and in establishing baseline data for swallow strength (see Clinical Corner 7-5). Submental muscle activity is associated with hyoid elevation and swallow initiation.[96] Both experienced and novice practitioners can use sEMG tracings to determine whether a swallowing event has occurred by looking at the visual representation.[97] Therefore measurement of swallow delay as detected by sEMG may be beneficial in determining the difference between normal and abnormal swallow responses because delay is associated with abnormality (Figure 7-13). Although there are no established normative data for the muscular strength needed to complete a swallow by bolus type or volume, sEMG technology can document the force needed to complete a successful swallow response.

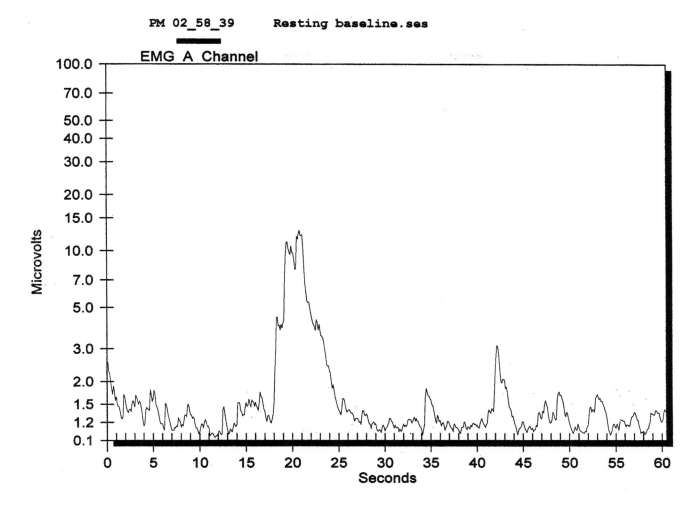

PM 02_58_39   Resting baseline.ses

Session Timing:
Continuous   Total session time: 60.5 sec.   or   1 min. 0.5 sec.

Overall Session Values:
Channel A					Tot	
Avg	Min	Max	StD	%S	%S	
1.81	1.00	12.9	1.83	0.00	0.00	

FIGURE 7-13 Tracing of a swallowing event using surface electromyographic electrodes fixed to the lateral neck. The force of the swallow is measured in microvolts (μV) (vertical axis). The horizontal axis shows muscle activity below 2 μV for 18 seconds until a peak (15 μV) of activity representing the swallow is seen at 20 seconds. After the swallow, muscle activity returns to below 2 μV as the muscles relax.

TAKE HOME NOTES

1. Patients often wait for long periods before they report their dysphagia.
2. Patients may not always be able to describe each element of their dysphagia.
3. Patients may not always realize that repeated bouts of pneumonia and weight loss may be a consequence of their dysphagia.
4. Symptoms are aspects of the swallowing process that the patient reports are problematic.
5. Signs are aspects of the swallowing process that are objectively measured and determined to connote a swallowing disorder.
6. Common dysphagic symptoms include the globus sensation, heartburn, loss of pleasure associated with eating, special preparation such as excessive chewing, regurgitation, and changes in diet level.

7. Common signs of dysphagia include drooling, choking, respiratory congestion after eating, increased need for suctioning, fatigue when eating, poor position when eating, loss of cognitive controls over the eating circumstance, undernutrition and muscle wasting, and the presence of feeding, tracheostomy, and endotracheal tubes.

8. The clinical examination of swallowing includes a review of the medical history, the physical evaluation and, if appropriate, test swallows.

9. The clinical examination may fail to detect all patients who aspirate and patients who do not aspirate.

10. The physical evaluation includes observations of the patient in eating and noneating situations, evaluation of mental status, and an evaluation of the cranial nerves needed for swallowing.

11. Water tests, measures of oxygen saturation levels, cervical auscultation, and the MEBD test have been proposed as supplemental clinical methods to detect aspiration.

12. Standardized tests for oropharyngeal dysphagia are the MASA and the MISA.

13. Standardized screening tests to detect oropharyngeal dysphagia include the MMASA, the TOR-BSST, the Barnes Jewish Hospital Dysphagia Screen, and the Emergency Physician Swallow Screening.

REFERENCES

1. Ravich WJ, Donner MW, Kashima H, et al: The swallowing center: concepts and procedures. *Gastrointest Radiol* 10:255, 1985.

2. Logemann JA, Veis S, Colangelo L: A screening procedure for oropharyngeal dysphagia. *Dysphagia* 14:44, 1999.

3. Smithard DG, O'Neill PA, Park C, et al: Complications and outcome after stroke: does dysphagia matter? *Stroke* 27:1200, 1996.

4. World Health Organization: *Principles and practices of screening for disease*, Geneva, 1968, World Health Organization.

5. Martino R, Pron G, Diamant N: Screening for oropharyngeal dysphagia in stroke. *Dysphagia* 15:19, 2000.

6. Serra-Prat M, Palomera M, Gomez C, et al: Oropharyngeal dysphagia as a risk factor for malnutrition and lower respiratory tract infection in independently living older persons: a population-based prospective study. *Age Aging* 41:376, 2012.

7. Daniels SK, Anderson JA, Wilson PC: Valid items for screening dysphagia risk in patients with stroke: a systematic review. *Stroke* 43:892, 2012.

8. Schepp SK, Tirschwell DL, Miller RM, et al: Swallowing screens after acute stroke. *Stroke* 43:869, 2012.

9. Antonios N, Carnaby-Mann G, Crary M, et al: Analysis of a physician tool for evaluating dysphagia on an inpatient stroke unit: the modified Mann assessment of swallowing ability. *J Stroke Cerebrovasc Dis* 19:49, 2010.

10. Martino R, Silver F, Teasell R, et al: The Toronto Bedside Swallowing Screening Test (TOR-BSST): development and validation of a dysphagia screening tool for patient with stroke. *Stroke* 40:555, 2009.

11. Wilson RH, Howe EC: A cost-effectiveness analysis of screening methods for dysphagia after stroke. *PM & R: J Inj Func Rehab* 4:273, 2012.

12. McCullough GH, Wertz RT, Rosenbek JC, et al: Clinicians' preference and practice in conducting clinical/bedside and videofluoroscopic examinations of swallowing in an adult neurogenic population. *Am J Speech Lang Pathol* 8:149, 1999.

13. Mathers-Schmidt BA, Kurlinski M: Dysphagia evaluation practices and inconsistencies in clinical assessment and instrumental examination decision making. *Dysphagia* 18:114, 2003.

14. McCullough GH, Wertz RT, Rosenbek JC, et al: Inter- and intrajudge reliability of a clinical examination of swallowing in adults. *Dysphagia* 15:58, 2000.

15. Ekberg O, Feinberg MJ: Altered swallowing function in elderly patients with dysphagia: radiographic findings in 56 cases. *AJR Am J Roentgenol* 156:1181, 1991.

16. Cook IJ, Kahrilas PJ: AGA technical review on management of oropharyngeal dysphagia. *Gastroenterology* 116:455, 1999.

17. Edwards DA: Discriminative value of symptoms in the differential diagnosis of dysphagia. *Clin Gastroenterol* 6:5, 1976.

18. Jones B, Ravich WJ, Kramer SS, et al: Pharyngoesophageal interrelationships: observations and working concepts. *Gastrointest Radiol* 10:225, 1985.

19. Logemann JA: *Evaluation and treatment of swallowing disorders*, ed 2, San Diego, 1998, Pro-Ed.

20. Lindgren S, Ekberg O: Swallowing complaints and cineradiographic abnormalities of the pharynx. *Dysphagia* 3:97, 1988.

21. Kim CH, Weaver AL, Hsu JJ, et al: Discriminant value of esophageal symptoms: a study of the initial clinical findings in 499 patients with dysphagia of various causes. *Mayo Clin Proc* 68:948, 1993.

22. DiPippo KL, Holas MMA, Resing MJ: The Burke Dysphagia Screening Test: validation of its use in patients with stroke. *Arch Phys Med Rehabil* 75:1284, 1994.

23. Manor Y, Gilada N, Cohen A, et al: Validation of a swallowing disturbance questionnaire for detecting dysphagia in patients with Parkinson's disease. *Mov Disord* 22:1917, 2007.

24. Wallace KL, Middleton S, Cook IJ: Development and validation of a self-report symptom inventory to assess the severity of oral-pharyngeal dysphagia. *Gastroenterology* 118:678, 2000.

25. McHorney CA, Robbins J, Lomax K, et al: The SWAL-QOL and SWAL-CARE outcomes tool for oropharyngeal dysphagia in adults: III. Documentation of reliability and validity. *Dysphagia* 17:92, 2002.

26. Silbergleit AK, Schultz L, Jacobson BH, et al: The Dysphagia Handicap Index. *Dysphagia* 27:46, 2012.

27. Belafsky P, Mouadeb DA, Rees CJ, et al: Validity and reliability of the eating assessment tool (EAT-10). *Ann Otol Rhinol Laryngol* 117:919, 2008.

28. Chen AY, Frankowski R, Bishop-Leone J, et al: The development and validation of a dysphagia-specific quality-of-life questionnaire for patients with head and neck cancer: the MD Anderson Dysphagia Inventory. *Arch Otolaryngol Head Neck Surg* 127:870, 2001.

29. Bjordalk K, Ablner-Elmquist M, Tollesson E, et al: Development of a European organization for research and treatment of cancer (EORTC) questionnaire module to be used in quality of life assessments in head and neck cancer patients. *Acta Oncol* 33:879, 1994.

30. Timmerman AA, Speyer R, Heijnen BJ, et al: Psychometric characteristics of health-related quality-of-life-questionnaires in oropharyngeal dysphagia. *Dysphagia* 29:183, 2014.

31. Jensen K, Lambertsen K, Torkov P, et al: Patient assessed symptoms are poor predictors of objective findings. Results from a cross sectional study in patients treated with radiotherapy for head and neck cancer. *Acta Oncol* 46:1159, 2007.

32. Ravich WJ, Wilson RF, Jones B, et al: Psychogenic dysphagia and globus: reevaluation of 23 patients. *Dysphagia* 4:35, 1989.

33. Moser G, Vacariu-Ganser GV, Schneider C, et al: High incidence of esophageal motor disorder in consecutive patients with globus sensation. *Gastroenterology* 101:1512, 1991.

34. Linden P, Kuhlemeir KV, Patterson C: Probability of correctly predicting subglottic penetration from clinical observations. *Dysphagia* 8:170, 1993.

35. McCulloch GH, Wertz RT, Rosenbek JC: Sensitivity and specificity of clinical/bedside signs for detecting aspiration in adults subsequent to stroke. *J Commun Disord* 34:55, 2001.

36. Daniels SK, McAdam CP, Brailey K, et al: Clinical assessment of swallowing and prediction of dysphagia severity. *Am J Speech Lang Pathol* 6:17, 1997.

37. McCullough GH, Rosenbek JC, Wertz RT, et al: Clinical swallowing examination measures for detecting aspiration post-stroke. *J Speech Lang Hear Res* 48:1280, 2005.

38. Chang HY, Torng PC, Wang TG, et al: Acoustic voice analysis does not identify presence of penetration/aspiration as confirmed by videofluoroscopic swallowing study. *Arch Phys Med Rehabil* 93:1191, 2012.

39. Waito A, Bailey GL, Molfenter SM, et al: Voice quality abnormalities as a sign of dysphagia: validation against acoustic and videofluoroscopic data. *Dysphagia* 26:125, 2011.

40. Steele CM, Cichero JAY: Physiological factors related to aspiration risk: a systematic review. *Dysphagia* 29:295, 2014.

41. Daniels SK, Ballo LA, Mahoney MC, et al: Clinical predictors and aspiration risk: outcome measures in acute stroke patients. *Arch Phys Med Rehabil* 81:1030, 2000.

42. Huggins PS, Tuomi SK, Young C: Effects of nasogastric tubes on the young, normal swallowing mechanism. *Dysphagia* 14:157, 1999.

43. Yorkston KA, Miller RM, Strand EA: *Management of speech and swallowing disorders in degenerative disease*, Tucson, AZ, 1995, Communication Skill Builders.

44. Leder SB, Suiter DM, Warner HL: Answering orientation questions, following single-step verbal commands: effect on aspiration status. *Dysphagia* 24:290, 2009.

45. Leder SB, Suiter DM, Murray J, et al: Can an oral mechanism examination contribute to the assessment of odds of aspiration? *Dysphagia* 28:370, 2013.

46. Yoshikawa M, Yoshida M, Tsuga K, et al: Comparisons of three types of tongue pressure measurement devices. *Dysphagia* 26:232, 2011.

47. Leder SB: Videofluoroscopic evaluation of aspiration with visual examination of the gag reflex. *Dysphagia* 12:21, 1997.

48. Langmore SE, Logemann JA: After the clinical bedside examination: what next? *Am J Speech Lang Pathol* 9:13, 1991.

49. Miller RM: Clinical examination for dysphagia. In Groher ME, editor: *Dysphagia: diagnosis and management*, Boston, 1997, Butterworth-Heinemann.

50. Groher ME, Crary MA, Mann GC, et al: The impact of rheologically controlled materials on the identification of airway compromise on the clinical and videofluoroscopic swallowing examinations. *Dysphagia* 21:218, 2006.

51. Takahashi K, Groher ME, Michi K: Methodology for detecting swallowing sound. *Dysphagia* 9:54, 1994.

52. Leslie P, Drinnan MJ, Finn P, et al: Reliability and validity of cervical auscultation: a controlled comparison using videofluoroscopy. *Dysphagia* 19:231, 2004.

53. Cichero JAY, Murdoch BE: Acoustic signature of the normal swallow characteristics by age, gender, and bolus volume. *Ann Otol Rhinol Laryngol* 111:623, 2002.

54. Cichero JAY, Murdoch BE: What happens after the swallow? Introducing the glottal release sound. *J Med Speech Pathol* 11:31, 2003.

55. Uyama R, Takahashi K, Michi Ken-ichi, et al: Objective evaluation using acoustic characteristics of swallowing and expiratory sounds for detecting dysphagic swallow. *J Jpn Stomatol Soc* 46:147, 1997.

56. Shirazi SS, Buchel C, Daun R, et al: Detection of swallows with silent aspiration using swallowing and breath sound analysis. *Med Biol Eng Comput* 50:1261, 2012.

57. Borr C, Hielscher-Fastabend M, Lucking A: Reliability and validity of cervical auscultation. *Dysphagia* 22:225, 2007.

58. Hamlet S, Penney DG, Formole J: Stethoscope acoustics and cervical auscultation of swallowing. *Dysphagia* 9:63, 1994.

59. Groher ME, McKaig TM: Dysphagia and dietary levels in skilled nursing facilities. *J Am Geriatr Soc* 43:1, 1995.

60. Splaingard ML, Hutchins B, Sulton LD, et al: Aspiration in rehabilitation patients: videofluoroscopy vs bedside clinical assessment. *Arch Phys Med Rehabil* 69:637, 1988.

61. Mann G, Hankey GJ: Initial clinical and demographic predictors of swallowing impairment following acute stroke. *Dysphagia* 16:208, 2001.

62. Edelman DA, Sheehy-Deardorff DA, White MT: Bedside assessment of swallowing is predictive of an abnormal barium swallow examination. *J Burn Care Res* 29:89, 2008.

63. Leder SB, Espinoza JF: Aspiration risk after acute stroke: comparison of clinical examination and fiberoptic endoscopic evaluation of swallowing. *Dysphagia* 17:214, 2002.

64. Bianchi C, Baiardi P, Khirani S, et al: Cough peak flow as a predictor of pulmonary morbidity in patients with dysphagia. *Am J Phys Med Rehabil* 91:783, 2012.

65. Shem KL, Castillo K, Wong SL, et al: Diagnostic accuracy of bedside swallow evaluation versus videofluoroscopy to assess dysphagia in individuals with tetraplegia. *Phys Med Rehab* 4:283, 2012.

66. DiPippo KL, Holas MA, Reding MJ: Validation of the 3 oz water test for aspiration following stroke. *Arch Neurol* 49:1259, 1992.

67. Garon B, Engle M, Ormiston C: Reliability of the 3 oz water test utilizing cough reflex as the sole indicator of aspiration. *J Neurol Rehabil* 9:139, 1995.

68. Suiter DM, Leder SB: Clinical utility of the 3-ounce water swallow test. *Dysphagia* 23:244, 2008.

69. Nathadwarawala KM, McGroary A, Wiles CM: Swallowing in neurological outpatients: use of a timed test. *Dysphagia* 9:120, 1994.

70. Mari F, Matei M, Ceravolo MG, et al: Predictive value of clinical studies in detecting aspiration in patients with neurological disorders. *J Neurol Neurosurg Psychiatry* 63:456, 1997.

71. Lim SH, Lieu PK, Phua SY, et al: Accuracy of bedside clinical methods compared with fiberoptic examination of swallowing (FEES) in determining the risk of aspiration in acute stroke patients. *Dysphagia* 16:1, 2000.

72. Tohara H, Saitoh E, Mays K, et al: Three tests for predicting aspiration without videofluoroscopy. *Dysphagia* 18:126, 2003.

73. Bours GJJW, Speyer R, Lemmens J, et al: Bedside screening tests vs. videofluoroscopy or fibreoptic endoscopic evaluation of swallowing

to detect dysphagia in patients with neurological disorders: systematic review. *J Adv Nurs* 65:477, 2009.

74. Schulheiss C, Nusser-Muller-Busch R, Seidl RO: The semisolid bolus swallow test for clinical diagnosis of oropharyngeal dysphagia: a prospective randomized study. *Eur Arch Otorhinolaryngol* 268:1837, 2011.

75. Murray J, Langmore SE, Ginsberg S, et al: The significance of accumulated oropharyngeal secretions and swallowing frequency in predicting aspiration. *Dysphagia* 11:99, 1996.

76. Crary MA, Sura L, Carnaby G: Validation and demonstration of an isolated acoustic recording technique to estimate spontaneous swallow frequency. *Dysphagia* 28:86, 2013.

77. Crary MA, Carnaby GD, Sia I, et al: Spontaneous swallowing frequency has potential to identify dysphagia in acute stroke. *Stroke* 44:3452, 2013.

78. Carnaby-Mann G, Lenius K: The bedside examination in dysphagia. *Phys Med Rehabil Clin North Am* 19:747, 2008.

79. Collins M, Bakheit A: Does pulse oximetry reliably detect aspiration in dysphagic stroke patients? *Stroke* 28:1773, 1997.

80. Sherman B, Nisenbaum JM, Jesberger ML, et al: Assessment of dysphagia with the use of pulse oximetry. *Dysphagia* 14:152, 1999.

81. Smith HA, Lee SH, O'Neill PA, et al: The combination of bedside swallowing assessment and oxygen saturation monitoring of swallowing in acute stroke: a safe and humane screening tool. *Age Aging* 29:495, 2000.

82. Colodny N: Comparison of dysphagics and nondysphagics on pulse oximetry during oral feeding. *Dysphagia* 15:68, 2000.

83. Thompson-Henry S, Braddock B: The modified Evan's blue dye procedure fails to detect aspiration in the tracheostomized patient: five case reports. *Dysphagia* 10:172, 1995.

84. Brady SL, Hildner CD, Hutchins B: Simultaneous videofluoroscopic swallow study and modified Evans blue dye procedure: an evaluation of blue dye visualization in cases of known aspiration. *Dysphagia* 14:146, 1999.

85. O'Neill-Pirozzi TM, Lisiecki DJ, Momose KJ, et al: Simultaneous modified barium swallow and blue dye tests: a determination of the accuracy of the blue dye test aspiration findings. *Dysphagia* 18:32, 2003.

86. Mann G: *MASA: The Mann assessment of swallowing ability*, Clifton, NY, 2002, Thomson Learning.

87. Lambert HC, Gisel EG, Wood-Dauphinee S, et al: *MISA: The McGill ingestive skills assessment and forms*, Ottawa, 2006, Canadian Association of Occupational Therapists ACE.

88. Lambert HC, Abrahamowicz M, Groher M, et al: The McGill Ingestive assessment predicts time to death in an elderly population with neurogenic dysphagia: preliminary evidence. *Dysphagia* 20:123, 2005.

89. Crary MA, Mann GDC, Groher ME: Initial psychometric assessment of a functional oral intake scale for dysphagic stroke patients. *Arch Phys Med Rehabil* 86:1516, 2005.

90. Vellas B, Guigoz Y, Garry PJ, et al: *The Mini Nutritional Assessment: MNA. Nutrition in the elderly*, ed 2, Paris, 1994, Serdi.

91. Allen CJ, Parameswaram K, Belda J, et al: Reproducibility, validity, and responsiveness of a disease-specific symptom questionnaire for gastroesophageal reflux disease. *Dis Esophagus* 13:265, 2000.

92. Shaw M, Dent J, Reebe T, et al: The Reflux Disease Questionnaire: a measure for assessment of treatment response in clinical trials. *Health Qual Life Outcomes* 6:31, 2008.

93. Revicki DA, Wood M, Wikland I, et al: Reliability and validity of the Gastrointestinal Symptom Rating Scale in patients with gastroesophageal reflux disease. *Qual Life Res* 7:75, 1998.

94. Bardhan KD, Stanghellini V, Armstrong P, et al: International validation of ReQuest in patients with endoscopy-negative gastroesophageal reflux disease. *Aliment Pharmacol Ther* 20:891, 2004.

95. Belafsky PC, Postma GN, Koufman JA: Validity and reliability of the reflux symptom index. *J Voice* 16:274, 2002.

96. Crary MA, Caraby Mann GD, Groher ME: Biomechanical correlates of surface electromyography signals obtained during swallowing by healthy adults. *J Speech Lang Hear Res* 49:186, 2006.

97. Crary MA, Carnaby Mann GD, Groher ME: Identification of swallowing events from sEMG signals obtained from healthy adults. *Dysphagia* 22:94, 2007.

CHAPTER 8

Imaging Swallowing Examinations: Videofluoroscopy and Endoscopy

Michael A. Crary

To view additional case videos and content, please visit the evolve website.

OBJECTIVES

1. Explain why it is important to image the swallowing mechanism and evaluate swallow function with an imaging study. List some basic guidelines to help determine whether any imaging swallowing examination is indicated.
2. Describe the basic components and potential modifications of a fluoroscopic swallowing examination and an endoscopic swallowing examination.
3. Describe some of the strengths and weaknesses of the fluoroscopic swallowing examination and the endoscopic swallowing examination. ·
4. Compare the endoscopic examination with the fluoroscopic examination, specifically regarding the identification of various dysphagia characteristics.

CONSIDERATIONS FOR AN IMAGING SWALLOWING EXAMINATION

Many instrumental procedures may be used to evaluate different aspects of swallowing function. This chapter addresses the two most commonly used imaging procedures: videofluoroscopy (also called videofluorography) and flexible endoscopy (also known as fiberoptic endoscopy or transnasal endoscopy). However, before these imaging evaluation procedures are detailed, they should be placed in the context of the overall clinical evaluation of the adult patient with dysphagia. Frequent questions about these procedures include "What are they intended to achieve?" and "When is an imaging procedure indicated?" The following information is derived largely from practice guidelines published by the American Speech-Language-Hearing Association.[1-4] The concept underlying the use of practice guidelines is that they result from the creative, clinical, and scientific input of many experienced professionals with thorough professional review. In that regard, although these views may change with the acquisition of new information at a given point in time, they represent a fair summary of existing knowledge and opinion.

Goals of Imaging Swallowing Evaluations

Imaging examinations of swallowing are only a part of the comprehensive examination of swallowing performance and function. In general, a thorough clinical examination (see Chapter 7) should precede any imaging examination. The clinical examination can be important in tailoring specific questions to be addressed in an imaging examination and provides a comprehensive clinical profile of patients in whom dysphagia is suspected. In fact, one survey[5] reported that of all patients referred for dysphagia evaluation, comprehensive clinical assessments were completed on 71% but imaging studies were completed on only 36%. However, in a separate survey,[6] 60% of clinicians reported that they routinely completed a fluoroscopic swallowing study prior to initiating dysphagia therapy. These two surveys suggest that imaging studies are not always indicated but that clinicians feel they are useful in planning dysphagia therapy. Imaging examinations of swallowing may accomplish any number of objectives depending on the patient and the clinical situation. These examinations (1) provide valuable information on the anatomy and physiology of structures and muscles used in swallowing, (2) evaluate the ability of a patient to swallow various materials, (3) assess secretions and the patient's reaction to them, (4) document the adequacy of airway protection and the coordination between respiration and swallowing, and (5) help evaluate the effect of compensatory maneuvers on swallowing function and airway protection. Although the fluoroscopic and endoscopic examinations of swallowing function are not mirror images, they do share many common functions. In addition, each imaging study has specific attributes that the other may not possess. Furthermore, because each examination provides a permanent record of the swallowing evaluation, both contribute to increased objectivity with enhanced documentation and the ability to review results of the respective studies.

Purposes of Imaging Swallowing Examinations

Box 8-1 summarizes various purposes attributed to imaging swallowing examinations. Perhaps the most overt purpose of any imaging swallowing examination is the ability to image the structures of the swallowing mechanism and the movement of those structures during swallowing and other movements that may help assess their functional integrity. This assessment involves the lips, tongue, jaw, velopharyngeal mechanism, pharynx, larynx, and esophagus. Evaluation of these structures should incorporate some indication of anatomic adequacy and movement capability. In some cases it is possible to assess or perhaps infer sensory integrity and motor functions. Beyond basic anatomy and movement of specific structures, coordinated movement among various components of the swallow mechanism should be assessed with reference to swallowing function. This assessment requires the patient to swallow materials of varying amounts and textures to allow inspection of adjustments (either positive or negative) within the swallowing mechanism. This component of the imaging examination can help identify misdirection (specifically entrance into the airway) of a bolus and postswallow residue as a result of inefficient swallowing. If aspiration is identified, the

---

BOX 8-1 MULTIPLE PURPOSES ATTRIBUTED TO AN IMAGING SWALLOWING STUDY

- Image structures of the upper aerodigestive tract: oral cavity, velopharynx, pharynx, larynx, pharyngoesophageal segment, and esophagus.
- Assess movement patterns of swallowing-related structures in the upper aerodigestive tract to formulate inferences regarding physiologic integrity (e.g., speed of movement, symmetry, range, strength, sensation, coordination).
- Assess swallowing-related movement patterns of structures in the upper aerodigestive tract (e.g., effectiveness and safety of the swallow, accommodation to varying materials).
- Identify and describe any airway compromise (e.g., aspiration, penetration) and the circumstances under which these events occur.
- Evaluate the effect of compensatory maneuvers to improve swallowing safety and efficiency.
- Identify and describe any pooled secretions within the hypopharynx and larynx (or potentially other areas). Description should include the patient's ability to move or clear pooled secretions with swallows or coughing and clearing activities.
- Complete a cursory evaluation of esophageal anatomy and physiology to identify any overt esophageal contributors to dysphagia symptoms.
- Assist in forming clinical recommendations, including route of nutrition or hydration intake (i.e., oral, nonoral), safest or most efficient dietary level, need to make feeding modifications, or therapeutic interventions.

---

imaging examination is helpful in differentiating situations when the patient is more likely to aspirate versus those when aspiration is less likely. By using a variety of swallowed materials and incorporating compensatory maneuvers, clinicians may make inferences regarding the safest and most efficient material to swallow and the need for any postural or other adjustments that improve swallowing safety or efficiency. Secretions pooled within the swallowing mechanism can be problematic for patients and contribute to respiratory complications. These fluids should be identified and described, including the patient's reaction to them and the patient's ability to remove them from the swallowing tract. In some situations the clinician may conclude that oral feeding is not safe or adequate and hence might use the results of imaging examinations to recommend nonoral feeding sources (or to recommend discontinuation of nonoral feeding sources with reestablishment of oral feeding). In short, imaging examinations of swallowing function provide objective imaging of the swallowing mechanism that assists dysphagia clinicians in determining the need for and the direction of swallowing rehabilitation. More details of the fluoroscopic and endoscopic swallowing examinations are provided in later sections.

Indications for Imaging Swallowing Examinations

Box 8-2 addresses three important questions: (1) When *is* an imaging swallowing examination indicated? (2) When *may* an imaging swallowing be indicated? and (3) When is an imaging swallowing examination not indicated?[1]

Perhaps the basic answer to when an imaging examination is indicated is "when the clinical examination fails to answer the relevant questions." If the patient reports specific problems that are not clarified by the clinical examination, an imaging examination is indicated. This examination may help clarify whether a significant dysphagia exists and delineate the parameters of that type of dysphagia—oral, pharyngeal, esophageal, or a combination of these components. Information from an imaging examination may clarify airway protection issues that are potentially related to respiratory compromise or may elucidate swallow efficiency issues potentially related to nutritional decline.

BOX 8-2 INDICATIONS FOR AN IMAGING SWALLOWING EXAMINATION

Examination Definitely Indicated
- The comprehensive clinical examination fails to thoroughly address the clinical questions posed by the patient or problem.
- Dysphagia characteristics are vague and require confirmation or better delineation.
- Nutritional or respiratory issues indicate suspicion of dysphagia.
- Safety or efficiency of swallowing is a concern.
- Direction for swallowing rehabilitation is needed.
- Help is needed to assist in identifying underlying medical problems that contribute to dysphagia symptoms.

Examination *May* Be Indicated
- The patient has a medical condition that has a high risk for dysphagia.
- Swallow function demonstrates an overt change.
- The patient is unable to cooperate for a clinical examination.

Examination *Not* Indicated
- The patient no longer has dysphagia complaints.
- The patient's condition is too medically compromised or the patient is too uncooperative to complete the procedure.
- The clinician's judgment is that the examination would not alter the clinical course or management plan.

As previously mentioned, the effect of compensatory maneuvers may be verified during imaging examination, and other information on swallowing movements may be garnered that facilitates direction in swallowing rehabilitation. Finally, in some instances information gained from an imaging study may contribute to a better understanding of the medical diagnosis contributing to dysphagia symptoms.

An imaging swallowing examination *may* be indicated for various reasons, most of which are related to the condition of the patient. For example, some medical conditions pose a high risk for swallowing difficulty or may be complicated by swallowing difficulties that may not prompt a significant complaint from the patient. An imaging examination provides an objective evaluation of swallowing ability that may facilitate early identification of problems and hence lead to improved care. In addition, clinical conditions may change over time because of changes in the underlying disease (i.e., progressive or recovering conditions) or changes in the patient (new treatments or new disease). Some patients present with clinical conditions that preclude adequate cooperation with a clinical examination (cognitive or communicative impairments). In this situation, an imaging examination may help address the questions posed regarding swallowing ability.

Finally, in some clinical situations an imaging examination is not indicated. Perhaps the most obvious is when the patient reports that he or she had difficulty in the past but no longer has any swallowing difficulty. Other situations might include the patient whose medical condition is too compromised to tolerate a procedure or who is too uncooperative to participate in a procedure. If the clinician judges that the patient's condition will result in an imaging examination that provides no useful information, a valid decision may be to delay the examination until the patient's condition facilitates completion of a useful examination. The value of clinical judgment should not be underestimated. At times clinicians may simply feel that given all available information, the addition of an imaging examination of swallowing function will not provide any further beneficial information.

Imaging swallowing examinations—specifically fluoroscopic and endoscopic procedures—add an objective and valuable component to the comprehensive assessment of the patient with dysphagic symptoms. However, these examinations should not be isolated from the information obtained from a thorough clinical assessment. The combination of these tools is expected to provide the most complete clinical picture of the dysphagic patient, leading to the best possible treatment. Imaging examinations of swallowing function address both the anatomy and physiology of structures within the swallowing tract and how movement of these structures may accommodate swallowing different materials. Clinicians also may assess the effect of immediate compensations with these examinations. Available guidelines offer suggestions for when an imaging examination should, may, or should not be used; however, no guideline can account for all clinical situations. The judgment of the clinician with direct knowledge of the comprehensive picture is valuable in deciding when and how to use an imaging examination of swallowing function.

The following sections address the videofluoroscopic and fiberoptic endoscopic swallowing examinations separately and subsequently compare the two procedures directly to help clinicians decide whether one, both, or neither of these procedures is appropriate in various clinical situations.

VIDEOFLUOROSCOPIC SWALLOWING EXAMINATIONS

What's in a Name?

Various authors and health care institutions use different terms for what is essentially the same examination. Box 8-3 lists several name variants for this procedure. This list is not comprehensive but is probably representative of the variation that exists in nomenclature. The term *modified barium swallow*, initially coined by Logemann,[7] can be interpreted literally. The traditional barium swallow is focused on the esophagus and stomach and uses large amounts of liquid barium **(contrast agent)** and still-frame pictures to image the expanded esophagus and evaluate gastric emptying or other upper gastrointestinal (UGI) functions. This examination is usually done with the patient in one or more combinations of lying positions. The adult patient with dysphagia is likely to be compromised both by the large amounts of liquid barium and by the lying position during swallowing attempts. Therefore this examination was modified to use smaller amounts of contrast material varying in amount and consistency and to examine the patient in an upright position (whenever physically possible) to resemble the position most typically associated with eating. This procedure has become known as the modified barium swallow *(MBS)*.

BOX 8-3 TERMINOLOGY USED TO DESCRIBE THE VIDEOFLUOROSCOPIC SWALLOWING STUDY

- Modified barium swallow (MBS)
- Upper gastrointestinal series with hypopharynx
- Videofluoroscopic swallow study (VFSS)
- Videofluoroscopic barium examination (VFBE)
- Videofluoroscopic swallow examination (VFSE)
- Rehabilitation swallow study

Some health care professionals and researchers held to different conventions in selecting a name for this relatively new procedure. Gastrointestinal (GI) radiologists often referred to the procedure as an upper GI series with hypopharynx. This term reflects the traditional esophagram view but with the addition of a study of the hypopharynx. Other terms in the literature include *videofluoroscopic swallow study*,[8,9] *videofluoroscopic barium examination*,[10] and *videofluoroscopic swallow examination*.[11] Presumably, each of these terms was intended to identify the unique radiographic procedure that evaluates oropharyngeal swallowing function. Clinicians in different areas may know or use other terms that refer to the same study (see Practice Note 8-1). This chapter uses the more generic name variant, *videofluoroscopic swallowing examination (VFSE)*.

Objectives of the Videofluoroscopic Swallowing Examination

The videofluoroscopic swallowing examination can have multiple objectives. The primary objective is to obtain a video image of the upper aerodigestive tract during the act of swallowing. By manipulating what is swallowed, how it is swallowed, and patient positioning, clinicians can complete a comprehensive assessment of swallowing ability. Box 8-4 lists the more overt objectives of a videofluoroscopic swallowing examination. Additional objectives may be appropriate for individual patients or problems.[12]

Evaluation of the swallowing mechanism is initially approached by identification and description of any deviations in the anatomy of structures within the swallowing tract. This presupposes the clinician's detailed knowledge of anatomy, including radiographic anatomy. Figure 8-1

PRACTICE NOTE 8-1

Different terms have been applied to the fluoroscopic evaluation of swallowing. Many clinicians who engaged in these examinations in the early 1980s may have been confused by the term *modified barium swallow*. In the author's experience, referring physicians would often order the more traditional "barium swallow" when they intended to order the "modified version." In an attempt to reduce confusion within the author's health care system, the term *rehab swallow* was adopted and later became the term *rehab barium swallow*. This term, negotiated between speech-language pathologists and radiologists, was meant to reflect the importance of this study in "determining the need for and the direction of swallowing rehabilitation." Inclusion of the word *rehab* helped ensure that a speech-language pathologist was involved in each of these studies presented to radiology. Both the medical and the rehabilitative objectives of this examination were met by performing these studies in conjunction with a radiologist.

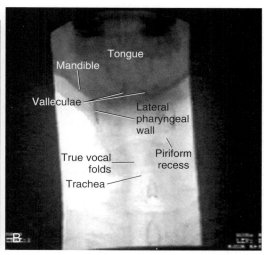

FIGURE 8-1   Lateral (*A*) and anterior (*B*) radiographic views of a normal swallowing mechanism. *PES,* Pharyngoesophageal segment.

BOX 8-4   OBJECTIVES OF THE VIDEOFLUOROSCOPIC SWALLOWING EXAMINATION

- Evaluate anatomy and physiology of the swallowing mechanism.
- Evaluate swallow physiology.
- Identify patterns of impaired swallow physiology.
- Identify consequences of impaired swallow physiology.
- Evaluate the effect of compensations.
- Confirm patient symptoms.
- Make prediction.

---

depicts both lateral and anterior radiographic views of a normal swallowing mechanism. Review of anatomic detail and examples of normal swallow physiology may be found in narrated Video 2-3 on the Evolve website that accompanies this textbook. *Basic physiology* of the swallowing mechanism may be evaluated by asking the patient to phonate, breath hold, perform a Valsalva maneuver, produce falsetto phonation, or perform other activities that facilitate movement of the structures within the swallowing tract. This component of the evaluation is helpful in identification of potential movement deficits that may contribute to oropharyngeal dysphagia and in selecting appropriate compensatory maneuvers.

Swallow physiology is evaluated by asking patients to swallow various amounts and textures of contrast materials. Knowledge of both normal and impaired swallow physiology is implicit in evaluating this component of the fluoroscopic examination. Abnormal aspects of physiology typically are detailed in terms of reduced or altered movement patterns. In addition, the consequences of physiologic impairments such as aspiration or residue are documented.

Finally, the effect of various compensations is evaluated. Compensatory postures or swallow maneuvers are useful both for introducing immediate improvement in the safety or efficiency of the swallow and for identifying potentially beneficial therapy strategies.

Symptom confirmation is an important objective of any imaging examination, including the videofluoroscopic swallowing examination. If a patient reports food sticking in the lower neck area, the fluoroscopic study should thoroughly evaluate that area. If nothing of consequence is identified there, other potential contributors to that symptom should be evaluated (in this specific case, the esophagus and lower esophageal sphincter should be thoroughly evaluated). Addressing this objective relies heavily on the clinician's skill in focusing on the patient's complaints and descriptions of dysphagia symptoms and in directing the fluoroscopic study to adequately evaluate those components of the swallowing mechanism that may contribute to a specific set of symptoms.

Given that the fluoroscopic swallowing examination is a time-limited event and cannot possibly sample all foods that a given patient might eat, a certain amount of prediction is involved in interpreting this examination. For this reason, we include "prediction" as an objective of the fluoroscopic swallowing examination. After a thorough evaluation of the structure and function of the swallowing mechanism, swallow physiology and consequences of impaired movement, and the effects of compensatory maneuvers, the clinician must engage in a series of educated decisions regarding the functional swallowing performance of each patient. Examples of such decisions include the potential for future health complications, such as aspiration-related pneumonias or nutritional deficits; the level of functional eating ability and any recommended diet level changes; the need for swallowing therapy and, if indicated, the specific direction of that therapy; whether additional clinical or imaging evaluations are indicated; and if consultations with other health care providers are needed to address the problems identified in the current examination. These are only a few of the potential areas of prediction in which clinicians may engage. Ultimately, questions of safe and adequate oral intake of food and liquid must be directly addressed and based in part on the results of this examination.

Procedures for the Videofluoroscopic Swallowing Examination

A standard protocol is highly recommended for the fluoroscopic study.[8,9,12] Standardizing the protocol increases consistency and reproducibility of examinations both within and across patients. The use of a standard protocol does not preclude individual variations that may be required for specific patients or problems; however, it does provide a consistent framework from which reasonable variations may be accomplished. Several factors within the protocol must be considered, including instructions to the patient, patient positioning, materials to be swallowed, sequence of attempted swallows, and what to look for, including interpretation and documentation of the findings.

Instructions to the Patient

As with any assessment, it is important that patients understand what is expected of them. Although this may not always be possible in patients with significant cognitive or communicative limitations, in general a brief set of instructions is provided to each patient being examined. Limited study has been directed at the role of patient instruction in the outcome of fluoroscopic swallowing studies. One aspect that has been considered is the role of verbal cues to swallow. Daniels et al.[13] evaluated the effect of verbal cues on bolus flow during swallowing in a small group of healthy older adults. Each subject self-administered 5 mL of liquid barium and either held the liquid in the mouth until cued to swallow or swallowed in the usual manner. Cued swallows differed from usual swallows in bolus position in the mouth (more posterior) and pharynx (bolus more advanced in superior pharynx) and they resulted in shorter swallows compared with noncued swallows. Nagy et al.[14] also reported timing and bolus location differences between cued and noncued swallows in healthy younger adults. Although interesting differences emerged in both of these studies between cued and noncued swallows, two additional observations must be considered. First, as reported by Martin-Harris et al.,[15] swallow timing and bolus position prior to the pharyngeal swallow is variable in healthy adults. Second, data obtained from healthy adults are not directly transferrable to performance in patients with swallowing impairment. Clinicians often must conduct these

---

PRACTICE NOTE 8-2

During a visit to Japan, I observed a particularly innovative positioning chair used for videofluorographic swallowing evaluations. The patient (in this specific instance, the patient had significant physical limitations after a stroke) was seated in what looked like a modified motorized wheelchair. The chair was then placed in the imaging field of a C-arm fluoroscope. By remote control, the examiner could raise or lower the patient, tilt the patient forward or backward, and tilt the patient from side to side. This chair was beneficial in this particular imaging examination in that positioning variants could be evaluated for their impact on swallow function. Without this special chair, position variants likely would not have been evaluated or would have been evaluated only with extreme burden on both the patient and the examiner.

---

examinations in response to the status of their patients but data such as reported in the Daniels[13] and Nagy[14] studies tell us that not all timing or bolus position results are the direct result of dysphagia. Instructions to the patient, or perhaps other contextual examination issues, can affect the results of fluoroscopic swallowing studies.

Patient Positioning

Positioning depends in large part on the physical abilities of the patient. In general, this study is accomplished with the patient in an upright, seated position with adequate support for the head and body. Patients with physical limitations from weakness, fatigue, disease, or other reasons may require special positioning systems during the examination (see Practice Note 8-2). Various commercial positioning chairs are available to assist in optimal positioning of patients with physical limitations. Before purchasing or building a positioning chair, it is important to know the physical dimensions of the specific fluoroscopic system to be used. Often there is a fixed maximum distance between the table and tower of the fluoroscope. In addition, this study is typically completed in lateral and anterior views. The selected chair or positioning system should be adaptable to accommodate both views. Finally, specifically for lateral views, large patients may not fit easily into the fixed space between the table and tower of the fluoroscope. In such cases, it is possible to turn the patient slightly toward an oblique orientation while maintaining a lateral perspective as much as possible.

Typically, the videofluoroscopic swallowing examination begins with the patient in a lateral (or semioblique) position in reference to the fluoroscopic image (Figure 8-2). This perspective affords an excellent view of the swallowing mechanism from the lips to cervical esophagus and provides the best view of the trachea separate from the esophagus. This view is beneficial in determining whether

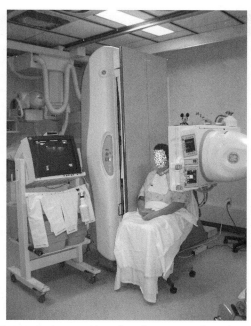

FIGURE 8-2 Patient positioned in fluoroscope for a lateral view image.

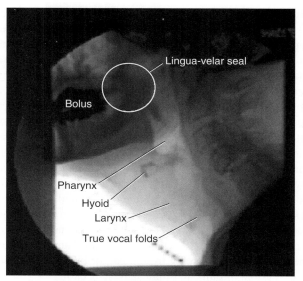

FIGURE 8-3 Lateral radiographic view with bolus held in mouth.

material enters the upper airway. After examination of the swallow in the lateral perspective, the patient is turned for an anterior view. This perspective permits excellent evaluation of symmetry along the swallowing mechanism. When the esophagus is imaged with the patient in a sitting position the extent of the view is often limited. In these situations, imaging is done with the patient in a standing or lying position depending on physical limitations of the patient or specific aspects of the dysphagia presentation. In fact, for some patients who can tolerate standing during the fluoroscopic examination without compromise, the entire examination can be done with the patient in a standing position. This situation permits a great degree of control in moving and positioning the patient.

Material Used in the Fluoroscopic Study

The key material used in the fluoroscopic swallow study is barium sulfate suspension. This is a positive contrast agent that is **radiopaque**. As a result, barium sulfate appears as black on the fluoroscopic image compared with negative contrast substances, such as air, which appear as varying shades of gray. Tissue and bone appear as shades of gray (darker than air) depending on their density. Figure 8-3 depicts the shades of the bolus in the mouth, various bony structures (including the hyoid bone), and the air spaces in the pharynx and the trachea.

A popular point of discussion and even argument among clinicians is whether to use barium sulfate in isolation or in combination with real food items. No firm answer has emerged from these discussions and proponents of both

perspectives have seemingly valid points. Individuals who focus on isolated barium products for this study claim that the range of food textures is so great that it would be impossible to image every possible food or liquid that a given patient might ingest. Another argument against using real food is the potential for complications resulting from aspiration of food products into the airway. Proponents of combining barium and real food items argue that barium products do not represent the consistencies noted in real food products. However, a study by Nagy, Steele, and Pelletier[16] reported that adding barium sulfate to liquids did not significantly alter examined swallowing parameters. Although taste intensity was affected by the addition of barium, lingual-palatal pressures and surface electromyographic amplitudes were not significantly impacted. Interestingly, taste has been shown to affect swallowing characteristics (see Chapter 10) and a separate study by Dietsch et al.[17] reported that addition of barium to various liquids suppressed taste intensity, reduced palatability, and increased rate of refusal to drink liquids a second time. These studies present interesting observations that begin to address the food-versus-barium argument, but additional research will be needed including a wider range of swallowed materials (e.g., more than liquids) and a focus on patients with dysphagia before any strong conclusions can be offered.

Regardless of the outcome of this food-versus-barium discussion, the importance of using a range of textures and volumes during the fluoroscopic swallowing study cannot be overstated. It is well known that a normal swallowing mechanism adjusts to changes in bolus volume and texture.[18-21] In the absence of this accommodation, a patient with dysphagia may demonstrate a variety of compensations or demonstrate the consequences of impaired physiology and the inability to compensate. Volumes used in fluoroscopic swallowing studies vary across published reports. One consideration is the average amount ingested in normal-swallowing adults. Published literature suggests that approximately 20 mL of liquid represents the average drink from a cup.[22] Moreover, an average teaspoon is approximately 5 mL. Therefore, based on a functional perspective, it seems reasonable that the majority of swallow attempts would include volumes somewhere within this range unless clinical indications exist to use less or more material. In fact, results of a recent study[23] suggested that swallows of a 5-mL bolus of thin barium liquid and a 5-mL bolus of nectar-thick barium liquid contributed the greatest amount of information to interpretation of 15 physiologic swallowing components. The author's standard protocol has been to use 5 and 10 mL of each material and then allow the patient to drink freely from a cup or by a straw whenever feasible or clinically indicated. This choice of volume and consistency is based in part on the functional considerations previously mentioned and in consideration of a study suggesting that when using standard materials, 5-mL and 10-mL volumes of thin and thick liquid demonstrated the strongest associations between clinical signs of aspiration and observed aspiration during the videofluoroscopic swallowing study.[24]

In addition to varying volume, consistency—or viscosity—is varied across swallows. General categories of viscosity or textures include thin liquid, thickened liquid, paste or pudding, and masticated material.[10] One barium product line has attempted to standardize the viscosity of barium sulfate liquids into thin, nectar, and honey. A paste material also is available in this product line. One benefit of these standardized barium products is consistency and reproducibility of repeated examinations both within and across patients. In short, use of standardized materials reduces variability across examinations that might result from use of different materials.

One final consideration in choice of materials to include in the fluoroscopic swallow study is the nature of symptoms reported by the patient (see Practice Note 8-3). For example, Madhavan et al.[25] evaluated which materials had the highest diagnostic yield (most frequently identified the underlying problem) in patients complaining of food sticking in their throat. In comparing liquids (thin and thick), pudding, a barium tablet, and half a nonmasticated marshmallow, these investigators reported that the marshmallow provided the highest diagnostic yield for this particular symptom. Thus for some patients presenting specific symptoms a modified approach to the fluoroscopic swallowing evaluation might be indicated.

Sequencing the Events in the Fluoroscopic Study

Different protocols have suggested different sequences of events during the fluoroscopic swallowing study. For

---

PRACTICE NOTE 8-3

In my clinical practice I have come to use two different approaches to the fluoroscopic swallowing examination. For patients with clinically identified oropharyngeal dysphagia who may be rehabilitation candidates I use what I term the *rehab* fluoroscopic protocol. In this protocol I measure volume of each bolus and present a range of materials from thin liquid to thick liquid to pudding. If the patient can manage these materials, I may add cup or straw drinking and masticated materials. Conversely, for patients with specific symptoms (such as food sticking in the throat) who are ingesting a wide range of food and liquids by mouth, I use a different approach. These patients are examined in the standing position and given a cup with the various materials and asked to drink or eat as they would at home. My reason for this distinction is a practical one. Given patients who are eating and drinking a wide range of food and liquids, small volumes of measured materials would likely increase the duration of the examination (and hence the radiation exposure) and likely not reveal any difficulties until larger volumes or thicker materials are evaluated. Likewise, given patients with significant oropharyngeal dysphagia, large (uncontrolled) volumes of these same materials may increase risks of airway compromise.

---

example, Logemann[12] recommends beginning with thin liquids in progressive sequential amounts (1 mL, 3 mL, 5 mL, 10 mL). Once thin liquid swallows are completed, pudding and then masticated materials are evaluated. Palmer et al.[8] began their fluoroscopic swallowing protocol with 5 mL of thick liquids (this category includes pudding material in their protocol), followed by thin liquid and then masticated materials. Martin-Harris et al.[23] initiated their protocol with 5 mL of thin liquid followed by thicker liquids, pudding, and a masticated material. However, this group did caution that larger, thicker, and masticated materials were given to patients only if they demonstrated adequate airway protection and pharyngeal clearance on the thin liquid materials. Jung et al.[26] evaluated order effects between liquids and semisolid foods using both fluoroscopy and endoscopy. They concluded that the order of test materials did not affect the accuracy of safety of either imaging study. The author agrees that a standard protocol is beneficial when completing the fluoroscopic swallowing study, but recommends flexibility in the sequence of events to maximize the "diagnostic outcomes" for each patient. At least two approaches might be considered when sequencing materials during a fluoroscopic swallowing study. Both of these approaches are detailed here. In the first approach materials are presented in a standard sequence regardless of the patient's swallowing ability. In the second approach materials are presented in a highly variable order in response to the individual patient's performance on the previous bolus. Both of these approaches typically begin with the patient seated and viewed from the lateral perspective. The first tasks typically are simple speech or phonation activities to facilitate an impression of movement of structures in the swallowing mechanism (lips, tongue, velum, and pharyngeal wall). Subsequently the initial barium bolus is provided to the patient.

In the standard sequence approach, unless there is significant dryness (xerostomia), weakness, or anatomic deviation in the oral cavity structures, the initial bolus is typically 5 mL of nectar-thickened liquid. The next material is 5 mL of thin liquid followed by 5 mL of pudding. This sequence is subsequently repeated with 10-mL volumes. The patient then is given a cup of thin liquid barium to drink freely and a masticated material coated with barium pudding (usually a cracker). Video 2-3 on the Evolve website shows examples of swallows of these and other materials by a healthy adult volunteer. Video 8-1 depicts examples of swallowing by patients with various dysphagia symptoms.

After this sequence of events is imaged from the lateral view, the patient is turned and viewed from the anterior perspective. From this view the patient is asked to sustain phonation or repeat the same vowel to visualize movement of the true vocal folds. Some patients are asked to phonate in a falsetto mode to evaluate medial movement of the lateral pharyngeal walls. Some are asked to perform a "trumpet" maneuver to evaluate potential weakness in the lateral pharyngeal walls. The trumpet maneuver is accomplished by asking the patient to lift the chin to provide a clear view of the entire pharynx. Then the patient is asked to puff the cheeks and blow as if playing a trumpet (Figure 8-4). Turning the head to each side during swallowing may assist in evaluating each hemipharynx and any effect on pharyngeal esophageal segment (PES) opening. Materials used in the anterior view depend largely on the results of swallows examined with the lateral view. In general, not all materials are repeated with the change in orientation, but sufficient swallows are evaluated to assess symmetry, physiology, and the consequences of impaired movement.

Either before or after the evaluation of the swallow from the anterior view, compensatory maneuvers might be introduced to evaluate their effect on any observed impairments in swallow physiology. Common compensatory maneuvers include the chin-down position, head turn, supraglottic swallow, and Mendelsohn maneuver (see Chapter 10). The effects of these maneuvers can be evaluated in terms of improved swallow safety (less aspiration or penetration) or efficiency (better timing or less residue).

Finally, the esophagus is evaluated whenever feasible. If the patient cannot be positioned appropriately or if the risk of aspiration is too great, esophageal inspection is not added to the standard oropharyngeal examination. Typically, a full

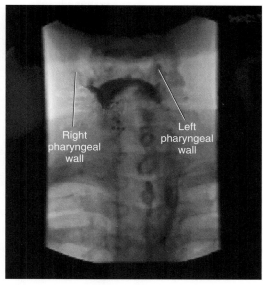

FIGURE 8-4 Anterior radiographic view of patient performing "trumpet" maneuver.

esophageal study is not completed at the same time as the oropharyngeal study. However, a cursory examination of the esophagus may be completed to rule out overt blockages or poor passage of material through the esophagus into the stomach. If the clinical presentation indicates potential for a significant esophageal-based dysphagia and the oropharyngeal examination does not identify any overt difficulties, a more thorough esophagram should be completed.

Clinicians must decide how much of the standard protocol to complete for any given patient. Continuing to provide material to a patient who is aspirating a significant amount of each attempted bolus is unwise and contraindicated. Similarly, a study should not be continued if a patient becomes excessively fatigued or is otherwise unresponsive. Following a standard protocol blindly without consideration for the individual needs of the patient is poor practice. Box 8-5 lists the materials and sequence of presentation that may be included in a standardized fluoroscopic swallow study.

The individualized sequence approach includes the same components as the standard sequence approach with the exception that the presentation of materials is patient performance dependent (see also Clinical Corner 8-1). In this approach, the clinician considers the patient's performance on each presented material before choosing the next material or volume (Figure 8-5). For example, if 5 mL of nectar-thick liquid is the initial bolus and the patient does not aspirate but excessive residue is noted, the clinician might chose to use 5 mL of thin liquids as the next material to reduce the amount of residue and determine if airway protection is maintained. If this outcome is obtained (less residue and no aspiration) then the next bolus might be 10 mL of thin

BOX 8-5 MATERIALS AND STANDARD SEQUENCE OF PRESENTATION THAT MAY BE INCLUDED IN A FLUOROSCOPIC SWALLOWING EXAMINATION

From Lateral View
- Short speech sample and vowel phonation
- 5 mL of thin liquid barium
- 5 mL of thick liquid barium
- 5 mL of barium paste (pudding)
- 10 mL of thin liquid barium
- 10 mL of thick liquid barium
- 10 mL of barium paste (pudding)
- Thin liquid taken freely from cup or through straw
- Masticated material (cracker coated with barium paste)
- Repeat thin liquid if residue from cracker

From Anterior View (Actual Material Depends on Results of Lateral View)
- Repeated vowel phonation and falsetto
- Swallow with head forward and turned

Compensatory Maneuvers
- May be introduced at any time in the examination as clinically indicated

Esophageal Evaluation
- Cursory examination for overt obstruction or dysmotility

CLINICAL CORNER 8-1: CHANGING PRESENTATION METHOD OF MATERIALS TO SWALLOW

Depending on the specific clinical presentation of the patient, it may be important to evaluate swallowing performance when the clinician provides the materials to be swallowed versus when the patient self-feeds. This includes smaller, measured amounts and self-selected volumes by spoon, cup, or straw. The difference in performance may be staggering for some patients, particularly those with cognitive or movement impairments attributable to neurologic deficits. For example, if a patient does not initiate a swallow when the clinician places a bolus in the mouth, the clinician should give the same material in a spoon placed in the patient's hand and assist him or her (if needed) in placing the spoon in the mouth. Although in some cases this simple modification is not informative, in others this adjustment may make a large difference in patient performance and hence clinical interpretation of the videofluoroscopic swallow study results.

Critical Thinking
1. What clinical disorders or impairments might contribute to an absent swallow initiation?
2. What neurologic or cognitive mechanisms might have an effect on a change in patient performance when self-feeding versus being fed?
3. What clinical implications would result when swallow performance does change when the patient engages in self-feeding?

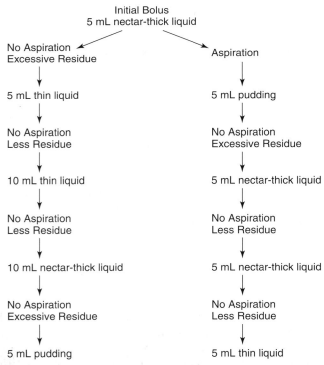

FIGURE 8-5 One example of how an individualized material sequence might be organized during a fluoroscopic swallowing study.

liquid. Conversely, if the initial bolus (5 mL of nectar-thick liquid) is aspirated, the next bolus might be 5 mL of pudding to determine if thicker materials are kept out of the airway. It is important to note that neither of these material sequence approaches has been empirically studied and thus it is unknown if one is superior to the other or if a completely different approach might be better than both of these options. They are presented here only for demonstration of options that clinicians might pursue during the fluoroscopic swallowing study. Beyond that caveat, the remaining components of this imaging study are recommended.

What to Look For

Despite recent attempts to "quantify" the interpretation of the videofluoroscopic swallowing study,[23,27-30] the prevailing interpretation for this imaging examination is to describe various events associated with swallowing different materials. As noted with materials and sequencing of events during this examination, suggestions for interpretation vary across clinicians and authors. The following text presents a general approach to interpretation of the videofluoroscopic swallowing study.

The "short form" of what to look for is anatomy and physiology underlying swallowing activity. Initially, anatomic detail and any deviations from normal are to be noted. This includes not only the oral cavity structures, velopharynx, pharynx, larynx, **pharyngoesophageal sphincter**, and cervical esophagus, but also the structure of the cervical spine. Depending on the clinical presentation of the patient, anatomy may be viewed from both lateral and anterior perspectives before any physiologic or swallowing assessment is initiated. The lateral view provides the best inspection of the movement within the swallowing mechanism. Box 8-6 summarizes the more salient observations obtained from both lateral and anterior views of the fluoroscopic study. Once the anatomy of the swallowing mechanism has been reviewed, basic movement patterns of structures within the swallowing mechanism should be evaluated without swallowing attempts. This practice aids in understanding any physiologic deficits within the mechanism that may contribute to swallowing problems. Typically this component of the examination is brief and involves short speech samples or vowel phonation. During these activities the clinician looks for appropriate movement of the lips, tongue, jaw, velum, larynx, and pharyngeal walls. Movement of the pharyngeal walls can best be evaluated by having the patient produce a falsetto phonation while viewed from the anterior perspective. The lateral pharyngeal walls typically move toward the pharyngeal midline with this maneuver.

After assessment of the anatomy and basic movement capabilities of the swallowing mechanism, the clinician subsequently advances to a direct inspection of swallowing activity. Often the patient is asked to hold a bolus in the mouth before attempting to swallow (but see previous text on the potential effect of verbal cues with this strategy). This affords the opportunity to evaluate lip seal anteriorly and lingual-velar seal posteriorly. Impairment in these functions results in anterior spillage of the bolus or posterior spillage potentially into an open airway. If a solid bolus is used, clinicians should observe the patient masticate the food material, form a cohesive bolus, and propel this material into the oropharynx. A larger masticated bolus may be swallowed in piecemeal fashion. In this pattern, the patient may deliver small amounts of masticated food into the pharynx while retaining the remaining food in the mouth for further preparation. Whether a liquid or solid bolus is used, the timing and efficiency of oral transit of the bolus should be documented. Poor temporal coordination of the oral component of swallowing might lead to entrance of material into an airway that has not yet closed. Alternatively, a prolonged oral component of swallowing may relate to prolonged mealtimes and thus reduced oral intake with increased nutritional risk for a patient. Reduced efficiency of oral transport might contribute to residue in and around the oral cavity after the swallowing attempt. This might result from poor motor coordination or from anatomic deficits.

Deficits in oral-nasal separation—whether from anatomic changes or physiologic deficits in velar movement patterns—can result in entrance of food or liquid into the nasal cavity. This finding is commonly termed nasopharyngeal reflux. The hyoid bone and larynx typically move as a functional unit during swallowing attempts. Although extensive variation has been described in hyolaryngeal movement, most investigators and clinicians agree that the basic movement is upward and forward (elevation followed by anterior movement of both structures). Although this might seem to be a simple activity, appropriate movement of the hyolaryngeal complex involves adequate tongue base function and function of the muscles in the pharyngeal wall. Collectively these events lead to opening of the PES. In addition, movement of the hyolaryngeal complex is

---

BOX 8-6   OBSERVATIONS THAT MAY BE OBTAINED FROM THE VIDEOFLUOROSCOPIC SWALLOWING EXAMINATION

Anatomy
- All structures

Nonswallow Movement (Speech or Vowel Phonation)
- Lips
- Tongue
- Mandible
- Velum
- Larynx (vocal fold movement from anterior view)
- Pharyngeal walls (falsetto)

Swallow Movement (Varies Depending on Bolus Size and Consistency)
- Oral containment of liquids anterior and posterior
- Mastication of semisolids and solids
- Oral transit of material into hypopharynx
- Oronasal separation
- Hyoid movement
- Laryngeal elevation and closure
- Pharyngeal constriction
- PES opening

Consequences of Impaired Swallow Physiology
- Spillage (anterior or posterior)
- Residue
- Misdirection of bolus and airway compromise

Effect of Compensatory Maneuvers (Varies Depending on Impairments)
- Postural adjustment
- Head position changes
- Swallow timing changes (e.g., Mendelsohn maneuver)
- Breath-hold maneuvers
- Bolus changes

PES, Pharyngoesophageal segment.

responsible for movement of the epiglottis during swallowing. This latter structure is positioned between the tongue base and the larynx. As the larynx elevates, the tongue base moves posteriorly and inferiorly, the superior pharynx constricts, and the epiglottis retroflexes to assist in airway protection. Deficits in this combined movement pattern (tongue base, hyoid and larynx, pharynx) often contribute to postswallow residue in the valleculae anterior to the epiglottis. In addition to elevating within the pharynx, the larynx also closes during the swallowing attempt to protect the airway from the entrance of unwanted materials. On the lateral fluoroscopic view, this may be seen as a forward tilting of the arytenoid cartilages approximating the petiole of the epiglottis. As the larynx elevates, the pharynx constricts and along with tongue base retropulsion facilitates passage of the bolus through the hypopharynx into the PES. The PES opens behind the larynx and permits passage of the bolus into the cervical esophagus. Deficits in pharyngeal constriction or PES opening typically result in postswallow residue along the pharyngeal walls and in the piriform sinuses.

If swallow physiology is impaired, clinicians should document the functional consequences of that impairment. Several consequences of impaired swallowing physiology were mentioned previously. Thorough descriptions of postswallow residue and airway compromise in the form of material entering the laryngeal vestibule or aspirated below the true vocal folds should be incorporated. These descriptions should include the reason for residue or aspiration, the timing of each event, and the patient's reaction (or lack thereof) to residue or aspirated material (see Practice Note 8-4). Finally, the effects of compensatory maneuvers should be investigated and documented. The effects of these maneuvers should be considered in terms of changes in observed swallow physiology (e.g., faster swallow, more movement) and the functional consequences of these maneuvers (e.g., less residue, improved airway protection). Common compensatory maneuvers are described as therapy techniques in Chapter 10.

Clinicians often adopt or develop checklists to assist in the interpretation of the videofluoroscopic swallowing study. This practice may help organize the interpretation process, but clinicians should use such checklists only as assistive devices. Interpretation of the videofluoroscopic swallowing study involves more than a summary of items checked off on a list. Various attempts have been made to assist in the interpretation of the videofluoroscopic swallowing study. The Dysphagia Outcome and Severity Scale (DOSS)[31] is a 7-point ordinal scale that addresses multiple domains of dysphagia, including degree of functional deficit, diet recommendations, level of patient independence with feeding, and type of nutrition. This scale demonstrates adequate interrater and intrarater reliability but has no demonstrated validity. Also, this scale invokes

PRACTICE NOTE 8-4

Aspiration of any material into the airway is a serious event. However, clinicians can take steps to better understand aspiration events and identify strategies to minimize or eliminate aspiration during imaging studies. In our "early" years most of us experienced the situation where a fluoroscopic swallow study was terminated when a patient aspirated any material. Obviously, this scenario does not benefit the patient as a prematurely terminated examination provides few if any useful answers to the clinical problem posed by the patient. Over years of clinical practice I have developed strategies to help evaluate aspiration events during imaging studies. First, I believe it is important to know how the patient responds to an aspiration event. Thus when a patient aspirates any material, I do not intervene immediately and also ask the radiologist to remain quiet. This practice affords the opportunity to determine if the patient will respond to the aspirant and the nature of the response. Second, unless the overall health status of the patient contradicts, the aspirated material is presented a second time to assess consistency of aspiration. If the material is not aspirated on the second attempt, a third trial is presented. Although far from perfect, I use a two-out-of-three rule to estimate potential aspiration risk of any material (thickness and volume). The bottom line is that aspiration is an inconsistent event and this simple strategy provides at least some measure of how consistent aspiration might be for any material in any given patient. Once I have an idea of how consistent aspiration might be for that material, I use compensatory postures or maneuvers or different materials and volumes to reduce or eliminate the aspiration.

a multiple domain approach in which information from many sources (not just the fluoroscopic study) is considered. As such, this scale is not a focused interpretation of fluoroscopic swallowing examinations. The Penetration-Aspiration scale[32] is a unidimensional ordinal scale that describes the depth of entrance of material into the airway and the patient's ability to clear any entered material. Clinicians must be aware that this "pen-asp" scale is not a dysphagia severity scale. The scale addresses only a single aspect of dysphagia—material entering the airway. As such, this scale is biased toward patients who demonstrate laryngeal penetration or aspiration. Many patients may demonstrate significant dysphagia in the absence of either laryngeal penetration or aspiration of material below the vocal folds. Like the DOSS, the Penetration-Aspiration scale has demonstrated reliability but has not been validated. Furthermore, as pointed out by Carnaby,[30] published literature using this scale reveals no consistent or consensus method for scoring and resulting scores (regardless of how obtained) do not relate to patient outcomes. Thus, the

Penetration-Aspiration scale may be appropriate to describe the depth and patient reaction to aspirated material on individual swallows, but that appears to be the extent of its clinical value.

More recently, Martin-Harris et al.[23] (Modified Barium Swallow Impairment Tool [MBSImp]), Han et al.[27,28] (Videofluoroscopic Dysphagia Scale [VDS]), and Carnaby (Computed Video Fluoroscopic Evaluation: C-VFE)[30] have attempted to systematically develop and validate protocols and scoring procedures for the videofluoroscopic swallowing study. Although none of these protocols are widely used in general clinical practice, all three protocols demonstrate excellent approaches to developing a standardized, validated protocol and scoring system for the videofluoroscopic swallow study. Table 8-1 presents the assessed items in each of these protocols. Note that although some items are represented in each protocol, clinically significant differences are apparent across all three. Nonetheless, the strength of these approaches to quantify evaluation of fluoroscopic swallowing studies lies within the psychometric validation inherent with each protocol. Readers are referred to the individual references for more details on each of these approaches. The application of such quantified assessments using validated protocols is anticipated to become commonplace in the near future. Additional measures of swallow performance have focused on timing aspects of swallowing. Logemann[12] recommended evaluation of the duration of bolus movement during a swallow and suggested evaluation of oral transit time, pharyngeal transit time, pharyngeal delay time, and esophageal transit time. She further defines a summary measure of swallowing function, the oropharyngeal swallow efficiency (OPSE) score, as the ratio of the percentage of material swallowed into the esophagus divided by oral plus pharyngeal transit times. Given imaging technology used to capture video images, the assessment of timing measures is relatively easy to complete. An additional form of measurement—**biokinematic** assessment—focuses on measuring the movement of various structures during swallowing events or combined movement with timing analysis. A variety of swallow movements have been reported with this approach, including maximal excursion of the hyoid bone and the larynx, maximal opening of the upper esophageal sphincter, and amount of pharyngeal constriction.[33-35]

Timing and movement assessments of swallowing do add an objective dimension beyond basic descriptions of swallowing patterns. However, as emphasized by McCullough et al.,[36] a need exists to validate many suggested measures and to reduce in number and define the multitude of measures that have been proposed for interpretation of the videofluoroscopic swallowing study. In the author's experience, clinicians formulate impressions of speed of movement of a bolus through the swallowing tract, but objective evaluation of specific timing components is not

TABLE 8-1 Comparison of Items Evaluated on Three Numerically Scored Videofluoroscopic Swallowing Examinations

MBSImp (Martin-Harris)	VDS (Han)	C-VFE (Carnaby)
Lip closure	Lip closure	Oral preparation
Hold position/tongue control	Bolus formation	Oral transit
Bolus preparation/mastication	Mastication	Pharyngeal initiation
Bolus transport/lingual motion	Apraxia	Hyolaryngeal elevation
Oral residue	Tongue-to-palate contact	Pharyngeal function
Initiation of pharyngeal swallow	Premature bolus loss	PES function
Soft palate elevation	Oral transit time	Aspiration
Laryngeal elevation	Triggering of pharyngeal swallow	
Anterior hyoid motion	Vallecular residue	
Epiglottic movement	Laryngeal elevation	
Laryngeal closure	Pyriform sinus residue	
Pharyngeal stripping wave	Coating of pharyngeal wall	
Pharyngeal contraction	Pharyngeal transit time	
PES opening	Aspiration	
Tongue base retraction		
Pharyngeal residue		
Esophageal clearance (upright position)		

C-VFE, Computed Video Fluoroscopic Evaluation; MBSImp, Modified Barium Swallow Impairment tool; PES, pharyngeal esophageal segment; VDS, Videofluoroscopic Dysphagia Scale.

commonplace in clinical practice. Perhaps future research will identify aspects of objective timing and movement evaluation that are most meaningful in the clinical interpretation of swallowing deficits.

Strengths and Weaknesses of the Fluoroscopic Swallowing Study

The videofluoroscopic swallowing examination is considered the gold standard in the clinical assessment of dysphagia (see also Clinical Corner 8-2). This examination has many strengths that merit this designation. It is a dynamic study that when recorded provides a thorough evaluation

---

CLINICAL CORNER 8-2: MORE IMAGING STUDIES FOR THE SWALLOW MECHANISM

Radiologists have various methods to image the swallowing/digestive system. Two common techniques include the standard barium swallowing study and scintigraphy. The first of these studies, the barium swallow study, may be referenced as the *upper gastrointestinal (UGI) examination* or an *esophagram*. The focus of this radiologic examination is on the esophagus. The hypopharynx and the stomach may also be imaged during this procedure. Although variations of this study have been described, the procedure is typically completed with the patient in a lying, usually prone, position. Liquid barium is ingested in large volumes through a straw. The radiologist views the dynamic study in real time but usually captures only still images that demonstrate specific pathologies in the esophagus.

The second study, scintigraphy, is actually a nuclear medicine procedure. Scintigraphic studies use a radionuclide, commonly technetium-99 sulfur colloid, mixed with another substance. In the author's facility this radionuclide is often mixed in an egg-white solution, and the study is known as a "tech-egg study." However, the radionuclide may be mixed with a variety of semisolid or thick liquid foods. In this study, radiation is emitted from the radionuclide and is measured by a scintillation camera and computer. In simple terms, the patient swallows a radioactive material (of very low dose) and stands, sits, or lies in front of a radiation detector. The benefit of this technique is that the timing, direction, and location of the swallowed materials or any objectively measured portion of the swallowed material can be assessed. Thus gastric emptying studies may be completed by this technique to determine how much of a swallowed material leaves the stomach in a specified period. This technique also can quantify the amount and depth of aspirated material. Although scintigraphy has been used in studies of oropharyngeal dysphagia, it is not routinely used in the clinical evaluation of this problem.

Critical Thinking

1. For what types of dysphagia symptoms is a UGI examination preferred over a videofluoroscopic swallowing study?
2. Discuss some limitations of conducting both a videofluoroscopic swallowing study and an esophagram during the same evaluation.
3. Discuss potential strengths and limitations of using scintigraphy in the evaluation of oropharyngeal dysphagia.

---

of the biomechanics of oropharyngeal swallowing with unlimited review capability. In addition, it provides a comprehensive perspective on swallowing from the lips through the esophagus. Finally, within the hospital setting it is typically readily accessible for both patient and clinician.

Despite these strengths of the fluoroscopic swallowing study, weaknesses and questions remain. A major concern regarding interpretation of the fluoroscopic swallowing examination is extensive variability among raters (also with raters). Both McCullough et al.[37] and Baijens et al.[38] report extensive interrater and intrarater variability in fluoroscopic swallow study interpretation. Both investigative teams strongly recommend application of a systematic training for clinicians who interpret these studies. The use of radiation may be of concern in some instances, especially when multiple, repeated studies are conducted. However, the amount of radiation in a single examination is quite small. The fluoroscopic examination also is not the best examination to evaluate pooled secretions because these will not be visualized with this procedure. Other concerns or areas of question include the following: documentation of aspiration but not the effects of aspiration, difficulty in appreciation of airway closure mechanisms, possibly limited access outside the hospital setting, examination of only a very short period in an abnormal environment and thus possibly not truly reflective of functional eating abilities, possible problematic transportation to the radiology department, and inconsistent interpretation among clinicians. This list is not intended to cast aspersions on the videofluoroscopic swallowing examination. Rather, it serves as a group of caveats that clinicians may consider when conducting and interpreting this imaging study.

ENDOSCOPIC SWALLOWING EXAMINATIONS

Differences between the Endoscopic Swallowing Examination and the Fluoroscopic Swallowing Examination

Like the fluoroscopic swallowing examination, the endoscopic procedure is referred to by a variety of names. *Videoendoscopic evaluation of dysphagia (VEED)*,[39] *videoendoscopic swallowing study (VESS)*,[40] and *fiberoptic endoscopic evaluation of swallowing safety (FEESS)*[41] have all been used to describe similar procedures. The American Speech-Language-Hearing Association[3,42] recommends use of the term fiberoptic endoscopic evaluation of swallowing (FEES) as the generic identifier of this procedure, with the exception of a specific procedure to assess upper airway sensitivity: *fiberoptic endoscopic evaluation of swallowing with sensory testing. (FEESST)*[43] However, in keeping with the discussion of the fluoroscopic examination, this chapter uses the generic descriptive term *endoscopic swallowing examination*.

The endoscopic swallowing examination is newer than the fluoroscopic examination in the clinical arena of

BOX 8-7 SIMILARITIES AND DIFFERENCES BETWEEN THE FLUOROSCOPIC AND ENDOSCOPIC SWALLOW STUDIES

Similarities
- Purpose
- Materials
- Process of evaluation

Differences
- Technique
- Image perspective
- Portability
- Repeatability
- Duration of examination
- Sensory assessment

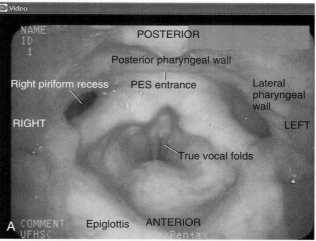

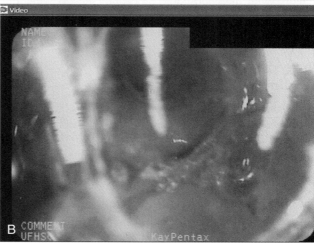

FIGURE 8-6 A clear endoscopic image of the pharynx (*A*), an image obscured by secretions on the endoscope (*B*), and an example of "whiteout" (*C*). *PES,* Pharyngoesophageal segment.

dysphagia and, as a result, is used by fewer professionals. This imaging examination is growing in popularity and application and shares both similarities and differences with the fluoroscopic study. Box 8-7 summarizes the more salient similarities and differences between these two imaging procedures to assess swallowing function.

Similarities

Both fluoroscopic and endoscopic procedures have a similar purpose in the assessment of swallowing. Each is intended to provide an objective assessment of the anatomy and physiology of the upper aerodigestive mechanisms used in swallowing. Although each procedure has distinct advantages or disadvantages over the other, both are intended for a similar purpose. Materials used in both examinations vary in amount and texture. The fluoroscopic study uses barium sulfate as a visible contrast agent, whereas the endoscopic study uses liquids and foods of natural or added color to be visible. Thus both studies use a range of liquid and solid foods designed to be easily visualized by the respective examinations. Finally, both studies use a similar assessment process. Both procedures can evaluate the anatomy and physiology of the upper swallow mechanism, swallow function, and the effect of compensatory maneuvers.

Differences

Aside from obvious technique differences, the resulting images from the respective procedures differ. Fluoroscopy is considered to provide the more comprehensive perspective, including structures from the lips to the stomach. Endoscopy has imaging capability focused on the pharynx from the nasopharynx to the hypopharynx. Oral cavity and esophageal structure and function are not part of the typical endoscopic swallowing examination. In addition, although the endoscopic image is lost at the peak of the swallow or when material covers the end of the endoscope, the fluoroscopic image suffers no similar limitations. Figure 8-6 compares a clear endoscopic image, an image impaired by secretions on the endoscope, and a "whiteout" image that occurs at the swallowing peak. Despite the potential for image degradation during the endoscopic examination, this procedure is superior to fluoroscopy in the evaluation of anatomy and pooled secretions within the swallowing mechanism. Another advantage of the endoscopic procedure is the potential for portability. Endoscopic systems are available that can be transported with relative ease to the patient in various locations, thus increasing access to this examination. Because endoscopy does not involve radiation, repeated examinations are not viewed with as much concern as repeated fluoroscopic examinations. Also, because no radiation is used individual examinations can be somewhat longer than a fluoroscopic examination. Finally, with the endoscopic procedure sensory functions may be tested, albeit crudely, by touching the mucosa and asking the patient to acknowledge the tactile stimulus.

Procedures for the Endoscopic Swallowing Study

The endoscopic swallowing study is ideally suited to visualize the pharynx from nasopharynx to hypopharynx, the base of tongue region, and the larynx. Although slight variations have been described for this imaging study, certain elements are common across all variations.[39,43-45] In general the endoscopic swallowing study includes five components: (1) assessment of pharyngeal anatomy (including laryngeal structures), (2) evaluation of movement and sensation of pharyngeal structures, (3) assessment of secretions, (4) direct evaluation of swallowing function with liquid and solid material, and (5) evaluation of the effect of compensatory maneuvers.

Specialized equipment is required for this procedure. The minimal requirements for an adequate endoscopic system for evaluation of swallowing function include a fiberoptic endoscope, a light source, and a camera. These basic elements are depicted in Figure 8-7. More advanced options include a recording device (videotape, DVD, or computer file), as seen in Figure 8-8. Video endoscopes are also available that provide excellent images as a result of

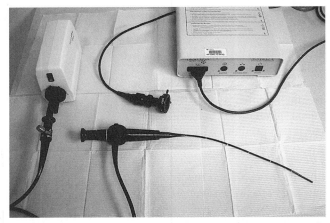

FIGURE 8-7 Basic equipment required for the endoscopic swallowing study: endoscope, light source, and camera.

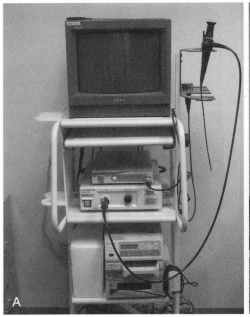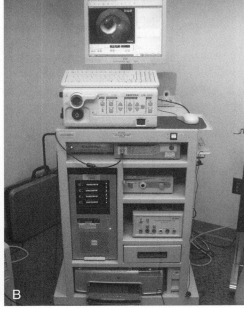

FIGURE 8-8 Complete endoscopy systems.

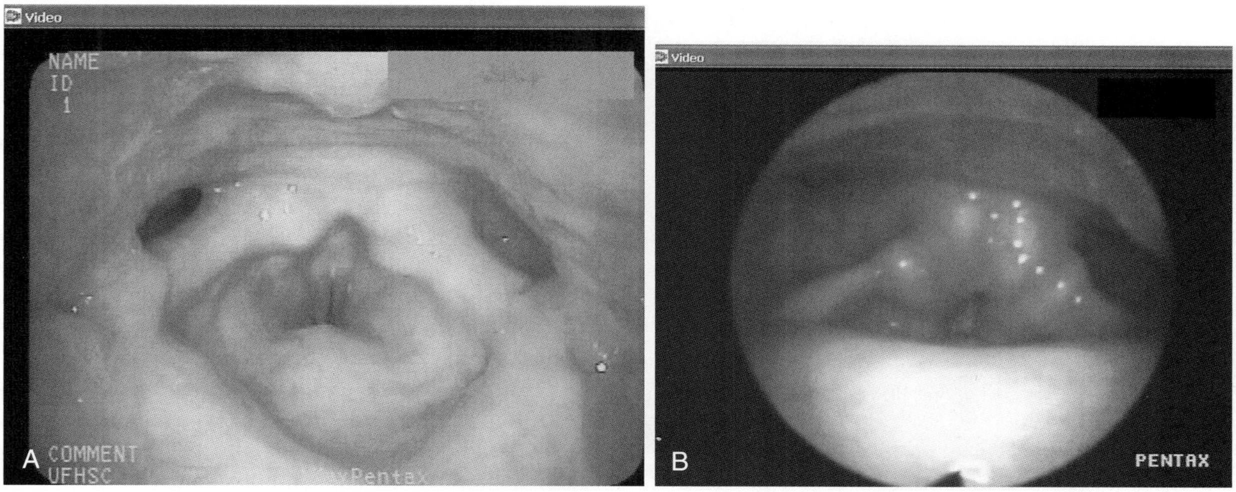

FIGURE 8-9 Examples of images from a videoscope (A) compared with a traditional scope (B).

placing the "camera" as a microchip at the distal end of the endoscope. Figure 8-9 shows comparison images from a regular endoscope and a videoscope.

The first step in the endoscopic procedure should be patient instruction. This is especially important for patients undergoing the examination for the first time. The transnasal endoscopic procedure is not painful, but it may be uncomfortable for some individuals. Whenever possible, the procedure should be thoroughly explained to the patient.

The next issue is whether to use nasal anesthesia. Historically, both a **vasoconstrictor** and anesthesia have been sprayed into the nose before the procedure (see Practice Note 8-5). Despite evidence that neither medication is required for most examinations,[46,47] at least one study[48] reported that a nasal spray anesthesia (1 mL of 4% lidocaine) reduced discomfort and pain and improved overall tolerance of the procedure. However, these "benefits" coexisted with greater impairment to swallow performance with nasal spray anesthesia. Conversely, Kamarunas et al.[49] reported that a gel anesthesia applied to the nose did not significantly affect swallow performance. Both of these investigations conclude that future studies are required to more thoroughly evaluate the effect of the type and dose of nasal anesthesia used during the endoscopic swallow study. If used, these medications should be applied only under medical supervision and with appropriate administrative approvals because all medications have potential side effects.

Initially, the fiberoptic endoscope is passed through one nasal passage with care taken by the examiner to ensure that the scope stays in the **inferior nasal meatus** and away from the nasal septum. Once the scope is in the nasal **choana**, it may be positioned to view the velopharynx. (NOTE: Experienced endoscopists realize that the optimal view of the velopharynx is obtained with the scope placed

PRACTICE NOTE 8-5

Like many speech-language pathologists, I learned endoscopic techniques under the mentorship of an otolaryngologist. While working in the otolaryngology clinic, it was customary to apply both a vasoconstrictor and topical anesthetic. Interestingly, many patients would tell me that this was the worst part of the examination and that the effects of the medications lasted well after the endoscopic examination was completed. Once I stopped using these medications, I would occasionally encounter patients who had been first examined by a physician who used this technique. At times, they would say "Aren't you going to spray me first?" My response was to assure them that if a gentle approach was used, no medications were needed. Most, if not all of these patients, learned that the "numbing medications" were not necessary to perform this examination.

As a teacher who has conducted workshops on the endoscopic swallowing examination, I believe that clinicians should undergo this procedure themselves before they are allowed to use it to evaluate patients. This experience, although not painful, usually gives the clinician a healthy respect for the gentle approach to transnasal endoscopy.

in the middle nasal meatus. However, this can contribute to increased patient discomfort.) The function of the velopharyngeal mechanism can be examined by asking the patient to hum, produce vowels and consonants, and speak short sentences. Initially, a dry (saliva-only) swallow is completed to assess velar movement during swallowing. If nasopharyngeal reflux is suspected, this can initially be evaluated by looking for saliva passage through the

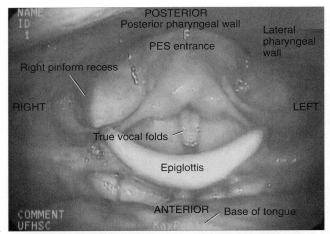

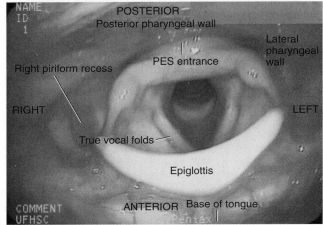

FIGURE 8-10 Normal endoscopic view of adducted (A) and abducted (B) larynx. PES, Pharyngoesophageal segment.

velopharyngeal port during the dry swallow. It is preferable not to give the patient material to swallow at this point but to wait until the airway is clearly visualized.

After inspection of the velopharyngeal mechanism, the scope is advanced into the oropharynx with the tip positioned below the uvula and above the epiglottis. From this position the pharynx, including laryngeal structures, should be well visualized. Figure 8-10 presents the normal anatomic view from this position of the abducted and adducted larynx. Refer to narrated Video 2-4 on the Evolve website for more detailed information on normal swallowing viewed endoscopically. Assessment techniques for pharyngeal activities include falsetto phonation, performing the Valsalva maneuver, and swallowing various materials. Falsetto phonation facilitates medial movement of the lateral pharyngeal walls. This activity is a good method to identify hemipharyngeal weakness. The wall with little or no movement is likely to be paretic. The Valsalva maneuver is a method to expand the pharynx. This view may be helpful in identifying subtle anatomic deviations or as an indication of weakness on one side of the pharynx.

Assessment of laryngeal function includes activities for adduction and abduction, diadochokinesis, breath hold, and cough–clear actions. Simple phonation is adequate for laryngeal adduction. The vowel "ee" is most often used because it elongates the larynx and enhances the endoscopic view. Abduction may be evaluated by forced inhalation or sniffing. Laryngeal diadochokinesis may be assessed by alternating phonation and sniffing or by repeated productions of the syllable "see" or "he." Breath-hold maneuvers should include both a simple breath hold ("hold your breath") and a forced breath hold ("hold your breath and bear down"). It is well recognized that many adults do not completely close the larynx with a simple breath hold. Laryngeal closure is typically achieved with forced breath hold (barring significant anatomic or physiologic deficit). When a breath-hold maneuver may be incorporated into a therapy program, it is important to know whether a simple breath hold will achieve glottal closure or whether a forced breath hold is indicated. Finally, it is important to ascertain the patient's ability to execute a voluntary cough and whether that cough is sufficient to clear any pooled secretions or mucus from the vocal folds and laryngeal vestibule.

Attempted swallows should be completed with a range of materials that are clearly visible under endoscopic inspection. The selection and sequential presentation of materials to be swallowed follow concepts similar to the selection and sequential presentation of materials during the fluoroscopic examination. The type of material swallowed and the number of swallows evaluated may affect the interpretation of this examination. For example, Butler et al.[50] evaluated aspiration in older healthy adults using different liquids taken by cup or straw. A major conclusion of this study was that milk resulted in more frequent aspiration than water in this population. Volume and delivery method also affected the degree of airway compromise. Baijens et al.[51] further reported that the number of swallows examined affected the identification of thin liquid aspiration events in both oncologic and neurologic patients with dysphagia. Results of these two studies suggest that multiple swallows of a variety of materials should be assessed to increase the identification of aspiration events. During each swallow, a period of whiteout occurs at the point of maximal pharyngeal constriction. After the swallow, the pharynx and larynx are again visible and assessment of airway compromise by penetration or aspiration and patterns of residue may be assessed. Again, although the view is different, the concepts of what to look for in the endoscopic examination are similar to those for the fluoroscopic examination. If impaired swallow physiology is identified, compensatory maneuvers may be implemented under endoscopic inspection to evaluate their effect on both the impaired physiology and the consequences of that impairment. Box 8-8 summarizes some salient techniques and observations to be

BOX 8-8 SUGGESTED TECHNIQUES AND OBSERVATIONS FOR THE ENDOSCOPIC SWALLOWING EVALUATION

Velopharynx
- Anatomic deviations
- Movement on phonation
- Movement on swallow
- Signs of material through sphincter during swallow

Pharynx
- Anatomic deviations
- Secretions
- Movement on falsetto (medial movement of lateral pharyngeal walls)
- Valsalva maneuver—expand pharynx (pouches or other anatomic deviations)

Larynx
- Anatomic deviations
- Secretions
- Movement on phonation—adduction
- Movement on breath hold/forced breath hold—adduction
- Movement on abduction—inhale or sniff
- Rapid alternating movement
- Cough

Swallow
- Vary volume and "consistency" of materials
- Oral containment: lingual-velar seal
- "Whiteout"—degree of pharyngeal constriction
- Residue
- Airway compromise—laryngeal penetration/aspiration
- Patient reaction to residue or airway compromise
- Effect of maneuvers and compensations

included in the endoscopic swallowing examination. Clinicians are encouraged to seek formal training in this technique because it is relatively new in the dysphagia evaluation arena and not performed routinely by all practicing clinicians.

What to Look For

Much like the videofluoroscopic swallowing study, interpretation of the endoscopic swallowing study also is dominated by description.[44,45] A sample of descriptive observations from this examination is presented in Box 8-8. In general, examining clinicians should evaluate the anatomic integrity of each "level" (velopharynx, pharynx, larynx) of the swallowing mechanism. Basic movement characteristics of each level should be documented with specific reference to absent or reduced movement. Also, the presence of secretions should be noted. Secretions should be described in terms of location in the pharynx or larynx, amount and consistency (watery, thick, and so on), and

movement during spontaneous swallows, throat clearing, or coughing. Once the basic anatomy and physiology of the swallow mechanism has been evaluated, swallow attempts may be assessed. Much like the fluoroscopic swallow study, the patient should be observed attempting to swallow materials of different volumes and consistencies. Movements of swallowing structures should be described during swallow attempts. Airway compromise and residue should be described along with the patient's reaction to penetration, aspiration, or residue. Video 8-2 on the Evolve website presents a variety of abnormal swallow characteristics observed during the endoscopic swallow study.

In addition to basic descriptions, scales such as the Penetration-Aspiration scale[19] that were initially developed for the videofluoroscopic swallowing study have been applied to interpretation of the endoscopic swallowing study.[52] Furthermore, similar to the fluoroscopic swallowing study, clinicians and investigators have considered a variety of timing measures to apply to the endoscopic swallowing study.[44] However, each measure presents the same strengths and limitations applied to the endoscopic swallowing study that were noted for the fluoroscopic swallowing study. Also similar to the videofluoroscopic swallowing study, recent attempts have emerged to quantify the interpretation of the endoscopic swallowing study and to identify those endoscopic observations that may be beneficial in clinical decision making about patients with dysphagia.[53-57] Still, as with recent similar attempts to quantify interpretation of fluoroscopic swallow studies, these protocols are not commonly used in general clinical practice.

Strengths and Weaknesses of the Endoscopic Swallowing Study

Like the fluoroscopic swallowing examination, the endoscopic procedure is a dynamic study that when recorded provides an objective examination of pharyngeal swallowing function with review capability. It provides a superior inspection of pharyngeal anatomy, sensation, laryngeal closure patterns, and secretions compared with fluoroscopy. Accessibility is deemed a strength of the endoscopic procedure because of the portability of equipment and no concern of x-ray exposure posed by repeated assessments. Some clinicians and researchers have used this technique in repeated applications as a biofeedback tool, often to teach patients airway protection strategies.[58-60] Finally, swallowing examinations with this procedure can be longer than with the fluoroscopic procedure because no radiation is involved.

Perhaps the biggest limitation of the endoscopic swallowing study is the relatively limited scope of view. Unlike the fluoroscopic study, this procedure does not provide imaging of the oral cavity, the PES, or the esophagus. The image and thus evaluation focus is clearly on pharyngeal

---

CLINICAL CORNER 8-3: ENDOSCOPY BEYOND THE PHARYNX

This chapter has focused on the fiberoptic endoscopic swallowing study (FEES) procedure because this is the most common endoscopic procedure completed by dysphagia clinicians, including physicians and speech-language pathologists. However, other procedures, such as the commonly termed esophagoscopy or esophagogastroduodenoscopy (EGD) are frequently completely by gastroenterologists. A more recent procedure, transnasal esophagoscopy (TNE), is becoming increasing popular among otolaryngologists. Both procedures have the potential to evaluate the esophagus by using a longer and larger endoscope than the one used for the FEES procedure. The EGD procedure involves sedation of the patient, whereas TNE does not. During TNE the physician can also evaluate bolus transit though the esophagus because the awake patient can swallow various materials. TNE also affords the otolaryngologist the opportunity to evaluate the pharynx and larynx as the endoscope is passed transnasally in the awake patient.

Dysphagia clinicians may also encounter additional procedures such as capsule or pill endoscopy. As the name implies, this technique requires the patient to swallow a capsule (approximately the size of a vitamin pill) containing a wireless camera that transmits pictures to a small device worn by the patient. Video images are captured as the pill moves through the esophagus. In the author's experience to date, this procedure is not frequently encountered by clinicians working within the scope of oropharyngeal dysphagia.

Critical Thinking

1. When would a patient benefit from a TNE procedure versus an FEES procedure?
2. Discuss specific symptoms that suggest one examination over the other.
3. Discuss the reverse preference for FEES over TNE.
4. What other endoscopic imaging techniques can you identify that may be appropriate for patients with swallowing difficulties?

---

aspects of swallowing (see also Clinical Corner 8-3). The issue of whiteout during the swallowing peak has been raised as a potential limitation of this procedure; however, in practice this brief period of image loss rarely affects the outcome of the evaluation and, in some instances, the absence of this normal finding implicates a weakened pharyngeal swallow.

Safety issues have been raised regarding this procedure; potential complications include nosebleed, laryngospasm, **vasovagal response**, and allergic reaction to medications when used. However, published reports of relatively large numbers of patients receiving this procedure have documented that it is a safe procedure with few complications.[44,61-65]

As mentioned earlier in this section, additional research has demonstrated that neither anesthetics nor vasoconstrictors are necessary to complete this procedure.[46,47] Still, patient safety must be a primary concern in any clinical setting. Patients who may be combative or demonstrate movement disorders that might preclude completion of a safe examination or those patients with bleeding disorders might increase any risk factor associated with this procedure.

One final limitation of the endoscopic swallowing study merits consideration. Before engaging in either the application or the interpretation of endoscopic swallowing studies, clinicians must avail themselves of an appropriate degree of supervised training (of course, this same concern should be addressed for the fluoroscopic study). Published guidelines are available from the American Speech-Language-Hearing Association that detail the knowledge and skills required to undertake this procedure and suggest mechanisms to obtain appropriate training.[42,66]

DIRECT COMPARISONS BETWEEN FLUOROSCOPIC AND ENDOSCOPIC SWALLOWING EXAMINATIONS

Several investigations have undertaken direct comparisons between fluoroscopic and endoscopic swallowing examinations. Some comparisons have been practical suggestions for application based on clinical experience,[39,40] whereas others have been more rigorous comparisons of specific findings on the respective procedures in common groups of patients with dysphagia.[44,67] Recall that one advantage of the fluoroscopic procedure was a more comprehensive evaluation of swallowing from the lips to the stomach. Based on this advantage, the fluoroscopic procedure has been advocated as the preferred procedure for initial swallowing assessments and for imaging assessment of dysphagia symptoms focused on the esophagus. Conversely, the endoscopic procedure provides a superior inspection of anatomy and secretions.[68] Based on this advantage, the endoscopic procedure has been advocated in cases involving paralysis secondary to cranial neuropathies, postsurgical or traumatic anatomic changes, or for any dysphagia in which the management or aspiration of secretions is problematic. Finally, because of the portability advantage of the endoscopic procedure and the absence of radiation exposure, this procedure has been advocated for patients who are not able to be transported (i.e., bedbound patients), for situations requiring repeated swallowing examinations, and for use as a biofeedback application in treatment. These advocated clinical preferences are summarized in Table 8-2.

Studies comparing specific findings between these two imaging procedures have consistently identified a high

TABLE 8-2 Relative Clinical Advantages and Uses of Fluoroscopic and Endoscopic Swallow Studies

Application	Advantage Fluoroscopy	Advantage Endoscopy
Initial evaluation	√	
Esophageal dysphagia	√	
Paresis/paralysis (cranial nerve)		√
Anatomic deviations		√
Evaluate secretions		√
Patient cannot be transported		√
Repeated use		√
Biofeedback		√

TABLE 8-3 Results of Two Studies Comparing Specific Findings of Fluoroscopic and Endoscopic Swallow Studies

Finding	Study 1	Study 2
Pharyngeal residue	80%	89%
Aspiration	90%	86%
Laryngeal penetration	85%	86%
Premature spillage (posterior)	66%	61%

Numbers reflect percent agreement between the two imaging examinations.

degree of agreement. In general, agreement between these two imaging evaluations ranges between 60% and more than 90% across various items of interest. Table 8-3 summarizes the results of two studies comparing the same swallowing deficits.[69,70] Findings of residue or airway compromise reveal agreement averaging from 80% to 90% between these two procedures. However, Crary and Baron[71] offered a note of caution. These investigators compared endoscopic findings that were directly observed with those inferred from other findings with matched results from videofluoroscopic studies completed for the same patients. For example, if material was observed entering the airway, this was a directly observed endoscopic finding. However, if residue was noted after a swallow on the endoscopic examination, the investigators may have inferred pharyngeal weakness, reduced laryngeal elevation, or reduced opening of the PES. Directly observed findings demonstrated much higher agreement with the fluoroscopic swallowing study than findings inferred from other endoscopic results. Crary and Baron concluded that when the endoscopic evaluation

is dominated by inferred findings, a fluoroscopic examination should also be completed for the same patient. Thus, depending on the requirements of the clinical situation, one procedure might be indicated over the other, or the two procedures might be used in a complementary fashion during the same dysphagia evaluation.

TAKE HOME NOTES

1. Imaging studies of swallowing provide objective imaging of the anatomy and physiology of the swallowing mechanism and swallowing biomechanics across varying bolus and patient conditions.
2. Imaging studies of swallowing should be strongly considered whenever a thorough clinical evaluation is insufficient to answer the pertinent clinical questions for a given patient. This may include delineation of dysphagia parameters, clarification of airway protection issues, the effects of compensatory maneuvers, and monitoring changes over time. These examinations may also provide information useful in understanding medical conditions that underlie dysphagia.
3. Commonalities exist between procedures for the fluoroscopic and endoscopic swallowing examinations. Both provide dynamic imaging of the swallowing mechanism and performance, use multiple bolus volumes and textures, and have the potential to evaluate the effect of compensatory maneuvers on swallowing safety and efficiency. In addition, each may be modified to address individual needs of specific patient groups or dysphagia characteristics.
4. Both imaging swallowing examinations have strengths and weakness that might affect their optimal use. The fluoroscopic study offers the more comprehensive perspective of the swallowing mechanism, whereas the endoscopic study offers the superior view of anatomy and secretions. Certain weaknesses are common to both procedures. They may document the presence of aspiration but do not address the consequences of aspiration. They evaluate swallowing performance in abnormal environments using procedures that do not resemble functional eating activities. Despite these potential criticisms, these examinations are important in the assessment of swallowing performance.
5. Published reports indicate strong agreement between the fluoroscopic and endoscopic swallowing studies—specifically, in the identification of individual dysphagia characteristics such as postswallow residue and aspiration. Agreement in the identification of specific clinical findings along with consideration of the relative strengths and weaknesses of each procedure will help with the appropriate application of either or both procedures.

CLINICAL CASE EXAMPLE 8-1

An 85-year-old woman was seen in the outpatient dysphagia clinic. The patient currently resides in a long-term care facility. The facility staff is concerned because the patient is declining food and is beginning to lose weight. In addition, she has been reported to cough during mealtimes. Her adult son has accompanied her to the evaluation and serves as the primary informant. He visits his mother at least twice each week and has observed mealtimes and participated in feeding her. The patient is unable to self-feed because of severe arthritis in her hands. She has moderate dementia but is able to communicate her preferences and dislikes with simple responses. She is receiving a total oral diet of pureed foods and thickened liquids. She indicates that she does not like this diet and that the food has no taste. On occasion the family has brought regular food to her and observed her eat it without difficulty. Clinical examination revealed no gross abnormality in cranial nerve function or any anatomic deviations in the oral structures. Voice was deemed appropriate for her age and medical condition. Volitional cough was intact. The patient was provided a range of material to swallow based on the report of her daily oral intake. Initially thickened liquids were presented with a spoon. The patient was able to swallow these without difficulty or postswallow voice change. Larger amounts of thickened liquid were provided from a cup. Again, no difficulties were detected. Subsequently thin liquid (fruit juice) was provided first by spoon, then by cup, then by straw. A single cough was observed after cup drinking. No difficulties were observed during straw drinking. Pudding was presented in spoon-size amounts. Lingual mastication was evident and no difficulties were observed. Subsequently, a cracker was presented. Mastication was obvious, but oral residue was observed after swallow attempts. Thin liquid was presented by a straw to clear the oral residue. No overt signs of aspiration were noted and the voice was clear after drinking. Oral residue was cleared with straw drinking.

Interpretation

This patient did not require any imaging examination for swallowing function. Clinical examination with swallowing evaluation was sufficient in addressing the concerns regarding her refusal of food and occasional coughing during meals. Recommendations for this patient included upgrading her diet to soft mechanical or further depending on preference and tolerance and allowing her to drink thin liquids. An occupational therapy consultation was generated to fashion a cup-holding device to allow the patient to drink thin liquids (specifically water) through a straw at her discretion. Follow-up with this patient indicated that the recommendations were implemented; food and liquid intake increased and no dysphagia-related complications were encountered.

CLINICAL CASE EXAMPLE 8-2

A 64-year-old man presented to a dysphagia clinic after radiation therapy for a tonsillar fossa carcinoma. The patient reported dry mouth (xerostomia), which made it difficult for him to swallow dry, solid foods, and moderate pain in his throat that was worse with any swallow. He had no overt cranial nerve deficits, but his voice was mildly hoarse (he reported that this was a result of the radiation therapy). He reported that he consistently coughed to clear thickened secretions from his throat.

Interpretation

This patient presented with several indications for completion of an endoscopic swallowing examination. He had received radiation therapy, which can contribute to xerostomia, mucositis, anatomic changes, and even physiologic changes in the pharyngeal structures used in swallowing. He demonstrated voice changes meriting inspection of the laryngeal valve, and he reported pooling of thickened secretions. Endoscopic swallowing study revealed thickened secretions bilaterally in the piriform sinuses and to a lesser degree within the laryngeal vestibule. The vocal folds were mobile but **edematous** and **erythematous**, suggesting irritation, and the left vocal fold was slightly bowed, creating a small glottal gap during phonation. Swallowing attempts of various consistencies revealed no difficulties with thin or thick liquids but mild postswallow residue in the hypopharynx for pudding and masticated materials. This residue was completely cleared with subsequent swallows of thin liquid. Based on the results of this examination no fluoroscopic study was completed. Recommendations were to continue total oral feeding, to moisten the mouth before ingestion of pudding or solid materials, to use liquids to clear residue from more solid foods, and to consult his oncologist for treatment of mucositis.

CLINICAL CASE EXAMPLE 8-3

A 76-year-old man reports swallowing difficulty after a hemispheric stroke. His primary complaint is that food sticks; he localizes the problem to the base of the neck just above the sternum. He complains of having excess saliva that causes him to cough. His cough is weak, and his voice is dysphonic and breathy.

Interpretation

This patient has dysphagia complaints that require both endoscopic and fluoroscopic swallowing examinations. Difficulty managing secretions, weak cough, and voice changes are indications for an endoscopic examination of pharyngeal and laryngeal functions. Reports of food sticking at the level of the neck base indicate the need to complete a fluoroscopic examination. Endoscopic examination revealed a left vocal fold paresis with incomplete glottal closure, and pooled "foamy" secretions throughout the hypopharynx and in the laryngeal vestibule. Falsetto maneuver revealed a paretic left hemipharynx. Swallow attempts revealed postswallow residue in the left piriform sinus that increased as the viscosity of the swallowed material increased. Fluoroscopic swallowing study confirmed a left hemipharyngeal paresis and incomplete opening of the PES with less opening on the left side. Recommendations initially focused on referral to an otolaryngologist for consideration of vocal fold medialization and procedures to improved PES opening.

REFERENCES

1. American Speech-Language-Hearing Association: Clinical indicators for instrumental assessment of dysphagia [guidelines]. Available at www.asha.org/policy.

2. American Speech-Language-Hearing Association: Guidelines for speech-language pathologists performing videofluoroscopic swallowing studies [guidelines]. Available at www.asha.org/policy.

3. American Speech-Language-Hearing Association: Role of the speech-language pathologist in the performance and interpretation of endoscopic evaluation of swallowing: guidelines [guidelines]. Available at www.asha.org/policy.

4. American Speech-Language-Hearing Association: Knowledge and skills for speech-language pathologists performing endoscopic assessment of swallowing functions [guidelines]. Available at www.asha.org/policy.

5. Martino R, Pron G, Diamant NE: Oropharyngeal dysphagia: surveying practice patterns of the speech-language pathologist. *Dysphagia* 19:165, 2004.

6. Carnaby GD, Harenberg L: What is "usual care" in dysphagia rehabilitation: a survey of USA dysphagia practice patterns. *Dysphagia* 28:567, 2013.

7. Logemann J: *Evaluation and treatment of swallowing disorders*, San Diego, 1983, College-Hill Press.

8. Palmer JB, Kuhlemeier KV, Tippett DC, et al: A protocol for the videofluorographic swallowing study. *Dysphagia* 8:209, 1993.

9. Martin-Harris B, Jones B: The videofluorographic swallowing study. *Phys Med Rehabil Clin North Am* 19:769, 2008.

10. Roberts MW, Tylenda CA, Sonies BC, et al: Dysphagia in bulimia nervosa. *Dysphagia* 4:106, 1989.

11. Peruzzi WT, Logemann JA, Currie D, et al: Assessment of aspiration in patients with tracheostomies: comparison of the bedside colored dye assessment with videofluoroscopic examination. *Respir Care* 46:243, 2001.

12. Logemann JA: *Manual for the videofluorographic study of swallowing*, ed 2, Austin, TX, 1993, Pro-ED.

13. Daniels SK, Schroeder MF, DeGeorge PC, et al: Effects of verbal cue on bolus flow during swallowing. *Am J Speech Lang Pathol* 16:140, 2007.

14. Nagy A, Leigh C, Hori SF, et al: Timing differences between cued and noncued swallows in healthy young adults. *Dysphagia* 28:428, 2013.

15. Martin-Harris B, Brodsky M, Michel Y, et al: Delayed initiation of the pharyngeal swallow: normal variability in adult swallows. *J Speech Lang Hear Res* 50:585, 2007.

16. Nagy A, Steele CM, Pelletier CA: Barium versus nonbarium stimuli: differences in taste intensity, chemesthesis, and swallowing behaviour in healthy adult women. *J Speech Lang Hear Res* 57:758, 2014.

17. Dietsch AM, Solomon NP, Steele CM, et al: The effect of barium on perceptions of taste intensity and palatability. *Dysphagia* 29:96, 2014.

18. Buchholz DW, Bosma JF, Donner MW: Adaptation, compensation, and decompensation of the pharyngeal swallow. *Gastrointest Radiol* 10:235, 1985.

19. Kahrilas PJ, Lin S, Logemann JA, et al: Deglutitive tongue action: volume accommodation and bolus propulsion. *Gastroenterology* 104:152, 1993.

20. Kahrilas PJ, Lin S, Chen J, et al: Oropharyngeal accommodation to swallow volume. *Gastroenterology* 111:297, 1996.

21. Kendall KA, Leonard RJ, McKenzie SW: Accommodation to changes in bolus viscosity in normal deglutition: a videofluoroscopic study. *Ann Otol Rhinolaryngol* 110:1059, 2001.

22. Adnerhill I, Eckberg O, Groher ME: Determining normal bolus size for thin liquids. *Dysphagia* 4:1, 1989.

23. Martin-Harris B, Brodsky MB, Michel Y, et al: MBS measurement tool for swallow impairment—MBSImp: establishing a standard. *Dysphagia* 23:392, 2008.

24. Groher ME, Crary MA, Carnaby-Mann GD, et al: The impact of rheologically controlled materials on the identification airway compromise on the clinical and videofluoroscopic swallowing examinations. *Dysphagia* 21:218, 2006.

25. Madhavan A, Hollen M, Shaw L, et al: *Food sticking in the throat during swallowing*. Presentation to the Annual Convention of the American Speech-Language-Hearing Association, Atlanta, Georgia, November, 2012.

26. Jung SH, Kim J, Jeong H, et al: Effect of the order of test diets on the accuracy and safety of swallowing studies. *Ann Rehabil Med* 38:304, 2014.

27. Han TR, Paik NJ, Park JW, et al: The prediction of persistent dysphagia beyond six months after stroke. *Dysphagia* 23:59, 2008.

28. Kim J, Oh BM, Kim JY, et al: Validation of the videofluoroscopic dysphagia in various etiologies. *Dysphagia* 29:438, 2014.

29. Mann (Carnaby) G, Hankey GJ, Cameron D: Swallowing disorders following acute stroke: prevalence and diagnostic accuracy. *Cerebrovascular Dis* 10:380, 2000.

30. Carnaby GD: *Relationships among videofluoroscopic scales and stroke outcome*. Presentation to the Dysphagia Research Society, Nashville, TN, March, 2014.

31. O'Neil KH, Purdy M, Falk J, et al: The dysphagia outcome and severity scale. *Dysphagia* 14:139, 1999.

32. Rosenbek JC, Robbins JA, Roecker EB, et al: A penetration-aspiration scale. *Dysphagia* 11:93, 1996.

33. Crary MA, Butler MK, Baldwin BO: Objective distance measurements from videofluorographic swallow studies using computer interactive analysis: technical note. *Dysphagia* 9:116, 1994.

34. Kendal KA, McKenzie S, Leonard RJ, et al: Timing of events in normal swallowing: a videofluoroscopic study. *Dysphagia* 15:74, 2000.

35. Kendall KA, Leonard RJ: Pharyngeal constriction in elderly dysphagic patients compared with young and elderly nondysphagic controls. *Dysphagia* 16:272, 2001.

36. McCullough GH, Wertz RT, Rosenbek J, et al: Clinicians' preferences and practices in conducting clinical/bedside and videofluorographic swallowing examinations in an adult, neurogenic population. *Am J Speech Lang Pathol* 8:149, 1999.

37. McCullough GH, Wertz RT, Rosenbek J, et al: Inter- and intrajudge reliability for videofluoroscopic swallowing evaluation measures. *Dysphagia* 16:110, 2001.

38. Baijens L, Barikroo A, Pilz W: Intrarater and interrater reliability for measurements in videofluoroscopy of swallowing. *Eur J Radiol* 82:1683, 2013.

39. Bastian RW: Videoendoscopic evaluation of patients with dysphagia: an adjunct to the modified barium swallow. *Otolaryngol Head Neck Surg* 104:339, 1991.

40. Bastian RW: The videoendoscopic swallowing study: an alternative and partner to the videofluoroscopic swallowing study. *Dysphagia* 8:359, 1993.

41. Langmore SE, Shatz K, Olsen N: Fiberoptic endoscopic examination of swallowing safety: a new procedure. *Dysphagia* 2:216, 1998.

42. American Speech-Language-Hearing Association: The role of the speech-language pathologist in the performance and interpretation of endoscopic evaluation of swallowing; [technical report]. Available at www.asha.org/policy.

43. Aviv J, Kim T, Sacco R, et al: FEESST: a new beside endoscopic test of the motor and sensory components of swallowing. *Ann Otol Rhinolaryngol* 107:378, 1998.

44. Langmore SE: *Endoscopic evaluation and treatment of swallowing disorders*, New York, 2001, Thieme.

45. Murray J: *Manual of dysphagia assessment in adults*, San Diego, 1999, Singular Publishing.

46. Leder SB, Ross D, Briskin KB, et al: A prospective, double blind, randomized study on the use of a topical anesthetic, vasoconstrictor, and placebo during transnasal flexible fiberoptic endoscopy. *J Speech Lang Res* 40:1352, 1997.

47. Singh V, Brockbank M, Todd G: Flexible transnasal endoscopy: is local anesthetic necessary? *Laryngol Otol* 111:616, 1997.

48. Lester S, Langmore SE, Lintzenich CR, et al: The effects of topical anesthetic on swallowing during nasoendoscopy. *Laryngoscope* 123:1704, 2013.

49. Kamarunas EE, McCullough GH, Guidry TJ, et al: Effects of topical nasal anesthetic on fiberoptic endoscopic examination of swallowing with sensory testing (FEESST). *Dysphagia* 29:33, 2014.

50. Butler SG, Stuart A, Leng X, et al: Factors influencing aspiration during swallowing in healthy older adults. *Laryngoscope* 120:2147, 2010.

51. Baijens LW, Speyer R, Pilz W, et al: FEES protocol derived estimates of sensitivity: aspiration in dysphagic patients. *Dysphagia* 29:583, 2014.

52. Colodny N: Interjudge and intrajudge reliabilities in fiberoptic endoscopic evaluation of swallowing (FEES) using the penetration-aspiration scale: a replication study. *Dysphagia* 17:308, 2002.

53. Farneti D: Pooling score: an endoscopic model for evaluating severity of dysphagia. *Acta Otorhinolaryngol Ital* 28:135, 2008.

54. Farneti D: Endoscopic scale for evaluation of severity of dysphagia: preliminary observations. *Rev Laryngol Otol Rhinol* 129:137, 2008.

55. Dziewas R, Warnecke T, Olenberg S, et al: Towards a basic endoscopic assessment of swallowing in acute stroke—development and evaluation of a simple dysphagia score. *Cerebrovasc Disord* 26:41, 2008.

56. Farneti D, Fattori B, Nacci A, et al: The pooling-score (p-score): inter- and intra-rater reliability in endoscopic assessment of the severity of dysphagia. *Acta Otorhinolarygol Ital* 34:105, 2014.

57. Warnecke T, Ritter MA, Kroger B, et al: Fiberoptic endoscopic dysphagia severity scale predicts outcome after acute stroke. *Cerebrovasc Dis* 28:283, 2009.

58. Denk DM, Kaider A: Videoendoscopic biofeedback: a simple method to improve the efficacy of swallowing rehabilitation of patients after head and neck surgery. *ORL J Otorhinolaryngol Relat Spec* 59:100, 1997.

59. Leder SB, Novella S, Patwa H: Use of fiberoptic endoscopic evaluation of swallowing (FEES) in patients with amyotrophic lateral sclerosis. *Dysphagia* 19:177, 2004.

60. Manor Y, Mootanah R, Freud D, et al: Video-assisted swallowing therapy for patients with Parkinson's disease. *Parkinsonism Relat Disord* 19:207, 2013.

61. Warnecke T, Teismann I, Oelenberg S, et al: The safety of fiberoptic endoscopic evaluation in acute stroke patients. *Stroke* 40:482, 2009.

62. McGowan SL, Gleeson M, Smith M, et al: A pilot study of fiberoptic endoscopic evaluation of swallowing in patients with cuffed tracheostomies in neurological intensive care. *Neurocrit Care* 6:90, 2007.

63. Aviv JE, Mury T, Zschommier A, et al: Flexible endoscopic evaluation of swallowing with sensory testing: patient characteristics and analysis of safety in 1,340 consecutive examinations. *Ann Otol Rhinol Laryngol* 114:173, 2005.

64. Cohen MA, Setzen M, Perlman PW, et al: The safety of flexible endoscopic evaluation of swallowing with sensory testing in an outpatient otolaryngology setting. *Laryngoscope* 113:21, 2003.

65. Warnecke T, Teismann I, Oelenberg S, et al: The safety of fiberoptic endoscopic evaluation of swallowing in acute stroke patients. *Stroke* 40:482, 2009.

66. American Speech-Language-Hearing Association: Knowledge and skills needed by speech-language pathologists providing services to individuals with swallowing and/or feeding disorders. *ASHA Suppl* 22:81, 2002.

67. Périé S, Laccourreye L, Flahault A, et al: Role of videoendoscopy in assessment of pharyngeal function in oropharyngeal dysphagia: comparison with videofluoroscopy and manometry. *Laryngoscope* 108:1712, 1998.

68. Schröter-Morasch H, Bartolome G, Troppmann N, et al: Values and limitations of pharyngolaryngoscopy (transnasal, transoral) in patients with dysphagia. *Folia Phoniatr Logop* 51:172, 1999.

69. Langmore SE, Shatz K, Olson N: Endoscopic and videofluoroscopic evaluations of swallowing and aspiration. *Ann Otol Rhinolaryngol* 100:678, 1991.

70. Wu CH, Hsiao TY, Chen JC, et al: Evaluation of swallowing safety with fiberoptic endoscope: comparison with videofluoroscopic technique. *Laryngoscope* 107:396, 1997.

71. Crary MA, Baron J: Endoscopic and fluoroscopic evaluations of swallowing: comparison of observed and inferred findings. *Dysphagia* 12:108, 1997.

CHAPTER 9

Treatment Considerations, Options, and Decisions

Michael A. Crary

To view additional case videos and content, please visit the evolve website.

CHAPTER OUTLINE

OBJECTIVES

1. Introduce the concept of how evidence-based practice guides treatment decisions.
2. Discuss general factors that influence therapy decisions.
3. Provide examples from the three major classes of therapeutic interventions for dysphagia.
4. Discuss how the evaluation results will affect treatment planning.
5. Present a decision tree for selecting and implementing dysphagia therapy.

EVIDENCE-BASED PRACTICE

The selection of any treatment for the patient with dysphagia should be based on the best available evidence from the published literature, the patient's wishes, and the clinician's experience with similar problems. The combination of these three variables in preparing a treatment plan is referred to as evidence-based practice (EBP). Given any individual patient, clinicians will assign different weights to each variable. For example, if the clinician has had excellent success with an unconventional form of therapy for which there is no research support, he or she may, with the patient's consent, choose to apply that treatment strategy. Or if a patient did not feel able to cooperate with a recommended plan of treatment, another course of action may need to be implemented. EBP differs from traditional clinical management because it does not rely solely on clinical intuition and experience but also values patient desires and a critical appraisal of published research.

In all fields of health care, clinicians have been challenged to evaluate and use available research evidence to solve clinical problems and provide the best patient care possible in the most cost-efficient manner. Examples of

---

PRACTICE NOTE 9-1

In 1998 the Dutch Neurological Society published guidelines for the treatment of neurogenic dysphagia developed from an evidence-based review. The following pathway of care was to be used when encountering a patient with dysphagia from a neurogenic source.

1. Dysphagia should be detected with 50 mL of water because this is the most useful screening test.
2. If dysphagia is present, a nasogastric tube should be placed.
3. If after 2 weeks dysphagia is still present, a percutaneous gastrostomy tube should be placed.
4. There is no scientific support for evaluation with videofluoroscopy.
5. There is no scientific support for swallowing therapy.

   Although these guidelines may seem stringent and not in the patient's best interest, at the time they were developed the published research supported this pathway of clinical care.

---

how EBP affects patient care are numerous (see for example Practice Note 9-1). For example, assume that a clinician had been using the tactile-thermal stimulation technique (see Chapter 10) with patients who show swallowing onset delay because of experimental evidence suggesting its application with that particular group of patients. However, when reviewing additional evidence in multiple studies with similar patients, the investigators reported that the effect was minimal. In this circumstance the clinician might be hesitant to apply the treatment. However, before changing practice, the clinician must evaluate the strength (believability) of the new evidence before he or she alters the treatment approach. Even in the face of strong evidence, some clinicians find it hard to abandon their own experience and intuition. Complete reliance on experimental evidence runs the risk of setting patient care guidelines and paths of care that experience suggests may not be in the patient's best interest (see Practice Note 9-1). The intersections of experimental evidence, clinical experience, and patient desires ultimately lead to the best treatment approach. When using an EBP model it is incumbent on the clinician to consult the research literature to evaluate treatment **effectiveness** or **efficacy** in patients similar to the one requiring evaluation or treatment.

Astute clinicians recognize that failure to implement EBP runs the risk of overusing familiar and comfortable treatments that might be less effective in achieving desired outcomes. Similarly, clinicians could be using what they perceive to be the most effective treatment strategy, but they are applying it incorrectly—for example, recommending that an exercise be done 10 times a day when the experimental evidence suggests that the best outcomes are achieved when it is done 100 times a day.

EVALUATING EVIDENCE

After the clinical and/or instrumental evaluation the clinician should be able to formulate questions (hypotheses) about which treatment approach might fit the patient's profile. For example, if the patient is having difficulty protecting the airway during the swallow sequence, could he or she benefit from learning a swallowing maneuver, and would a change in posture be beneficial? A more focused question might be "Does the combination of a postural change and a swallowing maneuver help protect the airway, or is one intervention better alone?" Another relevant question might be "How long does the patient need to maintain these interventions before complete swallowing safety is achieved?"

The search for answers to questions could come from multiple sources, including personal experience ("It worked before so I will try it again"), textbooks (although these are rarely opened once the course is completed), expert advice through continuing education opportunities ("the expert said it, so it must be true"), commercial sales ("this is exactly what you will need"), and journal articles (although research has shown that the frequency of professional reading declines with years away from the university). All these sources, with the exception of the published journal articles, represent information that can be gathered. Information is different from evidence, because evidence results from a controlled approach to a clinical question.

Assuming the clinician wants to review the evidence pertaining to a clinical question, the next step is to consult relevant databases using key search terms that might help answer those questions. Terms such as *posture, swallowing, outcomes,* and *treatment* might be used in the initial search. Finding the relevant evidence can be accomplished by using databases such as MEDLINE or PubMed, or websites that summarize data such as the Cochrane Library or the American College of Physicians. Typing terms in a web search such as *evidence based* and *clinical trials* can lead to other relevant databases. Government-based websites such as the National Guideline Clearinghouse (www.guideline.gov) can be a useful starting point in an evidence-based search. If the search is directed toward a specific disease such as Parkinson's, accessing a specific organization's official website also is a valuable point of departure.

After the evidence is accessed, the clinician must evaluate the relevance to the patient in question and its strength (believability) and clarity in guiding treatment. Judging the strength of the evidence is done through an analysis of the study's design characteristics. Some websites (e.g., the Cochrane Library) are designed to provide critical reviews of the extant evidence on a multitude of diagnostic and treatment questions. Because these systematic analyses are designed to gather and grade the strength of many studies on a single topic, they are very useful for the busy clinician who may not have the time to do an extensive search. In the small subspecialty of oropharyngeal swallowing

TABLE 9-1 Classification System for Grading Levels of Evidence

Evidence Grade	Level of Evidence	Type of Evidence
A	1a	Systematic review of RCTs
	1b	Individual RCT
	1c	All or none
B	2a	Systematic review of cohort studies
	2b	Individual cohort study
	2c	Outcomes research
	3a	Systematic review of case-control studies
	3b	Individual case-control study
C	4	Case series (and poor-quality case-control and cohort studies)
D	5	Expert opinion without critical appraisal or based on physiology or "first" principles

RCT, Randomized controlled trial.

Grading levels of evidence. The far right column shows the study design designations. Depending on the design of the study, it is assigned a strength level (middle column). The strongest designs are at level 1, and the weakest designs are level 5. Within each level the strength of evidence can be graded, such as levels 2a to 3b, with a study graded at 2a being stronger than 3b. Because it is not always possible to make fine distinctions between studies based on their design, investigators grade studies with more general categories such as A through D (far left column).

(Adapted from Oxford Centre for Evidence-Based Medicine, 2001.)

disorders, not every clinical question will have been reviewed systematically.

Because the study's design often determines the relative strength of the evidence, it is important to know what constitutes weak evidence for any given outcome and what constitutes stronger evidence for the same outcome. Table 9-1 presents a classification system for grading levels of evidence according to the study's design characteristics. For instance, the highest level of evidence (grade A or 1) is associated with study designs that are randomized controlled trials (RCTs). A lower grade (grade D or 5) is associated with studies that report on a series of patients. Investigators who use the RCT design to study a question are bound by much stricter criteria to answer their question. In general, these criteria try to eliminate any bias in the study that might shed doubt on the believability of the results. Some of these criteria include a large sample size in an experimental and control group with subjects assigned randomly, measurements made by investigators who are **blinded** to the study, and accounting for the outcomes of all study subjects at the end of the experiment. Study designs at levels B, C, and D may meet some of these criteria, but not all of them. The fewer criteria met, the weaker the evidence. In general, a clinician should have more confidence in studies graded at grade A than at grade D. Therefore the applicability of the findings from RCTs would be applied clinically with more confidence than findings from studies that reported on similar outcomes with a case series design. Such criteria can help the clinician decide which diagnostic or treatment approach might fit the patient and how much confidence to place in the outcome. An extensive discussion of each level of evidence and its corresponding characteristics is beyond the scope of this chapter. Readers are referred to The Handbook of Evidence-Based Practice in Communication Disorders for a thorough discussion.[1]

Recently we have noted an increase in systematic reviews and metaanalyses along with an increased number of randomized clinical trials relating to various aspects of dysphagia in adults. These changes in available literature create novel challenges for clinicians and others seeking to understand the evidence for any clinical issue. Perhaps the most basic question to ask about any published manuscript is, "Was it well done?" Levels of evidence make the assumption that research is well done or at the very least that consumers of research can tell which studies were well done (see Practice Note 9-2 for sources of evidence to avoid). Unfortunately, not all clinical research studies are completed with the same degree of control or accuracy. Randomized clinical trials can be evaluated by comparing the published details against the CONSORT (Consolidated Standards of Reporting Trials Document checklist (http://www.consort-statement .org). Other higher level forms of evidence also should follow rules to maintain the integrity of that specific format for evidence. For example, the PRISMA (Preferred Reporting Items for Systematic Reviews and Meta-Analyses) Statement provides guidelines for reporting (and hence evaluating) systematic reviews and metaanalyses (http:// prisma-statement.org). Still, any clinical research manuscript should be evaluated for its scientific rigor before serious consideration is afforded the results as contributing to the evidence base on that specific topic. Box 9-1 presents some simplified criteria by which published clinical research may be evaluated for scientific rigor (G Carnaby, personal communication). Stronger manuscripts will meet most or all of these criteria. Depending on the strength of the study design, stronger studies should garner more weight and credibility in making clinical decisions. The fewer criteria met (and it is the author's responsibility to overtly address these criteria) the weaker the evidence contribution of the manuscript.

Judgment of the strength of the experimental evidence must be complemented by other analytic methods. For example, were the relevant studies done with patients similar to the patient in question, or were the characteristics in the reference sample different—such as age or gender? Was the treatment protocol in the study described precisely enough so that it could be replicated? Do you have the skills needed to replicate the treatment? For example, if the treatment described the use of certain equipment, do you have the equipment and are you trained to use it? And finally, are the outcomes in the study similar to the ones you and

BOX 9-1 CRITICAL EVALUATION OF CLINICAL RESEARCH MANUSCRIPTS

Abstract
- Objectives of study and key results clearly described.
- Includes any tangential or unsubstantiated data or information (-ve item).

Introduction
- Statement of purpose: why was the study completed?
- Was background sufficient to understand the aims of the study?

Methods
- Methods presented in sufficient detail to permit replication.
- References provided for standard methods.
- Are procedures used valid and with demonstrated reliability?
- Modified or unique methods clearly described.
- Rationale provided for procedures employed.
- Statistical analyses clearly described.
- Is sample size sufficiently large and does the sample match your patient population?
- Do the procedures appropriately reflect the purpose and aims of the study?

Results
- Do the obtained results make sense in reference to the purpose and aims of the study?

- Are tables and figures easy to understand and clearly labeled?
- Are data in tables correct (e.g., do the numbers add up)?
- Were appropriate statistical methods followed and results clearly reported?

Discussion
- Are the key findings of the study clearly stated?
- Are the key results discussed in reference to published information?
- Is tangential information included or information not previously included
- Do the authors overspeculate beyond the scope of the results?
- Are the results both statistically and clinically significant or meaningful?
- Were strengths *and* limitations of the study clearly presented and discussed?
- Were future directions suggested?

References
- Are references appropriate for text comments and recent?
- Do the authors overcite their own work and exclude other relevant papers (-ve item)?

---

your patient envision? Even the best-designed, grade 1 study may not be applicable to your clinical question. One also must judge whether the study under scrutiny has clinical significance. That is, if the conclusion from a study was that technique "X" improved hyoid elevation by 2 mm in a group of acute poststroke patients, is that change clinically significant or was it only a statistically significant difference? In this example, unless the study reported that a 2-mm change in hyoid elevation actually made a difference in airway protection or in an improvement of dietary intake, one may choose to ignore the data even though statistically technique "X" made a difference. Furthermore, would the patient be pleased with a 2-mm change in hyoid movement if he or she was not able to eat or drink more? (see Practice Note 9-2).

GENERAL TREATMENT CONSIDERATIONS

Two common considerations inherent to all aspects of dysphagia are airway protection and nutrition and hydration. Clinicians often face the important question, "Can the patient safely resume or increase adequate oral intake?" Dissecting this question reveals critical considerations in dysphagia treatment. The primary concerns for patients with dysphagia may be found in the words *safe* and *adequate*. Safety is often expressed in terms of airway

PRACTICE NOTE 9-2

I came across a tongue-in-cheek article on EBP a few years ago in the *British Medical Journal*. The following list summarizes forms of evidence that we should **AVOID** but that may appear in a variety of scenarios.
- *Eminence:* the most gray hair makes the final decision.
- *Vehemence:* the loudest voice wins.
- *Eloquence:* the best dressed or the smoothest talker convinces everyone else.
- *Diffidence:* the level of gloom expressed determines the outcome.
- *Nervousness:* the fear of litigation determines the outcome.
- *Confidence:* the degree of bravado or "certainty" dominates the discussion.

Adapted from Isaacs D, Fitzgerald D: Seven alternatives to evidence-based medicine, *BMJ* 319:1618, 1999.

protection. Patients who aspirate most of any given bolus of food or liquid are not considered safe in reference to the risk of aspiration and subsequent respiratory infection or, possibly, the risk of airway obstruction from more solid foods. The reference to adequate refers to the individual's ability to ingest sufficient food or liquid by mouth to maintain (or increase, if required in the situation) nutrition and hydration. A patient who engages in total oral feeding only to ingest inadequate volumes of food or liquid is a patient who is at risk for future health problems. When patients are fed by nonoral routes, treatment should be focused on the potential to resume oral intake of food and liquid. If the patient is taking a total oral diet, the focus may be on expanding the amount of intake to enhance nutrition or on expanding the variety of the diet to improve social aspects of eating and presumably quality of life. In planning treatment, it is important to have a clear grasp of the patient's present situation and a clear vision of where both clinician and patient want to be in the future and the factors that may help or hinder that direction.

CLINICAL CASE EXAMPLE 9-1

A 69-year-old woman had a respiratory arrest after cardiac bypass surgery. After extubation she gained strength and a swallowing study was ordered. The videofluoroscopy revealed a delayed oral stage with good airway protection on all materials and volumes. It was recommended that she be given a soft mechanical diet with regular fluids and that the speech-language pathologist (SLP) monitor her at the bedside the next day. During breakfast it was noted that the patient ate half of her meal, complaining of fatigue and lack of appetite. The doctor ordered a 3-day calorie count because he was concerned about her nutritional and hydration status. The dietitian calculated that the patient's caloric need per day was 2000 calories. On the second day of oral feeding her respiratory status changed, as did her mental status. The calorie counts revealed that she was taking in only about 1100 of the 2000 calories needed. At that time the team believed that she could not sustain nutrition orally and that the secondary changes in respiratory and mental status were attributable to poor nutritional and hydration status. A nasogastric tube was placed so that nutrition and hydration could be maintained until her overall strength improved to the point where she could ingest enough calories to meet her metabolic needs.

In selecting any therapy, consideration must be given to the objective of that therapy. For example, in medicine one goal of therapy might be to cure a disease. How do clinicians "cure" dysphagia? Does curing dysphagia suggest that clinicians must return patients who are fed nonorally to oral feeding? This outcome is not always possible. Do clinicians want to prevent recurrence of a dysphagia-related **comorbidity**? One potential objective might be to diminish or eliminate recurrent chest infections. This goal certainly provides direction in treatment planning. In some situations clinicians may focus on limiting functional deterioration or facilitating recovery. To adopt this focus, clinicians must have a clear understanding of the underlying conditions contributing to dysphagia in individual patients. Certainly, clinicians hope that interventions do not contribute to later

---

BOX 9-2 TREATMENT CONSIDERATIONS FOCUSING ON THE NATURE OF THE SWALLOWING DEFICIT

- Feeding or swallowing deficits (or both)
- Voluntary or involuntary processes
- Stage of deficit
- Deficit or compensatory activity

---

complications and that they, in fact, contribute to prevention of complications such as chest infections and malnutrition.

Beyond specific goals of treatment, clinicians must consider the nature of the swallowing deficit and the treatment options available to them and the patient (NOTE: these are not always the same). Box 9-2 summarizes some issues that might be addressed regarding the swallowing deficit. A basic question might revolve around feeding versus swallowing processes: Are there physical or cognitive factors that preclude successful feeding but that do not interfere with swallowing function? Are both of these factors present and, if so, do they interact in a positive or negative manner? Certain dysphagia-causing diseases might demonstrate differences between voluntary or involuntary motor processes. If differences are present, are there swallowing activities that may be used to tap into voluntary versus involuntary motor processes? Stage of deficit is an artificial delineation often used for convenience. Are the swallowing deficits primarily located within the oral, oropharyngeal, pharyngeal, or esophageal component? Clinicians must also remember that not only are these "stages" artificial, but that the swallowing mechanism is interactive—events occurring in one anatomic area have the potential to affect performance in another area (see Chapter 2). A difficult clinical task can be attempting to separate the specific swallowing deficit from any compensatory activities used by individual patients. For example, consider the patient who attempts to swallow but immediately begins to expectorate, or a patient who demonstrates a pattern of multiple, incomplete swallows interspersed with throat clearing, resulting in only a minute amount of material actually swallowed. Does this pattern reflect a specific pattern of impaired physiology? Does it reflect the presence of compensations intended to protect the airway, or are there other possibilities? In some cases, this distinction may not be important. However, in others, it may be important to understand what might be changed as a result of therapy versus what might not be changed. This consideration may affect the decision to engage in therapy and, if so, the direction of therapy.

Another noteworthy point is that dysphagia treatment is rarely unifocal. Dysphagia is the result of underlying disease or disorder processes. Consequently, patients with dysphagia often receive therapies from medical, surgical, or behavioral realms. Clinicians who are treating patients

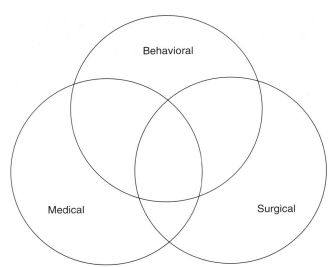

FIGURE 9-1 A schematic representation of potential interactions of behavioral, medical, and surgical treatment options in dysphagia.

PRACTICE NOTE 9-3

A 34-year-old patient had sustained severe burns to his head, neck, and upper torso. Because of the severe pain that typically accompanies such injuries, he was on narcotics that made it difficult for him to remain awake. He had improved to the point where his physician believed he could start to eat orally. During the clinical evaluation the SLP noted he could only remain totally alert for 5 minutes and questioned whether he could stay awake long enough to eat an entire meal. The clinical examination also showed that although he coughed on liquids, he did not cough if he held his breath through the entire swallow sequence. Because this method required concentration for each attempt, it was questionable if the patient's alertness level would allow this compensation. After reading the report, the physician decided to begin weaning the patient from his medications, keeping the patient on his nasogastric tube. After 1 week the patient was reevaluated by the SLP. His marked change in level of alertness made her confident that he now could tolerate oral feeding and cooperate with any needed compensations during the meal. This case illustrates how a change in medical management might affect the success of a behavioral intervention.

with dysphagia should be aware of concomitant treatments, as well as dysphagia treatments in other realms that may either work together or in place of behavioral treatment strategies the SLP may provide (see Practice Note 9-3). Figure 9-1 is a schematic reminder of how these therapy categories may interact. In certain clinical situations one category may comprise the primary or sole treatment approach. In other situations two or all three categories may interact to form the most beneficial intervention.

- Etiology (underlying cause, disease, or disorder)
- Severity
- Eating history
- Psychosocial factors
- Anticipated medical course
- Caregiver factors

PRACTICE NOTE 9-4

A 37-year-old woman came to the outpatient clinic with a diagnosis of suspected dysphagia secondary to multiple sclerosis (MS). She had just been discharged from the hospital, where she received the diagnosis of MS. Her modified barium swallow study showed minor penetration of the airway with a strong cough on thin liquids only. The SLP recommended that she continue the present diet; however, the focus of the appointment was on the possible progression of the MS and how that might affect swallowing. Because some types of MS show periods of exacerbation and remission, it was important to tell the patient that if swallowing became suddenly worse, it might be a signal of a new exacerbation; however, with medical and behavioral treatment, it should improve. Another area of discussion was whether the patient would ever want a feeding tube, and in which circumstances she would want it. The discussion of executing an advance directive to guide her future medical care was important because most likely she would have additional problems with swallowing in the future. The concept of an advance directive is discussed in Chapter 11.

PATIENT-SPECIFIC TREATMENT

Patients bring to any clinical situation a variety of unique circumstances. Box 9-3 provides a list of potential patient-related considerations that may have an effect on dysphagia treatment options and decisions. Because dysphagia is the result of underlying disease processes, the cause of dysphagia should be understood as best as clinically possible because the underlying disease presents a clinical course that has direct effect on swallowing function and benefits from various intervention strategies over time (see Practice Note 9-4).

The severity of dysphagia is a more complex concept than might first be imagined. How is the severity of dysphagia graded? Some clinicians and investigators have used impairment of swallowing physiology based on instrumental examination, whereas others have used more functional measures such as amount of food or liquid taken by mouth.[3,4]

25

Some clinicians may believe that patients who take no food by mouth also have the poorest swallowing physiology. Unfortunately, this is not always the case. Patient status may change over time, and some patients who receive only nonoral feeding may actually have adequate swallowing physiology to ingest some food or liquid by mouth. Thus severity of dysphagia should not be considered a unitary concept because many factors are involved.

Eating history may provide clinicians with some idea of a patient's motivation and willingness to push toward increased oral intake. This interacts directly with certain psychosocial considerations. For example, the patient who reports that he "lives to eat, not eats to live" and who engages in the practice of chewing food that cannot be swallowed just for the taste may be more compliant with a rigorous therapy plan than the patient who uses only nonoral sources and never attempts any oral intake of food or liquid. In addition, eating history may provide the clinician with cultural biases in food selection (i.e., the patient never ate that food or always ate that food) or limitations in specific food availability associated with the patient's environment. Social aspects of eating should also be considered in terms of the patient's current situation ("I attempt to eat alone in my room") and future goals ("I would like to eat in a restaurant"). Finally, for patients who engage in both oral and tube feeding, eating history may explain the timing of one form of feeding relative to the other. This factor may be important in reaching functional goals in therapy.

The patient's anticipated medical course is an essential factor for the clinician to understand. It may affect the consideration of whether to initiate therapy as well as which types of therapy to undertake. In some clinical scenarios it may be better to wait and monitor the patient's condition (e.g., stability, endurance). In other situations aggressive therapy is indicated. Clinicians must keep in mind that therapeutic strategies should change as the patient's underlying condition (and potentially dysphagia) changes (review Practice Note 9-3 and 9-4).

Caregiver considerations are an extension of patient considerations, especially for patients (at any age) who are unable to perform self-care (including feeding). Whether the caregiver is a nurse, other qualified health care provider, spouse or other family member, or friend, caregiver performance can have a direct effect (positive or negative) on the performance of the patient with dysphagia (review Practice Note 9-5). Mealtimes can become complicated by a caregiver who is uninitiated in proper feeding strategies for the dependent patient. Positioning of the patient, rate and manner of food presentation, and other variables need to be clearly understood by caregivers (see Practice Note 9-5).

The patient's residential environment also can affect the nature of dysphagia interventions (see Chapter 1). The needs of the patient in the intensive care unit are different from those of the individual receiving outpatient therapy. In

---

PRACTICE NOTE 9-5

A 78-year-old woman who lived alone had just had a second stroke that left her immobile and dysphagic. Her swallowing improved in the hospital to the point where she could safely eat a blended diet. She also needed oral supplements six times a day to receive a sufficient amount of calories. Her neighbor and best friend volunteered to take her home. Before leaving the hospital the neighbor received training from the dietitian on how to prepare the patient's food. After 6 months, the neighbor said that the time to prepare the food was becoming a burden and that her friend really could not afford the supplemental feedings. She did not want to put her friend in a nursing home. The physician, friend, and patient agreed that a gastrostomy would allow the patient to receive the majority of calories through her tube. It also was determined that a few of her favorite food items that did not require special preparation could be taken orally for pleasure.

---

addition, the resources available in different environments differ dramatically. Clinicians working in academic medical centers often have more resources available than do clinicians working in rural long-term care facilities.

APPROACH-SPECIFIC TREATMENT

Treatment techniques (including medical, surgical, and behavioral), like individual patients, require specific consideration in planning intervention. As previously mentioned, treatment options change as the patient's condition changes over time. From this perspective the decision of when to intervene, as well as how to intervene (choice of technique), changes according to the patient's condition. In general, treatment strategies may be considered in reference to the degree of interaction with the patient or the intent of treatment. A common approach to patients who are severely debilitated or in the acute phase of an illness is a prophylactic or preventative approach. Such approaches often tend to be passive, not requiring substantial activity from the patient. Oral hygiene, passive movements, and perhaps diet changes might be considered passive interventions. Active interventions are those in which the patient is required to engage in direct maneuvers or compensations to change some aspect of swallowing performance. Another dichotomy that may overlap with active versus passive interventions is that of patient-centered versus environment-centered interventions. Patient-centered interventions may be active or passive, but all focus on the patient. Environment-centered interventions are primarily passive, with the focus on changing some aspect of the patient's environment. Dining rooms or special mealtimes for patients with dysphagia are examples of environment-centered interventions.

Treatment Choices

Box 9-4 presents a list of considerations that apply in choosing any specific treatment technique. Clinicians must consider which treatment options are realistically available. In determining this, the following should be considered: the physical presence of technology and equipment required to use a specific technique (e.g., surface electromyography [sEMG] biofeedback), the clinician's knowledge of and skill in performing a specific technique, and the patient's acceptance of the technique. (Does the patient understand the instructions? Is he or she able to perform the technique? Can the patient afford the technique? What are the demands on the patient to adequately perform the technique?)

Clinical indicators address the question, "Why choose this particular technique?" For example, how does the technique under consideration relate to the specifics of the patient's dysphagic complaints or symptoms? Is the technique clinically and biologically plausible? Should the technique be performed in isolation or in combination with other techniques? These considerations are important in selecting any specific technique. Seeking the answers to these questions forms the basis of an evidence-based literature search.

Anticipated risks and benefits to the patient should be considered in reference to the immediate outcome of the proposed technique. Some techniques that appear to be relatively benign may complicate certain comorbid conditions in some patients. For example, techniques that emphasize a prolonged apneic pause during swallowing attempts might be problematic for some patients with significant respiratory diseases (see Chapter 6 for a discussion of respiratory-related issues). Techniques that require significant muscular effort during repeated swallow attempts might be counterproductive in certain patients with muscle wasting or weakness. In addition to identifying the risks, clinicians also must identify the potential immediate benefits to the patient from any given technique. Some techniques have been shown to be immediately effective in reducing or eliminating certain swallowing deficits (e.g., head turn to compensate for hemipharyngeal weakness leading to residue and aspiration; see Chapter 10). Clinicians should always consider the potential risks of any technique in reference to the potential benefits to the patient.

Functional outcome refers to the long-term benefit of the proposed technique. This is often considered in reference to the goal(s) of therapy. A technique that results in an immediate change in swallowing performance may or may not have a long-term positive effect or it may not be functional for the daily environment. Similarly, some techniques may not have an immediate effect but may produce long-term functional benefit after intensive practice. Therefore choice of technique should be considered in reference to long-term functional outcome in addition to the potential for immediate impact.

Patient empowerment may be interpreted in different ways. One focus of this term is patient involvement in the design of the treatment plan. Involving patients implies their understanding of the proposed plan of treatment and their willingness to participate in that particular plan. This process makes the patient a partner in treatment rather than only a recipient. Patients who are empowered in this process are known to be more compliant with treatment activities, hence increasing the probability for successful outcomes.

OVERVIEW OF TREATMENT OPTIONS

Clinicians should be aware of multiple options for dysphagia intervention, including medical, surgical, and behavioral treatment. Such knowledge increases pertinent communication with other health care providers and facilitates selection of the best treatment options for individual patients. This section provides a brief overview of some of the more recognized medical, surgical, and behavioral treatment options for dysphagia. Chapters 10 and 15 provide a more detailed review of behavioral treatment techniques.

Medical Options

Box 9-5 offers an introduction to common medical options for dysphagia intervention. Medical options in this context refer to dietary modifications or pharmacologic management.

BOX 9-4 CONSIDERATIONS IN CHOOSING A SPECIFIC TREATMENT TECHNIQUE

Options	→	What?
Clinical indicators	→	Why?
Anticipated risks and benefits	→	Immediate
Functional outcome	→	Long term
Patient empowerment	→	Compliance

BOX 9-5 COMMON MEDICAL OPTIONS FOR DYSPHAGIA TREATMENT

Dietary Modifications
- Special diets
- Regulation of nutrition and hydration
- Possible interaction with feeding route (oral vs. nonoral)

Pharmacologic Management
- Antireflux medications
- Prokinetic agents
- Salivary management

Dietary adjustments might seem a strange inclusion under medical treatment options; however, clinicians should be aware that the patient's diet (oral or nonoral route) may need to be modified to accommodate an underlying disease or condition. Common examples of this occur in diabetes or hypertension, which are both related to stroke. Other examples are found among patients who do not tolerate certain tube feedings well, resulting in diarrhea or constipation. A different example is the patient who requires a minimal (or maximal) amount of caloric intake or hydration for health reasons that may or may not be related to dysphagia. Even if the dietary requirements are tangentially related to the condition contributing to dysphagia, the fact that a specific regimen is required will interact with planning dysphagia intervention.

Pharmacologic management of dysphagia refers to the use of medications to improve some aspect of swallowing function. The most commonly encountered medications are those used to combat reflux, improve gastric motility, and alter secretions. A hierarchy of medications is available to combat reflux symptoms. On the lower end of the hierarchy are approaches such as over-the-counter antacids and certain chewing gum products. The next level of medication is the class of **histamine-receptor antagonists**. These medications are reported to eliminate approximately two thirds of stomach acid. The strongest level of medication is the proton-pump inhibitor. These medications are reported to eliminate nearly all stomach acid and represent the strongest pharmacologic approach to acid suppression (see Chapter 5). Multiple drugs are available within each class of medications, and often the choice of medication is based on patient tolerance (fewer side effects) and symptom reduction.

Few medications to improve gastric motility are available.[5] These so-called prokinetic agents are intended to improve esophageal motility, increase lower esophageal sphincter pressure, and promote gastric emptying.

Salivary secretions are important to swallowing functions. They provide important lubrication to the swallowing mechanism and contain important chemicals that protect the teeth and assist with digestive functions. In general, two components of saliva may be considered. One is the watery saliva that emerges from the sublingual and other salivary glands during chewing or other oral movements. The other is the thicker coating of the internal mucosa. Many medical conditions and medical treatments can alter saliva. Some medical treatments such as radiotherapy (see Chapter 4) and certain medications reduce the amount of watery saliva, leaving the patient with a dry mouth and reports of thick, adhering mucus in the mouth and throat. Depending on the cause of the condition, certain medications (mucolytics) might be used to thin the thicker secretions, making them easier to swallow (or expectorate if necessary). In addition, certain medications are available

BOX 9-6 COMMON SURGICAL OPTIONS FOR DYSPHAGIA TREATMENT

- Improved glottal closure
  - Medialization thyroplasty
  - Injection of biomaterials
- Protection of the airway
  - Stents
  - Laryngotracheal separation
  - Laryngectomy
  - Tracheostomy tubes
  - Feeding tubes
- Improved pharyngoesophageal segment opening
  - Dilatation
  - Myotomy
  - Botulinum toxin injection

that attempt to increase the volume of watery secretions. Alternatively, substances are available (most do not require prescription) that can provide lubrication to the mouth from external application. Medical conditions rarely increase salivary flow. Careful examination of the patient who reports excessive saliva often reveals a reduction in the frequency of swallowing as the cause for salivary retention in the mouth or pharynx.

Surgical Options

Box 9-6 summarizes common surgical interventions for dysphagia. Surgical interventions can be divided into three categories: those that improve glottal closure, those designed to protect the airway, and those designed to improve opening of the pharyngoesophageal segment (PES).

Improving Glottal Closure

Two basic approaches have become popular to improve glottal closure: medialization thyroplasty and injection of biomaterials. Before these techniques are described, it should be noted that which patients will benefit from these procedures is not always clear. Clinical experience has revealed that some patients who aspirate receive direct and immediate benefit from improving glottal closure, whereas others have negligible benefit even in combination with other therapies. In this regard, these techniques should be included within the conceptual background of the dysphagia clinician, but with the caveat that the techniques need to be considered realistically in the context of individual patients.

Medialization thyroplasty is a surgical technique that requires the patient to be sedated but not under general anesthesia. A small incision is made in the lower neck over the thyroid cartilage. A small window is made through the cartilage just behind the vocal fold. The vocal fold is moved toward the midline, and a small piece of medical-grade plastic is placed behind the vocal fold between it and the thyroid cartilage. Because the patient is awake during the procedure, transnasal endoscopy is used to monitor the degree of medialization of the vocal fold, and the patient may be asked to phonate so that the surgeon can assess glottal function for voice production. Using patient swallowing symptom report, Kraus et al.[6] found that all their patients reported improvement in swallowing function after thyroplasty. In a modified version of thyroplasty in 15 patients with vocal fold paralysis after thoracic surgery (see Chapter 6), all patients reported improvement in or a reduction of dysphagia symptoms.[7]

Biomaterials may be injected directly into a weakened vocal fold in an attempt to "bulk up" the tissue, thus improving glottal closure. Historically, Teflon was a common material injected into the vocal fold; however, in recent years Teflon has fallen out of favor and has been replaced by **autologous** fat taken from the patient's anterior belly or collagen (commercially available). Most commonly (although variations exist), materials are injected into the vocal fold while the patient is under general anesthesia. Typically, injection of biomaterials is used to reduce a smaller glottal gap, whereas medialization thyroplasty is used for larger gaps. However, different surgeons may prefer one technique over the other.

Protecting the Airway

Although glottal closure techniques are intended to enhance airway protection during swallowing, certain medical conditions may require more dramatic airway protection approaches. Some of these surgical approaches are intended for short-term use until a crisis passes, whereas others may be permanent. A laryngeal stent has been described as a "plug" within the larynx to prevent material from entering the airway. Because the glottis is blocked, this procedure requires a tracheostomy. Laryngotracheal separation is a self-describing surgical procedure. The trachea is surgically separated just below the larynx and brought forward to a tracheostoma, and the remaining trachea inferior to the larynx is sutured closed. Thus the larynx is in place but is separated from the airway. Both stents and laryngotracheal separation have been described as temporary surgical interventions until patients recover from acute aspiration risk.[8] However, data on the success of reversibility are mixed. In a series of patients with amyotrophic lateral sclerosis, Mita[9] reported a reduction in the rates of aspiration and rehospitalization; however, only 21% of the patients were able to eat orally. Pletcher et al.[10] performed laryngotracheal separation for a patient with severe aspiration after a brainstem stroke. The patient recovered to a point at which oral ingestion and voice could be restored, and the procedure was reversed. In a 5-year follow-up the patient continued to eat safely and had good voice. Zocratto et al.[11] provided follow-up data on 60 patients who underwent laryngotracheal separation, 12 of whom had surgical reversals. The complication rate in the group without reversals was 43%, although aspiration was successfully managed. In the group with reversals, the complication rate was 58%. The authors concluded that although the benefits of aspiration reduction were positive, the postsurgical complication rate was unacceptably high. A total laryngectomy represents a potential permanent surgical solution to dysphagia and aspiration. Although a dramatic approach, in some circumstances patients will have better overall function without the larynx (see Clinical Case Example 11-1). Permanent separation of the airway and food tracts may allow the individual to ingest food and liquid safely, and techniques for voice restoration in laryngectomy may facilitate spoken communication.

The use of tracheostomy tubes or feeding tubes in attempts to protect the airway from prandial aspiration has been questioned. Available research suggests that this may not be valid reasoning, and that in some patients tracheostomy tubes can further impair swallowing function and increase the risk of airway compromise (see Chapter 6). Placement of a feeding tube (nasogastric or gastrostomy) does not necessarily reduce aspiration and may increase the rate or severity of aspiration, often from reflux mechanisms (see Chapter 11). Therefore although both surgical options are valid and helpful in individual patients, caution and clear reasoning should be exercised in their consideration.

Improving Pharyngeal Esophageal Segment Opening

Three general surgical approaches are available to improve opening of the PES: stretching, cutting, or paralysis. Stretching is accomplished by the process of dilatation. Dilatation may be accomplished by more than one technique, but the goal is to stretch the lumen of the PES. If PES opening is restricted by scarring, dilatation tears tissue to create a larger opening. However, the risk is twofold: (1) The tear may extend beyond the esophageal tissue, and (2) the effect is often temporary, requiring repeated procedures and, at times, reaching a plateau of benefit. PES limitations resulting from physiologic processes may also respond to dilatation.[12] Although dilatation is used less often than other techniques, reports have demonstrated benefit from this procedure in cases of physiologic stenosis of the PES.

Surgical myotomy is a technique in which the fibers of the cricopharyngeal muscle within the PES are separated.[13] As with many surgical techniques, variations exist and little evidence suggests that one technique variation is superior to any other. Myotomy may be used in combination with other surgical techniques such as supraglottic laryngectomy or total laryngectomy. Applied judiciously to the appropriate patient, surgical myotomy may provide significant benefit to the individual with dysphagia.

Injection of botulinum toxin (Botox) has been described as an effective technique to "relax" the PES. Botulinum toxin works by the process of **chemodenervation**, in which the chemical communication between the motor nerve and the muscle is interrupted. The result is a paresis in the muscle. Injection of botulinum toxin has been shown to improve PES opening and hence swallowing function in selected patients.[14-16] A general rule for selecting patients for this technique (as well as for other techniques focusing on the PES) is that swallowing mechanics above the PES should be optimized. Significant esophageal reflux might be considered a contraindication to these techniques because weakening the PES may result in supraesophageal complications to voice and the airway.

Behavioral Options

More options exist for behavioral interventions for dysphagia than both medical and surgical options combined. Box 9-7 summarizes five general categories of behavioral intervention that may be used in dysphagia intervention. These categories are not meant to be either exhaustive or specific (see Chapters 10 and 15 for specifics on techniques); rather they are intended to serve as an overview to behavioral therapy approaches.

Food Modifications

Food modifications are among the most widely used behavioral interventions in dysphagia therapy. Food and liquid may be modified in many ways to compensate for a swallowing deficit or in an attempt to alter the swallow pattern toward the goal of improved function. Several aspects of food and liquid modifications may be considered.

Rheology

Modifying the rheologic properties of foods and liquids is a common strategy. Thickening liquids with commercial products or purchasing thickened liquids such as nectars is often done in an attempt to slow liquid-bolus transit and form a slightly more cohesive bolus. It is believed that these rheologic changes give patients a better opportunity to swallow without (or with less) airway compromise. This practice has attained a quasiscientific level at which multiple degrees of thickening have been advocated. The issue

---

BOX 9-7 FIVE GENERAL CATEGORIES OF BEHAVIORAL INTERVENTIONS FOR DYSPHAGIA

- Food modification
- Modifying feeding activity
- Patient modifications
- Swallow modification
- Mechanism modifications

---

also is complicated by the fact that the rheologic properties of test swallow materials used at the bedside are not the same as those used for the modified barium swallow studies.[17,18] Therefore swallowing success on materials used in the modified barium swallow study may not be a rheologic match with what the patient actually receives on the meal tray. Current evidence on the benefits of thickened liquids is limited, and there is some suggestion that patients may not enjoy, and thus may not comply with, a regimen of thickened liquids.[19] Solid foods may also be rheologically modified. A common example of this is pureed food. Experienced clinicians recognize that the concept of puree is highly variable. As one clinician commented, "One man's puree is another man's soup." Nonetheless, clinicians, caregivers, and patients chop, mix, blend, and puree foods to reduce the need for chewing, reduce the particulate nature of certain foods, and enhance the ease of swallowing. Another example in this category is the soft mechanical diet. This diet level requires mastication, but foods are soft and often form a cohesive bolus when swallowed. A related question is "How soft?" Some patients are able to masticate certain foods with their teeth or tongue without significant reduction in functional eating ability. Little evidence exists to help formulate guidelines to identify which patients should receive which diet level. Thus clinicians must consider this decision in reference to each individual patient. Dysphagia experts from the American Speech-Language-Hearing Association and the American Dietetic Association have developed the National Dysphagia Diet.[20] Liquid materials have been described with specific rheologic ranges (in **centipoise**) to define thin, nectar thick, and honey thick. Other recommendations on what types of semisolids and solids would be considered safe and unsafe for the patient are described.

Volume

Bolus volume modification is self-explanatory. Some patients require smaller bolus volumes to be able to control and safely transit the bolus through the swallowing mechanism with minimal postswallow residue. Others may require a larger bolus for various reasons, such as increased sensory input. The average bolus size (± 1 standard deviation) of a liquid bolus taken from a cup ranges from 15 to 26 mL and differs between men and women.[21,22] Bolus volume is one factor that may alter swallow physiology. Thus when small bolus volumes are used, either in assessment or in treatment, swallow physiology may be altered. The important clinical issue is to take all available steps to ascertain that physiology is altered in a positive direction to enhance swallow function through changes in bolus volume.

Temperature

Temperature manipulation is an interesting, multifocal consideration in dysphagia intervention. Cold materials are believed to enhance awareness of a bolus and may have an effect on oropharyngeal swallowing physiology. How cold a bolus should be is an unanswered question. Hot materials (and very cold materials) typically are ingested in smaller amounts and thus may interact with bolus volume. Both hot and cold materials may affect esophageal function. Anyone who has ingested either very hot or very cold materials recognizes the discomfort as that material passes through the esophagus. In those with **myotonia**, cold may interfere with the rapid musculature contraction need for sequential swallows. In diffuse esophageal spasm, extreme pain may be triggered by hot or cold materials within the esophagus. The presence of this condition (or other conditions) may be a contraindication for using hot or cold materials in dysphagia intervention. There are reports of swallow **syncope** (vasovagal reflex) triggering **bradycardia** associated with the temperature (hot) of the bolus.[23]

A different perspective on temperature is that of the patient who does eat by mouth but eats inefficiently. These individuals may face the inconvenience and frustration associated with a warm meal getting too cool before the meal is finished. Such patients often report that they use microwaves, ovens, hot plates, or other means to maintain a desired temperature of food over the course of a meal.

Taste and Smell

The senses of taste and smell are not part of the traditional evaluation of swallowing function, and patients are often left to the culinary skills of caregivers or kitchen staff in reference to the palatability of food. However, taste and smell are both essential features of eating. These senses are interrelated because the four basic tastes are supplemented by flavors (mediated by odor) to provide sensory input during meals. Taste and smell alterations may affect appetite, motivation, and swallowing physiology. Furthermore, taste enhancement (which is typically accomplished by increasing flavor) has been shown to have a positive effect on oral intake in older adults and in certain clinical populations.[24] Hence, taste and smell manipulation may contribute to changes in swallow physiology, appetite, motivation, and enjoyment of meals. The positive aspects of these sensory manipulations may be improved ingestion of food and liquid, contributing to improved health status. Figure 9-2 shows the same pureed meal presented in different aesthetic contexts. Inasmuch as a picture is worth a thousand words, these images should speak loudly.

What a patient sees on a plate might be as important as how it smells or tastes. Certain pureed foods can be visually unappealing and may depress or, at best, not facilitate appetite or motivation to eat. Although aesthetics of food presentation is still an aspect requiring clinical investigation, available clinical research has focused on enhancing the visual appeal of meals as a factor in improving intake.

Modify Feeding Activity

Mealtime activity may require modification to accommodate the needs of individual patients. Examples of mealtime modification include changing the meal schedule, oropharyngeal cleansing or hydration, and the use of feeding aids.

For some patients, the meal schedule may be extremely important—for example, the importance of timing meals to the maximal benefit cycle of medications in certain diseases such as Parkinson's disease. Other examples include the patient who is satiated with small amounts of food and requires multiple meals per day to maintain adequate nutrition. Finally, a common recommendation for timing of oral feedings in patients who are being weaned from feeding tubes is for the patient to ingest the oral meal before tube feeding to take advantage of biologic motivation (hunger) during the oral meals (see feeding tube weaning in Chapter 11).

Other mealtime adjustments may be warranted in various situations. For example, patients who reside in care facilities may require special dining arrangements to minimize distractions during meals. These "dysphagia dining rooms" often afford the patient a better caregiver–patient ratio and thus the potential for increased cueing or other strategies that may facilitate a positive meal experience.[25] This arrangement may interact with other mealtime modifications, including rate of feeding, specific placement of a bolus, and various clearing strategies to minimize residue and enhance airway protection. During mealtimes, these tactics may be more successful with enhanced clinician or caregiver supervision in an area with reduced distraction.[26]

Patients who have poor oropharyngeal clearance when swallowing certain foods may benefit from alternating food swallows with liquid swallows. The intent here is to use the subsequent liquid as a "wash" or cleansing mechanism to remove residue from the prior swallow. If a patient has xerostomia (dry mouth), preswallow hydration of the oral cavity may be beneficial. This may be accomplished by swallowing liquid, by sucking on gauze soaked in liquid, by spraying water into the mouth, or by using synthetic saliva.

Feeding aids may benefit patients with any number of physiologic or anatomic limitations. Occupational therapists (see Chapter 1) may be invaluable in fashioning devices to accommodate limitations in hand and limb function. Such devices may make the difference between the patient achieving independence as a self-feeder or remaining a dependent feeder. Other modifications may be required in cases of trauma or surgical restructuring of the oral mechanism. Possible alternatives may include the use of nipples, flow-controlled feeders, straws, specialized utensils (e.g., glossectomy spoons), or catheters.

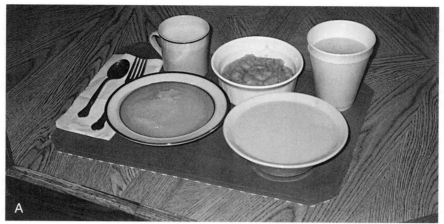

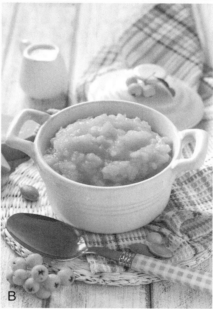

FIGURE 9-2   **A** and **B** are photographs of pureed meals with different aesthetic presentation. (Photo © istock.)

Patient Modifications

The most common strategies used in this category are positioning strategies. These might involve head-position strategies such as head-turn or chin-tuck maneuvers or whole-body–positioning strategies. Chapters 10 and 15 address head position strategies in more detail. This section addresses whole-body positioning.

An initial caveat is the reminder that for certain patients, changing body position may require the consultation of other dysphagia team members, specifically the physical therapist (see Chapter 1). In general, the patient should be positioned such that physical capabilities are maximized and accommodations to improve swallowing can be incorporated. With that in mind, common position adjustments might include the patient tilting to the side or back, side-lying, or maintaining an upright posture.

Patients with hemipharyngeal weakness may benefit from tilting the upper body such that the stronger side is lower and able to benefit from gravity to assist bolus transit. This positioning technique may be combined with a head turn toward the weaker side of the pharynx. An exaggerated example of this approach is the side-lying position. This technique may be used in circumstances in which patients want to maximize residual pharyngeal muscle function, while at the same time reducing bolus speed by removing the influence of gravity. If pharyngeal asymmetry exists, the stronger side is typically lower.

Tilting the patient backward may be beneficial when oral movements reduce transit of the bolus through the mouth or when significant residue remains in the piriform sinuses after a swallow. One consideration for this technique should be airway protection ability.

Upright posture may be an important consideration in patients with oropharyngeal or esophageal deficits. Residue in the proximal esophagus may reflux into the hypopharynx during or after meals. Keeping the patient upright adds the potential protective mechanism of gravity in an attempt to minimize the upward movement of esophageal residue. In cases of severe reflux, upright posture during and after meals may be important even if the patient receives nutrition from a gastrostomy tube. Finally, it is well known that elevating the head of the bed is beneficial in combating nocturnal reflux.[27]

Mechanism Modifications

Attempts to modify the swallowing mechanism include motor exercises, sensory stimulation, and prosthetic adjustments to compensate for physiologic or anatomic deficits. Motor exercises typically address one of five features of motor function: strength, range, tone, steadiness, or accuracy. Depending on the underlying disease and the overt movement dysfunction, various techniques may be applied. Common approaches to improve strength may include resistance activities in which the patient attempts to move against resistance. Range of movement may be increased by stretching activities. Stretching activities used by patients with trismus in an attempt to increase mouth opening are one example of increasing range of movement. Accuracy and steadiness affect coordination. Depending on the specific attributes of the movement dysfunction, various techniques may be used, ranging from altering the rheologic properties of swallowed materials to using a contained bolus manipulated around the mouth but not swallowed.

Sensory stimulation activities may involve changes in taste, temperature, or the application of pressure. Limited experimentation has occurred with the use of electrical stimulation as a sensory approach to improving movement associated with swallowing (see Chapter 10). Finally, improved oral hygiene, when indicated, may facilitate improved sensory functions and reduce disease risks.

Prosthetic management may be accomplished in conjunction with a maxillofacial prosthodontist as a member of the dysphagia team. Prosthodontists can fabricate palatal lifts, obturators, and other devices to fill anatomic deviations that might exist in certain patients with dysphagia.

Swallow Modifications

Swallow modifications focus primarily on altering the physiology of the attempted swallow. These activities often require active participation from the patient and intensive practice to induce movement change. Chapters 10 and 15 provide a detailed review of the more common behavioral techniques to modify swallow physiology in children and adults.

MAKING TREATMENT DECISIONS

Many approaches may be followed in developing intervention plans. This section offers a framework detailing steps in clinical decision making that may be helpful to dysphagia clinicians. Three aspects are considered: (1) sources of information used in treatment planning, (2) formation of meaningful clinical questions, and (3) development of individual treatment plans.

Sources of Information

Figure 9-3 presents a flowchart detailing potential sources of clinical information that may address treatment issues. In this depiction, treatment issues are divided into

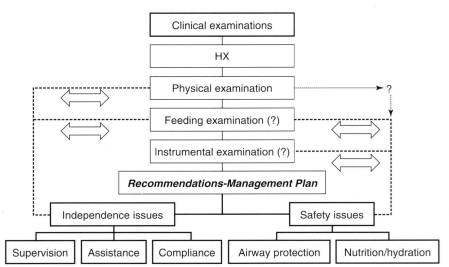

FIGURE 9-3 Flowchart depicting potential sources of treatment-planning information based on various components of the dysphagia evaluation. *HX*, Medical history.

	Patient or Problem	Therapy Technique	Other Options	Outcomes
Focus Your Question	Starting with your patient, ask: "How would I describe a group of similar patients?"	Ask: "Which technique am I considering?"	Ask: "What is the main alternative or option?"	Ask: "What can I hope to gain?"
		Be specific	Be specific	Be specific
Example	In patients with neurogenic pharyngeal dysphagia in nonprogressive disease with residue and aspiration . . .	"Would use sEMG biofeedback"	"Compared with only a Mendelsohn maneuver"	"Improve the functional outcome of therapy and decrease the number of therapy sessions"

FIGURE 9-4 One framework from which to pose meaningful clinical questions regarding best treatment options. *sEMG,* Surface electromyography.

"independence issues" and "safety issues." Independence issues include supervision, assistance, and compliance. Supervision refers to the patient's need for direct supervision during mealtime, perhaps to monitor food intake and use of compensations or for other reasons. Assistance refers to the use of direct physical assistance during mealtime. Compliance refers to the patient's adherence to an intervention plan. Safety issues include airway protection and nutrition and hydration. Airway protection refers to the overt presence of aspiration or the risk of aspiration from excessive residue or other factors. This term should also consider airway obstruction from solid foods. Nutrition and hydration refer to the patient's ability to ingest sufficient calories and fluids. Independence and safety issues often interact. For example, the patient who requires but does not receive adequate assistance may have reduced airway protection or may ingest insufficient amounts of food or liquid.

The diagram in Figure 9-3 attempts to estimate the sources of assessment information relative to independence and safety issues. Independence issues may be addressed more from the physical examination and the feeding examination. Instrumental examinations may not be needed to address independence issues. Conversely, instrumental examinations seem essential in making safety determinations, especially airway protection issues. Nutrition and hydration issues are better addressed through a combination of the instrumental examination and the feeding examination.

Forming Meaningful Questions

Once relevant clinical information has been gathered and organized into some conceptual framework (such as that

depicted in Figure 9-3), a next logical step is to pose the question "Which treatment techniques are best suited to this individual patient or problem?" This becomes part of an evidence-based approach to treatment of dysphagia. The framework depicted in Figure 9-4 offers one potential method from which to formulate meaningful clinical questions pertaining to treatment options.

Starting with the focus on the patient or problem, clinicians should first frame the question. The example in Figure 9-4 presents a patient with neurogenic pharyngeal dysphagia resulting from nonprogressive disease. This patient demonstrates residue and aspiration on examination. Based on the examination, a treatment option is considered—in this case, the use of sEMG biofeedback. Next, treatment alternatives are considered—in this case, teaching the Mendelsohn maneuver in isolation. Finally, expected outcomes are framed as a question. Can the use of biofeedback in addition to the clinical maneuver improve functional outcome (e.g., better swallow) while reducing the number of treatment sessions (i.e., increasing efficiency of therapy)? After forming this question, clinicians need to survey the evidence on these techniques to find the answer. For this specific example, evidence supporting the use of biofeedback includes research indicating that use of this technique enhanced functional outcomes of therapy with less time investment than therapy without this technique.[28-30] If such evidence was identified, the clinician should consider using this technique.

Planning Individual Therapy

Once the treatment question is formulated and treatment options have been systematically considered (based on

BOX 9-8 ONE FORMAT FOR DEVELOPING INDIVIDUAL TREATMENT PLANS FOR DYSPHAGIA

Goals
- Statement(s) of anticipated functional outcome

Objectives
- Target aspects of the swallow or patient that require change to reach the functional goal

Action Plans
- Activities in which the patient and clinician engage; procedures and progress monitors to be used in therapy are specified

---

available evidence), the individual treatment plan may be developed. One format for the treatment plan is depicted in Box 9-8. Goals are statements of anticipated outcome based on the patient's pretreatment functional level with consideration of the clinical examination results (presumably identifying some or all of the reasons for the pretreatment functional level). Beginning clinicians are encouraged to keep in mind that goals can change as the patient's status changes. In addition, it may be prudent clinical practice to focus on a single functional goal, especially in the initial aspects of therapy. Goals should be simple statements that are understood by the patient and caregivers (review Practice Note 9-6). For example, a goal statement for a patient who is taking no food or liquid by mouth may be "to establish the safe and consistent oral intake of any substance in any amount." Conceptually, if the patient cannot reach this functional level, further advances in oral intake are unlikely. Setting goals that are too ambitious may reduce patient (and clinician) motivation and compliance with a treatment program. Surpassing goals most likely will not contribute to that scenario (see Practice Note 9-6).

Objectives target items regarding the swallow or the patient that require change for the functional goal to be reached. These may be specific aspects of swallow physiology such as increased hyolaryngeal elevation or patient-related aspects such as rate of eating. If objectives are met, goals will be reached.

Action plans reflect activities in which the patient and clinician will engage. These are direct statements of procedures (review Clinical Corner 9-1). Action plans should include instructions to the patient reflecting technique, frequency of practice, amount to be swallowed, or other directly overt aspects of the therapy program. In addition, action plans should include techniques to monitor the immediate effect of the treatment technique(s). These monitors do not need to be elaborate, nor do they require repeated instrumental examinations to evaluate progress. However, often based on instrumental examinations,

PRACTICE NOTE 9-6

Two months after his brainstem stroke and being fed by gastrostomy, a patient came for an evaluation to determine whether he was a candidate for dysphagia treatment. The SLP thought the patient could begin therapy and in the discussion asked the patient what he hoped to achieve in therapy. The SLP used the 7-point Functional Oral Intake Scale (see Chapter 7) and asked the patient to point to a number on the scale that he believe would be a reasonable goal. Because he was completely tube fed at the time of the evaluation, the patient's current level was at 1. He immediately pointed to 7 (total oral diet with no restrictions). Having treated similar patients in the past and based on the current evaluation, the SLP believed that a total oral diet without restrictions was unreasonable. Instead she asked the patient if he would be satisfied as an initial goal to reach level 4 (total oral diet of one consistency). She pointed out that reaching that goal would mean he would be free of the tube feeding. The patient agreed that this goal would provide him great relief and add immensely to his quality of life. Use of the Functional Oral Intake Scale can be valuable in reaching agreement on therapist and patient expectations.

CLINICAL CORNER 9-1: CLINICAL PERFORMANCE AND EVIDENCE

A new clinician was told by her supervisor that patients who demonstrate swallow delay may benefit from the therapeutic intervention of a sour bolus. The clinician was told that the hospital kept a large supply of lemon ice on each floor for this purpose. The clinician was working with a patient who showed swallow delay as a result of a partial tongue resection secondary to cancer. After 6 days of therapy with the lemon ice, the clinician did not believe that the swallow delay had improved.

Critical Thinking
1. What are some potential reasons why the sour bolus did not help trigger a faster swallow in her patient?
2. Do a literature search on sour bolus and swallow delay and decide when, how, and with whom you would use this technique.

---

monitors may be behaviors that indicate change in the swallow performance (see also Clinical Corner 9-1 and 9-2). For example, consider the patient who expectorates after each swallowing attempt. One potential monitor of performance change in swallowing might be a reduction in the frequency of postswallow expectoration. Actions plans affect objectives, which in turn affect functional goals and therefore overt swallowing performance (review Clinical Corner 9-2).

FRAMEWORK FOR TREATMENT PLANNING

Figures 9-5 and 9-6 depict one organizational framework for planning dysphagia treatment. Using pharyngeal dysphagia as an example, these flowcharts present the general organization of the treatment planning concepts in this

---

CLINICAL CORNER 9-2: CLINICAL PERFORMANCE AND MEASUREMENT

After radiation treatment to the tongue base, the patient was working on hard swallow techniques to improve laryngeal elevation. Attempts in therapy using 5 and 10 mL of water showed considerable swallow delay, double swallows on most boluses to clear them from the oral cavity and pharynx, and considerable postswallow coughing with approximately 30 seconds between swallow attempts before the coughing subsided.

Critical Thinking

1. Physiologically, speculate on why the patient was coughing after the swallow.
2. In addition to measuring the number of expectorations, what other simple behavioral measurements could be made to show progress in therapy?

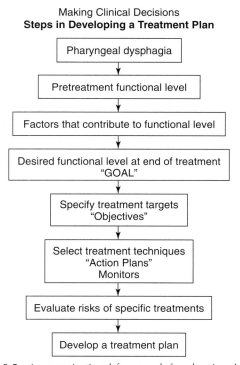

Making Clinical Decisions
Steps in Developing a Treatment Plan

Pharyngeal dysphagia

↓

Pretreatment functional level

↓

Factors that contribute to functional level

↓

Desired functional level at end of treatment
"GOAL"

↓

Specify treatment targets
"Objectives"

↓

Select treatment techniques
"Action Plans"
Monitors

↓

Evaluate risks of specific treatments

↓

Develop a treatment plan

FIGURE 9-5   An organizational framework for planning dysphagia treatment.

---

chapter, followed by a specific clinical example. At the top of the hierarchy (see Figure 9-5), pretreatment functional level is determined. As previously indicated, severity of dysphagia or functional level is a complex issue. One perspective might be to consider the amount and type of food and liquid a patient is safely ingesting by mouth at the time of evaluation. Although simplistic, this approach may be the most meaningful to the patient. Extending from this functional level are swallowing factors believed to be contributing to the reduced function. Next, a goal for therapy is established. This is an outcome statement and, whenever possible, it should be developed in conjunction with the patient and caregivers. Objectives and specific actions are selected as stepping stones by which the patient may reach the functional goal. Finally, risks of the respective treatment techniques are considered in reference to the anticipated benefits.

Figure 9-6, *A*, uses the example of pharyngeal dysphagia, and specific decisions that might be made during the planning process are detailed. Early in the planning process, the clinician must decide whether the patient is a good candidate for therapy. This decision involves a prognosis. Several considerations for treatment candidacy were discussed earlier in this chapter; however, prognosis for therapy response is not an exact science for dysphagia. The best course of action may be to overtly recognize the basis for any prognostic decision based on available evidence.

If the patient is considered a good therapy candidate, goals and objectives are developed. Figure 9-6, *A*, presents four objectives that may be considered in pharyngeal dysphagia: laryngeal elevation, pharyngeal contraction, airway protection, and PES opening. The next step is to select action plans for each of these objectives. Figure 9-6, *B*, takes one of the objectives— laryngeal elevation—and considers three potential action plans. The Mendelsohn maneuver facilitates sustained laryngeal elevation and thus is an appropriate action plan. On the negative side, this maneuver may prolong the apneic pause during swallowing and thus may be contraindicated for some patients with compromised respiratory function. In addition, it is difficult to teach this maneuver to certain patients. Clinicians should consider the available evidence supporting use of this maneuver for the specific problem and patient under consideration (see Chapters 10 and 15). Finally, the decision to use (or not to use) a technique is made along with any special considerations. An example of a special consideration for this maneuver is using biofeedback to help teach what may be a difficult maneuver. Similar considerations apply to the "hard swallow" technique and the surgical technique of laryngeal suspension. The clinician must consider the following questions: What is the intended effect of the technique? Are there any potential contraindications or risks? Is there any available evidence to support use of the technique?

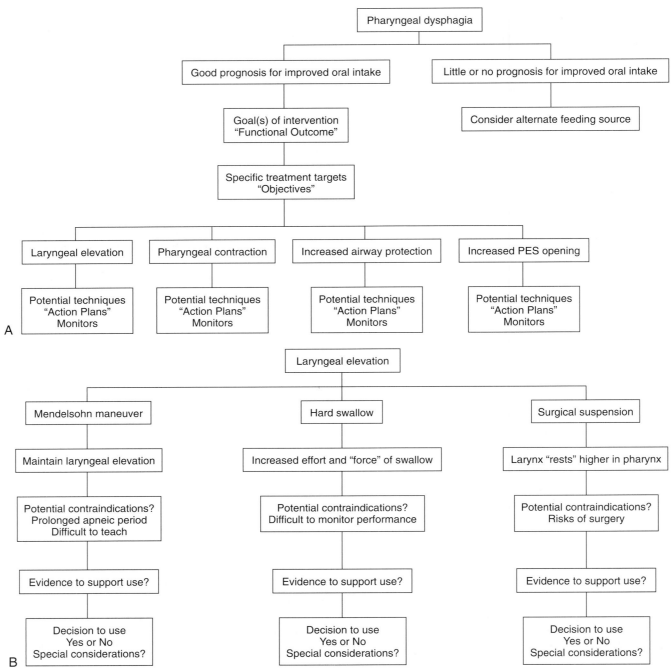

FIGURE 9-6 **A** and **B** show a specific example of an organizational framework for planning dysphagia treatment based on a hypothetical case of pharyngeal dysphagia. *PES,* Pharyngoesophageal segment.

CLINICAL CASE EXAMPLE 9-2

A 78-year-old woman had a left cerebrovascular accident 6 months ago and has no known family; she is now residing in a long-term care facility. She has a possible history of a prior stroke but no details are available. The patient is ambulatory with a walker and physical assistance; however, she spends most waking hours in a wheelchair or in bed. She is currently receiving a total oral diet, which is modified to pureed and thickened liquids. She is able to self-feed. She was referred for dysphagia evaluation and treatment because of continuing weight loss and reports of coughing during meals. A review of her chart indicates a recent history of repeated urinary tract infections. Clinical examination reveals a small woman who is interactive but with subtle signs of impaired mental status and possible mild aphasia. She demonstrates no overt corticobulbar deficits. The right arm and leg are paretic, with the leg more involved than the arm. When asked about swallowing, she replied that she swallows "just fine." When asked about the food at the facility, she indicated that it is "okay." Fluoroscopic swallowing evaluation indicated mild physiologic deviations, including slow oral transit, reduced hyolaryngeal elevation, reduced pharyngeal contraction, and reduced PES opening. Postswallow residue was noted in the valleculae and the piriform recesses, primarily on thicker materials. When liquid was used to remove residue, a minute amount of aspiration was noted after swallow. The patient demonstrated a consistent reactive cough with aspiration. Maneuvers such as the chin tuck or head turn had no effect on this pattern of swallowing. The patient was able to chew a cracker but had difficulty forming a cohesive oral bolus and removing the material from her mouth.

The first consideration for treatment planning is the current functional eating level of the patient. In this particular case, the patient is self-feeding and taking all food and liquid by mouth but with a restricted diet of pureed and thickened liquids. A primary concern is continuing weight loss. A related concern might be the recurring urinary tract infections.

The next consideration is that of factors that may contribute to the existing functional level. Both the weight loss and the recurring infections may relate to an insufficient intake of nutrition and hydration. This point should be addressed through communication with the long-term care facility. Predisposing factors may not always be overt and clear, so many issues should be considered. A few factors to consider in this case include swallow physiology, physical status, appetite, and the patient's environment. The clinician must consider the functional eating level in reference to the observed swallow physiology as seen fluoroscopically. This patient demonstrated slow transit and mild reduction in pharyngeal components of the swallow. She had more difficulty with dry, particulate materials (cracker). She did aspirate mildly in certain circumstances and had a strong reactive cough. This last observation may relate to the observed coughing during meals. The relation of the physiologic deviations to the functional eating pattern is more difficult to understand. Overall slowness may be related to prolonged mealtimes and thus to reduced food intake. Is it possible that this patient is demonstrating mild cognitive changes that may reflect early-stage dementia and the swallowing changes that may accompany the cognitive change (see Chapter 2)? This might be one area for further clinical examination.

Are there other possibilities that may help support or refute a possible relation between the observed swallow physiology and the functional eating pattern? Physical status may help explain some of the reduced intake of food and liquid. Recall that this patient is self-feeding. In addition, recall that she has some weakness in the right upper limb and may have had a previous stroke. It would be beneficial to observe her eating a meal to help determine the extent to which physical limitation may restrict intake of food and liquid. Appetite loss may be another factor in reduced intake. Although the patient described the food as "okay," she did not indicate high motivation for eating. This may be related to cognitive or environmental (social) issues. Depression should also be considered. The current dining situation may be distracting, noisy, or unpleasant to the patient. She may require cues to continue eating or other adjustments that are not provided in her current situation. Under these circumstances, she may have reduced intake. All these factors must be considered to derive the best possible intervention for this patient.

The primary goal for this patient might be to stop weight loss and subsequently to increase weight to appropriate levels. A related goal may be to reduce urinary tract infections (if these result from reduced hydration). To address these goals, the factors contributing to the current functional level must be addressed, and treatment objectives must be selected for factors that may be altered to improve functional status. One obvious objective is to increase the amount of nutrition and hydration taken by mouth. The methods by which this is accomplished should relate directly to those factors perceived to contribute to reduced oral intake.

Selecting specific action plans in this particular case may require a period of further observation under differing conditions. For example, it might be prudent to observe this patient eating a more rheologically complex meal, observe her eating meals of varying amounts, enhance taste properties, increase mealtime cues, or change the dining environment. The best intervention approach may be a combination of these strategies. One monitor for improvement might be the amount of calories and hydration consumed daily. The functional outcome is weight gain to appropriate levels and reduced urinary tract infections.

TAKE HOME NOTES

1. Evidence-based practice is the use of combinations of published research, clinician expertise, and patient wishes in establishing the most effective treatment plan.
2. Clinicians should become informed on the critical appraisal of published manuscripts as they may influence evidence on which clinical decisions are made.
3. Primary considerations for dysphagia treatment include airway protection and nutrition and hydration. These may be influenced by multiple factors related to the patient, the underlying disease or disorder, the clinician, and the health care environment.
4. Dysphagia treatment is often multifocal and multidisciplinary. Clinicians should be familiar with multiple treatment options across medical, surgical, and behavioral domains.
5. Choice of a specific therapy technique may depend on the specifics of the patient's health care status, the skills of the treating clinician, the health care environment, or other factors.
6. Clinicians must make sure to evaluate health care risks and potential obstacles when considering treatment options.
7. A comprehensive therapy plan should include a statement of functional goals, objectives to meet those goals, and specific actions to initiate for each objective.

REFERENCES

1. Dollaghan CA: *The handbook of evidence-based practice in communication disorders*, Baltimore, 2007, Paul H Brookes.
2. Leonard RJ, Kendall KK, McKenzie S, et al: Structural displacements in normal swallowing: a videofluoroscopic study. *Dysphagia* 15:146, 2000.
3. O'Neil KH, Purdy M, Ralk J, et al: The Dysphagia Outcome and Severity Scale. *Dysphagia* 14:139, 1999.
4. Crary MA, Carnaby GC, Groher ME, et al: Initial psychometric assessment of a functional oral intake scale for dysphagia in stroke patients. *Arch Phys Med Rehabil* 86:1516, 2005.
5. Storr M, Allescher HD: Esophageal pharmacology and treatment of primary motility disorders. *Dis Esophagus* 12:241, 1999.
6. Kraus PH, Orlikoff RF, Rizk SS, et al: Arytenoid adduction as an adjunct to type I thyroplasty for unilateral vocal fold paralysis. *Head Neck* 21:52, 1999.
7. Grant JR, Hartemink DA, Patel N, et al: Acute and subacute awake injection laryngoplasty for thoracic surgery patients. *J Voice* 22:245, 2008.
8. Isshiki N: Progress in laryngeal framework surgery. *Acta Otolaryngol* 120:120, 2000.
9. Mita S: Laryngotracheal separation and tracheoesophageal diversion for intractable aspiration in amyotrophic lateral sclerosis—usefulness and indications. *Brain Nerve* 59:1149, 2007.
10. Pletcher SD, Mandpe AH, Block MI, et al: Reversal of laryngotracheal separation: a detailed case report with long-term follow-up. *Dysphagia* 20:19, 2005.
11. Zocratto OB, Savassi-Rocha PR, Paixao RM, et al: Laryngotracheal separation surgery: outcome in 60 patients. *Otolaryngol Head Neck Surg* 135:571, 2006.
12. Scolapio JS, Gostout CJ, Schroder KW, et al: Dysphagia without endoscopically evident disease: to dilate or not? *Am J Gastroenterol* 96:327, 2001.
13. Kelly JH: Management of upper esophageal sphincter disorders: indications and complications of myotomy. *Am J Med* 108(Suppl):43S, 2000.
14. Crary MA, Glowasky AL: Using botulinum toxin A to improve speech and swallowing function following total laryngectomy. *Arch Otolaryngol Head Neck Surg* 122:760, 1996.
15. Murray T, Wasserman T, Carrau RL, et al: Injection of botulinum toxin A for the treatment of dysfunction of the upper esophageal sphincter. *Am J Otolaryngol* 26:157, 2005.
16. Shaw GY, Searl JP: Botulinum toxin treatment for cricopharyngeal dysfunction. *Dysphagia* 16:161, 2001.
17. Cichero JA, Jackson O, Halley PJ, et al: How thick is thick? Multicenter study of the rheological and material property characteristics of mealtime fluids and videofluoroscopy fluids. *Dysphagia* 15:188, 2000.
18. Groher ME, Crary MA, Carnaby Mann G, et al: The impact of rheologically controlled materials on the identification of airway compromise on the clinical and videofluoroscopic swallowing examination. *Dysphagia* 211:218, 2006.
19. Low J, Wyles C, Wilkinson T, et al: The effects of compliance on clinical outcomes for patients with dysphagia on videofluoroscopy. *Dysphagia* 16:123, 2001.
20. National Dysphagia Diet Task Force: *National dysphagia diet: standardization for optimal care*, Chicago, 2002, American Dietetic Association.
21. Adnerhill I, Ekberg O, Groher ME: Determining normal bolus size for thin liquids. *Dysphagia* 4:1, 1989.
22. Steele CM, Van Lieshout P: Influence of bolus consistency on lingual behaviors in sequential swallowing. *Dysphagia* 19:192, 2004.
23. Omi W, Murata Y, Yaegashi T, et al: Swallow syncope, a case report and review of the literature. *Cardiology* 105:75, 2006.
24. Schiffman SS: Intensification of sensory properties of foods for the elderly. *J Nutr* 130(Suppl):927S, 2000.
25. Shanley C, O'Loughlin G: Dysphagia among nursing home residents: an assessment and management protocol. *J Gerontol Nurs* 26:35, 2000.
26. Musson ND, Kincaid J, Ryan P, et al: Nature, nurture, nutrition: interdisciplinary programs to address the prevention of malnutrition and dehydration. *Dysphagia* 5:96, 1990.
27. de Carle DJ: Gastro-oesophageal reflux disease. *Med J Aust* 169:549, 1998.
28. Crary MA: A direct intervention for chronic neurogenic dysphagia secondary to brainstem stroke. *Dysphagia* 10:6, 1995.
29. Huckabee ML, Cannito MP: Outcomes of swallowing rehabilitation in chronic brainstem dysphagia: a retrospective evaluation. *Dysphagia* 14:93, 2002.
30. Crary MA, Carnaby Mann GD, Groher ME: Functional benefits of dysphagia therapy using adjunctive sEMG biofeedback. *Dysphagia* 19:160, 2004.

CHAPTER 10

Treatment for Adults

Michael A. Crary

To view additional case videos and content, please visit the evolve website.

CHAPTER OUTLINE

OBJECTIVES

1. Describe some of the basic differences between compensation strategies and rehabilitation strategies. Tell how this distinction applies to specific therapy techniques.
2. Describe the impact of various therapy techniques on the swallowing mechanism.
3. Identify the expected functional benefits associated with various behavioral treatment strategies.
4. Describe risks from specific therapy techniques that may be posed to patients.
5. Describe the concept of "prevention" in dysphagia management as it applies to negative outcomes and to dysphagia itself. Give specific examples of both applications.
6. Explain strategies that may be helpful in evaluating the appropriateness of existing or novel interventions for a specific patient.

WHICH TECHNIQUES AND WHAT TO CONSIDER

As indicated in Chapter 9, practicing clinicians should avail themselves of evidence supporting (or refuting) the application of any therapy technique. Beyond evidence, however, clinicians will benefit from a conceptual framework from which any clinical technique might be considered. Following this line of reasoning, some common questions to consider might include (1) "What is the purpose of the technique?" (2) "What are the details of the technique?" (3) "What is the impact on the swallowing mechanism?" and perhaps most importantly (4) "Does this technique fit the needs and limitations of my patient?"

Clinicians may have different intentions for applying various management strategies. The term *management* may be viewed as the umbrella approach to dysphagia. Within dysphagia management clinicians may opt for compensation strategies, rehabilitation strategies, or prevention strategies (Figure 10-1). Compensation approaches to dysphagia management might be chosen to maintain the status quo and reduce the risk of morbidity in patients with dysphagia. In this scenario, the clinician is not actively attempting to change the swallowing mechanism, but rather is using strategies to prevent the development of dysphagia-related complications while maintaining adequate nutrition and hydration. Compensations are considered to be short-term adjustments that facilitate improved swallowing function

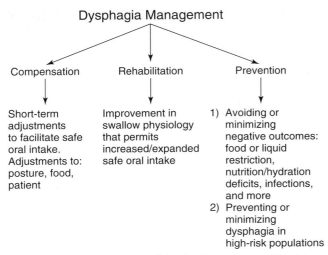

Dysphagia Management

Compensation — Rehabilitation — Prevention

Short-term adjustments to facilitate safe oral intake. Adjustments to: posture, food, patient

Improvement in swallow physiology that permits increased/expanded safe oral intake

1) Avoiding or minimizing negative outcomes: food or liquid restriction, nutrition/hydration deficits, infections, and more
2) Preventing or minimizing dysphagia in high-risk populations

FIGURE 10-1   Components of dysphagia management in adults.

BOX 10-1   LIST OF THERAPY TECHNIQUES

- Postural adjustments
  - Body posture
  - Head posture
- Modifying liquids and solids
- Oral motor exercises
- Supraglottic swallow
- Super-supraglottic swallow
- Mendelsohn maneuver
- Effortful swallow
- Multiple swallows
- Tongue-hold maneuver
- Head-lift exercise
- Thermal-tactile application
- Applying exercise principles
- Adjunctive modalities

but do not have a lasting effect on swallow physiology. Compensations might include adjustments to posture, food and liquid, or the swallow pattern. If a compensatory technique is not used, the patient will not be expected to swallow safely or in adequate amounts. Conversely, the term *rehabilitation* reflects an intervention intending to improve an impaired swallow mechanism by the systematic application of techniques focused at the specific impairments identified in the swallowing evaluation. Rehabilitation techniques are anticipated to enact lasting changes in swallowing performance that will remain even after a technique is discontinued. Given this distinction, clinicians may ask whether a technique is intended to have short-term or long-term effect, accommodate various bolus characteristics, change the swallow physiology, or have other influences on the patient or the swallow mechanism. Clinicians would use different techniques depending on the purpose or intent of the clinical intervention (compensate vs. rehabilitate). Finally, we must consider the concept of *prevention* in dysphagia management. Prevention may be considered from two points of view. First, prevention should focus on avoiding or minimizing negative outcomes. Examples of negative outcomes might include food or liquid restrictions, nutrition and hydration deficits, or infections. More recently, published research has highlighted another view of prevention: preventing or minimizing dysphagia in high-risk populations. Clinicians will want to consider both of these perspectives under the umbrella of dysphagia management.

Details of any technique are essential for appropriate clinical application. Even simple techniques may become confused by the clinician or the patient. For example, a recent survey[1] reported poor agreement in the details of the chin-down posture. This seemingly simple compensation may be more variable than conceived and variants have been described using different terminology. Variability may

be clinically important as different postures are likely to have different physiologic and hence functional effects on the swallow mechanism. Thus a basic question is whether published articles, presentations, or other sources of information provide clear descriptions on how to perform or teach the technique under consideration. This information might incorporate a clear description of the technique and specific instructions for how to apply the technique clinically. This information should include how often and under what conditions the technique should be used. Furthermore, it is important to determine whether the published evidence was gathered from a group of patients similar to the patient being considered for a given technique. For example, evidence supporting the use of a given technique for stroke patients may not be applicable to patients with head and neck cancer.

An additional consideration for any therapy technique would be to understand the intended effect on the swallow mechanism. The impact of any technique relates to the outcome of the intervention using that technique. Ultimately, intervention should result in functional benefit for any patient, but what are the specifics of the intended functional benefit? Following terminology from Chapter 9, the technique is the action plan used by the clinician. Techniques have expected physiologic effects on the swallow mechanism that are related to the objectives of treatment. If successful, the goal or functional outcome of therapy is realized. Thus it is important for the clinician to understand how the specific technique relates to the intended physiologic effect on the swallow mechanism and how this change will relate to the functional benefit sought by intervention.

Box 10-1 lists common swallow therapy techniques described in dysphagia treatment literature. Each technique has some degree of supporting evidence in subgroups of patients with dysphagia. The following information is presented (if available) for each technique: (1) purpose of the technique, (2) details of the technique, and (3) impact on the swallow mechanism.

MANAGING DYSPHAGIA SYMPTOMS: COMPENSATION, REHABILITATION, AND PREVENTION

As mentioned previously, compensation strategies are considered to be short-term adjustments or modifications to posture, food and liquid, or swallow patterns. Compensations can play an important role in dysphagia management for the right patient. In general, a compensation is appropriate if the patient is anticipated to improve to the point at which successful swallowing is possible in the absence of the compensatory strategy. Compensations are not expected to have a significant positive effect on swallow physiology (no rehabilitative impact) and no lasting effect on functional swallowing. Thus successful swallowing typically depends on appropriate use of the compensation technique. Clinicians must consider whether any compensation is indicated for a given patient and subsequently, based on swallowing assessment, choose the most effective compensation.

Body Posture Adjustments

Postural adjustments may involve the entire body or only the head. In general, changes in head or body posture are considered effective in reducing aspiration in various patient groups.[2,3] Reported results suggest that change in posture has the potential to redirect the bolus and may change the speed of bolus flow, thus giving the patient more time to adjust the swallow. In some clinical situations, notably in patients who have abnormal postures because of physical reasons, adjustments in body posture to facilitate safe swallowing may be long term. However, even in these situations, adjustments in body posture are considered compensations rather than attempts to change the dynamics of the abnormal swallow. Furthermore, Logemann[4] appropriately notes that no single posture improves swallowing function in all patients. Thus depending on the specific swallowing deficits presented by an individual patient, the treating clinician may use one or more compensatory postures to facilitate safer swallowing function. Beyond posture, clinicians may find it necessary to use additional compensations to facilitate safe swallowing function in some patients.[5]

Typically, body posture changes involve lying down or side-lying. Both changes are expected to reduce the effect of gravity either during the swallow or on postswallow residue. The side-lying technique may be applied when a

The effect of altering body posture on the swallow may be assessed during the swallow imaging examination. Because this compensation is often used to reduce or eliminate aspiration, the fluoroscopic swallowing study is well suited to evaluating the effect of postural adjustments. When considering side-lying or other lying-down positions, the patient may be appropriately positioned on the fluoroscope table to examine the effect of various "down" positions. Furthermore, fluoroscopy tables can be tilted to different degrees to determine whether a flat or inclined position provides the greatest benefit. One issue with inclined positions is how to make the transition from the radiology suite to the patient's daily environment. Clinical creativity is the best advice here.

When fluoroscopic evaluation is simply not possible, clinicians may attempt to evaluate the effect of altering body posture using endoscopy or by change(s) in clinical signs associated with aspiration. Endoscopy offers an advantage over use of clinical signs because the airway is observed before and after each swallow attempt. If clinical signs alone are used, we strongly suggest inclusion of cervical auscultation to monitor airway sounds before and after swallowing attempts. This clinical approach has several limitations, but in some instances it may be the only avenue available to assess the effect of postural alterations on swallow safety.

difference in pharyngeal function is noted between the right and left sides. In this situation, conventional wisdom suggests that the stronger side be the down side. This position uses gravity to direct the bolus (or residue) toward the stronger hemipharynx. The direct clinical effect of altering body posture on the swallow, specifically on airway protection, may be assessed during the swallowing imaging examination (see Practice Note 10-1). One physiologic result of lying down during swallowing may be increased hypopharyngeal pressure on the bolus, contributing to increased maximum opening of the pharyngoesophageal sphincter (PES) and reduced duration of sphincter opening during the swallow.[6] These physiologic changes may be helpful in strengthening the swallow in some patients.

Postural adjustments may not be the ideal intervention for patients who are at risk for noncompliance because of physical or cognitive limitations. Also, change in body posture, specifically any variant of lying down, may affect esophageal motor functions.[7,8] An additional functional consideration may be the effect of supine position on reflux episodes.[9] Patients with severe reflux (even those being fed via tube) may benefit from maintaining an upright posture during and after feeding. The upright posture helps reduce or prevent reflux that may contribute to aspiration. In addition, nocturnal head-of-bed elevation has long been

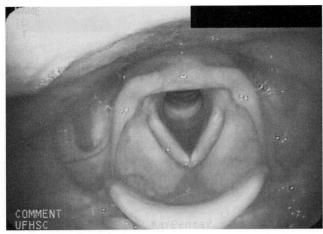

FIGURE 10-2 Oropharyngeal widening resulting from head extension (chin raise).

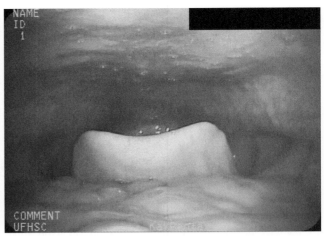

FIGURE 10-3 Oropharyngeal narrowing resulting from head flexion (chin tuck).

advocated for patients with nocturnal reflux. This simple postural adjustment is highly effective in promoting acid clearance from the esophagus.[10] Thus clinicians should evaluate the impact of body posture variations on esophageal functions during the swallow imaging examination. This guideline especially applies to patients with clinical symptoms or signs of esophageal deficit.

Head Posture Adjustments

Changes in head posture may include extension, flexion, or rotation. Each of these postural adjustments is considered compensatory and hopefully used for a limited time. Although in the same category of intervention, each adjustment has a different impact on the swallow mechanism and thus each is used for a range of specific clinical indications. Videos 10-1 through 10-4 show endoscopic and fluoroscopic examples of each head posture adjustment.

Head Extension

Head extension may be accomplished by raising the chin. This has the anatomic effect of widening the oropharynx (Figure 10-2) and may be helpful in moving a bolus from the mouth into the pharynx when oral or lingual deficits are present. Thus patients who have received a glossectomy, other oral resection, reconstruction, or patients who have significant lingual paralysis may benefit from use of a head-extension technique. The basic concept is to elevate the chin and use gravity to assist in oral bolus transit toward the pharynx. The patient should be determined to have adequate pharyngeal function and adequate laryngeal closure for airway protection. Clinical benefit (reduced aspiration) from the head-extension posture used during the fluoroscopic swallow examination has been demonstrated in a small number of patients treated for oral cancer.[2] Conversely, with head extension, defective laryngeal closure

was observed in approximately one third (10/35) of patients demonstrating normal laryngeal closure during swallowing in a head-neutral position.[11]

Head extension may also affect the PES and the coordination between pharyngeal and PES activity. Specifically, head extension increases **intraluminal** pressure (less relaxation), decreases duration of relaxation in the PES, and changes the temporal coordination between pharyngeal and PES swallow pressures as measured manometrically.[12] These changes may complicate an existing swallowing problem. Thus head extension may be a useful clinical technique in patients with difficulty transporting a bolus from the mouth to the pharynx, but it may contribute to swallowing difficulties in patients who have airway protection or PES deficits. Like most compensatory maneuvers, the effect of head extension on swallow function may be evaluated during the swallow imaging examination.

Head Flexion–Chin Tuck

Head flexion has been suggested as a technique to facilitate improved airway protection in patients who demonstrate deficits in airway protection during swallowing.[11] Flexing the head (chin tuck) has the anatomic effect of improving laryngeal vestibule closure,[12] narrowing the oropharynx[13] (Figure 10-3), and reducing the distance between the hyoid bone and the larynx.[14]

The physiologic effects of head flexion (chin tuck) in patients with dysphagia are reported as minimal. In patients with pharyngeal dysphagia, no manometric differences were found between control swallows and swallows using the chin-tuck maneuver.[14,15] However, in a small sample of healthy volunteers, weaker pharyngeal contractions were observed during swallows using the chin-tuck position.[16] Moreover, the combination of a reclining posture (60 degrees) with a chin tuck (60 degrees) may significantly increase the duration of **swallowing apnea**.[17] This change in respiratory pattern may contribute to increased respiratory stress in some patients. At the very least, clinicians should monitor pharyngeal residue and any respiratory changes induced by introduction of the chin tuck or any swallowing maneuver.

Clinical benefit from the chin-tuck maneuver has been described primarily in reference to improved airway protection. Shanahan et al.[18] reported elimination of aspiration with the chin tuck in 15 patients with dysphagia resulting from neurologic damage. These investigators also reported that this postural maneuver was not useful for patients who demonstrated delay in swallow initiation and postswallow residue in the piriform recesses. From a larger, heterogeneous sample, Rasley et al.[3] reported that the chin-tuck position eliminated aspiration on all tested volumes in 21 of 84 (25%) patients. Logemann, Rademaker, and Pauloski[2] reported that five of six (83%) patients with head and neck cancer–related dysphagia were able to eliminate aspiration on at least one bolus volume of liquid barium during the fluoroscopic swallowing study. Lewin et al.[19] reported elimination of aspiration for liquids using the chin-tuck position during the fluoroscopic swallow examination in 17 of 21 patients after esophagectomy. Finally, Logemann et al.[20] conducted a large randomized study to evaluate the effectiveness of the chin-down posture (chin tuck) compared with thickened liquids in the reduction of aspiration in patients with dysphagia related to dementia or Parkinson's disease. Results indicated that the chin-down posture was less effective than thickening liquids in reducing aspiration events during the fluoroscopic swallow examination.

Note that each of these studies evaluated the effect of the chin-tuck position within the confines of the fluoroscopic swallow examination. Thus each study describes the effect of this posture as an immediate compensation. Zuydam et al.[21] reported that compensatory maneuvers (chin tuck and supraglottic swallow) used as therapy techniques were effective in only 50% of patients who aspirated. In a companion paper to the effect study of chin tuck versus thickened liquids,[19] Robbins et al.[22] monitored a subgroup of the original patients for 3 months after the initial swallow examination. Patients were randomly assigned to one of the three interventions (chin tuck for thin liquids, nectar-thick liquids, or honey-thick liquids) as a management strategy and the rate of new pneumonia (**incidence**) was evaluated as the primary outcome. Results indicated no significant differences in the rates of pneumonia across the three interventions.

The chin-tuck position may be helpful in reducing or eliminating aspiration in some patients with dysphagia. However, it does not produce benefit in all patients and may be inferior to thickened liquids in some patients. Although anatomic adjustments have been demonstrated in response to this posture, physiologic changes reportedly are minimal

and may be contraindicated in some cases. Furthermore, at least one study raises the possibility that this posture, especially combined with a reclining body position, may alter the coordination of swallow and respiration. Finally, it is possible that this technique may need to be combined with other strategies, including other postures or bolus changes, to produce maximum benefit.[2] Because this is such a simple task to perform, its effect on appropriate patients should be evaluated during swallow imaging studies.

In this chapter we have used the term *chin-tuck* to refer to a specific compensatory posture. We have also used terms from published descriptions including head flexion and chin-down posture. This variability in terminology is given a practical focus by the survey results of Okada et al.,[1] who remind us that different postures may result in different physiologic or functional results. Thus what may seem simple to clinicians may be confusing to patients. In evaluating research on any technique, clinicians need to look beyond the terminology and be certain of the technique and how to teach that technique to patients. When evaluating the effect of any technique or instructing patients, clarity and consistency are very important.

Head Rotation–Head Turn

Head rotation or the head-turn maneuver is another postural adjustment that can function as an effective short-term compensation to improve swallowing function. The head-turn posture has been advocated primarily in cases of unilateral pharyngeal deficit.[23,24] Conventional wisdom suggests that patients turn the head toward the weaker side in cases of hemilateral impairment. The anatomic result of this postural maneuver is a narrowing or closing off of the swallowing tract on the side toward which the head is turned. This effect is demonstrated in Figure 10-4 in which the head is turned to each side with the corresponding change in oropharyngeal configuration. However, this closure effect may not extend throughout the hypopharynx but may be restricted to the level of the hyoid bone at the superior hypopharynx, which leaves the inferior aspects of the pharynx open in some patients.[25]

Physiologic effects of head rotation include a drop in PES pressure and corresponding increase in PES opening.[24,26] Additional physiologic effects of the head-turn position include increased pharyngeal manometric swallow pressures on the side of the pharynx toward which the head is turned, a drop in PES resting pressure opposite the direction of head turn, and a delay in PES closure (e.g., longer relaxation of the PES).[27] These physiologic findings suggest that the head rotation technique should be considered for patients with reduced PES opening. The combined anatomic and physiologic changes resulting from turning the head are anticipated to facilitate an increase in the amount swallowed with less residue and reduced risk of airway compromise.

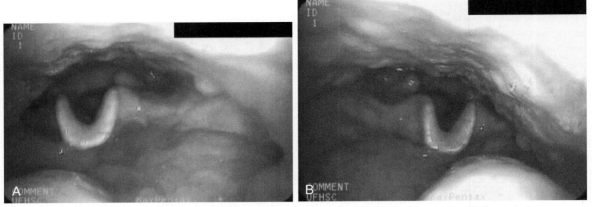

FIGURE 10-4   Changes in oropharyngeal configuration resulting from head rotation. **A**, Right; **B**, Left.

Clinical benefit from the head-turn position has been reported in a variety of patient groups. Logemann et al.[24] reported improved swallow function (larger amount of bolus swallowed with less residue) in all five (100%) patients with dysphagia after lateral medullary stroke. Within a sample of patients with various causes of dysphagia, Rasley et al.[3] reported that liquid aspiration was eliminated for all tested volumes in 20 of 77 (26%) patients. In a group of postsurgical head and neck cancer patients, Logemann, Rademaker, and Pauloski[2] reported 75% effectiveness (9/12 patients) in the elimination of liquid aspiration in at least one volume.

Like many postural maneuvers, head rotation should be considered a compensatory technique, not a lifelong adjustment in swallowing. Also, like other techniques in this category, effectiveness may be reduced by compliance, cognitive factors, physical factors, or the presence of multiple swallowing deficits (see Practice Note 10-2). Moreover, this postural adjustment may be combined with other compensations or maneuvers to improve swallow function.[2] Finally, the functional effects of a head-turn maneuver may be checked easily during either the fluoroscopic or endoscopic swallow examinations.

Thickening Liquids and Modifying Diets

Thickened Liquids: Pros and Cons

Alterations in liquid viscosity (specifically meaning "thickness") have been advocated in both the evaluation and treatment of patients with dysphagia.[28-30] Two major foci seem to emerge in relation to the use of thickened liquids: (1) thicker liquids result in less aspiration among patients with dysphagia and (2) thicker liquids have a physiologic effect on the swallow mechanism. In a 2005 survey of speech-language pathologists experienced in dysphagia intervention,[31] the most commonly reported reasons for the use of thickened liquids included delayed onset of swallowing and impaired oral control of thin liquids. Reduction of

---

PRACTICE NOTE 10-2

Evaluating the impact of head rotation (or any head posture) during either the fluoroscopic or endoscopic swallow examinations is helpful not only in identifying potential benefit from the posture, but also in identifying the degree of rotation (or flexion). The endoscopic swallow examination may have a slight advantage over the fluoroscopic study in the head-turn position in that the clinician can identify factors that may limit or negate potential benefit from the compensation. For example, years ago we evaluated a patient who had extensive left hemipharyngeal and laryngeal paralysis secondary to resection for a jugular foramen tumor. In addition to tenth cranial nerve deficits extending from the velum to the larynx, this patient also had a twelfth cranial nerve paralysis that impaired movement and atrophy in the left side of the tongue. A head-turn position toward the left was attempted under endoscopic inspection. The technique failed as material was observed to collect in the posterior oral cavity on the left side, spill over the epiglottis, and enter the airway. Further evaluation of this examination revealed that the lingual atrophy in the left tongue created an anatomic deficit much like a small cup or bowl toward which all liquid (thin and thick) would flow. Subsequently, when a swallow was attempted, this material was already on the left side of the swallow mechanism and, combined with a weakened left pharynx, liquids would simply pass over the epiglottis and migrate toward the airway. Fortunately, other compensations were beneficial for this patient.

---

aspiration was not specifically reported among the most frequent reasons for use of thickened liquids. However, this lack of focus on aspiration seems to be the result of the survey questions, which did not include direct reference to aspiration reduction as a rationale for use of thickened liquids in adult patients with dysphagia. In this survey, the perception of patients' acceptance of thickened liquids was influenced by the degree of "thickness." Honey and spoon-thick liquids were considered less accepted (strong dislike) than nectar-thick liquids. Furthermore, these initial negative perceptions either worsened or remained the same with continued use over time. These patterns of patient acceptance also are reflected in the use patterns of thickened liquids among patients in skilled nursing facilities.[32] Results of a national review of thickened-liquid application in skilled nursing facilities indicated that approximately 8% of all patients (from a total sample of 25,470) received thickened liquids—60% received nectar-thick liquids, 33% received honey-thick liquids, and 6% received pudding or spoon-thick liquids. Thus thickened liquids are used frequently in the management of adult dysphagia with the most frequent being nectar or syrup consistency.

The frequent use of thickened liquids occurs in the relative absence of strong evidence that they provide significant clinical benefit to adult patients with dysphagia. In the 2005 survey,[31] nearly 85% of responding clinicians indicated that they believed thickening liquids was an effective management compared with only 5% who disagreed with this position. These opinions reflect clinicians' positive perception, but until recently, only scant empirical support existed for this clinical practice. Kuhlemeier, Palmer, and Rosenberg[33] studied bolus factors that influenced aspiration rates among 190 patients with dysphagia and reported that thickness of liquid (thin, thick, ultrathick) and manner of presentation (spoon versus cup) had a direct effect on the rates of aspiration during the fluoroscopic swallowing examination. Ultrathick liquids presented by spoon resulted in the lowest aspiration rates, followed by thick liquids presented by spoon, then by cup with thin liquids resulting in the highest rates of aspiration during the fluoroscopic study. To date, the strongest evidence that liquid viscosity affects aspiration during the fluoroscopic swallowing examination comes from a large randomization trial of techniques to reduce liquid aspiration in patients with dementia or Parkinson's disease.[20] The results of this study support those from the earlier report from Kuhlemeier, Palmer, and Rosenberg.[33] Aspiration rates were lowest for honey-thickened liquids (thickest liquid evaluated) and greatest for thin liquids (accompanied by a chin-down posture). Aspiration rates for nectar-thickened liquids were between the two other viscosities and significantly different from both. Interestingly, the reported benefit from honey-thick liquids was not maintained when this viscosity was presented last among the materials examined. The investigators suggested that patient fatigue may have been a factor in this result. Certainly, clinicians should consider patient endurance (converse of fatigue) when interpreting the results of the swallowing evaluation and in making clinical recommendations based on any evaluation.

The study by Kuhlemeier, Palmer, and Rosenberg[33] implied that manner of bolus presentation may influence

TABLE 10-1 Potential Interaction Between Viscosity and Volume in Rates*

Aspiration

Amount	Thin	Nectar-Thick	Pudding
5 mL	20%	5%	5%
10 mL	20%	15%	20%

Residue

Amount	Thin	Nectar-Thick	Pudding
5 mL	65%	70%	80%
10 mL	65%	80%	90%

*Percent of aspiration and residue during the fluoroscopic swallowing examination.

the occurrence of aspiration in addition to viscosity. Other bolus characteristics also may affect aspiration rates. For example, in an unpublished study of aspiration and residue rates in adult patients evaluated in the acute care environment, we learned that bolus thickness and volume may interact. Table 10-1 summarizes the rates of aspiration and residue seen during fluoroscopic examination among 20 patients who swallowed 5 versus 10 mL of thin, nectar-thick, and pudding viscosities of barium sulfate contrast agent. Note that different clinical impressions result depending on both the thickness and the volume of the material swallowed. For example, the rates of aspiration and residue are the same for thin liquid across both volumes. However, although thickening material results in reduction or aspiration rates for 5 mL (20% to 5% to 5%), the benefit is not the same for 10 mL (20% to 15% to 20%). The rate of aspiration for 10 mL of pudding is as high as that for 5 or 10 mL of thin liquid. In addition, the rate of residue in the valleculae increases more for the larger volume as the swallowed material is thickened. This type of pattern implicates the need to evaluate more than just thickness of swallowed material. Therapy and perhaps diet recommendations would differ based on the pattern presented by an individual patient.

Although studies such as those reviewed suggest that thickening liquids reduces aspiration rates in groups of patients, clinicians must remember that these are not treatment studies. These studies evaluate the immediate effect of thickening liquids during the fluoroscopic study and do not speak directly to the effectiveness of using thickened liquids as an intervention or longer-term management strategy. In one clinical trial[22] of older adult patients with dementia or Parkinson's disease no significant differences in pneumonia rates were reported across patients who used thickened liquids versus a chin-down posture to reduce aspiration during a 3-month period. Conversely, Karagiannis, Chivers, and Karagiannis[34] evaluated the effect of thickened liquids on hospital inpatients. In a clinical trial they randomly assigned patients to either thickened liquids only or water plus thickened liquids. They concluded that more severely ill patients (severe neurologic dysfunction or immobility) were more likely to develop lung complications (e.g., pneumonia) when allowed to drink water in addition to thickened liquids. Although these results need to be supported by additional research, this initial study shows potential benefit from thickening liquids and offers guidelines for which patients might benefit from this strategy. Overall, clinical benefit, especially long-term benefit from continued use of thickened liquids as a management strategy, is unclear. Moreover, continued use of thickened liquids may impose other health risks to adult patients with dysphagia. A primary concern is the risk of dehydration from reduced fluid intake. Older adult patients, especially those with dysphagia, are considered at increased risk for dehydration secondary to reduced fluid intake.[35] Combining this potential risk with the results of surveys indicating a high rate of dislike of thickened liquids among adult patients with dysphagia suggests that reduced fluid intake, especially of thickened liquids, may further the risk of dehydration in this patient population. In one small randomized clinical trial,[36] stroke patients with dysphagia were assigned to receive thickened liquids or thickened liquids plus water. Patients in the combination liquid condition (water plus thickened liquids) ingested less-thickened liquids and had greater daily fluid intake than those in the thickened-liquid–only condition. Neither group experienced significant respiratory complications. Related to this study are the clinical experiences of more than 20 years from the Frazier Rehabilitation Institute.[37] This single rehabilitation hospital has allowed patients with dysphagia, including those considered to aspirate thin liquids, access to water between meals. They have experienced impressive outcomes with few instances of dehydration (5/234 or 2.1%) or chest infection (2/234 or 0.9%) among a large sample of patients ($N = 234$) who followed this protocol over an 18-month period. These single-center results are supported by the more recent clinical trial from Karagiannis, Chivers, and Karagiannis.[34] Patients who demonstrate good mobility and adequate cognitive ability are expected to benefit from application of the Frazier Water Protocol.[38] A note of caution, however—the Frazier Water Protocol is more complex that just providing water to patients with dysphagia. Clinicians are advised to review thoroughly the complete protocol before implementing this strategy.

These clinical and research examples are consistent in describing a reduced rate of aspiration as thickness of swallowed material is increased. In addition, the mode of presentation, volume, and patient fatigue may modify any clinical benefit from thickening liquids. Also important is that most of these studies are not therapeutic studies. Many are immediate effect studies that indicate a reduction of aspiration rates during the fluoroscopic swallowing examination. At least one clinical study supports the application of thickened liquids for more ill patients suggesting that not all patients require this strategy. Thus clinicians should continually monitor patient compliance, potential benefit, and potential complications in patients in whom thickened liquids are used as a therapeutic intervention.

Additional Effects of Thickened Liquids on the Swallow Mechanism

Thickening liquids also may affect swallow physiology. For example, increasing liquid viscosity has been shown to increase lingual-palatal contact pressures during swallowing by healthy volunteers.[39] Furthermore, increasing liquid viscosity may slow the transit of a bolus[40,41] and increase pharyngeal pressure and upper esophageal sphincter relaxation.[41,42] These studies and others implicate the tendency of the healthy swallow mechanism to accommodate to different bolus characteristics—in this specific instance, liquid viscosity. However, aside from timing alterations, few studies have evaluated bolus accommodation to varying liquid viscosities in adults with dysphagia, and at least one study has suggested that increasing liquid viscosity did not affect the timing or bolus propulsive force of swallows performed by adults with neurogenic dysphagia.[43] Thus differences may exist in bolus accommodation between healthy adults and adults with dysphagia. Given the prevalence of liquid modifications in clinical management, the effect of thickening liquids on swallow physiology in adult patients seems an important area of clinical investigation.

Other Liquid Modifications

In the preceding section bolus volume, viscosity, and method of presentation were introduced as variables that may affect a patient's performance relative to aspiration of liquids during the fluoroscopic swallowing study. Another liquid variable was evaluated by Bülow et al.[44] These investigators evaluated the potential benefit of carbonated liquids in the rate of penetration or aspiration, the speed of swallowing (pharyngeal transit time), and postswallow residue. Carbonated thin liquid resulted in less penetration into the airway than noncarbonated thin liquid, faster pharyngeal transit than thick liquid, and less residue than thick liquid. Sdravou, Walshe, and Dagdilelis[45] expanded on the observations of Bülow et al.[44] reporting that improved airway protection (less aspiration and penetration) resulted from carbonated liquids in both 5-mL and 10-mL volumes in patients with neurogenic dysphagia. However, unlike the prior study, no timing differences resulted from use of carbonated liquids. Furthermore, patient acceptance of carbonated liquids was high with only a single patient reporting dislike for this fluid. Krival and Bates[46] reported that carbonated liquids result in greater lingual-palatal pressure traits during swallowing in healthy adult women. They attributed these effort increases to **chemesthetic** stimulation of oral mucosa. Likewise, Morishita et al.[47] reported reduced duration of laryngeal elevation in older adult inpatients with no swallowing problems (but not younger subjects) when swallowing carbonated beverages. However, they reported no significant effect of carbonated beverages on pharyngeal reaction time or muscle activation (e.g., effort) during swallowing. They interpreted reduced laryngeal elevation duration in older subjects to reflect improved swallow physiology. Like Krival and Bates,[46] these investigators identified chemesthesis from carbonic acid in the beverage as a direct sensory nerve stimulant that may facilitate swallow changes. These findings are intriguing, but clinicians must remember that these studies, like those described in the preceding section, evaluate the immediate effect of carbonated liquids during the fluoroscopic or other physiologic swallowing examinations and do not necessarily translate directly into a proven benefit from use of carbonation as a treatment approach.

Taste may be another bolus characteristic with the potential to affect swallowing performance. Logemann et al.[48] were among the first to evaluate the effect of taste on swallowing performance in adults with dysphagia. In a comparison of a sour bolus (50% lemon juice and 50% barium liquid) with a regular barium bolus they reported that patients with neurogenic dysphagia demonstrated faster oral onset of the swallow (all patients), decreased pharyngeal delay (stroke patients), and reduced frequency of aspiration (other neurogenic causes). Subsequently, Pelletier and Lawless[49] evaluated the effect of citric acid (a sour bolus) and citric acid plus sucrose (a sweet-sour bolus) on the swallowing performance of nursing home residents with dysphagia. They reported that the citric acid solution (2.7%) reduced aspiration and penetration compared with water and that both taste stimuli resulted in increased spontaneous dry swallows following the initial bolus swallow. Additional studies of the effect of taste stimuli on swallowing have focused on healthy volunteers. Chee et al.[50] reported that glucose (sweet), citrus (sour), and saline (salty) liquids reduced swallowing speed in healthy adults. Palmer et al.[51] compared swallows of sour liquid with water in healthy volunteers and reported that muscle contraction increased (greater electromyographic activity) with the sour bolus but that timing aspects of the swallow did not change across taste conditions. Finally, Pelletier and Dhanaraj[52] reported that moderate sucrose (sweet) and high citric acid (sour) and salt concentrations resulted in significantly higher lingual swallowing pressures compared with water. A different outcome is reported in a study from Miyaoka et al.[53] These investigators reported no motor changes in swallowing by healthy volunteers resulting from altering taste (sweet, salty, sour, bitter, umami).

Thickening liquids may alter the taste of the liquid. Matta et al.[54] reported that adding starch-based or gum-based thickeners to common liquids (coffee, milk, apple and orange juice) added either a starchy, grainy, or slick flavor or texture to the liquid and suppressed the base flavor of the beverage. These effects were more pronounced with thicker liquids such as honey-thick consistencies. This observation might help explain the dislike of thick liquids, especially thicker liquids, by adult patients with dysphagia.[31] At least, such observations should encourage clinicians to consider taste and other sensory attributes when recommending thickened liquids for patients with dysphagia.

Thickening liquids is a common practice in the management of adult dysphagia. Common reasons for introduction of thicker liquids appear to revolve around clinician perceptions of the patient's ability to manage liquids orally and to protect the airway from aspiration of thin liquids. Unfortunately, little evidence exists to support this practice. Available evidence does indicate a reduction of aspiration rates in groups of patients when thin liquids are thickened to nectar or honey consistencies during the fluoroscopic swallowing study.[20,33] However, evidence also exists suggesting that thickening liquids as a management strategy does not necessarily reduce pneumonia rates.[22] Furthermore, evidence also exists that aspiration of thin liquids during the fluoroscopic swallowing study does not necessarily relate to the subsequent development of pneumonia in older adult patients with dysphagia.[55] Finally, growing experience with the Frazier Water Protocol[37] suggests that patients who aspirate thin liquids may be able to safely drink water with positive health benefit (with the noted exception of severely ill and immobile patients). Remember that the recipient of thickened liquid strategies is the patient with dysphagia. Available evidence indicates increasing dislike for thick liquids as the degree of thickness increases. Also, limited patient compliance research suggests that nearly 50% of patients prescribed thick liquids do not actually use them routinely.[56] These clinical and research observations emphasize the need for careful evaluation and continued monitoring of any patient for whom thickened liquids is recommended as a dysphagia management strategy. Clinicians should also consider other liquids modifications such as carbonation and taste variations when contemplating liquid modification as a component of dysphagia management.

Texture-Modified Diets

Similar to liquids, foods may be modified to accommodate perceived limitations in swallowing function in adults with dysphagia. Foods consumed by mouth may be modified for many reasons. Logemann[4] describes a study in which patient diet choices were examined. Patients who had been treated for oral cancer were monitored over a 6-month period. Patients tended to eliminate food consistencies that required too much time to eat or consistencies that they were prone to aspirate. These clinical observations suggest that patients will self-modify diet items that are difficult to swallow. Curran and Groher[57] described a strategy to modify a hospital's regular menu to reduce aspiration in patients with dysphagia. Similarly, O'Gara[28] and Pardoe[29] describe diet modifications intended to promote safe swallowing (minimize aspiration) and adequate nutrition. However, despite the optimism depicted in these early clinical descriptions, more recent clinical research has raised questions about the nutritional adequacy of modified diets. Wright et al.[58] reported that older hospital patients eating a texture-modified diet had lower nutritional intake (energy and protein) than patients consuming a normal diet. These investigators speculated further that other nutrients may also be deficient as a result of the texture-modified diet. Conversely, Germain et al.[59] reported nutritional benefit of texture-modified diets over traditional diets in institutionalized older adult patients. Although these two studies focused on different patient groups and evaluated nutritional intake over different periods, the apparent discrepancy between the results suggests that modifying diets for aspiration reduction should not be done in the absence of nutritional consultation. Crary et al.[60] reported that texture-modified diets can increase the risk of dehydration in acute stroke patients, even more than thickened liquids. Potential reasons for this association are not reported, but the observation that acute stroke patients on pureed diets had significantly greater indications for dehydration warrant further clinical and research attention. Thus dysphagia clinicians who recommend diet modifications should consult with nutritional specialists to ascertain nutrition and hydration adequacy of the modified diet.

Few guidelines exist to aid dysphagia clinicians in recommending a texture-modified diet or in establishing the optimal level of diet modification. Groher and McKaig[61] evaluated swallowing abilities and the type of texture-modified diet in 212 residents in two skilled nursing facilities; 31% of these patients were using a mechanically altered diet. Based on a swallowing examination the investigators recommended changes to oral diets with patient follow-up for 30 days to evaluate response to the new diet level. These investigators reported that 91% of patients examined had been consuming overly restrictive diets. Specifically, these patients could safely ingest diet levels higher (less modified) than they had been consuming on a regular basis; 4% of the patients were on diet levels above what they could safely tolerate, and only 5% were judged to be at the appropriate dietary level. These findings speak directly to two important program management points: (1) A qualified dysphagia clinician should be directly involved in any decision to modify an oral diet, and (2) patients should be monitored and reevaluated at regular intervals to ascertain whether they need diet modification or whether the prescribed level of diet modification remains optimal

> **BOX 10-2** FOUR LEVELS IN THE NATIONAL DYSPHAGIA DIET
>
> **Level 1: Dysphagia Pureed**
> Homogeneous, very cohesive, puddinglike; requires bolus control, no chewing required
>
> **Level 2: Dysphagia Mechanically Altered**
> Cohesive, moist, semisolid foods; requires chewing ability
>
> **Level 3: Dysphagia Advanced**
> Soft-solid foods that require more chewing ability
>
> **Level 4: Regular**
> All foods allowed

for the patient's swallowing abilities. Although this study indicates that modifying a diet level may be more complex than evaluation of airway protection, the results still do not offer clinical guidelines on selecting an appropriate modified diet level.

In an attempt to standardize menus and decision processes in the application of modified diets for adults with dysphagia, the National Dysphagia Diet was proposed in 2002.[62] The task force developing this diet suggested four standardized levels of diet modification based on assessment of food textures. These four levels are listed in Box 10-2. The task force developing these recommendations performed well in their attempt to recommend a standardized diet modification strategy. In their report they refer to the use of standard assessment tools, provide specific food recommendations for each diet level, describe foods to avoid at each level, describe food preparation approaches, and offer suggestions to enhance patient acceptance of modified diets. The task force also recommended a standard description of thickened liquids to include thin, nectar-like, honey-like, and spoon-thick. However, the efforts of this group did not include specific clinical strategies for use of thickened liquids.

Similar to the application of thickened liquids discussed previously, the National Dysphagia Diet represents a solid attempt to provide a standard approach to an important clinical problem, but it also lacks clinical research validation. To date, no significant study has compared the benefits of this standardized approach with other diet modification strategies. However, one study has raised an important question regarding the application of this standardized diet. Strowd et al.[63] reported a poor relation between dysphagia foods recommended in the National Dysphagia Diet and the barium materials used to assess patients with dysphagia. Specifically, the viscosity of barium test materials was much greater than the corresponding food recommendations in the National Dysphagia Diet. This observation questions, but does not invalidate, the apparent prescriptive value of National Dysphagia Diet recommendations. Until a high degree of correspondence is developed between the evaluation materials used to make diet recommendations and the food encompassed within those recommendations, clinicians are well advised to follow the advice of Groher and McKaig.[61] Patients receiving modified diets should be carefully monitored for acceptance and reevaluated periodically both for safety of the diet (here meaning airway protection) and nutrition and hydration adequacy. The core message is that diet modification for adults with dysphagia is not a simple adjustment. The decisions and processes inherent in diet modification demand input, cooperation, and ongoing communication from a team of qualified individuals.

One final point merits consideration. Like thickened liquids, texture-modified diets may not be pleasing or acceptable to adults with dysphagia. The National Dysphagia Diet task force acknowledged some of these issues and offered suggestions for improving acceptance. If food looks good, smells good, tastes good, and is presented at the appropriate temperature, it seems logical that patients will be more likely to eat it. The design of "altered foods" for adults with dysphagia is likely to become an important aspect of clinical science and practice. In fact, recently a German company has produced modified foods using a 3D printer! (http://www.engadget.com/2014/05/29/smoothfood-performance-eu-3d-printed-food-project/?a_dgi=aolshare_facebook). Studies evaluating food characteristics, such as particle size and other physical properties along with specific food content and other factors that may influence food quality, will likely be helpful in developing safe, nutritious, and pleasing diets for adult patients with dysphagia.[64]

CHANGING THE SWALLOW: REHABILITATION APPROACHES

As mentioned earlier in this chapter, rehabilitation approaches should result in functional benefit to the patient, but also physiologic improvement in the swallow mechanism. Many, if not most, dysphagia rehabilitation approaches implicate exercise components. However, the systematic application of exercise principles is relatively recent in dysphagia rehabilitation. Still, many historical and traditional activities do involve a degree of exercise and as such have the potential to physiologically improve the impaired swallow mechanism. In this section, these historical, traditional approaches are reviewed initially followed by more recent strategies that attempt to systematically incorporate exercise principles into dysphagia-rehabilitation strategies. Throughout the remainder, the focus of each technique or approach is on describing the technique, evidence for functional benefit to the patient, and evidence for physiologic improvement of the impaired swallow mechanism.

Improving the Mechanism: Oral Motor Exercises

The concept of exercises to stretch, strengthen, or otherwise improve the basic motor properties of muscles in the speech–swallow mechanism is not new.[65] Logemann[4] indicates that if the patient is aspirating significantly, oral motor exercises may be a better strategy than directly working on swallow function. The rationale for this position is logical. If a patient is continually aspirating, swallow attempts are not maximized (and the patient experiences continued failure). Logemann terms this approach to swallow rehabilitation *indirect therapy* and offers three foci: (1) exercises to improve oral motor control, (2) stimulation of the swallow reflex, and (3) exercises to increase adduction of tissues at the top of the airway (airway closure). Oral motor exercises include tongue range of motion, tongue resistance, and bolus control activities. Swallow reflex stimulation is advocated via cold thermal-tactile stimulation of the faucial pillars. Airway closure activities incorporate various phonation and "pushing" activities.

Thermal-tactile stimulation to elicit a swallow response has generally fallen out of favor (see later in this chapter). However, oral motor exercises represent a frequent therapy approach used by dysphagia clinicians. In an unpublished 2007 survey, Crary and Carnaby used case problem-solving scenarios to describe therapy strategies for adult patients with dysphagia after stroke. Sixty clinicians were surveyed. Oral motor exercises were recommended for all of the cases presented and were the most frequently recommended technique for each case even though each case depicted a different swallowing problem. In a more recent case-based survey[66] oral motor exercises were not the most frequently applied therapy strategy but they remained among the top one third of the most frequently applied dysphagia therapy strategies. Furthermore, Carnaby and Harenberg identified great variability in reported dysphagia therapy techniques for a single video-supported case, claiming that they could not identify a "usual care pattern" for dysphagia therapy. The results of these surveys suggest that dysphagia clinicians may not be selective in applying therapy strategies to different patients and that oral motor exercises remain frequently used, possibly because they posed little aspiration risk. This interpretation is speculative but does raise questions on the decision-making process used in selecting any therapy for patients with dysphagia.

Some available evidence does support the value of oral motor exercises. Lazarus et al.[67] demonstrated that tongue-pushing (resistance) exercises completed with either an Iowa Oral Performance Instrument (IOPI) or tongue blade produced lingual strength increases in young, healthy volunteers. Robbins et al.[68] reported that a systematic program of lingual resistance exercise improved lingual isometric and swallow pressures (e.g., strength) in a group of 10

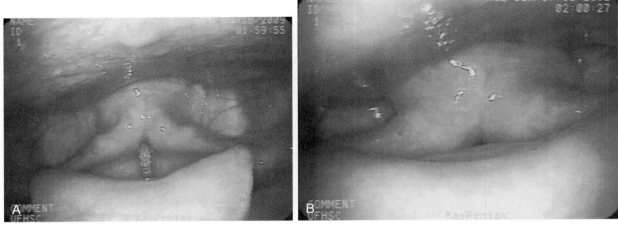

FIGURE 10-5 Laryngeal configurations associated with normal breath hold (*A*) and effortful breath hold (*B*).

healthy older adults. Subsequently, these investigators[69] demonstrated that a systematic program of lingual resistance exercise resulted in both increased lingual strength and swallowing ability in a group of 10 poststroke patients with dysphagia. Hagg and Anniko[70] demonstrated that a program of resistive lip training improved lip strength and swallow ability in stroke patients with dysphagia. These studies represent evidence that oral motor exercises, specifically lingual and labial resistance exercises, have the potential to strengthen weak swallowing musculature and improve swallow function. To date, little or no evidence has emerged to support other aspects of oral motor exercise. However, as described later in this chapter, exercise principles are being increasingly applied to dysphagia therapy in a variety of approaches.

PROTECTING THE AIRWAY: BREATH HOLD AND SUPRAGLOTTIC AND SUPER-SUPRAGLOTTIC SWALLOWS

The voluntary breath hold, supraglottic swallow, and super-supraglottic swallow maneuvers are techniques designed to protect the airway from aspiration of food and liquid by closing the airway before swallowing. In the case of the two supraglottic swallow techniques, a voluntary cough is executed after the swallow to clear any residue from the vocal folds. The difference between these two maneuvers is the degree of effort in the preswallow breath hold. As implied by the name, the super-supraglottic swallow requires an effortful breath hold, whereas the supraglottic swallow requires a breath hold with no extra effort. The extra effort in the super-supraglottic maneuver is needed to facilitate glottal closure. Glottal closure is one of the earliest aspects of the swallow[71]; thus techniques that facilitate

glottal closure in patients who aspirate may contribute to reduced aspiration.

Endoscopic inspection has revealed that healthy adults may not completely close the glottis during a voluntary breath-hold maneuver. Estimates range from 57% to 82% of healthy volunteers who completely close the glottis with a voluntary breath hold.[72-74] Adding effort or vocalization to the voluntary breath-hold maneuver increases the likelihood that the glottis will be closed.[72,74,75] Figure 10-5 demonstrates the difference in glottal closure patterns between a simple breath-hold maneuver and a forced or effortful breath-hold maneuver. Figure 10-5, *A*, demonstrates the glottal closure pattern associated with a simple breath-hold maneuver (e.g., voluntary breath hold or supraglottic swallow). The primary feature is the horizontal (right to left) movement of the arytenoid cartilages and vocal folds to close the airway. When complete, this pattern may be effective in accomplishing airway protection during swallowing attempts. Adding effort to the breath-hold maneuver increases the probability of complete glottal closure. Figure 10-5, *B*, demonstrates the glottal closure pattern associated with a forceful breath-hold maneuver (e.g., super-supraglottic swallow). Note that in addition to the horizontal closure pattern observed in the supraglottic swallow, the arytenoids move anteriorly approximating the petiole of the epiglottis. This movement results in more complete closure of the entire supraglottis rather than closure at the level of the vocal folds only. Of interest is the observation that these two glottal closure patterns (horizontal and anterior) reflect stages in glottal closure in the normal swallow. As demonstrated in Video 10-5, slow-motion analysis of the normal swallow reveals that the glottis is initially closed by the horizontal (medial) movement of the vocal folds. Subsequently, with laryngeal elevation the arytenoid cartilages move forward to approximately the petiole of the epiglottis. Magnetic resonance imaging has demonstrated that complete closure of the larynx is obtained at the point of maximum laryngeal elevation in the normal swallow.[76] These closure patterns are reflected respectively in the voluntary breath-hold, supraglottic, and super-supraglottic swallow maneuvers.

The physiologic effects of the supraglottic swallow maneuver have been assessed in both normal and dysphagic adults. Different studies report varied findings ranging from no difference between the supraglottic swallow and a control (normal) swallow to prolonged airway closure, increased anterior laryngeal movement, increased tongue base movement, and increased PES opening. In a study of eight healthy volunteers Bülow et al.[16] reported no movement or manometric pressure difference between the supraglottic swallow and normal swallows. These investigators noted that healthy volunteers varied in their ability to perform the supraglottic swallow and suggested that substantial training of this technique may be required for patients to perform this maneuver appropriately. This same clinical research team also reported no manometric alterations in peak amplitude or duration of intrabolus pressure[15] or number of misdirected swallows[14] among eight patients who used the supraglottic swallow. Furthermore, they noted that three of eight patients could not perform this technique. Bodén, Hallgren, and Hedström[77] reported a weaker peak contraction in the upper esophageal sphincter (also termed the *PES*) when healthy volunteers swallowed using the supraglottic swallow. These authors claimed that this decreased peak pressure is unlikely to improve swallow efficiency or decrease aspiration in patients with dysphagia. On the more positive side, Ohmae et al.[78] reported earlier and longer laryngeal closure, prolonged opening of the PES, and longer duration of hyoid and laryngeal movement in healthy volunteers who attempted the supraglottic and super-supraglottic swallow maneuvers. These observations were more pronounced in the super-supraglottic technique. Other research also supports increased physiologic effects of the super-supraglottic swallow over the supraglottic swallow. For example, Miller and Watkin[79] reported longer duration of pharyngeal wall movement in healthy volunteers who swallowed with the super-supraglottic swallow technique. This finding implicates a longer swallow duration when this technique is used. This implication is supported by data from Bodén et al.,[77] who reported longer bolus transit time in healthy volunteers who performed the super-supraglottic swallow technique compared with normal or supraglottic swallows. These changes might be considered detrimental to some patients with dysphagia by increasing the duration of the swallow and postswallow residue in patients with existing poor PES relaxation. However, the super-supraglottic swallow also has been reported to result in positive swallow changes in some

patient groups. Lazarus et al.[80] reported longer base-of-tongue contact with the posterior pharyngeal wall in combination with higher manometric pressures at this contact point in three patients with dysphagia after treatment for head and neck cancer. Logemann et al.[81] reported earlier base-of-tongue movement, a higher position of the hyoid bone at swallow onset, and overall increased hyoid movement during swallowing in five patients with head and neck cancer after radiotherapy who used the super-supraglottic swallow. These same patients also demonstrated reduced maximum opening of the PES but little change in pharyngeal wall movement as a result of the maneuver.

Despite multiple studies evaluating the physiologic effect of these airway protection maneuvers on the swallow, few studies have documented clinical benefit. Hamlet et al.[82] identified reduced aspiration in a single patient who used this technique after supraglottic laryngectomy. However, the patient reported very prolonged mealtimes with this technique and thus modified the technique to reduce mealtimes. Lazarus et al.[83] reported that the supraglottic and super-supraglottic maneuvers prolonged airway closure but did not eliminate aspiration in a single patient after surgical treatment for head and neck cancer. The Mendelsohn maneuver (see next section), however, was successful for this patient. This case report emphasizes the importance of verifying the clinical effect of any maneuver before using it as a therapeutic technique. Lazarus[84] reported 100% elimination of aspiration using the super-supraglottic swallow during the fluoroscopic swallow examination in four patients who were within 6 months of completing radiotherapy intervention for head and neck cancer. However, she indicated that three of the four patients required multiple swallows per liquid bolus even with use of this swallow maneuver.

One of the few (if only) studies to evaluate these airway protection maneuvers on stroke patients reached a negative conclusion based on patient safety concerns. Chaudhuri et al.[85] evaluated the cardiovascular effects of the supraglottic and super-supraglottic swallow maneuver in stroke patients with dysphagia. Three groups of patients were evaluated during the poststroke period of inpatient rehabilitation. Group 1 included patients with dysphagia and a history of coronary artery disease. Group 2 patients had dysphagia but did not have a history of coronary artery disease. Group 3 patients were considered a control group and were selected from among orthopedic patients without dysphagia or a history of coronary artery disease. In all patients more than 1 week had passed since their stroke. All patients received training on the supraglottic and super-supraglottic swallow maneuvers and subsequently used these maneuvers in a dysphagia treatment session. Cardiac findings were monitored by a **Holter monitor** during treatment sessions and during subsequent routine daily activities. Results indicated cardiovascular abnormalities in 82% (9 of 11) of patients in group 1 and in 100% (4 of 4) of patients in group 2 during training and treatment sessions in which these airway protection maneuvers were used. No obvious cardiac differences were noted between the maneuvers. The authors attribute these cardiovascular changes to a modification of the Valsalva maneuver that occurs with physical exertion. They concluded that these maneuvers should not be used in stroke patients with dysphagia especially if they have a history of cardiac arrhythmia or coronary artery disease. These results raise many important questions regarding application of these maneuvers or, for that matter, any maneuver that might affect bodily functions beyond the swallow. Like all studies, questions may be raised about this research, but until additional research confirms or refutes the findings of the Chaudhuri study,[85] clinicians should be cautious when applying these maneuvers in the acute stroke population.

Both variants of the supraglottic swallow maneuver appear to prolong airway closure and may have other physiologic effects on swallow performance. However, the available data on clinical benefit are restricted to small groups of patients; mostly those with dysphagia after treatment for head and neck cancer. An important study of clinical effect in stroke patients suggests that patients in acute stroke rehabilitation may be at risk for cardiovascular events from these maneuvers. These implications and suggestions that these techniques might require substantial clinical training warrant a focused look at potential clinical benefits compared with potential risks from these techniques. These maneuvers would be considered compensatory in that they may contribute to improved swallowing function when applied correctly. Although, short-term physiologic change has been documented using these maneuvers, evidence of a lasting positive effect on swallowing once the maneuver is no longer applied (rehabilitative function) is limited.

Prolonging the Swallow: The Mendelsohn Maneuver

The Mendelsohn maneuver is achieved by asking the patient to suspend the swallow at the peak of hyolaryngeal excursion and pharyngeal constriction and to prolong this posture for a few seconds before relaxing and allowing the swallowing tract to return to the preswallow position. The result of this maneuver is to prolong and extend hyolaryngeal excursion.[86] Figure 10-6 presents a lateral fluoroscopic view of a swallow with the patient in the resting position and during the elevated and constricted position of the Mendelsohn maneuver. Video 10-6 depicts this maneuver performed by a healthy adult volunteer. Some investigators have suggested that, in addition to prolonged hyolaryngeal excursion, this maneuver also prolongs PES opening[86]; however, this is not a consistent finding across studies of normal swallowing.[87] Other physiologic changes in the normal swallow facilitated by this maneuver include (1) longer duration of lateral pharyngeal wall movement[79]; (2) increased pharyngeal peak contractions along with prolonged duration of pharyngeal peak contraction and increased bolus transit time[77]; (3) increased amplitude and duration of surface electromyographic (sEMG) signals (increased effort and duration), especially in the submental muscle group (Clinical Corner 10-1),[88] and increased tongue-palate pressure duration.[89] Moreover, a related pair of studies using high-resolution manometry to evaluate pharyngeal[90] and esophageal[91] response to the Mendelsohn maneuver reported increased velopharyngeal sphincter pressure and decreased preopening upper esophageal

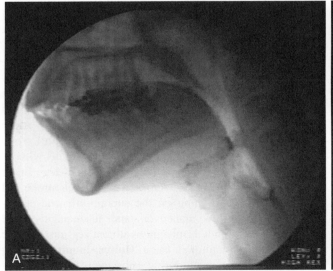
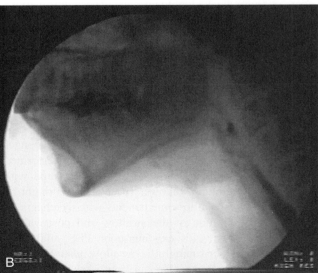

FIGURE 10-6 Pharyngolaryngeal configuration at rest (A) and with Mendelsohn maneuver (B).

CLINICAL CORNER 10-1: PHYSIOLOGICAL EFFECTS OF SWALLOW MANEUVERS

Lazarus et al.[80] reported on the effects of four voluntary swallowing maneuvers (effortful swallow, supra-superglottic swallow, Mendelsohn maneuver, and tongue-hold maneuver) in three patients who had been treated for head and neck cancer with various medical and surgical interventions. Their results suggest that all maneuvers increased both the duration and pressure of the base of tongue to posterior pharyngeal wall contact. They also reported less upper pharyngeal residue when using each maneuver. Their results are descriptive with no analytic statistical comparison.

Critical Thinking

1. What is the benefit of small sample-size research in understanding the value of clinical techniques?
2. What are some limitations that must be considered when small samples are used to study clinical techniques?
3. How should clinical practitioners interpret and use this information?

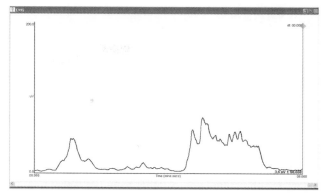

FIGURE 10-7   sEMG trace depicting a "normal" swallow (*left*) and a swallow using the Mendelsohn maneuver (*right*).

sphincter but decreased esophageal peristalsis with this maneuver in healthy adults.

Physiologic swallow changes resulting from the Mendelsohn maneuver have also been reported in small studies of patients with dysphagia. Physiologic swallow changes in a small group (*N* = 3) of head and neck cancer patients include increased duration of base-of-tongue and posterior pharyngeal wall contact and increased pressure of this contact.[80] In addition, McCullough and Kim[92] reported increased hyoid maximum elevation following therapeutic intervention with the Mendelsohn maneuver in a group of poststroke patients with dysphagia. Maximum width of upper esophageal sphincter opening increased following therapy but not significantly.

This maneuver has been used extensively as a therapy technique and may serve both compensatory and rehabilitative functions. The compensatory function is indicated in studies that report reduced postswallow residue or aspiration with this maneuver.[80,83] The rehabilitative function is indicated in the studies that report improved swallowing function after use of this technique and without dependence on the technique. For example, Lazarus et al.[83] reported improved swallow timing coordination in a single patient who used this maneuver. Neumann et al.[93] reported successful therapy outcome (defined as total oral feeding) in two thirds of 58 tube-fed patients with neurologic deficit as the primary cause for dysphagia. Nearly half of these patients used the Mendelsohn maneuver during therapy. Crary[94] used a technique termed *sustained pharyngeal contraction* (similar to the Mendelsohn maneuver) in an intensive therapy program with six tube-dependent brainstem stroke patients. This technique was taught to patients with the assistance of sEMG biofeedback. After an average of 3 weeks of daily treatment, five of the six patients with chronic, severe dysphagia returned to total oral feeding without complications. Changes in swallow physiology reflected improved coordination and effort during swallow attempts. In a follow-up paper, Crary et al.[95] reported increased safe oral intake in 87% of 45 patients with chronic dysphagia in an average of 10 therapy sessions. Huckabee and Cannito[96] also reported significant improvement in swallowing function over 10 therapy sessions within a single week. These investigators used the Mendelsohn maneuver as part of their treatment regimen.

In general, positive outcomes in swallow function have been reported after use of the Mendelsohn maneuver in dysphagia therapy (refer to Video series 4-9, *B-D,* for an example of patient performance on this maneuver over time). However, one clinical concern about this technique is that it can be difficult to teach patients to complete the maneuver. For example, in the study by Ding et al.,[88] healthy adult volunteers required between one and nine practice trials to adequately learn the Mendelsohn maneuver. Some clinical investigators have reported successful use of adjunctive biofeedback, primarily sEMG, to address the difficulty learning the Mendelsohn maneuver.[94-96] This adjunctive modality provides patients with immediate physiologic information on muscle activity during attempts at the maneuver. Figure 10-7 depicts a trace of sEMG activity from a normal swallow (left side or first event) compared with a swallow using the Mendelsohn maneuver (right side or second event). The different configurations are obvious and hence use of sEMG biofeedback may facilitate enhanced learning of this swallowing maneuver (see description later in this chapter). Another clinical concern with this maneuver is that, if done correctly, the prolongation of the swallow increases the apneic phase of the swallow. This prolonged cessation of respiration may be contraindicated in patients with respiratory disease or

PRACTICE NOTE 10-3

The Mendelsohn maneuver increases swallowing-related apnea. Over the course of a treatment session or if used during meals, this effect could be cumulative and have a negative effect on a patient's respiratory status. As a simple tool to assess the impact of this maneuver on respiratory function, I simply ask the patient to hold his or her breath. I then count to 4 (sometimes 5!) and ask the patient to breathe. If the respiratory stress of a simple breath hold is not dramatic (e.g., no increase in respiratory rate), then I will consider application of the Mendelsohn maneuver (or other maneuvers that might prolong the apneic pause). However, if I note significant respiratory changes (rapid or prolonged deep breathing) I will avoid all maneuvers that prolong swallow apnea and search for other strategies with less negative effect on the patient.

severe incoordination between swallowing activity and respiration (see Practice Note 10-3).

Increasing Force: The Effortful Swallow

The effortful swallow technique, sometimes referred to as the hard swallow or the forceful swallow, represents a volitional attempt by the patient to increase the force applied to the bolus from structures within the swallowing mechanism. Pouderoux and Kahrilas[39] demonstrated a fourfold increase in tongue propulsive force in forceful swallows of healthy volunteers. Asking patients to "swallow harder" may induce several physiologic changes compared with a "normal" swallow. Bülow et al.[16] reported reduced hyoid and laryngeal-mandibular distances (hyoid and laryngeal elevation) before an effortful swallow completed by healthy volunteers ("swallow very hard while squeezing the tongue in an upward-backward motion toward the soft palate"). As a result of this preswallow posture, less hyoid and laryngeal elevation occurred during the effortful swallows. No pharyngeal pressure increases were observed via manometry during effortful swallows produced by these healthy volunteers. Conversely, Hind et al.[97] reported that during effortful swallows healthy volunteers demonstrated increased elevation of the hyoid bone. These investigators also reported increased lingual pressures (pressure of tongue against hard palate during swallows) and increased swallow durations, including duration of hyoid excursion, duration of laryngeal closure, and duration of PES opening. Pressure increases combined with prolonged airway closure suggest that the effortful swallow technique may help certain patients clear a bolus through the swallow mechanism while reducing the risk of airway compromise via penetration or aspiration. Huckabee and colleagues[98-102] have completed a series of interesting investigations on the effortful swallow technique performed by healthy volunteers that expand the

initial results of Pouderoux and Kahrilas[36] and Hind et al.[97] In the initial study,[98] this group reported greater pharyngeal pressures and lower PES pressures (more relaxation) during effortful swallows completed by healthy volunteers. In addition, sEMG amplitudes were higher with effortful swallows, implying greater overall effort during these swallow attempts. Hiss and Huckabee[99] compared the timing of pharyngeal and PES pressure onsets across effortful versus normal swallows. Their results indicated delayed onset of effortful swallows (delayed increase in pharyngeal pressures or relaxation in PES) combined with an overall increased duration of these swallows. These results suggest that the effortful swallow technique may be contraindicated in patients with delayed onset of the pharyngeal component of the swallow, but it may help with pharyngeal clearance via increased pharyngeal pressures and greater PES relaxation. These initial results were further examined in a follow-up study by Witte et al.[102] These investigators evaluated the effect of a bolus (saliva versus 10 mL of water) on effortful versus normal swallows. In general, saliva swallows produced higher upper pharyngeal pressures during both types of swallows, but PES relaxation was greater for effortful swallows of saliva compared with water. These results were supported in a high-resolution manometry study by Takasaki et al.,[103] also demonstrating increased velopharynx, mid-hypopharynx, and upper esophageal sphincter pressures with effortful swallows, especially with effortful saliva swallows. Consistent with increased pharyngeal pressures during swallowing, Fritz et al.[104] reported reduced preswallow pharyngeal area and prolonged pharyngeal closure during effortful swallows. Together, these studies implicate a positive effect of the effortful swallow on pharyngeal pressure increase and PES relaxation—an effect that may be enhanced during saliva swallows.

In a pair of related reports Huckabee and Steele[100,101] evaluated the influence of orolingual pressure on amplitude and timing of pharyngeal pressures during normal and effortful swallows performed by healthy volunteers. These investigators reported that providing instructions that emphasize increased tongue-palate pressure during effortful swallows ("push hard with your tongue" versus "do not use your tongue to increase swallow force") resulted in increased sEMG amplitudes, tongue-palate pressures, and pharyngeal pressures. Conversely, only minimal timing differences were observed as a result of the effortful swallow with emphasis on tongue-palate pressure. In a study comparing the effortful swallow to the Mendelsohn maneuver, Fukuoka et al.[105] reported that the effortful swallow was more effective in increasing tongue-palate pressures over a wide area of the hard palate. Finally, Clark and Shelton[106] demonstrated increased anterior lingual-palatal pressures during effortful swallows versus noneffortful swallows in healthy adults. Moreover, following a 4-week effortful swallow training program, these same pressures increased with greater increases associated with effortful swallows. These investigations support prior results and interpretations that as a result in increased swallow-related pressures, the effortful swallow technique may be beneficial in facilitating pharyngeal bolus clearance in certain patients with oropharyngeal dysphagia.

One additional aspect should be mentioned in reference to the physiologic effect of the effortful swallow in healthy volunteers. Lever et al.[107] reported increased peristaltic amplitudes in the distal, but not the proximal, esophagus during effortful swallows. In addition, lower esophageal sphincter (LES) residual pressure was lower for women but not men with the effortful swallow technique. Nekl et al.[108] completed an expanded replication of the Lever study using solid-state manometry with intraluminal impedance. Their results indicated enhanced esophageal peristalsis and bolus clearance within the entire esophagus with the effortful swallow versus a noneffortful swallow. O'Rourke and colleagues[109] further demonstrated that the effortful swallow contributed to greater esophageal peristalsis compared with the Mendelsohn maneuver (which contributed to reduced esophageal peristalsis). Although these studies do not evaluate the effortful swallow as a treatment for reduced esophageal peristalsis, collectively, they have implications for pharyngoesophageal interactions including potential behavioral therapy strategies for patients who have reduced esophageal motility and clearance.

As reflected in the preceding paragraphs, the majority of investigations on the physiologic effect of the effortful swallow technique have been conducted with healthy adults, mostly young healthy adults. It is appropriate to make inferences on clinical applications from such investigations, but direct extension to performance in patients with dysphagia is considered over interpretation. Thus it is important to study both the physiologic effect and treatment outcomes of this technique (or for that matter, any technique) in patients with dysphagia.

A presumption based on studies of healthy volunteers is that the effortful swallow technique increases movement and lingual-palatal and pharyngeal pressures during swallows. Potential benefits of these kinematic and physiologic changes are improved airway protection and less postswallow residue. However, few reports have addressed the physiologic impact of this "maneuver" on swallowing in adults with dysphagia or documented the effect of this technique on swallowing change after therapy. In patients with pharyngeal dysfunction the effortful swallow reportedly had no effect on the number of misdirected swallows (frequency of penetration or aspiration) or degree of pharyngeal residue, but it did reduce the depth of penetration of swallowed material into the larynx and trachea.[14] These same authors reported that four of the eight patients in this study had difficulty performing the technique, likely because of lingual weakness (although this was not studied

directly in this study). In a separate study, this group of investigators examined manometric intrabolus pressure (defined as the manometric pressure when the pressure sensor was completely within the bolus) at the inferior pharyngeal constrictor in eight patients with pharyngeal dysphagia.[15] Results indicated no alteration in either peak pressure or duration of intrabolus pressure with use of the effortful swallow technique. Conversely, Lazarus et al.[80] reported increased swallow pressure (base of tongue to posterior pharyngeal wall) and increased duration of contact (base of tongue to posterior pharyngeal wall) in three patients with dysphagia secondary to treatment for head and neck cancer. These discrepant reports may result from a focus on different points in the swallow mechanism (upper pharynx versus lower pharynx) or from different causes contributing to dysphagia (six stroke patients and two patients with head and neck cancer versus three patients with head and neck cancer). Additionally, the variability noted across patients may exaggerate the findings from any small sample study of patient groups (Clinical Corner 10-2).

Treatment outcomes from use of the effortful swallow technique in adults with dysphagia are more difficult to identify. Some clinical investigators have used the effortful swallow as part of a treatment program and thus the results from these treatment studies are not focused on the effortful swallow technique. Crary[94] used sEMG biofeedback to teach patients to swallow "harder and longer" during therapy. Five of six patients demonstrated dramatic functional improvement (feeding tube removal) and physiologic improvement in swallowing after therapy. Physiologic change in swallowing included increased amplitude and duration of the sEMG signal measured during bolus swallows. These changes mirror those reported in healthy volunteers who use this technique. Carnaby-Mann and Crary[110] reported significant clinical improvement and enhanced hyolaryngeal excursion in five patients who completed a 3-week course of therapy (McNeill Dysphagia Therapy Program [MDTP]; see later in this chapter for additional information) using a technique that instructed them to swallow hard and fast for each bolus. These two studies suggest that the effortful swallow technique may produce positive clinical and physiologic change in patients with dysphagia. Still, no study has examined this technique thoroughly from a clinical point of view.

The effortful swallow technique may facilitate improved swallowing by increasing force applied to the bolus and extending the duration of the swallow. Outcomes may include stronger and more coordinated swallows but this clinical effect requires more investigation. Available literature suggests that the nature of instructions given to the patient and the type and amount of material swallowed may have an effect on the immediate effect and the treatment outcome of this technique. Another variable to consider is

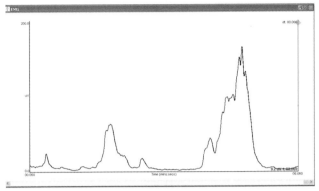

FIGURE 10-8 sEMG trace depicting a "normal" swallow (*left*) and an effortful swallow (*right*).

biofeedback may be an important adjunct in teaching patients the proper application of this clinical technique. More information on this modality is presented later in this chapter.

The therapy strategies just reviewed are considered more "traditional" strategies. Liquid and diet modifications, along with postural adjustments and swallow maneuvers, represent the large majority of dysphagia interventions used for several years. Table 10-2 summarizes the primary postural adjustments and swallow maneuvers with a brief description of how they are performed, their intended effects, the expected physiologic changes, and anticipated functional outcomes for each technique. Note that each postural adjustment and swallowing maneuver represents a form of "abnormal" swallowing. Thus, except in extreme situations, patients are not expected to use these swallowing interventions for long periods. Clinicians should view these techniques as either short-term compensations or, in some cases, as techniques to change and hopefully improve an impaired swallow mechanism.

Additional Techniques to Change the Swallow

Multiple Swallows as a Therapy Technique

At one time or another most individuals engage in multiple swallows to clear a single bolus. Similarly, clinicians often ask patients with dysphagia to "swallow again." Presumably this strategy is used to clear residue from the initial swallow. However, little evidence exists to either support or refute the application of multiple swallows as a therapy strategy. Multiple swallows are frequently seen in adults with dysphagia[111-113] and may be more frequent in healthy adults with increasing age.[114] Also, multiple swallows may be elicited by texture[112,113] or taste[49] in both healthy adults and in adult patients with dysphagia.

No data are available to evaluate the effectiveness of a multiple-swallow strategy as a therapy technique. A

the ability of the patient and the clinician to monitor the swallow performance using this technique. As mentioned for the Mendelsohn maneuver, sEMG biofeedback may be a valuable asset to help the patient use the technique effectively and to provide the clinician with immediate information on the patient's performance. Figure 10-8 depicts a normal dry swallow (right side of image) compared with an effortful dry swallow (left side of image). Like the Mendelsohn maneuver, the differences are obvious to even the untrained eye. Thus the visual display of sEMG

TABLE 10-2 Summary of Behavioral Swallowing Maneuvers Commonly Used in Dysphagia Therapy

Technique	Performance	Intent	Physiology	Outcomes
Side-lying	Lie down with stronger side lower	Slows bolus Provides time to adjust and protect airway	Emphasizes pharyngeal contraction	Less aspiration
Chin-up	Elevate chin	Propel bolus to back of mouth	Widens oropharynx Increases PES pressure	Better oral transport
Chin-down	Lower chin	Improves airway protection	Narrow oropharynx	Reduced aspiration
Head-turn	Turn head to right or left	Reduces postswallow residue and aspiration	Redirects bolus to stronger side of pharynx Lowers PES pressure	Increased amount swallowed Less residue and lower risk of aspiration
Supraglottic swallow	Hold breath Swallow Gentle cough	Reduces aspiration by increasing glottal closure	Horizontal glottal closure Increased movement of swallowing structures	Reduced aspiration Increased laryngeal excursion
Super-supraglottic swallow	Hold breath Bear down Swallow Gentle cough	Reduces aspiration by increasing glottal closure	Horizontal and anteroposterior glottal closure Increased movement of swallowing structures	Reduced aspiration Increased laryngeal excursion
Mendelsohn maneuver	Squeeze swallow at apex	Improves swallowing coordination	Increased and prolonged hyolaryngeal excursion	Improved swallowing coordination Less postswallow residue Less aspiration
Effortful swallow	Swallow harder	Increases lingual force on bolus	Increased tongue-palate pressures Increased duration of swallow Increased tongue base movement	Less residue

PES, Pharyngoesophageal sphincter.

common rationale for use of multiple swallows may be to clear residue from various points within the swallow mechanism after the initial bolus swallow. However, application of a multiple-swallow strategy, specifically excessive use of multiple swallows (either for a single bolus or after each bolus) may create a degree of inefficiency in a patient's functional eating ability (see also Clinical Corner 10-3). Logic dictates that using multiple swallows per bolus increases mealtime and thus may contribute to reduced oral intake. Also, excessive use of multiple swallows during functional eating may induce patient fatigue with negative consequences on oral intake or airway protection. Given the absence of objective data on the benefit or risk of a multiple-swallow strategy in dysphagia therapy, clinicians should take steps to evaluate the effect of this strategy on individual patients prior to inclusion in any therapy program.

The Tongue-Hold Maneuver

The posterior pharyngeal wall has a tendency to "bulge" forward during swallowing, contacting the tongue base and thus creating a pressure source to help push the bolus through the pharynx. When the tongue base is not able to move posteriorly toward the pharyngeal wall, and if the pharyngeal wall is physiologically capable, it may increase the degree of anterior "bulge" in a presumed attempt to compensate for the reduction in tongue base–pharyngeal wall contact. This effect is demonstrated in Video 10-7. The patient in this video sustained neck trauma that increased the distance from the base of the tongue to the posterior pharyngeal wall. On swallowing, the posterior pharyngeal wall moves aggressively forward—presumably to increase contact with the base of the tongue, resulting in a functional swallow.

The initial clinical observations of the tongue-hold maneuver were from a group of patients with oral cancer who demonstrated surgical anchoring of the anterior tongue, thereby limiting posterior tongue movement.[115] These individuals demonstrated anterior bulging of the posterior pharyngeal wall. Subsequently, healthy young adults were asked to perform a maneuver that attempted to mimic the anterior anchoring of the tongue.[116] These healthy subjects held the anterior tongue (slightly posterior to the tongue tip)

CLINICAL CORNER 10-3: MULTIPLE SWALLOWS

A common practice technique is to ask a patient to swallow again. Often this strategy is accompanied by the request to "swallow hard." During fluoroscopic or endoscopic swallow examinations this request is typically triggered by the observation of postswallow residue. During therapy this request is typically triggered by clinical signs that the patient has postswallow residue—often voice changes, throat clearing, or a cough. Despite these common practices the use of multiple swallows may introduce a degree of "inefficiency" into functional swallowing. As reviewed in this chapter, little evidence exists to either support or refute the use of multiple swallows as a therapy technique. This raises questions about the application of this strategy.

Critical Thinking
1. What are considered benefits from the application of a multiple-swallow technique in dysphagia therapy?
2. What difficulties or "inefficiencies" might be encountered by asking a patient to use a multiple-swallow strategy during functional eating?
3. What strategies might a clinician use during assessment or therapy in an attempt to decide whether a multiple-swallow strategy might help a patient?

---

between the teeth while swallowing. Fluoroscopic inspection indicated that with this swallow maneuver, healthy adults demonstrate an increased anterior bulging of the posterior pharyngeal wall.

Swallowing with this anterior tongue-hold maneuver does appear to contribute to increased anterior movement of the posterior pharyngeal wall during swallowing; however, at least three negative consequences of this maneuver during swallowing have been identified: (1) reduced duration of airway closure, (2) increased postswallow residue, and (3) increased delay in the initiation of the pharyngeal component of the swallow.[117] In some patients, each of these consequences, alone or in combination, could contribute to an increased possibility of airway compromise (penetration or aspiration). This observation necessitates a cautionary note for this maneuver: the Masako or tongue-hold maneuver should not be used with a bolus. Furthermore, no evidence currently exists supporting the clinical benefits of this swallow maneuver.

Physiologic swallow changes resulting from the tongue-hold maneuver are receiving increased evaluation. In a small sample of three patients with dysphagia secondary to treatment for head and neck cancer, Lazarus et al.[80] reported that the tongue-hold maneuver increased both the duration and pressure of tongue base–pharyngeal wall contact compared with swallowing with no maneuver. The tongue-hold maneuver also reportedly reduced postswallow residue in these same patients. This observation is in direct contrast to those offered by Fujiu-Kurachi,[117] who identified increased postswallow residue. Although little relevant research on the tongue-hold maneuver has been conducted in patients with dysphagia, recent work has evaluated manometric changes associated with this maneuver in healthy adult volunteers. Doeltgen et al.[118] reported that swallows performed by 40 healthy young adults resulted in lower pharyngeal contraction pressures, shorter pharyngeal pressure durations, but greater relaxation in the upper esophageal sphincter than control swallows. In a follow-up study, Doeltgen et al.[119] reported that the oropharyngeal and pharyngeal pressure changes with this maneuver were consistent across age, but that upper esophageal sphincter pressure increased (less relaxation) in older healthy subjects. These findings in part support the clinical observations of Fujiu-Kurachi.[117] Reduced pharyngeal pressures (and less upper esophageal sphincter relaxation in older adults) may contribute to increased postswallow residue. In related work, Hammer et al.[120] identified increased muscle activation in lingual and pharyngeal constrictor muscles before and during swallows with two degrees of tongue protrusion. However, they did not identify any change in pharyngeal swallow pressures associated with degrees of tongue protrusion during swallowing. Fujiu-Kurachi et al.[121] further reported that with increased tongue protrusion patterns of tongue pressure against the hard palate became increasingly variable. They suggested that the degree of lingual flexibility (measured as the degree of maximal tongue protrusion) may have influenced their results. Although still limited in number, available studies of the tongue-hold maneuver (mostly completed with healthy adults) indicate that pharyngeal pressures are reduced during swallowing and, specifically in older subjects, upper esophageal sphincter relaxation may be reduced. These physiologic changes associated with the tongue-hold maneuver question its use as a potential swallow rehabilitation technique (see Practice Note 10-4).

The tongue-hold maneuver may have clinical application when an increased anterior bulging of the posterior pharyngeal wall at the level of the tongue base is desired. However, the type of patient, specific dysphagia characteristics, and specific anticipated outcomes need to be further detailed in reference to this technique. Without further study and clarification of effect and functional benefit, the tongue-hold maneuver remains an unknown and potentially risky technique for use in dysphagia therapy.

The Head-Lift Exercise

The head-lift exercise, sometimes referred to as the Shaker technique, is an activity intended to improve opening of the PES by increasing the "strength" of muscle groups

PRACTICE NOTE 10-4

In discussing the potential benefits and risks to patients from application of the tongue-hold maneuver, clinicians often respond that they use this maneuver as a swallow exercise without a bolus. The problem with this point of view is that no data exist supporting potential exercise-related benefits of the tongue-hold maneuver. Clinicians have indicated that they feel swallowing muscles working harder when they swallow with the tongue-hold maneuver. Unfortunately, this feeling does not equate to acceptable exercise, and data such as those reported by Doeltgen et al.[118] seem to indicate a reduction in pharyngeal motor performance resulting from the tongue-hold maneuver. Thus the author's impression is that the tongue-hold maneuver may be a helpful technique, but currently there are no systematic data that support its clinical or physiologic benefit to adult patients with dysphagia.

that contribute to PES opening. During swallowing, the suprahyoid (and other) muscle groups help the hyolaryngeal complex to move up and forward, exerting an upward and anterior pull on the PES. This is an important physiologic component of PES opening. Strengthening of weakened suprahyoid muscle groups would be expected to have a positive effect on PES opening via these mechanisms. The head-lift technique is intended to strengthen these muscles by having the patient lie supine and raise the head (but not the shoulders) sufficiently to see the toes. This head posture is maintained for a defined period and repeated on a prescribed schedule.[122] Patients are asked to lie in the supine position and complete three head lifts sustained for 1 minute each. A 1-minute rest period occurs between each sustained head lift. Immediately following the sustained head lifts, patients are asked to complete 30 consecutive head lifts without sustaining the lifted position. This series of head-lift exercises is completed 3 times each day for a period of 6 weeks. Contraindications for this activity may include cervical spine deficits, reduced movement capability of the neck (as in some patients with head and neck cancer), or cognitive limitations or other factors that might contribute to poor compliance with the prescribed routine.

Numerous studies have evaluated the clinical benefit and the physiologic bases of the head-lift technique. Shaker et al.[122] demonstrated increased anterior laryngeal excursion and upper esophageal sphincter opening during swallowing in a group of healthy older adult subjects who completed this exercise. Similar physiologic changes in swallowing were not observed in a group of adults performing a sham exercise. A follow-up study evaluated both physiologic and clinical changes resulting from the head-

lift exercise in a group of adult patients who required tube feedings because of an abnormal upper esophageal sphincter opening.[123] After the head-lift exercise program, patients demonstrated improved anterior laryngeal excursion, improved upper esophageal sphincter opening, and less postswallow aspiration. A **systematic review** by Antunes and Lunet[124] identified a total of nine studies evaluating the head-lift technique. Most of these studies focused on physiologic change in the swallow mechanism associated with the technique and the majority included only small numbers of subjects. These authors concluded that while the head-lift technique holds promise for dysphagia rehabilitation, future studies are required to provide a sound evaluation of the effectiveness of this technique.

The main premise of clinical improvements observed after the head-lift exercise is that this exercise program strengthens the suprahyoid muscles. Two small studies on this technique reported that both the suprahyoid and infrahyoid muscle groups fatigued after the head-lift exercise.[125,126] Muscle fatigue is accepted as evidence for muscle activity or exercise. Another study reported enhanced thyrohyoid shortening (less distance between the hyoid bone and thyroid cartilage) after the head-lift exercise.[127] Collectively, these results are interpreted as evidence that the head-lift exercise strengthens muscles that aid in opening of the upper esophageal sphincter by elevation and anterior excursion of the hyolaryngeal complex. The primary muscles considered responsible for this action are the suprahyoid muscles. The primary measurement techniques have been biokinematic measures from videofluoroscopy or physiologic measures from sEMG. A related study by Yoshida et al.[128] compared submental (suprahyoid) muscle activity measured with sEMG between the head-lift and the tongue-press (tongue pushed against hard palate) exercises. These investigators reported no differences in the amplitude of sEMG signals obtained between the two exercises from a group of 53 healthy young adults. In fact, in the sustained posture condition, submental sEMG activity was higher during the tongue-press exercise. These investigators suggested that perhaps the tongue-press activity may accomplish similar physiologic goals as the head-lift exercise but with fewer physical demands on patients. Likewise, Watts[129] reported that a jaw-opening against resistance exercise generated greater hyolaryngeal muscle activation than the head-lift technique. Yoon et al.[130] also reported that a chin tuck against resistance activity generated greater sEMG activity in suprahyoid musculature compared to the head-lift exercise. Finally, Wada et al.[131] reported that a maximum and sustained jaw-opening activity (without resistance) completed as a therapy over a 4-week period resulted in increased hyoid excursion and increased opening of the upper esophageal sphincter in adults with dysphagia. These reports suggest that the goal of strengthening the suprahyoid musculature with an associated increase in upper esophageal opening might be accomplished with a variety of techniques.

The physical demands of the head-lift exercise should not be underestimated, especially in older or weaker patients with dysphagia. In a single study evaluating compliance with the demands of the head-lift exercise,[132] 26 older adults without dysphagia participated in the head-lift exercise as prescribed. Only 50% of these adults completed the **isokinetic** (repetitive lifts) portion of the exercise program, and 70% completed the isometric (sustained lift) portion. Most who withdrew from this exercise program did so within the first 2 weeks. These findings implicate the importance of compliance monitoring whenever the head-lift exercise program is used as a dysphagia therapy technique.

Thermal-Tactile Application

This therapy technique is perhaps one of the "grandparents" of dysphagia therapy. It has been used for years and has been revised and revisited in many treatment-related and swallow physiology studies. Logemann[4] is credited with introducing this technique in her 1983 text as a technique to stimulate the swallow reflex. Her suggestion to stroke the anterior faucial pillar with a cold stimulus (#00 or #0 laryngeal mirror) is believed to originate from the work of Pommerenke,[133] who identified the anterior faucial pillars as one of the more sensitive oral areas for initiating the swallow reflex. The primary outcome measure of success for this technique is a reduction in the delay in the initiation of swallowing, primarily the pharyngeal phase. By logical reasoning then, this technique may be suitable for those patients who demonstrate delayed initiation of the pharyngeal aspect of swallowing. Lazzara et al.[134] reported faster pharyngeal and total transit times for swallows after thermal stimulation in patients with dysphagia from neurologic deficit. The change in swallow response time was evaluated fluoroscopically for single swallows. They concluded that their results support the position that thermal stimulation to the anterior faucial pillars triggers the swallow response. Regan, Walshe, and Tobin[135] also demonstrated faster pharyngeal transit of liquid and paste materials in a small cohort of patients with dysphagia secondary to Parkinson's disease. These studies suggest that thermal-tactile stimulation within the posterior oral cavity can produce a short-term effect on swallow timing. However, immediate effects are not equivalent to therapy outcomes.

Rosenbek et al.[136] evaluated this technique (which they termed thermal application) as a therapy technique in seven adult patients with dysphagia after at least two strokes. Subjects received thermal application therapy daily for 1-week periods alternating with no treatment periods of a week. A total of 2 weeks of thermal application therapy was provided to each patient within this alternating treatment design. Despite an immediate effect of thermal application during the baseline fluoroscopic swallowing evaluation, these investigators did not find strong support for a therapy effect from this proposed intervention. Furthermore, aspiration and penetration were not improved as a result of thermal application, and any short-term therapy effects were not maintained at 1 month after therapy. In a follow-up study, Rosenbek et al.[137] reported that thermal application reduced the *duration of stage transition (DST)* in stroke patients with dysphagia. DST is the time interval between the arrival of the bolus at the posterior edge of the ramus of the mandible and the initiation of hyoid bone elevation. Smaller DST values represent less delay in the initiation of the pharyngeal component of the swallow. Thus, similar to the studies by Lazzara et al.[134] and earlier by Rosenbek et al.,[136] this study supports the presence of an immediate effect of cold application to the anterior faucial pillars—a reduction in the delay of the pharyngeal response during the swallow. Finally, Rosenbek and a large group of investigators[138] evaluated the intensity of treatment on the results of thermal application (which they now termed tactile-thermal application). Patients received 2 weeks of tactile-thermal application therapy and were randomly assigned to 150, 300, 450, or 600 trials per week. A trial included three or more strokes of both faucial pillars with an ice stick (similar to a popsicle). This investigative team reported that no frequency of treatment was superior to any other. Furthermore, the higher-intensity treatments (450 and 600 trials) were not fully completed during therapy (less than the target number of trials). Finally, changes in swallow timing and airway protection (penetration or aspiration) were observed but these were not consistent across different boluses evaluated in this study.

Studies of thermal stimulation in healthy adult volunteers have produced even more variable results than those in adult patients with dysphagia. Kaatzke-McDonald et al.[139] evaluated cold and taste (sugar versus salt) on swallow latency in healthy adult women. They reported that only the cold stimulus resulted in a reduction in swallow latency. Conversely, Sciortino et al.[140] reported that only the combination of mechanical, cold, and gustatory (sour) contributed to a reduction in swallow latency compared with a no-stimulation condition. Furthermore, this group reported that any stimulation effect lasted for only a single swallow. Finally, neither Knauer et al.[141] nor Ali et al.[142] identified any significant swallow changes resulting from application of a cold stimulus in healthy adult volunteers.

Studies evaluating functional benefits such as reduction in aspiration from application of a cold stimulus to the anterior faucial pillars have not provided positive results. The primary effect identified, but inconsistently, is reduced swallow delay. Thus this technique may be applicable for patients demonstrating delays in swallowing activity but not for patients who demonstrate airway compromise.

NEW REHABILITATION DIRECTIONS: EXERCISE PRINCIPLES AND MODALITIES

Many of the techniques described in this chapter may be envisioned as forms of exercise for the muscles encompassing the swallowing mechanism. In fact, various forms of exercise have been used for years in the rehabilitation of speech and swallowing functions.[65] Yet in recent years clinicians and clinical researchers have borrowed from exercise physiologists and related professions in an attempt to develop effective therapy programs based on systematic application of exercise principles. As noted later in this chapter, this application is relatively new and not fully developed. Many suggestions exist but only a few feasible applications have been developed and evaluated.

The use of adjunctive modalities also is growing in the area of dysphagia rehabilitation. Two adjunctive modalities that have received the most attention have been sEMG biofeedback and neuromuscular electrical stimulus (NMES). The term *adjunctive* specifies that the modality is used to support the benefits from the primary therapy. Neither sEMG biofeedback nor NMES provides maximum benefit to patients in the absence of a well-developed treatment program, but both modalities have the potential to enhance the benefits of good therapy.

Exercise Principles and Dysphagia Therapy

Reviews of exercise principles that may apply to dysphagia rehabilitation have focused primarily on strength training.[143,144] Although a comprehensive review of exercise principles is beyond the scope of this chapter, common exercise principles related to dysphagia rehabilitation have been reviewed by Crary and Carnaby (Table 10-3).[145] Clinicians should at least consider the principles of intensity and specificity when selecting any dysphagia rehabilitation program. Intensity may be increased in many ways. Increasing the resistance to movement is a common method to increase intensity. For example, lifting heavier weights adds increased resistance to a weight-lifting exercise. Intensity may also be increased by frequency of exercise. More repetitions of an exercise completed in a fixed period result in a more intense exercise. Increasing the intensity of exercise facilitates muscle change and results in greater strength. Conversely, when exercises are ceased or reduced in intensity, the principle of reversibility or a detraining effect may be seen. In simple terms, *reversibility* means that strength gains may be lost if exercise is reduced and if a maintenance program is not used.

The concept of specificity refers to the observation that certain exercises are more likely to benefit specific tasks. For example, extreme weight lifting would not be viewed as the most beneficial exercise routine for a long-distance runner. Different muscle groups are involved with different requirements to the neuromuscular system from the target activity (in this case, long-distance running). A common phrase used by dysphagia clinicians is paraphrased as follows—"the best way to rehabilitate swallowing is to have the patient swallow." This phrase represents the principle of specificity. However, a related concept should be mentioned—cross-system effect or transference. The cross-system effect occurs when exercise intended for one function produces benefits in a different function. Because muscles of the swallowing mechanism also are used in

TABLE 10-3 Definitions and Application Suggestions for Basic Exercise Principles That May Be Incorporated into Dysphagia Rehabilitation Programs

Principle	Definition	Application
Overload	Exercise at sufficient intensity, time, and frequency to challenge muscle and create muscle change	Increase total time or load used in training.
Progression	Systematically increasing the intensity (load) and demands (time/frequency) spent in exercise	Continually and gradually increase the demands of the exercise activity applied—perform more repetitions, increase the load, go faster.
Intensity	The load used in an exercise	Alter the amount pushed, pulled, or lifted in exercise.
Adaptation	Repeatedly practicing a movement, skill, or task to alter muscle condition	Use continued (regular) practice of a particular exercise pattern.
Reversibility	The effect of exercise training on muscle will be lost with lack of activity	"If you don't use it, you lose it"—a maintenance plan is needed to prevent detraining.
Specificity	Exercise should be specific to the goal	If your goal is to be a runner, then exercise should include running.
Recovery	Rest between repetitions of movement or sets of strength-training exercises	Ensure sufficient rest between activity to reduce fatigue and stabilize muscle.

(From Crary MA, Carnaby GD: Adoption into clinical practice of two therapies to manage swallowing disorders: exercise-based swallow rehabilitation and electrical stimulation, *Curr Opin Otolaryngol Head Neck Surg* 22:172, 2014, with permission.)

TABLE 10-4 Depiction of Exercise Goals and Incorporated Exercise Principles in Three Exercise-Based Dysphagia Rehabilitation Programs

Program	Goal	Principles Utilized
Lingual resistance	Development of lingual strength to improve swallowing	Progression Overload Adaptation Intensity Recovery
Shaker head lift	To strengthen suprahyoid musculature and improve upper esophageal sphincter opening	Adaptation Recovery
MDTP	Progressive development, strengthening, and refinement of the muscular components of the swallowing process	Progression Overload Adaptation Intensity Reversibility Specificity Recovery

MDTP, McNeill Dysphagia Therapy Program.
(From Crary MA, Carnaby GD: Adoption into clinical practice of two therapies to manage swallowing disorders: exercise-based swallow rehabilitation and electrical stimulation, *Curr Opin Otolaryngol Head Neck Surg* 22:172, 2014, with permission.)

speech and voice production, it seems logical that exercise directed at improving speech or voice functions may have a cross-system effect on swallowing function (or vice versa). Although this cross-system effect has not been well studied in relation to dysphagia rehabilitation, published examples do support the potential for exercises involving the swallowing mechanism to affect other functions of the upper aerodigestive tract.[146-148] Table 10-4 presents an interpretation of three current exercise-based dysphagia interventions (lingual resistance, head lift, MDTP) relative to inclusion of common exercise principles.

Positive functional benefits have been reported from exercise-based dysphagia therapy. Robbins et al.[68,69] were among the first to use specific exercise-based criteria to establish a dysphagia rehabilitation program. The focus of the therapy was to increase tongue strength using a tongue-press activity in which the tongue was pressed against the hard palate. Robbins and her colleagues progressively increased the intensity of the tongue-press activity by using the Iowa Oral Performance Instrument (IOPI) to measure the force of the tongue push and to provide patients feedback on how hard they were pushing. She incorporated the concept of 1-RM (1 repetition maximum or the greatest effort the patient can exert) to systematically increase resistance in the exercise (e.g., 60%, 70%, 80% of 1-RM). She also used a fixed period in which to complete therapy (8 weeks). Results from two studies showed increased

tongue strength during volitional tongue-push activity and swallowing, improvement in airway protection during swallowing, and increased lingual muscle size. These results are encouraging because they demonstrate that a simple, swallow-related exercise can increase strength in key muscle groups used in swallowing with some functional benefit to patients.

The McNeill Dysphagia Therapy Program (MDTP)[110,149] incorporates the exercise principles of specificity and intensity with frequent therapy sessions and variety to facilitate enhanced coordination during swallowing. Patients receive daily therapy sessions that are structured to evoke mass practice of swallowing. Swallowed materials are introduced sequentially to facilitate progressive resistance or speed and coordination of swallowing. Clinicians follow specific rules to advance patients during treatment based on patient performance. Following MDTP, patients demonstrated improved functional oral intake but also positive changes in swallowing effort and timing.[150,151] Results from this therapy program suggest that it is effective with patients with chronic dysphagia in whom other therapies have failed[110] and that MDTP produces clinical results superior to more traditional swallow maneuvers (e.g., Mendelsohn maneuver) taught with adjunctive biofeedback.[149] In addition, results of a randomized clinical trial in a stroke rehabilitation hospital indicate that MDTP produces superior functional outcomes to traditional therapy or to MDTP paired with transcutaneous electrical stimulation.[152] Initial results from MDTP intervention are encouraging but additional evaluation will help clarify issues of patient selection, frequency of intervention, and duration of intervention. MDTP represents an exercise-based therapy incorporating more than strength training alone.

What Do Adjunctive Modalities Offer the Patient?

Surface Electromyographic and Other Forms of Biofeedback

Many of the swallowing maneuvers discussed in this chapter require motor learning by the patient. Furthermore, many of these adjustments represent novel motor patterns that may be difficult to learn. Application of biofeedback as an adjunct to therapy may be valuable in enhancing the rate of motor learning, thereby resulting in reduced time in therapy. Biofeedback has been beneficial in teaching new movements, unfamiliar movements, or movements that are otherwise difficult to monitor.[153] Many swallowing therapy maneuvers fit into one or more of these categories. In addition, biofeedback may be useful in helping a patient monitor swallow performance. A simple example of this involves the effortful swallow. Asking a patient to "swallow harder" may not result in a significant increase in swallow effort. However, use of sEMG biofeedback to monitor the amplitude of the sEMG signal increases the probability that the patient has increased the effort involved in the swallow (see Figure 10-8). sEMG biofeedback is the process of monitoring and displaying muscle activity to a patient. Not only does this feedback help the patient to monitor effort, it also is immediate to the patient and the treating clinician and thus facilitates support or reinstruction from the clinician to the patient. A more comprehensive review of the application of sEMG biofeedback to dysphagia rehabilitation is offered by Crary and Groher.[154]

Several reports have advocated the use of sEMG biofeedback as an adjunct to dysphagia therapy. This form of biofeedback has been used to teach relaxation, strengthening, and coordination activities. Studies specific to dysphagia therapy have suggested that this form of biofeedback can reduce the amount of therapy time while producing favorable outcomes even in patients with chronic dysphagia.[94,155-158] A recent innovative application of sEMG biofeedback has been described by Athukorala et al.[159] Their "skill training" program required patients to swallow with sufficient precision and control to place the sEMG trace of their swallow within a randomly placed colored square on a computer screen. A group of 10 patients with dysphagia secondary to Parkinson's disease demonstrated selective improvement in swallow timing and sEMG characteristics. Additional work with this innovative paradigm may suggest novel directions for application of sEMG biofeedback.

Other forms of biofeedback may be applicable to swallow therapy. Having the patient watch swallow attempts on the monitor during a fluoroscopic examination has been suggested as a way to teach certain maneuvers.[160] Obviously, this application is time limited but potentially valuable for certain patients. In a similar manner, endoscopic biofeedback has been suggested as a mechanism to teach appropriate breath-hold maneuvers such as the supraglottic and super-supraglottic swallows.[161] If available, endoscopic biofeedback may be a valuable adjunct in teaching certain maneuvers. Less invasive than either fluoroscopy or endoscopy is the use of cervical auscultation as a biofeedback approach (see Chapter 9). Although this approach has not been formally evaluated, having patients listen for specific sound patterns associated with the swallow or the respiratory pattern surrounding the swallow may facilitate more rapid change in the swallowing pattern.

Regardless of the biofeedback form that is chosen, it is important for clinical practitioners to remember that biofeedback alone is not therapeutic (see Practice Note 10-5). As an adjunct to a well-conceived plan of therapy, judiciously applied biofeedback can have a positive effect. The key word is adjunct. The key concept is "What change is intended to be facilitated by biofeedback?" Clinicians should develop a strong therapy plan based on the individual characteristics of the patient, the problem, and the

---

PRACTICE NOTE 10-5

Many years ago I was asked to see a 4-year-old boy who had survived treatment for a brainstem tumor. Like many adults with brainstem difficulties, he had a significant dysphagia. I was actively studying the application of sEMG biofeedback at that time and decided that because of good results with survivors of adult brainstem stroke, I would try a similar approach with this child. We used a laptop computer to provide visual feedback. The software program featured a car on a hill that would go up the hill to a familiar yellow "M," a common symbol for a popular food chain. The harder the child swallowed, the closer the car got to the "M." The longer he maintained his swallow contraction, the longer the car stayed at the restaurant.

Therapy started with a bang! This boy was doing much better than anyone would have expected. He hit his goals almost immediately. Then I realized a critical mistake on my part. I did not verify that the movement driving the sEMG biofeedback was, in fact, a swallow. As it turned out, this little man was simply pushing his tongue against his palate and figured out that this would make the "car go." Clever!

I realized I needed to find a way to link the boy's attempts at swallowing with the biofeedback signal, so I made a second biofeedback source. I took a stethoscope head from a toy medical kit and connected it to a small microphone using rubber tubing. Then I plugged the microphone into a portable battery-operated speaker. I put the stethoscope head against my throat and swallowed hard. The sounds were clearly audible from the speaker and I asked the boy to do what I did. After he was trying to swallow on request on a consistent basis, I reintroduced sEMG biofeedback. His success level was not as dramatic this time. Eventually he did gain some functional swallowing ability with the combined biofeedback approach.

The lesson? Be sure of the movement for which you are providing biofeedback.

---

underlying disease and then decide whether and how to apply biofeedback to support this plan.

Neuromuscular Electrical Stimulation

NMES is a relatively new adjunctive modality in dysphagia rehabilitation. As a result of the novelty of NMES, many clinicians may not fully appreciate its implications or potential applications. An in-depth discussion of NMES principles is beyond the scope of this chapter, but a basic review of the principles and data addressing application to dysphagia rehabilitation is appropriate.

NMES is intended to facilitate improved contraction of weakened muscles when the peripheral nerve supply to those muscles is intact.[162] Electrical stimulation to muscles via NMES may be accomplished through electrodes placed on the skin (transcutaneous), with intramuscular placement (percutaneous), or with fully implanted devices. NMES may be viewed as a subset of functional electrical stimulation, which implies that electrical stimulation is applied during the performance of a functional movement or task. Multiple examples from various fields of physical rehabilitation indicate that NMES can enhance a functional activity, change physiology to support function without overt functional change, and contribute to a motor relearning effect.[162] Specific to dysphagia rehabilitation, NMES application has been studied primarily in reference to improved function or physiologic effect on the muscle groups involved in swallowing.

NMES was the most frequently recommended treatment technique in the 2013 case-based survey of dysphagia therapies conducted by Carnaby and Harenberg.[66] This result is a bit surprising in the face of conflicted evidence regarding the benefit of this modality. Several published studies have reported functional improvement in swallowing ability after dysphagia therapy with adjunctive NMES.[110,163-171] These reports of functional gain are also reflected in a large national survey of electrical stimulation in dysphagia rehabilitation.[172] Results from that survey indicated that nearly 80% of responding clinicians believed more than half of the patients they treated with NMES showed swallowing improvement. The primary gains reported by these clinicians included advances in the oral diet, reduced aspiration, and reduced reliance on tube feedings. Conversely, other studies reported no significant differences between outcomes of dysphagia therapy with and without adjunctive NMES.[173-175] Different patient samples, different electrical stimulation protocols, or different behavioral therapies combined with NMES may have contributed to discrepant outcomes across studies. In fact, a metaanalysis completed by Tan et al.[176] concluded that NMES outcomes were not different from traditional therapy in stroke patients, but when looking at dysphagia from various etiologies (non-stroke), NMES appeared to contribute to enhanced outcomes. Thus the status of NMES application in dysphagia in not clear. Perhaps the most rigorous study of NMES combined with behavioral therapy was reported by Carnaby et al.[177] This double-blind randomized clinical trial compared three treatment approaches in stroke patients receiving dysphagia therapy during subacute rehabilitation: MDTP with motor level NMES, MDTP with sham NMES, and traditional dysphagia therapy. Patients receiving the behavioral therapy (MDTP) with sham NMES demonstrated the best outcomes. NMES did not enhance clinical outcomes in this controlled study.

Studies investigating nontherapeutic effects of NMES on both healthy adults and adults with dysphagia also produce conflicting results. Suiter, Leder, and Ruark[178] evaluated the effect of 2 weeks of daily NMES without exercise in 10 healthy adult men. The investigators measured sEMG activity from the submental muscles before and after the 2 weeks of NMES and found no differences in swallow-related muscular activity. Humbert et al.[179] reported laryngeal and hyoid descent at rest and reduced laryngeal and hyoid elevation during swallowing when healthy adult subjects received electrical stimulation to the anterior neck. In a related study,[180] patients with chronic poststroke dysphagia demonstrated hyoid—but not laryngeal—descent at rest with the introduction of electrical stimulation to the anterior neck. Interestingly, in that study the degree of hyoid lowering during rest was inversely related to scores of swallow function during a videofluoroscopic swallow examination. Thus greater hyoid descent during electrical stimulation at rest related to better swallowing. In fact, Park et al.[181] used this effect in a novel treatment paradigm in which they combined the hyoid lowering effect from NMES with an effortful swallow, which resulted in increased laryngeal elevation posttherapy. Any physiologic effect of transcutaneous NMES might be affected by a number of variables. For example, Berretin-Felix et al.[182] reported interactions between NMES amplitude and age in healthy adults. Specifically, older adults demonstrated a decrease in certain physiologic aspects of swallowing with motor level (higher amplitude) stimulation. Nam et al.[183] reported that different electrode placements have a differential effect on swallow physiology in adult patients with dysphagia. Furata et al.[184] demonstrated an increase in spontaneous swallowing frequency in healthy adults using interferential current at a sensory stimulation level (lower amplitude). Heck, Doeltgen, and Huckabee[185] identified no immediate effect of submental muscle NMES but did report a delayed effect (lasting up to 1 hour) in decreased hypopharyngeal contraction but increased relaxation in the upper esophageal sphincter. This latter result is consistent with results from Jungheim et al.[186] who reported a 10% increase in upper esophageal sphincter relaxation duration.

As with many techniques, the available data on the potential benefits or risks associated with the application of NMES for dysphagia rehabilitation are not clear. Although many studies report positive gains, some report no benefit from the addition of NMES to behavioral therapy. Whereas some studies suggest movement of swallowing structures during application of NMES, other structures do not appear to be influenced. Most of these studies are limited by some common variables. With few exceptions, most studies have incorporated small numbers of subjects and many have weak scientific designs. Furthermore, many, if not most, have evaluated the clinical effect of NMES using unvalidated measurement tools. Given the positive clinical outcomes reported across several studies in the absence of reported complications, the application of NMES for dysphagia rehabilitation should be classified as promising but unclear until future, more rigorous studies contribute to our knowledge of the potential for this adjunctive modality.

PREVENTION IN DYSPHAGIA MANAGEMENT

Conceptually, prevention in dysphagia management can be viewed from two perspectives. A common goal of any dysphagia management (compensation or rehabilitation) is the avoidance or minimization of negative outcomes. From a broad perspective negative outcomes might include food or liquid restrictions, nutrition or hydration deficits, infections, and the more general category of reduced quality of life. In short, any dysphagia intervention should focus to improve functional oral intake while at the same minimizing (or completely avoiding) these negative outcomes.

The second perspective on prevention in dysphagia management is the prevention of dysphagia in high-risk populations. Initial work in this area has focused on preventing (or minimizing) dysphagia in patients treated with radiotherapy for head/neck cancer. Carroll et al.[187] reported improved swallowing mechanics after head and neck cancer treatment in patients who completed a simple program of swallowing exercises before receiving chemoradiotherapy. Carnaby-Mann et al.[188] reported preserved swallow function, less weight loss, preserved muscle mass, less xerostomia, and other health-related benefits in patients completing a simple swallow exercise program during the course of chemoradiation for head and neck cancer. Van der Molen et al.[189] did not identify the extent of benefit as patients in the Carnaby-Mann study but they did report that preventive exercises resulted in fewer patients on feeding tubes following medical therapy. Finally, Kotz et al.[190] reported no benefit from prophylactic swallowing exercises immediately but enhanced oral intake at 3 and 6 months following medical treatment. By 9 and 12 months following medical treatment, patients who did not perform prophylactic swallowing exercises were similar to those who did the exercises. These reports not only reflect the potential for positive benefits to be gained from exercise-based swallowing therapy, but they also represent a shift in dysphagia treatment. These reports strongly suggest the potential for exercise-based swallowing therapy to prevent or minimize dysphagia in clinical populations who are at risk to develop significant swallowing difficulties. Future efforts evaluating adherence with prophylactic therapy,[191] adequate amount of prophylactic swallowing therapy,[192] and other influential factors may lead to a broader approach to preventive swallowing intervention in a wider range of at risk populations.

Potential Future Directions

Much information has been presented in this chapter. Unfortunately, even this amount of information is likely insufficient to address the rich and growing body of information that pertains to the treatment of dysphagia. Clinical and translational research continues to yield new ideas that may be relevant to dysphagia therapy. Three focus points for future efforts in research surrounding dysphagia therapy might include the following areas. First, researchers and clinicians need to continue to evaluate the benefits and risks of traditional therapy techniques. More knowledge about techniques such as the chin tuck, Mendelsohn maneuver, effortful swallow, and others will give practicing clinicians much needed ammunition to select and apply these techniques on a best-practice basis. Second, further evaluation of exercise-based strategies for dysphagia rehabilitation is needed. Many swallowing difficulties are related to muscle weakness, but it is unlikely that all problems will respond to a single therapy. A better understanding of the exercise principles best suited for specific swallowing difficulties will help clinicians select the best available interventions for individual patients. Third, the potential applications of adjunctive modalities need to be considered and evaluated. Use of modalities is a relatively new aspect of dysphagia rehabilitation. Thus there is much to learn about which modalities may (or may not) be helpful to different aspects of dysphagia rehabilitation.

Other avenues of clinical research will emerge to help clinicians provide the best possible care to patients with dysphagia. As the evidence base for various clinical tools increases, the clinicians' skills and clinical outcomes will improve for many patients with dysphagia.

FINAL COMMENTS ON USING EVIDENCE

Information is not the same as evidence. Evidence is information that has been filtered systematically through scientific processes and meets minimum standards of rigor. The term evidence-based practice has become commonplace in the field of dysphagia rehabilitation. Earlier in this chapter clinically relevant questions regarding application of evidence were discussed. The concept of levels of evidence is discussed in Chapter 9 with details in Box 9-1. Although levels of evidence were not provided for each technique discussed in this chapter, most techniques are supported by some degree of evidence: primarily case reports, case control studies, or small cohort studies. This is a start; as a profession, speech-language pathologists are moving toward obtaining stronger evidence for therapeutic endeavors.[193] Clinicians can focus on simple but important questions in helping to choose appropriate clinical interventions. Perhaps the first consideration is whether information is published in credible journals or other formats. If so, does more than one publication exist? Replication of clinical findings is an important component of building supportive evidence. If information is not obtained in a published format, is it based on credible publications? This initial step provides some indication of the degree of scientific review. The levels of evidence described in Chapter 9 can be referenced in determining the strength of evidence supporting a given technique. However, given the overt recognition that most techniques have not been subjected to the highest levels of evidence, clinical practitioners still need to rely on some system to evaluate whether a given technique might be appropriate for a specific patient. The following questions, adapted from Sackett et al.,[194] may help with this process. These questions are not meant to be exhaustive. Rather they are intended as a starting point from which clinicians may evaluate information and evidence on the appropriateness of therapy techniques for specific patients. When reading available literature the following questions may be helpful in choosing a therapy technique:

1. Are the patients in the study similar to my patient?
2. Is the technique described in sufficient detail that I may use it in the same way?
3. Is the technique applied in an environment similar to the environment in which I practice (hospital, outpatient clinic, long-term care facility, other)?
4. Does the technique require technology that is available (or unavailable) to me?
5. Are the outcomes obtained in the study the same as (or similar to) those I want to obtain for my patient? What were the benefits to patients?
6. Are failures and reasons for failure described in the study? What are the risks to my patient?
7. Do I have the clinical skills to apply this technique as it is described in the study or is specific training required?

CLINICAL CASE EXAMPLE 10-1

A 70-year-old man had a brainstem stroke 2 years ago. The patient is receiving all nutrition by percutaneous gastrostomy (PEG) tube but attempts to swallow some liquids with reported intermittent success. Fluoroscopic evaluation indicates reduced pharyngeal constriction, reduced hyolaryngeal movement, and reduced PES opening. No aspiration is noted, and the patient is able to clear residue effectively by throat clearing and expectoration.

In searching for information on how to best approach the chronic dysphagia in this patient, you discover three published articles describing therapeutic experiences with long-term dysphagia in brainstem stroke. Two of the articles are from different centers and use slightly different approaches, although both incorporate a modification of the Mendelsohn maneuver and both use sEMG biofeedback to teach this technique and monitor physiologic progress. The third article is a summary of a retrospective outcome study from one of the centers reporting on a larger number of patients. Not all of these patients had brainstem strokes.

Interpretation

The strength of evidence in this case is a level IV. The first two studies are case series using the patients as historical controls. Both include a small number of patients and are retrospective. The fact that different centers reported similar results with similar patient groups reflects a degree of replication that strengthens the evidence.

An initial question is whether the patients described in these studies resemble your patient. This depends in large part on the detail of description of the patients in the articles and on the evaluation completed on your patient. This is essential if you are to apply the described techniques to your patient. Do the evaluation results, functional eating profile, chronicity, and other descriptive characteristics of the published patient groups resemble your patient? Also, was the technique applied in an environment similar to that of your patient? If your patient matches the published descriptions, the technique may be appropriate for your patient.

A second question might be whether the outcomes described in the articles are the same as those you want to achieve for your patient. How were these outcomes measured? Do you understand and can you use similar outcome measures? Did these outcome measures make sense in terms of the problems presented by your patient?

The next question might be, "Did I understand the treatment technique?" This depends on the details of the provided description in the publications. Did the therapy protocol make sense to you? Were specific steps described, including the frequency and number of repetitions for each application? In this instance, sEMG biofeedback was used. Is this equipment available to you? Do you have the skills to use this technology, or can you acquire them in a time frame that will allow you to use them with this specific patient? Was the application of the biofeedback to the therapy technique clearly explained in the articles? Can your patient use this technique as described in the articles?

A final consideration might be whether treatment failures were reported and described. Clinicians are acutely aware that not all treatments result in the same degree of improvement. It is important to know the characteristics of patients in whom therapy did not result in improvement and if possible, why there was no improvement.

It may not be possible to address all these questions based on the published literature. Practitioners face the task of addressing as many of these questions as possible before application of any technique. The closer the individual patient fits the profile of published descriptions, the stronger the argument in favor of applying that specific technique.

8. Is the technique pragmatically appropriate for my patient and environment (e.g., does it have time demands or intensity demands that exceed the reality of my workload or my patient's endurance or compliance)?

TAKE HOME NOTES

1. Evidence-based practice offers practitioners a systematic approach to improve clinical practice and enhance the care of individual patients. This approach involves finding, evaluating, and using scientific information.

2. Although most evidence supporting dysphagia intervention is not at the strongest levels, evidence does exist that can guide clinical practice and facilitate improved individual patient care.

3. Compensatory techniques are those intended for short-term use and that provide an adjustment to the swallowing pattern that has an immediate positive effect on safe, efficient swallowing. Rehabilitative techniques may not have an immediate effect but they contribute to reorganization of the impaired swallow, leading to improved functional swallowing once the technique is no longer applied. Prevention is a critical outcome of dysphagia therapy. Prevention may focus on minimizing negative outcomes or on preventing or minimizing dysphagia in at-risk populations.

4. Many factors should be considered before applying a therapy technique, including the technique, the patient, the environment, and the clinician. Not all techniques have been studied to the point of providing information on all of these factors. Clinical practitioners should consider many factors even in the face of limited evidence before applying a given therapy technique.

5. The functional effect of some therapy maneuvers is overtly evaluated during imaging studies. Others may require additional, adjunctive procedures (such as biofeedback) to evaluate, teach, and monitor the effect of the technique.

REFERENCES

1. Okada S, Saitoh E, Palmer JB, et al: What is the chin-down posture? A questionnaire survey of speech language pathologists in Japan and the United States. *Dysphagia* 22:204, 2007.
2. Logemann JA, Rademaker AW, Pauloski BR: Effects of postural change on aspiration in head and neck surgical patients. *Otolaryngol Head Neck Surg* 110:222, 1994.
3. Rasley A, Logemann JA, Kahrilas PJ, et al: Prevention of barium aspiration during videofluorographic swallowing studies: value of change in posture. *AJR Am J Roentgenol* 160:1005, 1993.
4. Logemann J: *Evaluation and treatment of swallowing disorders*, San Diego, 1983, College Hill Press.
5. Ohmae Y, Karaho T, Hanyu Y, et al: Effect of posture strategies on preventing aspiration. *Nippon Jibiinkoka Gakkai Kaiho* 100:220, 1997.
6. Johnsson F, Shaw D, Gabb M, et al: Influence of gravity and body position on normal oropharyngeal swallowing. *Am J Physiol* 269:G653, 1995.
7. Bernhard A, Pohl D, Fried M, et al: Influence of bolus consistency and position on esophageal high-resolution manometry findings. *Dig Dis Sci* 53:1198, 2008.
8. Tutuian R, Elton JP, Castell DO, et al: Effects of position on oesophageal function: studies using combined manometry and multichannel intraluminal impedance. *Neurogastroenterol Motil* 15:63, 2003.
9. Portale G, Peters J, Hsieh CC, et al: When are reflux episodes symptomatic? *Dis Esophagus* 20:47, 2007.
10. Johnson LF, DeMeester TR: Evaluation of elevation of the head of the bed, bethanechol, and antacid form tablets on gastroesophageal reflux. *Dig Dis Sci* 26:673, 1981.
11. Ekberg O: Posture of the head and pharyngeal swallowing. *Acta Radiol Diagn* 27:691, 1986.
12. Castell JA, Castell DO, Schultz AR, et al: Effect of head position on the dynamics of the upper esophageal sphincter and pharynx. *Dysphagia* 8:1, 1993.
13. Welch MV, Logemann JA, Rademaker AW, et al: Changes in pharyngeal dimensions effected by chin tuck. *Arch Phys Med Rehabil* 74:178, 1993.
14. Bülow M, Olsson R, Ekberg O: Videomanometric analysis of supraglottic swallow, effortful swallow and chin tuck in patients with pharyngeal dysfunction. *Dysphagia* 16:190, 2001.
15. Bülow M, Olsson R, Ekberg O: Supraglottic swallow, effortful swallow, and chin tuck did not alter hypopharyngeal intrabolus pressure in patients with pharyngeal dysfunction. *Dysphagia* 17:197, 2002.
16. Bülow M, Olsson R, Ekberg O: Videomanometric analysis of supraglottic swallow, effortful, and chin tuck in healthy volunteers. *Dysphagia* 14:67, 1999.
17. Ayuse T, Ayuse T, Ishitobi S, et al: Effect of reclining and chin-tuck position on coordination between respiration and swallowing. *J Oral Rehabil* 33:402, 2006.
18. Shanahan TK, Logemann JA, Rademaker AW, et al: Chin-down posture effect on aspiration in dysphagia patients. *Arch Phys Med Rehabil* 74:736, 1993.
19. Lewin JS, Hebert TM, Putnam JB, Jr, et al: Experience with the chin tuck maneuver in postesophagectomy aspirators. *Dysphagia* 16:216, 2001.
20. Logemann JA, Gensler G, Robbins J, et al: A randomized study of three interventions for aspiration of thin liquids in patients with dementia or Parkinson's disease. *J Speech Lang Hear Res* 51:173, 2008.
21. Zuydam AC, Rogers SN, Brown JS, et al: Swallowing rehabilitation after oro-pharyngeal resection for squamous cell carcinoma. *Br J Oral Maxillofac Surg* 38:513, 2000.
22. Robbins J, Gensler G, Hind J, et al: Comparison of 2 interventions for liquid aspiration on pneumonia incidence: a randomized trial. *Ann Intern Med* 148:509, 2008.
23. Kirchner JA: Pharyngeal and esophageal dysfunction: the diagnosis. *Minn Med* 50:921, 1967.
24. Logemann JA, Kahrilas PJ, Kobura M, et al: The benefit of head rotation on pharyngoesophageal dysphagia. *Arch Phys Med Rehabil* 70:767, 1989.

25. Tsukamoto Y: CT study of closure of the hemipharynx with head rotation in a case of lateral medullary syndrome. *Dysphagia* 15:17, 2000.

26. McCulloch TM, Hoffman MR, Ciucci MR: High-resolution manometry of pharyngeal swallow pressure events associated with head turn and chin tuck. *Ann Otol Rhinol Laryngol* 119:369, 2010.

27. Ohmae Y, Ogura M, Kitahara S, et al: Effects of head rotation on pharyngeal function during normal swallow. *Ann Otol Rhinol Laryngol* 107:344, 1998.

28. O'Gara JA: Dietary adjustments and nutritional therapy during treatment for oral-pharyngeal dysphagia. *Dysphagia* 4:209, 1990.

29. Pardoe EM: Development of a multistage diet for dysphagia. *J Am Diet Assoc* 93:568, 1993.

30. Penman JP, Thomson M: A review of the textured diets developed for the management of dysphagia. *J Hum Nutr Diet* 11:51, 1998.

31. Garcia JM, Chambers E, Molander M: Thickened liquids: practice patterns of speech-language pathologists. *Am J Speech Lang Pathol* 14:4, 2005.

32. Castellanos VH, Butler E, Gluch L, et al: Use of thickened liquids in skilled nursing facilities. *J Am Diet Assoc* 104:1222, 2004.

33. Kuhlemeier KV, Palmer JB, Rosenberg D: Effect of liquid bolus consistency and delivery method on aspiration and pharyngeal retention in dysphagia patients. *Dysphagia* 16:119, 2001.

34. Karagiannis MJ, Chivers L, Karagiannis TC: Effects of oral intake of water in patients with oropharyngeal dysphagia. *BMC Geriatr* 11:9, 2011.

35. Whelan K: Inadequate fluid intakes in dysphagic acute stoke. *Clin Nutr* 20:423, 2001.

36. Garon BR, Engle M, Ormiston C: A randomized control study to determine the effects of unlimited oral intake of water in patients with identified aspiration. *J Neurol Rehabil* 11:139, 1997.

37. Panther K: *Frazier Water Protocol: safety, hydration, and quality of life*, Rockville, MD, 2008, American Speech-Language-Hearing Association.

38. Karagiannis M, Karagiannis TC: Oropharyngeal dysphagia, free water protocol and quality of life: an update from a prospective clinical trial. *Hell J Nucl Med* Suppl 1:26, 2014.

39. Pouderoux P, Kahrilas PJ: Deglutitive tongue force modulation by volition, volume, and viscosity in humans. *Gastroenterology* 108:1418, 1995.

40. Chi-Fishman G, Sonies BC: Effects of systematic bolus viscosity and volume change on hyoid movement kinematics. *Dysphagia* 17:278, 2002.

41. Dantas RO, Dodds WJ, Massey BT, et al: The effect of high- vs low-density barium preparations in the quantitative features of swallowing. *AJR Am J Roentgenol* 153:1191, 1989.

42. Butler SG, Stuart A, Castell D, et al: Effects of age, gender, bolus condition, viscosity, and volume on pharyngeal and upper esophageal sphincter pressure and temporal measurements during swallowing. *J Speech Lang Hear Res* 52:240, 2009.

43. Clavé P, de Kraa M, Arreola V, et al: The effect of bolus viscosity on swallowing function in neurogenic dysphagia. *Aliment Pharmacol Ther* 24:1385, 2006.

44. Bülow M, Olsson R, Ekberg O: Videoradiographic analysis of how carbonated thin liquids and thickened liquids affect the physiology of swallowing in subjects with aspiration of thin liquids. *Acta Radiol* 44:366, 2004.

45. Sdravou K, Walshe M, Dagdilelis L: Effects of carbonated liquids on oropharyngeal swallowing measures in people with neurogenic dysphagia. *Dysphagia* 27:240, 2012.

46. Krival K, Bates C: Effects of club soda and ginger brew on linguapalatal pressures in healthy swallowing. *Dysphagia* 27:228, 2012.

47. Morishita M, Mori S, Yamagami S, et al: Effect of carbonated beverages on pharyngeal swallowing in young individuals and elderly inpatients. *Dysphagia* 29:213, 2014.

48. Logemann JA, Pauloski BR, Colangelo L, et al: Effects of a sour bolus on oropharyngeal swallowing measures in patients with neurogenic dysphagia. *J Speech Hear Res* 38:556, 1995.

49. Pelletier CA, Lawless HT: Effect of citric acid and citric acid-sucrose mixtures on swallowing in neurogenic oropharyngeal dysphagia. *Dysphagia* 18:231, 2003.

50. Chee C, Arshad S, Singh S, et al: The influence of chemical gustatory stimuli and oral anaesthesia on healthy human swallowing. *Chem Senses* 30:393, 2005.

51. Palmer PM, McCulloch TM, Jaffee D, et al: Effects of sour bolus on the intramuscular electromyographic (EMG) activity of muscles in the submental region. *Dysphagia* 20:210, 2005.

52. Pelletier CA, Dhanaraj GE: The effect of taste and palatability on lingual swallowing pressure. *Dysphagia* 21:121, 2006.

53. Miyaoka Y, Haishima K, Takagi M, et al: Influences of thermal and gustatory characteristics on sensory and motor aspects of swallowing. *Dysphagia* 21:38, 2005.

54. Matta Z, Changers E, Mertz Garcia J, et al: Sensory characteristics of beverages prepared with commercial thickeners used for dysphagia diets. *J Am Diet Assoc* 106:1049, 2006.

55. Feinberg MJ, Kneble J, Tully J: Prandial aspiration and pneumonia in an elderly population followed over 3 years. *Dysphagia* 11:104, 1996.

56. Shim JS, Oh BM, Han TR: Factors associated with compliance with viscosity-modified diet among dysphagic patients. *Ann Rehabil Med* 37:628, 2013.

57. Curran J, Groher ME: Development and dissemination of an aspiration risk reduction diet. *Dysphagia* 5:6, 1990.

58. Wright L, Cotter D, Hickson M, et al: Comparison of energy and protein intakes of older people consuming a texture modified diet with a normal hospital diet. *J Hum Nutr Diet* 18:213, 2005.

59. Germain I, Dufresne T, Gray-Donald K: A novel dysphagia diet improves the nutritional intake of institutionalized elders. *J Am Diet Assoc* 106:1614, 2006.

60. Crary MA, Carnaby GD, Shabbir Y, et al: *Clinical factors impacting dehydration risk in acute stroke*. Presentation to the World Stroke Congress, Istanbul, Turkey, October, 2014.

61. Groher ME, McKaig N: Dysphagia and dietary levels in skilled nursing facilities. *J Am Geriatr Soc* 43:528, 1995.

62. National Dysphagia Diet Taskforce: *The National Dysphagia Diet: standardization for optimal tare*, Chicago, 2002, American Dietetic Association.

63. Strowd L, Kyzima J, Pillsbury D, et al: Dysphagia dietary guidelines and the rheology of nutritional feeds and barium test feeds. *Chest* 133:1397, 2008.

64. Hall G, Wendin K: Sensory design of foods for the elderly. *Ann Nutr Metab* 52(Suppl 1):25, 2008.

65. Stathopoulos E, Duchan JF: History and principles of exercise-based therapy: how they inform our current treatment. *Semin Speech Lang* 27:227, 2006.

66. Carnaby GD, Harenberg L: What is "usual care" in dysphagia rehabilitation: a survey of USA dysphagia practice patterns. *Dysphagia* 28:567, 2013.

67. Lazarus C, Logemann JA, Huang CF, et al: Effects of two types of tongue strengthening exercises in young normals. *Folia Phoniatr Logop* 55:199, 2003.

68. Robbins J, Gangnon RE, Theis SM, et al: The effects of lingual exercise on swallowing in older adults. *J Am Geriatr Soc* 53:1483, 2005.

69. Robbins J, Kays SA, Gangnon RE, et al: The effects of lingual exercise in stroke patients with dysphagia. *Arch Phys Med Rehabil* 88:150, 2007.

70. Hagg M, Anniko M: Lip muscle training in stroke patients with dysphagia. *Acta Otolaryngol* 128:1027, 2008.

71. Shaker R, Dodds W, Dantas R, et al: Coordination of deglutitive glottic closure with oropharyngeal swallowing. *Gastroenterology* 98:1478, 1990.

72. Mendelsohn M, Martin RE: Airway protection during breath holding. *Ann Otol Rhinol Laryngol* 102:941, 1993.

73. Hirst LJ, Sama A, Carding PN, et al: Is a "safe swallow" really safe? *Int J Lang Commun Disord* 33(Suppl):279, 1998.

74. Donzelli J, Brady S: The effects of breath-holding on vocal fold adduction: implications for safe swallowing. *Arch Otolaryngol Head Neck Surg* 130:208, 2004.

75. Martin BJ, Logemann JA, Shaker R, et al: Normal laryngeal valving patterns during three breath hold maneuvers: a pilot investigation. *Dysphagia* 8:11, 1993.

76. Flaherty RF, Seltzer S, Campbell T, et al: Dynamic magnetic resonance imaging of vocal cord closure during deglutition. *Gastroenterology* 109:843, 1995.

77. Bodén K, Hallgren A, Witt Hedström H: Effects of three different swallow maneuvers analyzed by videomanometry. *Acta Radiol* 47:628, 2006.

78. Ohmae Y, Logemann JA, Kaiser P, et al: Effects of two breath-holding maneuvers on oropharyngeal swallow. *Ann Otol Rhinol Laryngol* 105:123, 1996.

79. Miller JL, Watkin KL: Lateral pharyngeal wall motion during swallowing using real time ultrasound. *Dysphagia* 12:125, 1997.

80. Lazarus C, Logemann JA, Song CW, et al: Effects of voluntary maneuvers on tongue base function for swallowing. *Folia Phoniatr Logop* 54:171, 2002.

81. Logemann JA, Pauloski BR, Rademaker AW, et al: Super-supraglottic swallow in irradiated head and neck cancer patients. *Head Neck* 19:535, 1997.

82. Hamlet S, Mathog R, Fleming S, et al: Modification of compensatory swallowing in a supraglottic laryngectomy patient. *Head Neck* 12:131, 1990.

83. Lazarus C, Logemann JA, Gibbons P: Effects of maneuvers on swallowing function in a dysphagic oral cancer patient. *Head Neck* 15:419, 1993.

84. Lazarus C: Effects of radiation therapy and voluntary maneuvers on swallowing function in head and neck cancer patients. *Clin Commun Disord* 3:11, 1993.

85. Chaudhuri G, Hildner CD, Brady S, et al: Cardiovascular effects on the supraglottic and super-supraglottic swallowing maneuvers in stroke patients with dysphagia. *Dysphagia* 17:19, 2002.

86. Kahrilas PJ, Logemann JA, Krugler C, et al: Volitional augmentation of upper esophageal sphincter opening during swallowing. *Am J Physiol* 260:G450, 1991.

87. Jaffe DM, Van Daele DJ, Rao SSC, et al: Contribution of cricopharyngeal muscle activity to upper esophageal sphincter manometry in the normal swallow and Mendelsohn's maneuver [abstract]. *Dysphagia* 15:101, 2001.

88. Ding R, Larson CR, Logemann JA, et al: Surface electromyographic and electroglottalgraphic studies in normal subjects under two swallow conditions: normal and during the Mendelsohn maneuver. *Dysphagia* 17:1, 2002.

89. Fukuoka T, Ono T, Hori K, et al: Effect of the effortful swallow and the Mendelsohn maneuver on tongue pressure production against the hard palate. *Dysphagia* 28:539, 2013.

90. Hoffman MR, Mielens JD, Ciucci MR, et al: High-resolution manometry of pharyngeal swallow pressure events associated with effortful swallow and the Mendelsohn maneuver. *Dysphagia* 27:418, 2012.

91. O'Rourke A, Morgan LB, Coss-Adame E, et al: The effect of voluntary pharyngeal swallowing maneuvers on esophageal swallowing physiology. *Dysphagia* 29:262, 2014.

92. McCullough GH, Kim Y: Effects of Mendelsohn maneuver on extent of hyoid movement and UES opening post-stroke. *Dysphagia* 28:511, 2013.

93. Neumann S, Bartolome G, Buchholz D, et al: Swallowing therapy of neurologic patients: correlation of outcome with pretreatment variables and therapeutic method. *Dysphagia* 10:1, 1995.

94. Crary MA: A direct intervention program for chronic neurogenic dysphagia secondary to brainstem stroke. *Dysphagia* 10:6, 1995.

95. Crary MA, Carnaby-Mann GD, Groher ME, et al: Functional benefits of dysphagia therapy using adjunctive biofeedback. *Dysphagia* 19:160, 2004.

96. Huckabee ML, Cannito MP: Outcomes of swallowing rehabilitation in chronic brainstem dysphagia: a retrospective evaluation. *Dysphagia* 14:93, 1999.

97. Hind JA, Nicosia MA, Roecker EB, et al: Comparison of effortful and noneffortful swallows in healthy middle-aged and older adults. *Arch Phys Med Rehabil* 82:1661, 2001.

98. Huckabee ML, Butler SG, Barclay M, et al: Submental surface electromyographic measurement and pharyngeal pressures during normal and effortful swallowing. *Arch Phys Med Rehabil* 86:2144, 2005.

99. Hiss SG, Huckabee ML: Timing of pharyngeal and upper esophageal sphincter pressures as a function of normal and effortful swallowing in young healthy adults. *Dysphagia* 20:149, 2005.

100. Huckabee ML, Steele CM: An analysis of lingual contribution to submental surface electromyographic measures and pharyngeal pressure during effortful swallow. *Arch Phys Med Rehabil* 87:1067, 2006.

101. Steele CM, Huckabee ML: The influence of oralingual pressure on the timing of pharyngeal pressure events. *Dysphagia* 22:30, 2007.

102. Witte U, Huckabee ML, Doeltgen SH, et al: The effect of effortful swallow on pharyngeal manometric measurements during saliva and water swallowing in healthy participants. *Arch Phys Med Rehabil* 89:822, 2008.

103. Takasaki K, Umeki H, Hara M, et al: Influence of effortful swallow on pharyngeal pressure: evaluation using a high-resolution manometry. *Otolaryngol Head Neck Surg* 144:16, 2011.

104. Fritz M, Cerrati E, Fang Y, et al: Magnetic resonance imaging of the effortful swallow. *Ann Otol Rhinol Laryngol* 123:786, 2014.

105. Fukuoka T, Ono T, Hori K, et al: Effect of effortful swallow and the Mendelsohn maneuver on tongue pressure production against the hard palate. *Dysphagia* 28:539, 2013.

106. Clark HM, Shelton N: Training effects of the effortful swallow under three exercise conditions. *Dysphagia* 29:553, 2014.

107. Lever TE, Cox KT, Holbert D, et al: The effect of an effortful swallow on the normal adult esophagus. *Dysphagia* 22:312, 2007.

108. Nekl CG, Lintzenich CR, Leng X, et al: Effects of effortful swallow on esophageal function in healthy adults. *Neurogastroenterol Motil* 24:252, 2012.

109. O'Rourke A, Morgan LB, Coss-Adame E, et al: The effect of voluntary pharyngeal swallow maneuvers on esophageal swallowing physiology. *Dysphagia* 29:262, 2014.

110. Carnaby-Mann GD, Crary MA: Adjunctive neuromuscular electrical stimulation for treatment-refractory dysphagia. *Ann Oto Rhinol Laryngol* 117:279, 2008.

111. Robbins JA, Logemann JA, Kirshner HS: Swallowing and speech production in Parkinson's disease. *Ann Neurol* 19:283, 1986.

112. Dziadziola J, Hamlet S, Michou G, et al: Multiple swallows and piecemeal deglutition; observations from normal adults and patients with head and neck cancer. *Dysphagia* 7:8, 1992.

113. Leslie P, Drinnan MJ, Ford GA, et al: Swallow respiration patterns in dysphagia patients following acute stroke. *Dysphagia* 17:202, 2002.

114. Nilsson H, Ekberg O, Olsson R, et al: Quantitative aspects of swallowing in an elderly population. *Dysphagia* 11:180, 1996.

115. Fujui M, Logemann JA, Pauloski BR: Increased postoperative posterior pharyngeal wall movement in patients with anterior oral cancer: preliminary findings and possible implications for treatment. *Am J Speech Lang Pathol* 4:24, 1995.

116. Fujui M, Logemann JA: Effect of a tongue holding maneuver on posterior pharyngeal wall movement during deglutition. *Am J Speech Lang Pathol* 5:23, 1996.

117. Fujui-Kurachi M: Developing the tongue holding maneuver. *Dysphagia* 11:9, 2002.

118. Doeltgen SH, Witte U, Gumbley F, et al: Evaluation of manometric measures during tongue-hold swallows. *Am J Speech Lang Pathol* 18:65, 2009.

119. Doeltgen SH, Macrae P, Huckabee ML: Pharyngeal pressure generation during tongue-hold swallows across age groups. *Am J Speech Lang Pathol* 20:124, 2011.

120. Hammer MJ, Jones CA, Mielens JD, et al: Evaluating the tongue-hold maneuver using high-resolution manometry and electromyography. *Dysphagia* 29:564, 2014.

121. Fujiu-Kurachi M, Fujiwara S, Tamine K, et al: Tongue pressure generation during tongue-hold swallows in young healthy adults measured with different tongue positions. *Dysphagia* 29:17, 2014.

122. Shaker R, Kern M, Bardan E, et al: Augmentation of deglutitive upper esophageal sphincter opening in the elderly by exercise. *Am J Physiol* 272:G1518, 1997.

123. Shaker R, Easterling C, Kern M, et al: Rehabilitation of swallowing by exercise in tube-fed patients with pharyngeal dysphagia secondary to abnormal UES opening. *Gastroenterology* 122:1314, 2002.

124. Antunes EB, Lunet N: Effects of the head lift exercise on the swallow function: a systematic review. *Gerodontology* 29:247, 2012.

125. Ferdjallah M, Wertsch J, Shaker R: Spectral analysis of surface EMG of upper esophageal sphincter opening muscles during head lift exercise. *J Rehabil Res Dev* 37:335, 2000.

126. White KT, Easterling C, Roberts N, et al: Fatigue analysis before and after shaker exercise: physiologic tool for exercise design. *Dysphagia* 23:385, 2008.

127. Mepani R, Antonik S, Massey B, et al: Augmentation of deglutitive thyrohyoid muscle shortening by the shaker exercise. *Dysphagia* 24:26, 2009.

128. Yoshida M, Groher ME, Crary MA, et al: Comparison of surface electromyographic (sEMG) activity of submental muscles between the head lift and tongue press exercises as a therapeutic exercise for pharyngeal dysphagia. *Gerodontology* 24:111, 2007.

129. Watts CR: Measurement of hyolaryngeal muscle activation using surface electromyography for comparison of two rehabilitative dysphagia exercises. *Arch Phy Med Rehabil* 94:2542, 2013.

130. Yoon WL, Khoo JKP, Liow SJR: Chin tuck against resistance (CTAR): a new method for enhancing suprahyoid muscle activity using a Shaker-type exercise. *Dysphagia* 29:243, 2014.

131. Wada S, Tohara H, Iida T, et al: Jaw-opening exercise for insufficient opening of upper esophageal sphincter. *Arch Phy Med Rehabil* 93:1995, 2012.

132. Easterling C, Grande B, Kern M, et al: Attaining and maintaining isometric and isokinetic goals of the Shaker exercise. *Dysphagia* 20:133, 2005.

133. Pommerenke W: A study of the sensory areas eliciting the swallowing reflex. *Am J Physiology* 84:36, 1928.

134. Lazzara GL, Lazarus C, Logemann JA: Impact of thermal stimulation on the triggering of the swallowing reflex. *Dysphagia* 1:73, 1986.

135. Regan J, Walshe M, Tobin WO: Immediate effects of thermal-tactile stimulation on timing of swallow in idiopathic Parkinson's disease. *Dysphagia* 25:207, 2012.

136. Rosenbek J, Robbins J, Fishback B, et al: Effects of thermal application on dysphagia after stroke. *J Speech Hear Res* 34:1257, 1991.

137. Rosenbek J, Roecker EB, Wood JL, et al: Thermal application reduces the duration of stage transition in dysphagia after stroke. *Dysphagia* 11:225, 1996.

138. Rosenbek J, Robbins J, Willford WO, et al: Comparing treatment intensities of tactile-thermal application. *Dysphagia* 13:1, 1998.

139. Kaatzke-McDonald MN, Post E, Davis PJ, et al: The effects of cold, touch, and chemical stimulation of the anterior faucial pillar on human swallowing. *Dysphagia* 11:198, 1996.

140. Sciortino K, Liss JM, Case JL, et al: Effects of mechanical, cold, gustatory, and combined stimulation to the human anterior faucial pillars. *Dysphagia* 18:16, 2003.

141. Knauer CM, Castell JA, Dalton CB, et al: Pharyngeal/upper esophageal sphincter pressure dynamics in humans: effects of pharmacologic agents and thermal stimulation. *Dig Dis Sci* 35:774, 1990.

142. Ali GN, Laundl TM, Wallace KL, et al: Influence of cold stimulation on the normal pharyngeal swallow response. *Dysphagia* 11:2, 1996.

143. Clark HM: Neuromuscular treatments for speech and swallowing: a tutorial. *Am J Speech Lang Pathol* 12:400, 2003.

144. Burkhead LM, Sapienza C, Rosenbek J: Strength-training exercise in dysphagia rehabilitation: principles, procedures, and directions for future research. *Dysphagia* 22:251, 2007.

145. Crary MA, Carnaby GD: Adoption into clinical practice of two therapies to manage swallowing disorders: exercise-based swallow rehabilitation and electrical stimulation. *Curr Opin Otolaryngol Head Neck Surg* 22:172, 2014.

146. LaGorio LA, Carnaby-Mann GD, Crary MA: Cross-system effects of dysphagia treatment on dysphonia: a case report. *Cases J* 1:67, 2008.

147. Easterling C: Does exercise aimed at improving swallow function have an effect on vocal function in the healthy elderly? *Dysphagia* 23:317, 2008.

148. El Sharkawi A, Ramig L, Logemann J, et al: Swallowing and voice effects of Lee Silverman Voice Treatment (LSVT): a pilot study. *J Neurol Neurosurg Psychiatry* 72:31, 2002.

149. Carnaby-Mann GD, Crary MA: *A case-control evaluation of the McNeill Dysphagia Therapy Program (MDTP)*. Presented at the Dysphagia Research Society, New Orleans, March 2009.

150. Crary MA, Carnaby GD, LaGorio L, et al: Functional and physiological outcomes from an exercise-based dysphagia therapy: a pilot investigation of the McNeill Dysphagia Therapy Program. *Arch Phys Med Rehabil* 93:1173, 2012.

151. Lan Y, Ohkubo M, Berretin-Felix G, et al: Normalization of temporal aspects of swallowing physiology after the McNeill Dysphagia Therapy Program. *Ann Otol Rhinol Laryngol* 141:525, 2012.

152. Carnaby G, LaGorio L, Miller D, et al: *A randomized, double blind trial of neuromuscular electrical stimulation+ McNeill Dysphagia Therapy (MDTP) after stroke (ANSRS)*. Paper presented at Dysphagia Research Society. Toronto CA, March 8, 2012.

153. Mulder T, Hulstyn W: Sensory feedback therapy and theoretical knowledge of motor control and learning. *Am J Phys Med* 63:226, 1984.

154. Crary MA, Groher ME: Basic concepts of surface electromyographic biofeedback in the treatment of dysphagia: a tutorial. *Am J Speech Lang Pathol* 9:116, 2000.

155. Haynes SN: Electromyographic biofeedback treatment of a woman with chronic dysphagia. *Biofeedback Self Regul* 1:121, 1976.

156. Lichstein KL, Eakin TL, Dunn ME: Combined psychological and medical treatment of oropharyngeal dysphagia. *Clin Biofeedback Health Int J* 9:9, 1986.

157. Bryant M: Biofeedback in the treatment of a selected dysphagic patient. *Dysphagia* 6:140, 1991.

158. Crary MA, Carnaby-Mann GD, Groher ME, et al: Functional benefits of dysphagia therapy using adjunctive sEMG biofeedback. *Dysphagia* 19:160, 2004.

159. Athukorala RP, Jones RD, Sella O, et al: Skill training for swallowing rehabilitation in patients with Parkinson's disease. *Arch Phys Med Rehabil* 95:1374, 2014.

160. Logemann JA, Kahrilas PJ: Relearning to swallow after stroke—application of maneuvers and indirect biofeedback: a case study. *Neurology* 40:1136, 1990.

161. Denk DM, Kaider A: Videoendoscopic biofeedback: a simple method to improve the efficacy of swallowing rehabilitation of patients after head and neck surgery. *ORL J Otorhinolaryngol Relat Spec* 59:100, 1997.

162. Sheffler LR, Chae J: Neuromuscular electrical stimulation in neurorehabilitation. *Muscle Nerve* 35:562, 2007.

163. Freed ML, Freed L, Chatburn RL, et al: Electrical stimulation for swallowing disorders caused by stroke. *Respir Care* 46:466, 2001.

164. Leelamint V, Limsakul C, Geater A: Synchronized electrical stimulation in treating pharyngeal dysphagia. *Laryngoscope* 112:2204, 2002.

165. Blumenfeld L, Hahn Y, LePage A, et al: Transcutaneous electrical stimulation versus traditional dysphagia therapy: a noncurrent cohort study. *Otolaryngol Head Neck Surg* 135:754, 2006.

166. Shaw GY, Sechtem PR, Searl J, et al: Transcutaneous neuromuscular electrical stimulation (VitalStim) curative therapy for severe dysphagia: myth or reality? *Ann Otol Rhinol Laryngol* 116:36, 2007.

167. Oh BM, Kim DY, Paik NJ: Recovery of swallowing function is accompanied by the expansion of the cortical map. *Int J Neurosci* 117:1215, 2007.

168. Baijens LW, Speyer R, Roodenburg N, et al: The effects of neuromuscular electrical stimulation for dysphagia in opercular syndrome: a case study. *Eur Arch Otorhinolaryngol* 265:825, 2008.

169. Ryu JS, Kang JY, Park JY, et al: The effect of electrical stimulation therapy on dysphagia following treatment for head and neck cancer. *Oral Oncol* 45:665, 2009.

170. Kushner DS, Peters K, Eroglu ST, et al: Neuromuscular electrical stimulation efficacy in acute stroke feeding tube-dependent dysphagia during inpatient rehabilitation. *Am J Phys Med Rehabil* 92:486, 2013.

171. Bhatt AD, Goodwin N, Cash E, et al: Impact of transcutaneous neuromuscular electrical stimulation on dysphagia in head and neck cancer patients treated with definitive chemoradiation. *Head Neck* 2014. [epub ahead of print].

172. Crary MA, Carnaby-Mann GD, Faunce A: Electrical stimulation therapy for dysphagia: descriptive results for two surveys. *Dysphagia* 22:165, 2007.

173. Kiger M, Brown CS, Watkins L: Dysphagia management: an analysis of patient outcomes using VitalStim therapy compared to traditional swallow therapy. *Dysphagia* 21:243, 2006.

174. Bülow M, Speyer R, Baijens L, et al: Neuromuscular electrical stimulation (NMES) in stroke patients with oral and pharyngeal dysphagia. *Dysphagia* 23:302, 2008.

175. Baijens LW, Speyer R, Passos VL, et al: Surface electrical stimulation in dysphagia Parkinson patients: a randomized clinical trial. *Laryngoscope* 123:E38, 2013.

176. Tan C, Liu Y, Li W, et al: Transcutaneous neuromuscular electrical stimulation can improve swallowing function in patients with dysphagia caused by non-stroke diseases: a meta-analysis. *J Oral Rehabil* 40:472, 2013.

177. Carnaby GD, LaGorio L, Miller D, et al: *A randomized double blind trial of neuromuscular electrical stimulation + McNeill dysphagia therapy (MDTP) after stroke (ANSRS)*. Presentation to the Dysphagia Research Society Annual Meeting, Toronto, Canada, March 2012.

178. Suiter DM, Leder SB, Ruark JL: Effects of neuromuscular electrical stimulation on submental muscle activity. *Dysphagia* 21:56, 2006.

179. Humbert IA, Poletto CJ, Saxon KG, et al: The effect of surface electrical stimulation on hyolaryngeal movement in normal individuals at rest and during swallowing. *J Appl Physiol* 101:1657, 2006.

180. Ludlow CL, Humbert IA, Saxon K, et al: Effects of surface electrical stimulation both at rest and during swallowing in chronic pharyngeal dysphagia. *Dysphagia* 22:1, 2007.

181. Park JW, Kim Y, Oh JC, et al: Effortful swallowing training combined with electrical stimulation in post-stroke dysphagia: a randomized controlled study. *Dysphagia* 27:521, 2012.

182. Berretin-Felix G, Carnaby GD, et al: *NMES immediate effects on swallow physiology in younger vs older healthy volunteers.*

Presentation to the Dysphagia Research Society Annual Meeting, San Antonio, Texas, March, 2011.

183. Nam HS, Beom J, Oh BM, et al: Kinematic effects of hyolaryngeal electrical stimulation therapy on hyoid excursion and laryngeal elevation. *Dysphagia* 28:548, 2013.

184. Furuta T, Takemura M, Tsujita J, et al: Interferential electric stimulation applied to the neck increases swallowing frequency. *Dysphagia* 27:94, 2012.

185. Heck FM, Doeltgen SH, Huckabee ML: Effects of submental neuromuscular electrical stimulation on pharyngeal pressure generation. *Arch Phys Med Rehabil* 93:2000, 2012.

186. Jungheim M, Janhsen AM, Miller S, et al: Impact of neuromuscular electrical stimulation on upper esophageal sphincter dynamics: a high-resolution manometry study. *Ann Otol Rhinol Laryngol* 124:5, 2015.

187. Carroll WR, Locher JL, Canon CL, et al: Pretreatment swallowing exercises improved swallow function after chemoradiation. *Laryngoscope* 118:39, 2008.

188. Carnaby-Mann GD, Crary MA, Schmalfuss I, et al: "Pharyngocise": randomized controlled trial of preventative exercises to maintain muscle structure and swallowing function during head-and-neck chemoradiotherapy. *Int J Radiat Oncol Biol Phys* 83:210, 2012.

189. Van der Molen L, van Rossum MA, Burkhead LM, et al: A randomized preventive rehabilitation trial in advanced head and neck cancer patients treated with chemoradiotherapy: feasibility, compliance, and short-term effects. *Dysphagia* 26:155, 2011.

190. Kotz T, Federman AD, Kao J, et al: Prophylactic swallowing exercises in patients with head and neck cancer undergoing chemoradiation: a randomized trial. *Arch Otolaryngol Head Neck Surg* 138:376, 2012.

191. Shinn EH, Basen-Engquist K, Baum G, et al: Adherence to preventive exercises and self-reported swallowing outcomes in postradiation head and neck cancer patients. *Head Neck* 35:1707, 2013.

192. Carnaby GD, Crary MA, Amdur R, et al: *Dysphagia prevention exercises in head neck cancer: pharyngocise dose response study.* Presentation to the Dysphagia Research Society, Toronto, Canada, March 2012.

193. Carnaby G, Madhavan A: A systematic review of randomized controlled trials in the field of dysphagia rehabilitation. *Curr Phys Med Rehabil Rep* 1:197, 2013.

194. Sackett DL, Haynes RB, Guyatt GH, et al: *Clinical epidemiology: a basic science for clinical medicine*, ed 2, Boston, 1991, Little, Brown.

CHAPTER 11
Ethical Considerations

Michael E. Groher

To view additional case videos and content, please visit the evolve website.

CHAPTER OBJECTIVES

1. Present the basic principles of medical ethics as they relate to the swallowing-impaired patient.
2. Discuss the risks and benefits of alternative types of feeding.
3. Highlight the differences between factors that predict aspiration and those that predict aspiration pneumonia.
4. Present an approach for weaning from feeding tubes.
5. Present examples of ethical dilemmas resulting from the placement or retention of alternative forms of feeding.

MEDICAL ETHICS

The Patient Self-Determination Act took effect on December 1, 1991. The act established guidelines to allow patients to participate fully in decisions regarding their health care, particularly decisions made in circumstances of severe or terminal illness. The act strives to establish a patient–physician interaction that allows both parties to balance individual morals and values against the known risks and benefits of proposed medical care. For example, patients might want to decide under which circumstances they would want to be resuscitated or whether they would want to be nourished by a feeding tube to sustain life. Counseling patients, families, and caregivers on the risks and benefits of tube feeding may involve the expertise of the dysphagia specialist.[1] One study found that speech-language pathologists (SLPs) who manage patients with dementia are involved in the decision making in 65% of cases when the recommendation is made for some type of alternative nutrition.[2]

Medical ethics is a subspecialty of medical care that brings together patients, caregivers, and nonmedical and medical professionals in an effort to make the best decision regarding a health care issue. The decision rests on the understanding that it is finalized by balancing data from individual and societal morals and values, evidence-based medical knowledge, and legal precedent. Ethical dilemmas result when balance is not achieved—when one party is not in agreement with the plan of care. For example, a patient may not agree to the short-term use of a nasogastric tube (NGT) for feeding because of religious objections, although the medical team is convinced that it may save or prolong the patient's life. These dilemmas need to be resolved and may be referred to the medical center's ethics committee. Solutions generally are possible with a rational analysis of (1) how the patient came to establish his or her health care preferences; (2) the medical risks and benefits of a proposed intervention; (3) the burdens that medical intervention might bear on the patient and family; (4) the effect on the patient's and family's quality of life; and (5) any legal constraints, such as the patient being incapable of making an informed decision.

Advance Directives

The advance directive (AD) is a statement made by a person with decision-making capacity indicating his or her preferences for receiving medical treatment or not receiving medical treatment under certain circumstances. When a person is admitted to a medical setting, the patient is automatically given the option to execute an AD. Admission is not contingent on signing an AD, and patients frequently do not. Any member of the health care team may initiate the document if he or she thinks it will facilitate the patient's care. If an AD has already been executed, either from another admission or as a document the patient executed in the past, it will be placed prominently in the medical record so the medical team can be guided by the patient's wishes in the event of a medical crisis. Most often an AD is specific to end-of-life decisions or circumstances when an individual's medical condition is futile. Typically, the AD has two parts: a living will and a durable power of attorney for health care. The living will is a written request to forego some type of medical treatment in a terminal or irreversible medical condition. The durable power of attorney for health care appoints a person (**surrogate**) to act in the patient's behalf on end-of-life or irreversible conditions should the patient be in a state that he or she is not competent to make an informed decision. It is understood that the surrogate will have prior knowledge of the patient's desires and therefore will act in the patient's best interest. Patients with terminal, progressive diseases should be encouraged to execute an AD while they are competent and free from severe disease to facilitate end-stage medical care. Making decisions about tube feeding when the patient is in a crisis often clouds a rational decision and may complicate medical care (Review Clinical Corners 11-1 and 11-2).

TUBE FEEDING

Because most ethical dilemmas that the swallowing specialist faces center on the use or denial of tube feeding, it is important to understand the risks and benefits of this intervention. Tube feeding entails psychological and medical risks and benefits.

There are two major categories of nonoral nutritional provision: enteral and parenteral. Nonoral parenteral feedings are sometimes collectively referred to as hyperalimentation.

Enteral Nutrition

The major types of enteral tube feeding include nasogastric, gastrostomy, and jejunostomy. Specially prepared high-

---

> **CLINICAL CORNER 11-1: STOP FEEDING?**
>
> A patient's surrogate told the medical care team that she wants to discontinue her husband's oral feeding because she has noticed as she assists him at mealtime that he has considerable choking episodes. Based on the patient's clinical and imaging swallowing evaluations, the treatment team believes that he should be able to continue eating orally.
>
> **Critical Thinking**
> 1. What is the next step for the treatment team? What are some options?
> 2. If the wife and the treatment team disagree after reviewing the case, who will make the final decision?

> **CLINICAL CORNER 11-2: ALS AND ASPIRATION**
>
> A 58-year-old man has a 3-year history of amyotrophic lateral sclerosis. A swallowing study has shown that he aspirates with a weak cough on all consistencies. Although the patient does not have an AD, he is adamant that he wants to continue eating orally.
>
> **Critical Thinking**
> 1. You are the SLP. Make a case for letting the patient continue to eat.
> 2. If the patient becomes ill in the future and takes you to court for encouraging him to eat, what defense will you have, and how will you prove it?

calorie formulas are delivered through the tube into the feeding site. They are delivered from a syringe, a plastic bag that hangs above the level of the tube site, or a mechanical pump.

Nasogastric Tubes

Tubes that are inserted through the nose and into the stomach can be used to deliver nutrients or suction unwanted secretions. Tubes that provide nutrition are NGTs. They range in diameter from 8 to 18 Fr. Usually the larger the diameter (18 Fr), the stiffer and more uncomfortable the tube is in the nose and throat. Larger NGTs are necessary for passing medications and pureed foods. They do not clog as much with these materials as do smaller bore tubes. Smaller bore tubes take thin liquid formulas, sometimes are prone to clogging and dislodgment, and generally are more comfortable in the aerodigestive tract. Smaller bore tubes that are weighted on the tip for ease of passage are called Dobhoff tubes.

The NGT is inserted through the nostril into the pharynx, through the pharyngeal esophageal segment (PES) into the esophagus, and finally through the lower esophageal segment into the stomach. In some cases it is passed beyond the stomach, through the pyloric valve, and into the jejunum as a method to avoid complications from gastric reflux. A special radiograph (kidney-ureter-bladder) is ordered to ensure that the tube is positioned correctly in the aerodigestive tract before feeding begins. NGTs are used in acute medical situations that render the individual unable to swallow or to sustain nutrition orally. An NGT is used for feeding when the medical care team believes that the patient's medical status has a good chance to improve in a short period. Although the length of time for use of an NGT is not prescribed, if a patient requires enteral feeding for longer than 3 or 4 weeks, another enteral feeding method usually is selected. More permanent options that are still reversible include gastrostomy or jejunostomy feeding tubes. These tubes can be placed surgically (usually requiring general anesthesia for the patient) or endoscopically (requiring light anesthesia). Endoscopic placements are called percutaneous endoscopic gastrostomy (PEG) or **percutaneous endoscopic jejunostomy**.

Gastrostomy and Jejunostomy Tubes

The gastrostomy tube is placed directly into the stomach with the assumption that the digestive processes of the stomach are intact. Formula is passed through a catheter that sits on the outside of the stomach. If the stomach is not functioning, the feeding tube may need to be placed into the jejunum of the small intestine. Because the stomach is bypassed, specialized, predigested formulas are required for jejunal tube feedings. Some clinicians argue that jejunal placement reduces the risk of reflux of the tube-fed material into the pharynx because the pyloric valve provides an additional barrier to retropulsion of stomach contents into the esophagus. However, the experimental evidence does not clearly support this contention.[3] Marik and Zaloga did a **systematic review** of eight studies that compared pre- and postpyloric feedings.[4] Their review showed no differences in pneumonia rates, mortality, percentage of caloric goals achieved, and intensive care admissions between the two groups. Table 11-1 summarizes the medical risks and benefits of enteral tube feeding.

Parenteral Nutrition

Parenteral nutrition is indicated when the gastrointestinal tract cannot be used because of medical complications such as gastroparesis, obstruction, or bleeding. Total parenteral nutrition (TPN) is a specialized formula that most commonly is delivered into a central vein (subclavian or internal jugular). Although there are potential medical complications from this therapy, such as **pneumothorax**, patients can be supported nutritionally with this formula for 4 to 6 weeks if necessary.[5] Peripheral parenteral nutrition (PPN) is a form of nutritional support delivered through a peripheral vein. Because of potential medical complications, this therapy can be used effectively for only 7 to 10

TABLE 11-1 Medical Risks and Benefits Associated with Enteral Tube Feeding

Risks	Benefits
Nasogastric	
Uncomfortable	Easy insertion
Poor cosmesis	No anesthesia
Distends PES and LES; may promote reflux	Tube can be small bore; well tolerated
Nasal ulceration	Good short-term nutrition
Sinusitis	Patient can eat with tube in place
Delays swallow	
May trigger vagal bradycardia Easy for patient to dislodge	
Gastrostomy	
Requires surgical placement	Good long-term option
Infection and care at tube site	Out of visual sight
Tube may fall out	Easy tube replacement
Reflux if stomach fills too fast	Easily removed
Diarrhea	Patient can eat with tube in place
Jejunostomy	
Requires surgical placement	May reduce reflux
Needs continuous drip feeding	Out of visual sight
Requires hospital visit if dislodged	Good nutrition if stomach not available
Intolerance of special formula	Low risk of blockage compared to NG tube
PEG or Jejunostomy	
Aspiration during procedure	Inserted under local anesthesia
Infection at tube site	Generally well tolerated
Potential for reflux	Operating room time not needed

NG, Nasogastric; *PES,* pharyngoesophageal segment; *UES,* upper esophageal sphincter.

days.[5] Intravenous feeding is a common form of parenteral nutrition, usually providing hydration and medication only rather than more complex elements such as amino acids. Hypodermal clysis is a form of parenteral nutrition that is given for hydration through the subcutaneous tissues in the chest, thigh, or abdomen. Table 11-2 summarizes parenteral and enteral alternative nutrition and hydration.

REASONS FOR TUBE FEEDING

The three most common reasons for placing a feeding tube include (1) the patient's inability to sustain nutrition orally, although the swallow response is safe; (2) the requirement for sufficient calories on a short-term basis to overcome an acute medical problem; and (3) the risk of tracheal aspiration if the patient is allowed to eat orally.

TABLE 11-2   Summary of Potential Methods of Providing Nutrition

Type of Nutrition Delivery	Route of Delivery	Method of Delivery	Indications for Use	Types of Formula	Possible Complications
Simple IV/ CTPN	IV (small vein; catheter inserted or surgically placed for CTPN in deep central vein)	Continuous or cyclic infusion by pump	Supplemental hydration; restoration of fluid and electrolyte balance, need for complete parenteral nutrition or long-term CTPN	Simple IV solutions (% dextrose and saline, electrolytes) Complete solutions: amino acids, dextrose, fatty acids, vitamins, minerals, trace elements, IV lipid solutions	Simple IV: Infection, edema, bleeding, burn at insertion site; weakened and collapsed veins Central line: Air embolism, pneumothorax, myocardial perforation, phlebitis, blood clot, infection, sepsis
Nasogastric tube	Catheter/tube placed transnasally to the stomach	Intermittent or continuous drip by pump	Short-term alternative to oral intake (approximately 2 weeks); transnasal insertion, easily removed	Commercial nutritionally complete (standard, hydrolyzed, modular) supplements; regular liquids	Misplacement into the airway; irritation to nasal, pharyngeal, esophageal mucosa; discomfort; negative cosmesis; may affect swallow function; may contribute to reflux and aspiration
G-tube/PEG	Feeding tube inserted directly into the stomach	Bolus or gravity (syringe); drip by infusion pump	Option for long-term alternative to oral intake; does not necessarily preclude oral intake in certain cases	Commercially prepared nutritionally complete enteral formulas; fiber supplements, supplemental and regular liquids, select medications; some individuals may liquefy table foods	Nausea, vomiting, diarrhea, constipation, reflux, clogged tube, skin irritation at gastrostomy site; aspiration
J-tube/PEG	Feeding tube inserted directly into the jejunum (small intestine)	Bolus or gravity syringe; drip by infusion pump	Does not require stomach for digestion; allows enteral nutrition earlier after stress or trauma; less risk of reflux and aspiration	Commercially prepared nutritionally complete enteral formulas; fiber supplements, supplemental liquids	Loss of controlled emptying of the stomach; misplacement; diarrhea, dehydration
Hypodermal clysis	Subcutaneous; common infusion sites are the chest, abdomen, thighs, and upper arms	Injection (3 L in 24 hours/two sites)	Hydration supplement for mild to moderate dehydration	Saline; half saline/ glucose; potassium chloride can be added	Mild subcutaneous edema

CTPN, Central total parenteral nutrition; *IV*, intravenous; *PEG*, percutaneous endoscopic gastrostomy.
(Reprinted from Krival K, McGrail A, Kelchner L: Frequently asked questions about alternate nutrition and hydration (ANH) in dysphagia care, Rockville, MD, 2006, American Speech-Language-Hearing Association.)

CLINICAL CORNER 11-3: FAMILY DILEMMA

A 90-year-old woman has a history of multiple bilateral strokes with poor oral intake. She is difficult to evaluate formally with either a clinical or instrumental evaluation. The reason for her poor intake is not known. She is slightly below her ideal body weight and has not responded to behavioral efforts to improve her oral intake. The team has decided she needs a gastrostomy tube to maintain nutrition. Her daughter, who is acting on her behalf, agrees that it was necessary but feels uncomfortable providing consent because in the past her mother told her she never wanted a feeding tube.

Critical Thinking
1. Do you think the dysphagia team should press the daughter for an alternative feeding route when they know that the resident did not want such an intervention?
2. If the patient were your mother, what would you do?

CLINICAL CORNER 11-4: CHOKING RISK

The dysphagia team is in total agreement that a gastrostomy tube should be placed in a mentally incompetent poststroke patient who is 89 years old. The family member who is the legal surrogate is against placement and asks that his mother be fed despite the risks. Some of the nursing assistants who were helping feed her have refused because they believe they are hastening her death. The family member has threatened to sue the hospital for negligence because it is his perception that his mother is not receiving good care and that the team is "against him" for not taking their advice.

Critical Thinking
1. What should be the next step in solving this dilemma, and who should initiate this step?
2. Can the medical care team continue to ethically provide care they feel is not warranted? What are their rights?

The decision to place a feeding tube can be controversial and may precipitate ethical dilemmas that involve the entire medical care team (review Clinical Corner 11-3). In general, no clear guidelines exist for long-term feeding tube placement; in most cases, the wishes of the patient or family guide the decision. For patients who are too ill to swallow and whose medical status is expected to improve, the decision to provide enteral feeding is apparent and usually proceeds without controversy. The decision is more difficult for the patient who is eating safely but cannot eat enough, particularly if the patient has an AD that states an unwillingness to be tube fed. In this situation, the patient may be putting himself or herself at medical risk from the consequences of undernutrition and dehydration. Bourdel-Marchasson et al.[6] did a retrospective study on 58 patients in long-term care who received a PEG because of their dysphagia and 50 patients who were dysphagic but refused a PEG. Controlling for age and medical needs, they followed patients for 1 year. At 2 months, the survival rate for those with PEGs was 81% compared with 58% of those who did not receive a PEG. Palecek et al.[7] argued that patients with advanced dementia who have made it clear they do not want a feeding tube may want to choose "comfort feeding only." Using this approach, the patient is hand fed substances that do not cause distress or excessive coughing episodes with the intent of providing maximum comfort and satisfaction, rather than a sufficient amount of calories. Placing a feeding tube in a patient who is at risk for tracheal aspiration to avoid the consequences of aspiration (e.g., life-threatening aspiration pneumonia) also is controversial. The literature suggests that for patients with chronic, terminal diseases that gastrostomy or jejunostomy does not reduce the incidence of aspiration pneumonia.[3,8,9] Furthermore, these measures do not prolong life

---

CLINICAL CORNER 11-5: REPEATED PNEUMONIA

A 64-year-old resident in a nursing home has a past history of multiple strokes with aphasia and dysphagia with multiple admissions to the hospital for aspiration pneumonia. After her treatments for pneumonia she returned to oral feeding. Periodic chest radiographs revealed some lung **infiltrates**, but she continued to eat her mechanical soft diet. The SLP watched the patient eat and noticed that for the first 10 minutes she appeared to be eating well but then started to choke on most items. The family refused an attempt to get a modified barium swallow study because their insurance would not pay for it. Because of the resident's prior history of aspiration pneumonia and the lack of a modified barium swallow study, the SLP believed the patient should not be eating orally. The physician disagreed with that recommendation, stating that tube feeding was not in the patient's best interest because of a lack of serious symptoms of dysphagia and her good appetite.

Critical Thinking
1. Should the disagreement between the SLP and physician be addressed? Whose position is more valid? Make a case for each.
2. At what point in this patient's medical scenario might it be appropriate to place a feeding tube?

---

beyond expected limits.[10,11] For patients with longer life expectancies or patients with dementia who are not interested in eating, tube feeding may extend their lives without undue risk. The decision to place a feeding tube in a patient must be carefully considered, and the patient's or surrogate's wishes must be weighed against the medical risks and benefits (review Clinical Corner 11-4 and Clinical Corner 11-5).

WEANING FROM FEEDING TUBES

Although much discussion and research have focused on patients who require feeding tubes, little effort has been directed toward which tube-fed patients can make the transition to oral feeding. At a minimum, tube-fed patients with dysphagia who are candidates to return to oral feeding must demonstrate a safe and efficient swallow on a consistent basis. In addition, they must be able to consume adequate amounts of food or liquid to support nutritional requirements. Their cognitive status also must be at a level at which they can follow single-stage commands and remain alert long enough to finish a meal. Respiratory stability is important because the work required during attempts at oral ingestion may induce fatigue. Fatigue may predispose patients to interruption between the required time needed to protect the airway during the swallow sequence, thereby increasing the possibility of aspiration (see Chapter 6). Finally, the ability to self-feed or cooperate fully with feeding assistance is desired.

Buchholz[12] has presented a clinical algorithm specific to patients with acquired brain injury or stroke that offers valuable suggestions for transition of tube-fed patients to oral feeding. The initial phase of weaning from tube feeding is termed the preparatory phase. This phase focuses on physiologic readiness for oral nutrition and incorporates medical and nutritional stability, implementation of intermittent attempts at tube feeding, and a complete swallowing assessment. The second phase, weaning, is described as a graduated increase in oral feeding with corresponding decreases in tube feeding. Placement of an NGT for feeding does not preclude patients from attempts at oral feeding, although attempts at oral feeding should be done on a schedule when the patient has not recently been fed through the tube. Avoiding attempts at oral feeding with a full stomach helps stimulate the hunger drive, which in turn may facilitate oral intake. Once a patient is able to consume 75% or more of his or her nutritional requirements consistently by mouth for 3 days, all tube feedings are discontinued. Specific clinical parameters to evaluate weaning success include weight gain, adequate hydration, a normal swallow, and no respiratory complications. No data are presented to support the specifics of this weaning approach in this population. However, data are available from other populations that pursue different recommendations and criteria for tube removal.

Naik et al.[13] evaluated predictors of feeding tube removal (and return to oral feeding) in cancer patients before and after PEG tube placement. Four clinical variables predicted PEG removal and return to oral feeding in these patients: age greater than 65 years, localized head and neck cancer, serum albumin level 3.75 g/dL or higher, and a serum creatinine level of less than 1.1 mg/dL. In the **multivariate analyses**, only age and localized head and neck cancer predicted resumption of oral feeding with PEG removal.

Clinical reality dictates that patients vary in terms of the need for feeding tube placement and in terms of readiness and success of feeding tube removal. In fact, not all tube-fed patients seek feeding tube removal. In addition, the transition process from tube feeding to oral feeding can be cognitively and physically challenging. Patients with feeding tubes typically consider the removal of the tube to be their primary goal, although some patients prefer to continue tube feedings even if return to some degree of oral intake is deemed possible. For some, oral intake can become a burden, whereas the implementation of tube feedings requires little effort. However, the transition process from tube to oral feeding should be thoroughly discussed and a plan of action outlined. For example, patients may be too aggressive when returning to oral feeding, experience failure, and then cease any efforts to resume an oral diet. Others are less aggressive and require more guidance and structure until the transition is complete. Discussion of patient-specific goals (see Chapter 9) for transitioning to oral feeding is advisable. One example for the initial goal might be oral intake of a single material to the point of nutritional adequacy with that item. At this point, the feeding tube might be removed with subsequent goals focused on the expansion of the oral diet.

The choice of the initial materials to restart oral feeding in the tube-fed patient is complex and based on findings from the clinical and instrumental swallowing examinations.[14] Key considerations focus on the patient's ability to control the material in the mouth and to move this material to the pharynx. For example, stroke patients with oral weakness may have difficulty controlling a liquid material, which may leak anteriorly from the lips or posterior to the pharynx and into an open airway. Conversely, patients recovering from treatment for head and neck cancer sometimes perform better with thin liquids as a result of xerostomia. Beyond the oral stage of swallow, the SLP is concerned with the patient's ability to protect the airway during the swallow and the potential for aspiration of postswallow residue associated with ineffective transport. As a result of clinical and instrumental evaluations with various materials, the SLP is likely to recommend a specific initial material for oral intake as well as some basic intervention strategies, such as specific postures or swallowing adaptations that increase airway protection or reduce postswallow residue (see Chapters 9, 10, and 15).

Once nutritional goals and the appropriate behavioral interventions have been identified, the patient is ready for oral intake. The clinician must remember that swallow safety does not always predict whether the patient can ingest a sufficient number of calories for feeding tube removal.[14] Therefore careful documentation of the amount of food the patient ingests orally is important. If the patient

---

BOX 11-1 SUGGESTIONS FOR THE TRANSITION OF TUBE-FED PATIENTS TO ORAL FEEDING

1. Identify a safe oral bolus.
2. Provide intermittent tube feedings.
3. Ingest oral feedings before a tube feeding.
4. Reestablish a normal meal routine.
5. Provide a specific diet in the initial transition stages.
6. Document the type and amount of all materials taken orally.
7. Keep track of the time it takes to consume a meal.
8. Document any complications with the oral diet.
9. Involve the patient and family in preferences for advancing the diet.
10. Monitor swallow safety, nutrition, hydration, and respiratory status.

---

has been receiving continuous tube feedings (delivered by a bedside pump), an intermittent schedule should be instituted to reinvolve normal hunger cycles.[12] Ideally, these intermittent feedings should be well tolerated before attempts at oral ingestion.[15] Attempts at oral feeding should begin with the patient fully upright and alert. For patients with fluctuating mental status, attempts at oral ingestion should be timed when their pattern of alertness is at its best. It is common for the return to oral ingestion to involve only short periods, once or twice per day. The number and type of food items received on the patient's tray are established during the clinical and instrumental examination and communicated to the dietitian or other medical staff. As tolerance improves, more challenging items can be introduced in larger bolus sizes. Box 11-1 summarizes some simple considerations in developing a strategy for the transition of tube-fed patients to oral feeding.

ASPIRATION PNEUMONIA

Aspiration pneumonia is a lung infection that may result from three primary sources: aspiration during swallowing, including saliva; retention of swallowed contents that eventually are aspirated; or aspiration of gastroesophageal contents. Aspiration of gastric contents with subsequent medical complications is called **aspiration pneumonitis**. Part of the discussion for Critical Thinking Case 6 concerns the importance of ascertaining the difference between the two. Physical signs of aspiration pneumonia include shortness of breath with a rapid heart rate, acute mental confusion, incontinence, and infection. Some patients have a fever and an increase in sputum with cough. The precise mechanisms of how one develops an aspiration pneumonia are unknown.[16] Older adult patients in skilled nursing facilities may have aspiration pneumonia with few of these overt signs.[17] Chest radiographs may show diffuse infiltrates,

usually in the posterior and right lower segments of the lung. If the source of the infection is thought to be related to oropharyngeal dysphagia, the patient is kept from eating while antibiotics are used to treat the infection. If the source is believed to be in the gastrointestinal tract, medications and posturing may be used to reduce the threat of recurrence.

Risk Factors

Aspiration pneumonia does not develop in all patients who aspirate material into the lung. For example, some patients frequently aspirate their saliva and do not become ill. This may be explained by the fact that their oral hygiene is sufficient to not allow bacteria to colonize and, in turn, infect the lung tissue. An aggressive oral care program is important for any patient with oropharyngeal dysphagia. When material is misdirected into the upper airway during swallow attempts, the first line of defense is cough at the level of the vocal folds. If the cough is sufficiently strong, most of the material may be expelled back into the pharynx to be swallowed while only a small amount enters the trachea below the level of the vocal folds. Even if material does enter the lung, it may trigger a secondary cough response that further protects the lower airway spaces. Specialized cells in the tissue of the lung work to engulf, absorb, and transport foreign fluid and food from the lung spaces. Other cells produce a chemical reaction that neutralizes aspirants that are acidic. For example, the acid in gastric reflux is particularly virulent in the lungs. The upper and lower airway defense systems are most active when the patient's immune system is strong. Therefore patients with an acute medical problem or older patients with chronic, multiple medical problems, particularly if they are immobile, may be at increased risk for aspiration pneumonia.

No studies in human beings have been able to link the amount and type of an aspirant to the development of pneumonia. Clinical practice suggests that although some patients aspirate and do not develop pneumonia, other similar patients do contract pneumonia. The ability to differentiate patients in whom pneumonia might develop from their aspirants might allow the clinician more latitude to not restrict patients from eating even in the circumstance of documented aspiration. Silver and Van Nostrand[18] studied 15 poststroke patients who were restricted from eating because they showed signs of aspiration on videofluoroscopic examination. They were subsequently studied with a nuclear medicine test known as scintigraphy. During scintigraphy the patient swallows a large radionuclide-labeled bolus with scanning immediately after and at hourly intervals (typically up to 3 hours) for any residue in the lung fields or digestive tract. They found that although some patients did aspirate the marker, after a short period the residue in the lungs was not detected by the scanner. This suggested that the lung defense mechanisms were active and therefore diminished the chances for the development of pneumonia. Eight of the patients with positive lung clearance were fed despite the evidence of aspiration on videofluoroscopy.

Although the data are not strong, some preliminary evidence suggests certain clinical signs are predictive of aspiration, whereas other variables (mostly historical) are more predictive of those in whom aspiration pneumonia will develop. In other words, aspiration pneumonia does not develop in all patients who aspirate, either on the clinical or instrumental examination. Interestingly, no data exist to support that clinical indicators from the clinical examination (such as dysphonia, dysarthria, wet-hoarse voice after trial swallows, and failure on the 3-oz water test) that predict aspiration (see Chapter 7) also predict aspiration pneumonia.

Studies of the factors that predict those in whom aspiration pneumonia will develop have focused on those most at risk—older adults. The following factors have emerged as predictive of development of aspiration pneumonia: diagnosis of congestive heart failure and chronic obstructive pulmonary disease; use of multiple medications, especially sedatives; feeding dependence; poor oral hygiene; smoking; prior history of aspiration pneumonia; neck hyperextension while eating; use of suctioning; bedbound state; and having a feeding tube in place.[19-21] Although not confirmed experimentally, it might be assumed that the greater the number of factors, the greater the risk for patients to develop pneumonia from their aspirants. Interestingly, although the presence of dysphagia was a predictor in some studies, it was not a strong predictor.

NONMEDICAL RISKS AND BENEFITS

In addition to being informed about the medical risks associated with tube feeding, clinicians, patients, and caregivers need to be informed of the nonmedical risks and benefits to make an informed decision regarding whether enteral feedings are in the patient's best interest.

Nonmedical Benefits

Some patients with dysphagia continually struggle to maintain sufficient oral nutrition and hydration. Similarly, caregivers who assist patients in their nutritional needs also may be challenged to maintain nutritional levels. Family members often are troubled that their loved one is losing weight. Weight loss leads to a decrease in energy levels and mobility may be decreased. Poor nutritional levels also may precipitate mental confusion. All these factors are viewed by the patient and family as a diminution in the quality of life. This realization often is accompanied by situational depression. Providing the patient with sufficient calories by

---

PRACTICE NOTE 11-1

I had been monitoring a patient with multiple sclerosis and dysphagia for 3 years. He had continued to eat orally, although mealtimes were prolonged and the special preparations required in his diet were becoming an unwanted burden. We had never discussed his thoughts about a feeding tube, but it seemed appropriate that this might be the time. I suggested that it was clear to me that oral feeding was becoming a burden and that a gastrostomy might be a choice because it would relieve the burden of the oral intake by providing calories to maintain his health. Food items that he enjoyed and did not require special preparation could be continued orally. This option brought an immediate smile to his face and a consultation request was sent to gastroenterology to evaluate him for a percutaneous gastrostomy. It is important for the clinician to assess the burden of oral alimentation because even though patients may want to maintain that level of function, offering options may be in their best interest.

---

enteral feeding may relieve the burden of trying to maintain nutrition orally (see Practice Note 11-1). In turn, the quality of life for the patient and caregivers improves. Bannerman et al.[22] studied two cohorts (55 and 54 patients) who received a PEG at least 16 months before their quality of life was measured.[22] Both patients and caregivers reported an increase in the quality of life; 55% in the first cohort reported improvement, and 80% in the second. Lost functions may return because nutrition and hydration levels can return to normal. Although the patient and caregivers may have to familiarize themselves with the mechanics and care of the enteral feeding route, in some instances enteral feeding can provide both physical and psychological relief from dysphagia.

Nonmedical Risks

Patients who no longer eat by mouth or must consider not eating by mouth may feel threatened because they are losing one of life's basic pleasures. Thus social withdrawal and depression may be a consequence of their decision. Patients with dementia who require enteral feeding may need to be sedated and physically restrained because they attempt to dislodge the feeding tube. Sedation and restraint during enteral feedings often is considered as a risk because it further erodes the patient's quality of life.

ETHICAL DILEMMAS

Ethical dilemmas surrounding eating may develop when physicians, patients, and families consider the need for tube feeding. Ethical dilemmas usually result when the patient or caregiver does not agree with or fails to understand the medical care team's plan. Such dilemmas usually only develop when there are misunderstandings between the medical team and the patient or family. Therefore they can be avoided with frequent and accurate information on the benefits and risks of tube feeding. The decision to start or stop artificial feeding is "ethically neutral" and only invokes an ethical dilemma if the decision is in conflict with the patient's goals, values, or wishes.[23] However, when dilemmas do occur, usually they can be resolved by reviewing the circumstances that led to the decision. Such a review entails an in-depth discussion with the key members of the medical team, the patient, and the family. If the dilemma is not resolved in this meeting, a request for resolution is sent to the medical center's ethics committee. In general, this committee is composed of physicians, nurses, a psychologist or social worker, a chaplain, and a member from the community. Swallowing specialists or dietitians may be asked to be a part of the committee if the issues require their expertise. In some cases, a clinician who deals extensively with swallowing disorders is a member of the committee.

Ethical issues in medicine surface for a number of reasons. First, the patient or family member is not convinced that they have received sufficient evidence to support the conclusions. Second, determinations of the best course of care, as well as who is the final arbiter making that decision, may not be clear. For example, the patient may have been told the best course of care by the attending physician but may have also received an opposing opinion from an outside consultant whom the patient trusts. Third, the medical care team and the patient may have personal biases that interfere with rational decision making. Fourth, it may not be clear who is acting in the patient's behalf and whether that person is acting in accordance with the patient's best interest. Finally, it may not be clear what the patient or surrogate considers a desirable outcome to the dilemma. In a large randomized control trial aimed toward providing information about decision making and feeding options in patients with dementia, surrogates who received training prior to the need to make decisions were better prepared and more comfortable with their decisions than those who received information about feeding options during a crisis situation. This study supports the need to involve caregivers early with patients who are at anticipated risk for severe dysphagia caused by progressive disease.[24]

It is the task of the medical ethics committee to resolve ethical dilemmas that surface when the medical team recommends a feeding tube and the patient or family refuses, or when the patient wants a feeding tube and the medical care team thinks it is not necessary. The committee performs a thorough, nonbiased review of the medical and nonmedical risks associated with tube feeding in an effort to resolve the dilemma. In most cases, the committee does

CLINICAL CASE EXAMPLE 11-1

A 55-year-old man had been in a skilled nursing facility for 10 years with an unknown, progressive disease of the basal ganglia. It affected all the muscles of the head, neck, and limbs. Because he was counseled early in the disease that it would progress and lead to a premature death, he signed an AD that stated he did not want any "heroic" measures when he became terminally ill. This included a statement that he did not want to be fed through a tube in his stomach. His disease progressed to the point where he could not produce intelligible speech because of weakness in the muscles of articulation. He used an electronic communication board to compensate for the loss of communication skills. He continued to eat orally but choked violently at every meal as the nurses were feeding him. At the time of the consultation to speech pathology, he had been treated for six episodes of aspiration pneumonia in the previous 18 months. His videofluorographic swallowing examination showed aspiration on all bolus volumes and types, ranging from thin liquid to a semisolid. He was capable of transferring the bolus from the mouth to the pharynx. He was asked numerous times if he wanted to change his mind regarding the possibility of feeding tube placement to perhaps lessen the risk of developing pneumonia, but he refused.

The patient's refusal of a feeding tube became a serious issue when the nursing assistants banded together and said they did not want to continue to feed him because they believed they were contributing to his death. The patient did not have a family member in the vicinity who might have been available to provide feeding assistance. A consultation was sought from the ethics committee to resolve the dilemma.

The ethics committee reviewed the entire medical history and established that the patient fully understood his medical condition. They found him competent to make decisions about his health based on the medical care team communications regarding the risks and benefits of continued oral feeding and those of tube feeding. It was clear from the SLP's report that dietary compensations and behavioral swallowing treatment strategies were not successful in reducing the patient's risk of aspiration. It also was apparent that the nurses were not willing to cooperate with his feeding, leaving the patient at nutritional risk. After extensive discussion, the surgeon on the committee asked if it would be prudent to perform an elective laryngectomy, effectively separating the airway and food way to avoid the risk of aspiration. This would sacrifice vocal fold function. Because his speech was already unintelligible, it seemed like a reasonable option to sacrifice voice for swallow safety. This option was explained to the patient, who agreed to the procedure.

its best to honor the patient's wishes within accepted legal and ethical boundaries.

One of the most commonly encountered dilemmas that the swallowing specialist faces is the patient who is known to aspirate and has decided that under no circumstances does he or she want a feeding tube. A dilemma may arise when the medical team has decided that the patient's risk of aspiration pneumonia during continued oral feeding is greater than the risk of aspiration pneumonia with enteral feeding. If the medical care team is convinced that the patient and family understand all the risks associated with continued oral feeding, they most likely will honor the patient's wishes under the Patient Self-Determination Act and allow the patient to continue to eat. At this point a number of dilemmas may surface. The physician may have allowed the patient to continue to eat, although convinced it was not in the patient's best interest and may believe he or she is sacrificing professional responsibility. Furthermore, the physician may feel liable for legal action if aspiration pneumonia develops and the patient dies. In this case, it is important that specific documentation be placed in the medical record regarding the medical team's recommendations and the patient's refusal of those recommendations. Some institutions require the patient to acknowledge that he or she has refused the medical team's advice in a separate written document. These documents have not been challenged in the courts, so their validity remains questionable. However, because the medical record is a legal document, it is crucial that all conversations with the family about the risks and benefits of tube feeding, and the patient education they received on those issues, be thoroughly documented. Impressions regarding whether the family fully understood the team's recommendations also should be recorded.

The swallowing specialist whose evaluation might have helped the team make the decision that oral feeding was contraindicated also may believe that his or her professional ethics are at risk, particularly if asked to continue to assist the patient by providing the "safest" way to feed. Some clinicians argue that they would be contributing to the patient's demise and would be liable to court action if the family chooses to pursue it. In this case clinicians have the right to sign off the case and pass it to another colleague who may have a different perspective.[25] Other colleagues may believe they can provide safe feeding instructions without compromising their professional or personal ethics. In most cases the swallowing specialist provides additional care if convinced that the patient and family were fully informed of the continued risk and it was properly documented in the medical record. Furthermore, staying involved with the family and patient can allow for reassessment during times of change that may alter the original decision for oral or enteral feeding (review and discuss Clinical Corners 11-6, 11-7, and 11-8).

CLINICAL CORNER 11-6: FEED/NO FEED DECISIONS

You are confronted with Patient 1, who has the following clinical signs from your evaluation and from the patient's medical history: terminal medical illness, family desires to prolong life, history of multiple cases of aspiration pneumonia, uncooperative with any testing, good cough response, no dysphonia, frequent choking episodes with meals, multiple medications, and pulling of feeding tube because of poor cognition. Patient 2 has the following clinical factors: trace aspiration on thin liquids; pharyngeal stasis on thicker materials with airway penetration; multiple, chronic medical conditions; no AD; prior history of aspiration pneumonia; good cognition; good oral hygiene; ongoing weight loss; and undernourishment.

Critical Thinking

1. Would you orally feed Patient 1? Justify your answer based on how you evaluate the importance of each clinical finding.
2. Would you orally feed Patient 2? Justify your answer based on how you evaluate the importance of each clinical finding.

CLINICAL CORNER 11-7: CONFUSED ASPIRATOR

The patient has a history of repeated aspiration pneumonias for which he has a gastrostomy. Unfortunately, he continues to pull the tube out because of his mental confusion. The physician wants to try oral feeding and wants to know the risk of aspiration. Only under ideal conditions did the modified barium swallow study show that the patient was not aspirating. The physician is worried that the family will place blame for a subsequent bout of pneumonia if the patient returns to oral feeding.

Critical Thinking

1. What advice would you give to the physician?
2. What things does the family need to know and respond to that might affect the final decision?

CLINICAL CORNER 11-8: WIFE VERSES TEAM

A patient attempted suicide 3 years ago and now has considerable frontal lobe injury. He stopped eating, has lost 16 pounds, and his health will deteriorate unless a feeding tube is placed. He is ambulatory and responsive but is considered incompetent to understand his situation. The medical care team believes that an NGT would improve his current condition, but the family refuses. Interestingly, his wife instructed the team to do everything possible to save his life at the time of the suicide attempt. Her refusal now is based on the fact that she says this is his way of saying he wants to die and she is honoring that wish.

Critical Thinking

1. What other information might be gathered to solve this dilemma?
2. Should the medical care team follow the wife's wishes? Make a case for each answer.

CLINICAL CASE EXAMPLE 11-2

A 90-year-old man had bilateral strokes that left him dysphagic with dementia. During his last hospitalization he had respiratory distress and a tracheostomy was performed. Although his prognosis was poor, he steadily recovered to the point that his physician wondered if he could once again eat orally. The SLP completed a clinical evaluation that revealed (1) poor mental status, but the ability to follow simple commands and stay alert; (2) generalized weakness of the tongue, lips, and velum; and (3) a weak and hoarse voice when his tracheotomy tube was occluded. On swallowing trials of 5 and 10 mL of thin and thick liquid, the patient coughed on each bolus. Pudding pooled in the oral cavity but was swallowed with delay and postswallow cough. Because of his fragile medical status and based on the results of the clinical evaluation, the SLP recommended that the patient continue NGT feeding and suggested the family consider gastrostomy. The daughter, acting on the patient's behalf, objected to this recommendation, stating that eating was his only pleasure in life. The SLP explained that the examination suggested he was aspirating and could die from aspiration pneumonia if he tried to eat. After asking questions about the definitions of aspiration and aspiration pneumonia, the daughter was not convinced he was aspirating because it could not be seen on a physical examination. She pressed the physician for a modified barium swallow study that she attended (Video 11-1 on the Evolve site). The patient was given 10 mL of a thickened liquid that pooled in the vallecula with residue above the PES. Although the hyoid bone moved, vallecular pooling and PES residue were consistent with tongue weakness. On subsequent boluses, material penetrated the airway with evidence of cough. Some material eventually went below the vocal folds without cough. On multiple swallows penetration was noted; however, eventually the pharynx was cleared. On the final swallows of a pudding-thick bolus, the patient was able to swallow without delay or pharyngeal residue with only trace penetration. The SLP believed that this examination showed that the patient was still at risk of aspiration, although considering his age, the presence of a tracheotomy tube, and the patient's general health, attempts at oral ingestion seemed warranted. The final decision to start oral feeding was based on evidence from the clinical and instrumental examinations as well as the daughter's implied stance that she did not want her father to have a gastrostomy. The patient started a soft mechanical diet but on the third day developed signs and symptoms consistent with aspiration pneumonia. Oral feedings were stopped while he was treated for suspected aspiration pneumonia. The daughter continued to argue for oral feeding and the team agreed to try again. This time he ate successfully for 5 days, and the decision was made to remove the tracheotomy tube. The patient left the hospital eating a regular diet with no restrictions.

TAKE HOME NOTES

Medical ethics is a subspecialty of medical care that brings together patients, caregivers, and nonmedical and medical professionals in an effort to make the best decision on a health care issue. It is driven by a congressional mandate called the Patient Self-Determination Act.

1. An AD is a statement made by a patient that provides guidance to health care professionals regarding the patient's wishes for treatment or no treatment in certain medical circumstances.
2. The two broad categories of nonoral feeding include enteral and parenteral.
3. The major enteral feeding routes are nasogastric, gastrostomy, and jejunostomy.
4. Feeding tubes do not necessarily reduce the risk of aspiration pneumonia or prolong life.
5. Aspiration pneumonia does not develop in all patients who aspirate. Some clinical factors are more predictive than others in identifying aspirators in whom pneumonia will develop.
6. Ethical dilemmas regarding the use and acceptance of tube feeding may result in conflicts between the patient and the medical care team. Most of these dilemmas can be resolved with a review of the patient's wishes and a detailed review of the course of medical care.
7. Professional ethics can be threatened if a patient refuses to follow medical advice. Asking another professional to assume the care of the patient is within a practitioner's right.

REFERENCES

1. Groher ME: Ethical dilemmas in providing nutrition. *Dysphagia* 9:12, 1990.
2. Sharp HM, Bryant KN: Ethical issues in dysphagia: when patients refuse assessment or treatment. *Semin Speech Lang* 24:285, 2003.
3. Lazarus BA, Murphy JB, Culpepper L: Aspiration associated with long-term gastric versus jejunal feeding: a critical analysis of the literature. *Arch Phys Med Rehabil* 70:46, 1990.
4. Marik PE, Zaloga GP: Gastric versus post-pyloric feeding: a systematic review. *Crit Care* 7:R46, 2003.
5. Griggs B: Nursing management of swallowing disorders. In Groher ME, editor: *Dysphagia: diagnosis and management*, Boston, 1997, Butterworth-Heinemann.
6. Bourdel-Marchasson I, Dumas F, Pinganaud G, et al: Adult percutaneous gastrostomy in long-term enteral feeding in a nursing home. *Int J Qual Health Care* 9:297, 1997.
7. Palecek EJ, Teno JM, Casarett DJ, et al: Comfort feeding only: a proposal to bring clarity to decision-making regarding difficulty with eating for persons with advanced dementia. *J Am Geriatr Soc* 58:580, 2010.
8. Feinberg MJ, Knebl J, Tully J, et al: Aspiration in the elderly. *Dysphagia* 5:61, 1990.
9. Finucane TE, Christmas C: Aspiration pneumonia. *N Engl J Med* 44:1869, 2001.

10. Finucane TE, Christmas C, Travis K: Tube feeding in patients with advanced dementia: a review of the evidence. *JAMA* 13:1365, 1990.

11. Regnard C, Leslie P, Crawford DM, et al: Gastrostomies in dementia: bad practice or bad evidence? *Age Ageing* 39:282, 2010.

12. Buchholz AC: Weaning patients with dysphagia from tube feeding to oral nutrition: a proposed algorithm. *Can J Diet Pract Res* 59:208, 1998.

13. Naik AD, Abraham NS, Roche VM, et al: Predicting which patients can resume oral nutrition after percutaneous endoscopic gastrostomy tube placement. *Aliment Pharmacol Ther* 21:1155, 2005.

14. Crary MA, Groher ME: Reinstituting oral feeding in tube-fed adult patients with dysphagia. *Nutr Clin Pract* 21:576, 2006.

15. Groher ME, McKaig TN: Dysphagia and dietary levels in skilled nursing facilities. *J Am Geriatr Soc* 43:528, 1995.

16. Van der Maarel-Wierink CD, Vanobbergen JNO, Schols JMGA, et al: Meta-analysis of dysphagia and aspiration pneumonia in frail elders. *J Dent Res* 90:1398, 2011.

17. Fein AM: Pneumonia in the elderly: special diagnostic and therapeutic considerations. *Med Clin North Am* 78:1015, 1994.

18. Silver KH, Van Nostrand D: The use of scintigraphy in the management of patients with pulmonary aspiration. *Dysphagia* 9:107, 1994.

19. Peck A, Cohen CE, Mulvibill MN: Long-term enteral feeding of aged demented nursing home patients. *J Am Geriat Soc* 38:1195, 1990.

20. Langmore SE, Terpenning MS, Schork A, et al: Predictors of aspiration pneumonia: how important is dysphagia? *Dysphagia* 13:69, 1998.

21. Langmore SE, Skarupski KA, Park PS, et al: Predictors of aspiration pneumonia in nursing home residents. *Dysphagia* 17:298, 2002.

22. Bannerman E, Pendlebury J, Phillips F, et al: A cross-sectional and longitudinal study of health-related quality of life after percutaneous gastrostomy. *Eur J Gastroenterol Hepatol* 12:1101, 2000.

23. Groher M, Groher T: When safe feeding is threatened: end-of-life options and decisions. *Top Lang Disorders* 32:149, 2012.

24. Hanson LC, Carey TS, Caprio AJ, et al: Improving decision making for feeding options in advanced dementia: a randomized, controlled trial. *J Am Geriatr Soc* 59:2009, 2011.

25. Beauchamp TL, Childress JF: *Principles of biomedical ethics*, ed 5, New York, 2001, Oxford University Press.

Part III
Dysphagia in Infants and Children

CHAPTER 12

Typical Feeding and Swallowing Development in Infants and Children

Pamela Dodrill

To view additional case videos and content, please visit the evolve website.

CHAPTER OUTLINE

OBJECTIVES

1. List relative differences in the head and neck anatomy of infants and adults.
2. Discuss the development of body systems involved in feeding.
3. Describe various feeding reflexes.
4. Identify motor and cognitive skills involved in early feeding.
5. Understand the benefits of breastfeeding.
6. Describe the mechanics of infant fluid extraction from the breast or bottle.
7. Discuss the motor skills required for the introduction of solid foods of various textures.
8. Understand the developmental stages in the transition to mature mealtime behavior.
9. Display an understanding of nutrition and growth considerations in infants and children.

DEVELOPMENT OF HEAD AND NECK ANATOMY

Oral feeding relies on the actions of the facial muscles and muscles of mastication, as well as the lingual, pharyngeal, and laryngeal muscles. In addition, oral feeding relies on the structures of the head and neck themselves, including

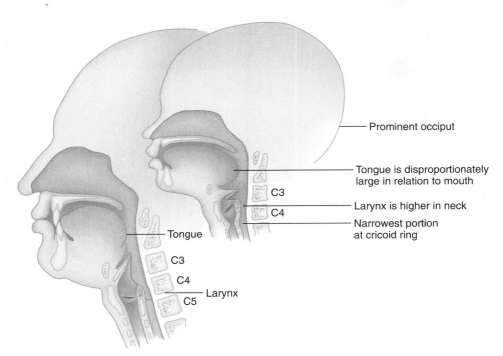

FIGURE 12-1 Comparison of the head and neck region of infants and adults. (From Finucane BT: Principles of Airway Management, 3rd edition, New York, 2003, Springer).

the lips, tongue, teeth, hard and soft palate, mandible, pharynx, and larynx.

Infant Head and Neck Development

The relative size and function of the head and neck region of newborns differs somewhat from that of older children and adults, which offers some degree of assistance to neonates and infants while they are developing their oral feeding skills (Figure 12-1). Specifically, compared with the older child or adult, the newborn oral cavity is smaller. The jaw is smaller, the tongue is relatively larger, and newborns have larger buccal fat pads. Together this arrangement assists the newborn to attach to the breast (or bottle) effectively, and minimizes the space available for the tongue to move, thereby reducing the coordination required to control tongue movements. In addition, relative to the older child and adult, the newborn larynx is positioned higher in the cervical spine region, and the uvula and epiglottis are in contact, providing additional protection for the airway against aspiration.

Branchial Arches

In utero, feeding structures develop from a series of paired arches at the top of the neural tube known as branchial (or pharyngeal) arches. Each arch develops its own blood vessels and nerves that supply a distinct group of muscles and skeletal and cartilage structures. The paired arches are numbered 1 through 6 (arch 5 exists only transiently) and grow and unite anteriorly (Table 12-1). The reader is advised to review the muscles involved in swallowing and their neural innervations as presented in Chapter 2.

DEVELOPMENT OF OTHER BODY SYSTEMS INVOLVED IN FEEDING

Typical human fetal gestation is approximately 40 weeks (range = 37-42 weeks). Infants born before 37 weeks gestational age (GA) are considered **preterm** (or premature).

Gut Development

Anatomic development of the fetal gut is essentially complete by 20 weeks GA.[1-4] However, maturation of physiologic function does not occur until later in gestation, and extends throughout the early postnatal period.[2-4] Gastrointestinal function that is immature at birth increases the risk of specific gut disease, such as necrotizing enterocolitis (see Chapter 13 for more information about this condition), malabsorption (failure to fully absorb nutrients ingested), and malnutrition. Functional and anatomic maturation is evidenced by improvements in esophageal motility, function of the lower esophageal sphincter (which acts to control gastroesophageal reflux), gastric emptying, intestinal motility, and development of the absorptive surface area of the gut.[2-4]

TABLE 12-1 Branchial Arches

Branchial Arch	Cranial Nerve	Bone and Cartilage	Muscles
1	V	Maxilla, mandible, malleus, incus	Muscles of mastication, anterior belly of the diagastric, mylohyoid, tensor veli palatini, tensor tympani
2	VII	Stapes, styloid process, hyoid (upper part of body and lesser horn)	Facial muscles, posterior belly of the diagastric, platysma, stylohyoid, stapedius
3	IX	Hyoid (lower part of body, greater horn), thymus, inferior parathyroids	Stylopharyngeus
4	X—SLN	Thyroid cartilage, epiglottis, superior parathyroids	Cricothyroid, levator veli palatini
6	X—RLN	Cricoid cartilage, arytenoid cartilage, corniculate cartilage	Intrinsic laryngeal muscles (other than cricothyroid)

RLN, Recurrent laryngeal nerve; *SLN,* superior laryngeal nerve.

Lung Development

The lungs are amongst the latest organ systems to reach an ex-utero survival threshold. By 23 weeks GA, some terminal sacs (primitive alveoli) are present and are vascularized enough that the respiratory system is able to perform basic gas exchange and ex-utero respiration is possible.[2-4] This is part of the reason that 23 weeks' GA is considered the limit of viability for premature neonates. By 28 weeks' GA, more terminal sacs are present and vascularization is better developed, allowing for greater gas exchange. Type I alveolar cells start to be replaced with type II alveolar cells, which secrete **surfactant**.[2-4] Surfactant acts to increase pulmonary compliance (ease of expansion of the lungs) and prevent atelectasis (collapse of parts of the lung). Neonates with insufficient surfactant require exogenous (transplanted) surfactant treatment until endogenous (self-developed) production is established. By 32 to 34 weeks' GA, alveolar development reaches a structural and functional stage at which respiration is generally more efficient. Gas exchange may be developed sufficiently that well neonates at this age will not require any ventilatory assistance. By 37 weeks' GA, immature alveoli have developed and surfactant production is generally sufficient for normal respiration. Alveoli numbers continue to develop over the first 2 years of life.[2-4]

Neurologic Development

The central nervous system matures in a peripheral to central (bottom-up) sequence. During the first trimester of gestation, early synapses begin forming in a fetus's spinal cord.[3-5] In the second trimester, the brainstem begins to mature.[3-5] Brainstem-mediated reflexes, such as breathing movements (i.e., rhythmic contractions of the diaphragm and chest muscles) and primitive sucking and swallowing, begin to emerge. The brainstem also controls other basic life functions, such as heart rate, blood pressure, digestion,

and sleep. The brainstem provides autonomic function support by the end of the second trimester, which allows some infants to become capable of survival in the ex-utero environment. In the third trimester, the cerebral volume and surface area increase markedly.[3-5] The cerebral cortex is responsible for most of what we think of as functional life (i.e., voluntary actions, thinking, remembering). Premature infants show only very basic electrical activity in the primary sensory regions of the cerebral cortex (those areas that perceive touch, hearing, and vision), as well as in primary motor regions.[3] Some simple learning is possible during the third trimester, as shown by the fact that newborn term infants often respond to familiar odors and sounds that they were exposed to in utero.[3-5]

Although infants are born with a number of survival reflexes, they are still very much dependent on their caregivers, partly because cerebral maturation is incomplete and their cortex is still quite immature. The brainstem is the most highly developed area of the brain at birth and controls all life-sustaining reflexes (including breathing and suckling) and basic life functions. In contrast, the cerebral cortex operates at a very primitive level at birth. It is the gradual maturation of this complex part of the brain that explains much of an infant's cognitive and emotional maturation in the first few years of life. Although all of the neurons in the cortex are produced before birth, they are poorly connected.[3-5] In contrast to the brainstem and spinal cord, the cerebral cortex produces many of its synaptic connections after birth, in a massive burst of synapse formation known as the *exuberant period.*[5] These new connections allow an infant to achieve his or her many developmental milestones. By 2 years of age, a toddler's cerebral cortex contains more than one hundred trillion synapses.[5] This period of synaptic proliferation varies in different parts of the cerebral cortex: it begins earlier in primary sensory regions (e.g., primary sensory cortex, visual cortex), and develops later in brain areas involved in higher cognitive and emotional functions (e.g., frontal and temporal lobes).[5] The number of synapses remains at a peak level in all areas of the cerebral cortex throughout middle childhood (4-8 years of age),[5] when it begins to gradually decline (through pruning) to adult levels.

Besides synapse formation and pruning, the other most significant event in postnatal brain development is myelination. The brain of a newborn contains very little myelin (fatty sheaths that insulate neurons and allow clear, efficient electrical transmission).[3-5] This lack of myelin is the main reason infants and young children process information so much more slowly than adults. Myelination of the cerebral cortex begins in the primary sensory and motor areas, then progresses to higher-order association areas that control more complex, executive processes (e.g., integration of perception, thoughts, feelings, memories).[3-5] Myelination is a drawn-out process, and myelination of some of the more complex areas continues throughout adolescence and into early adulthood. However, unlike synaptic pruning, myelination appears to be largely hard-wired, and its sequence is very predictable in most children.[5]

DEVELOPMENT OF FEEDING REFLEXES

The function of feeding or eating can be broken down into four main components:
1. Oral phase (i.e., mastication)
2. Triggering of the swallowing reflex
3. Pharyngeal phase
4. Esophageal phase

In older children and adults, mastication is a **voluntary** activity, relying on appropriate sensory registration of the bolus and a coordinated motor response, and is influenced by cognitive thought processes.[5,6] Triggering of the swallowing reflex is generally an involuntary reflexive activity, although it can be controlled voluntarily, whereas the pharyngeal and esophageal phases are involuntary activities. In neonates and young infants, all four components of feeding are **involuntary,** and it is only later in infancy that the oral phase comes under voluntary control[1,6] (Table 12-2). As a result, young infants display a number of brainstem-mediated oral reflexes that assist them with oral feeding.

Oral reflexes can be broken down broadly into **adaptive** and **protective** reflexes.

Adaptive reflexes assist the infant to direct feeds into the gut. Although reflexive in response to the appropriate stimulation, these actions can be affected by the infant's level of alertness or hunger.[1,7] These reflexes diminish over time and are replaced by more sophisticated, voluntary skills. The main adaptive reflexes are rooting and suckling.

Rooting occurs when tactile stimulation occurs to the side of the lips or cheek. In response, the infant will turn

TABLE 12-2 Comparison of Involuntary (Reflexive) and Voluntary (Volitional) Feeding Periods	
Reflexive Period	**Volitional Period**
Oral phase is reflexive.	Oral phase is volitional.
Intake is single consistency (fluid).	Intake is of variable consistencies (fluids and solids).
Plane of tongue movement is unidirectional.	Plane of tongue movement is multidirectional.
Suckling movement is brainstem mediated, using a CPG.*	Greater cortical input is required to control complex masticatory movement patterns for biting and chewing.

CPG, Central pattern generator.
*See Box 13-21 in Chapter 13 for further discussion of CPGs.

the head laterally toward the stimulus and open his or her mouth. This allows the infant to locate the source of the feed (e.g., the mother's breast). This reflex emerges in utero during the third trimester and continues to approximately 3 to 6 months of age, when it diminishes.[1,7] This generally occurs earlier in infants who are bottle fed compared with breastfed infants.

A **suckling** reflex is seen when tactile stimulation occurs to the top of the tongue or middle of the hard palate. In response, the infant will move the tongue in a forward-backward motion in the horizontal plane. This allows the infant to draw milk from the nipple. This reflex emerges early in the third trimester and continues to approximately 3 to 6 months of age,[1,7] at which point the *suckle reflex* integrates into a more mature, voluntary *sucking* pattern.

Note: Sometime the words *suckling* and *sucking* are used interchangeably, but this isn't fully correct use of terminology. The term **suckling** refers to the *reflexive* oral pattern used by young infants to feed from the breast or bottle and to self-soothe. The suckling period is the time when young infants only take milk as their sole source of fluid and nutrition. The term **sucking** refers to the *volitional* oral pattern used by older infants, children, and adults to draw fluids into the mouth. Both involve similar oral movements, but one is reflexive and the other is under voluntary control. The transition from the suckling reflex to sucking occurs as a result of cortical maturation (allowing infants to make decisions and voluntarily control their motor patterns), improvements in gross motor skills and postural stability (allowing infants to sit more upright during feeds), and enlargement of the oral cavity (allowing separation of jaw and tongue movements and more room for the tongue to move within the mouth). The transition from suckling to sucking allows infants to start beginner solids (i.e., purees) that are sucked off the spoon.

TABLE 12-3 Comparison of Nutritive and Nonnutritive Suckling

Nutritive Suckling	Nonnutritive Suckling
Used during feeding.	Used to soothe.
Suck: swallow ratio = approximately 1:1 initially (high milk flow), then 2:1 or 3:1 by end of feed.	Suck: swallow ratio = approximately 6:1 to 8:1 (less frequent, as there is no milk to swallow).
Suck rate = approximately 1 per second.	Suck rate = approximately 2 per second (faster, as no milk is being drawn in).
Initial continuous suckling for approximately 60-90 seconds at start of milk flow. Duration of sucking bursts decreases and length of pauses increases as feed proceeds. By end of feed, only 2-3 sucks per burst with 4-5-second pauses.	Repetitive patterns of bursts and pauses. Usually 7-8 sucks per burst and several-second pauses between bursts.

Another set of terms that clinicians working with infants need to be aware of is *nutritive suckling* and *nonnutritive suckling*. **Nutritive suckling** is the type of suckling used for feeding (i.e., fluid is drawn into the mouth), whereas **nonnutritive suckling** is the type of suckling used during soothing (i.e., no fluid is drawn into the mouth). See Table 12-3 for a comparison on both types of suckling.

Protective reflexes assist the infant to keep feeds out of the airway. Most protective reflexes diminish over time and are replaced by voluntary skills, but some continue into adulthood.[1,7] The main protective reflexes are tongue protrusion, tongue lateralization, phasic bite, gag, and cough.

The **tongue protrusion** reflex occurs in response to tactile stimulation to the anterior part of the tongue. The reflex consists of anterior propulsion of the tongue, which serves to protect the infant's airway by pushing food out of the mouth when the infant's oral skills are not mature enough to masticate food. This reflex is present late in the third trimester and diminishes by 3 to 6 months of age,[1,7] enabling the introduction of (beginner) solid foods.

The **tongue lateralization** reflex occurs in response to tactile stimulation of the lateral surface of the tongue. The reflex consists of the tongue moving toward the stimulus, and serves to protect the infant's airway by pushing food to the side of the mouth where it can be held between the gums or chewed. This reflex emerges late in the third trimester and, by 6 to 9 months of age, is integrated into more refined, voluntary tongue movements for chewing.[1,7]

The **phasic bite** reflex occurs in response to tactile stimulation of the gums, and consists of crude jaw movements to bite and release. This reflex serves to protect the infant's airway by holding food between the gums and breaking up large food particles. This reflex emerges late in the third trimester and diminishes by 9 to 12 months of age,[1,7] when it is integrated into more refined, voluntary biting and chewing patterns.

The **gag** reflex is demonstrated by infants in response to tactile stimulation to the posterior two thirds of the tongue and the pharyngeal wall. The reflex involves tongue protrusion and pharyngeal contraction to eject the bolus from the pharynx, and soft-palate elevation to prevent nasal regurgitation. The gag reflex emerges in the third trimester and is retained through adulthood. However, the gag reflex generally diminishes around 6 to 9 months of age, such that it only occurs in response to stimulation of the posterior one third of the tongue,[1,7] which assists in the introduction of textured solids. It is acknowledged that the sensitivity of the gag response can be highly variable between individuals, however, and largely depends on individual sensory experience.[8]

Coughing occurs in response to the presence of a material in or near the entrance to the laryngeal vestibule. In response, the vocal folds close momentarily before opening again to allow air to be expelled from the lungs forcefully to clear the larynx. This reflex emerges early in the third trimester and continues into adulthood.[1,7]

In young infants, **apnea** events may also occur in response to the presence of a material in or near the entrance to the laryngeal vestibule. In this situation, the vocal folds close for a prolonged period before opening again, presumably to protect the lungs from the potential damage of aspirated material. This reflex is often referred to as the **laryngeal chemoreflex.**[9] This reflex emerges early in the third trimester, but generally diminishes in the early months postnatally.[9]

The **swallow** reflex has both adaptive and protective roles. Swallowing occurs in response to the presence of a bolus in the posterior oral cavity (e.g., saliva, fluid, food). During the normal swallow, the entrance to the airway closes over via superior and anterior laryngeal excursion, epiglottic deflection, and vocal fold closure. At the same time, the upper esophageal sphincter is pulled open, and the bolus is propelled through the pharynx and esophagus. This allows the feed to be delivered to the gut and not into the airway. This reflex emerges early in the third trimester and continues into adulthood.[1,7,8]

Suck-Swallow-Breath Coordination

Within the pharynx, swallowing and breathing share a common space. This dual role of the pharynx underlies the difficulties observed when suckling, swallowing, and breathing are not well coordinated. Problems in any one of these processes, or a lack of synchronization among these processes, can have a detrimental effect on the infant's oral feeding abilities. Although both the suckling and swallowing reflexes emerge early in the third trimester, it is generally late in the third trimester before the infant's suckling and swallowing skills are strong enough and suckling, swallowing, and breathing patterns are coordinated enough to be able to meet all nutritional requirements by mouth.

DEVELOPMENT OF MOTOR AND COGNITIVE SKILLS INVOLVED IN EARLY FEEDING

During infancy, a child progresses from being fully dependent on a feeder through a period of semidependence in which he or she begins to take on some responsibility and make some choices related to feeding. Later still, children learn to feed themselves with complete independence.

Early neurologic development allows the transition from brainstem-mediated suckling reflexes to complex, volitional oral movements during eating, which require higher cortical input.[7,10,11] Anatomic changes result in an enlarging of the oral cavity, allowing more space for food to be manipulated within the mouth. In addition, developmental gains in the area of gross motor skills allow the infant to sit upright with decreasing amounts of support, and bring the hands to the mouth for self-feeding.

Postural support is an important prerequisite for the introduction of solids, as gross motor control of the trunk and neck is needed to support the fine motor skills involved in chewing and biting.[1] As infants mature, their trunk control, neck control, and jaw control all mature in a sequential process.[1] An optimal feeding position is characterized by orientation around midline, neutral anterior-posterior alignment of the head and neck, neutral alignment of the trunk, and flexed hips and knees (Figures 12-2, 12-3).

BREASTFEEDING

Breastfeeding is the natural and ideal method for infants to feed. There are a number of benefits of breast milk and breastfeeding for infants (Box 12-1).

Infants may breastfeed (or receive breast-milk feeds) for variable amounts of time, depending on a variety of child, maternal, and other environmental factors. Infants are **exclusively breastfed** or breast-milk fed if they receive breast milk and no other fluid or food (complementary feeds). Infants are **partially breastfed** or breast-milk fed if they receive breast milk in addition to complementary feeds (which may be formula, other fluids, or solids). Overall, research supports that any breastfeeding or breast-milk feeding offers benefits to most infants.[12-18] Infants who may not be able to have breast-milk feeds include those with allergies or intolerances to components of breast milk,

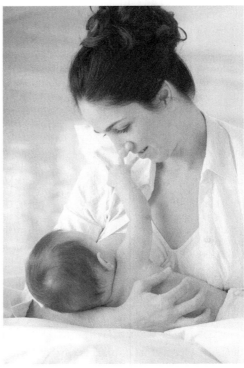

FIGURE 12-2 Good feeding position for infants. (From Stillerman E: *Parental Massage*, Mosby, St. Louis, 2008.)

infants with metabolic conditions that affect their digestion of milk (e.g. **galactosemia**), and those who are at risk because of maternal substance abuse or transmittable diseases.[16]

Health professionals working in the area of pediatric feeding and dysphagia management should be familiar with current breastfeeding guidelines. One should regularly check the websites of government and leading nongovernment organizations for up-to-date information. Examples include:

- World Health Organization (WHO): http://www.who.int/topics/breastfeeding/en/
- American Academy of Pediatrics (AAP): http://pediatrics.aappublications.org/content/129/3/e827
- European Society for Paediatric Hepatology, Gastroenterology and Nutrition (ESPHGAN): http://journals.lww.com/jpgn/Fulltext/2009/07000/Breast_feeding__A_Commentary_by_the_ESPGHAN.18.aspxEl

Special training is available for health professionals who are working with infants who are breastfeeding and their mothers. See the International Lactation Consultants Association (ILCA) website for details at http://www.ilca.org/.

At a minimum, the WHO recommends that all health staff who come in contact with pregnant mothers and

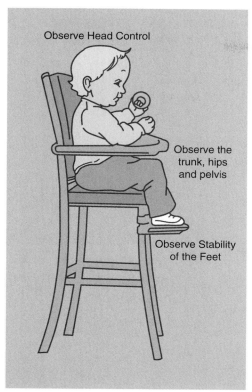

Observe Head Control

Observe the trunk, hips and pelvis

Observe Stability of the Feet

FIGURE 12-3 Good feeding position for a child ages 6 to 24 months, showing hip flexion, trunk in midline, and head in midline. Good foot support with a stool should continue throughout childhood. (From Mahan LK, Raymond J, Escott-Stump S: Krauses's Food & Nutrition Therapy, ed. 12, Saunders, St. Louis, 2008).

mothers of newborns should be aware of the "10 Steps to Successful Breastfeeding"[18] (Box 12-2).

Implementing the "10 Steps to Successful Breastfeeding" is part of the criteria for a hospital to be accredited in the **Baby Friendly Hospital Initiative (BFHI).** For further details, see the following websites:

WHO: http://www.who.int/nutrition/topics/bfhi/en/
United Nations Children's Fund: http://www.unicef.org/programme/breastfeeding/baby.htm
American BFHI: https://www.babyfriendlyusa.org/about-us/baby-friendly-hospital-initiative

Note: These guidelines are intended for healthy, full-term infants. It is recognized that there may be challenges for preterm and other medically high-risk infants in attaining these goals. See Practice note 15-10 in Chapter 15 for a discussion of the use of pacifiers in preterm infants.

BOTTLE FEEDING

Many infants receive expressed breast milk (EBM) or formula from a bottle for a variety of reasons, including maternal difficulty breastfeeding, infant difficulty breastfeeding, infant-mother separation (as occurs during prolonged hospitalization of the infant or maternal return to work), or family choice.

A variety of different bottles and artificial nipples are available (see Chapter 15).

BOX 12-1	BENEFITS OF BREAST MILK AND BREASTFEEDING
Breast milk	Breast milk contains the optimal mixture of energy for growth, nutrients for development, and immune factors for health.[12-18] Infant formula attempts to replicate breast milk and, although many improvements have been made to infant formula to make it closer to breast milk, no formula contains all of the many benefits of breast milk.
Breastfeeding	Breastfeeding is convenient and economical. Bottle feeding requires the purchase of feeding equipment (bottles and artificial nipples, as well as formula if expressed breast milk is not used), thorough cleaning and decontamination of feeding equipment for each use, and safe storage and preparation of feeds (formula or expressed breast milk). Breastfeeding allows the infant to self-regulate his or her appetite. Infants who are breastfed tend to feed on demand, taking feeds when they are hungry and only feeding until they are full. In contrast, infants who are bottle fed are often fed on a schedule (e.g., every 3 hours) and tend to be encouraged to feed until the bottle is finished. Learning to self-regulate appetite is important for healthy lifelong eating patterns.[12-18]
Benefits for infants	Breastfeeding and breast-milk feeding have been associated with reduced fat mass proportion and a reduced risk of allergy and intolerances, gastroenteritis, respiratory infections, otitis media, SIDS, and type II diabetes later in life.[12-18]
Benefits for mothers	Breastfeeding and breast-milk feeding have been associated with reduced risk of type II diabetes, ovarian cancer, and breast cancer.[12-18] Breastfeeding is also associated with improved postpregnancy weight loss and control of fertility.[14-18]

SIDS, Sudden infant death syndrome.

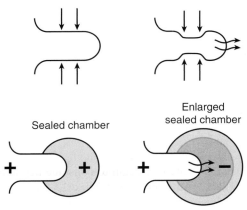

Sealed chamber   Enlarged sealed chamber

FIGURE 12-4 Compression and suction during suckling and sucking. (From Wolf LS, Glass RP: *Feeding and swallowing disorders in infancy: assessment and management,* Tucson, AZ, 1992, Therapy Skill Builders.)

During suckling and sucking at the breast or bottle, most infants use a combination of **positive pressure (compression)** and **negative pressure (suction)** to obtain milk from the nipple (Figure 12-4). Provided there is adequate lip seal around the nipple, and that the walls of the oral cavity are intact (i.e., no cleft lip or palate), the oral cavity acts as a sealed chamber. In this sealed chamber, downward movement of the tongue and jaw away from the palate enlarges the oral cavity, creating negative pressure and suction. Because of this negative pressure difference, milk is passively drawn out of the end of the nipple. Positive pressure is created by upward movement of the tongue and jaw toward the palate, which compresses the nipple, actively forcing fluid out of the end of the nipple. Infants who have difficulty generating either positive or negative pressure during suckling/sucking will likely be inefficient feeders, and may need to use specialized feeding equipment or strategies to assist them in obtaining sufficient milk flow.

INTRODUCTION OF SOLIDS

For infants to feed competently during the suckling period, they need to display functional suckling and swallowing skills, as well as the ability to coordinate suckling, swallowing, and breathing. Later, during the transitional feeding period, infants also need to learn to competently chew and bite so that they can safely consume solid foods. Increasing levels of oral motor skill are required to progress from breastfeeding and bottle feeding on to beginner (pureed) solid foods that are taken from a spoon, and then on to mashed and soft solid pieces that can be broken with the tongue, and later soft- and hard-mechanical food textures that require biting and chewing (Table 12-4).[1,7] Increasing oral motor skills are also required to move from drinking from the breast or bottle to drinking via a spout or straw cup and then an open cup.[1,7]

Note: See Practice note 15-11 in Chapter 15 for discussion of the "baby-led weaning" approach.

Infants generally begin weaning onto solid foods at the same time that they begin to be able to sit in an upright position and bring their hands to their mouth. Supportive seating, as well as manipulation of the size and firmness of food pieces offered by the caregiver, assists to maximize the child's ability to eat efficiently and safely.[1,7]

Developmental Milestones for Feeding

Newborns require full postural support during feeds. From birth to 4 months of age, an infant's diet consists entirely of fluid, taken in the form of breast- or bottle feeds. Young infants rely on adaptive oral reflexes (i.e., rooting and suckling) to locate and ingest feeds and display a forward-backward tongue pattern while feeding. Young infants are unable to consume or effectively digest any solid foods[13] and display protective oral reflexes (e.g., tongue protrusion, phasic bite, and strong gag reflexes) to protect their airway. As infants mature, changes in positioning, self-feeding, and oral skills occur (Table 12-5).

TABLE 12-4 Transitional Food Textures

Texture	Direction of Oral Movements Required to Consume Texture	Mastication
Fluids (e.g., breast milk, formula, water)	Bolus suckled from the breast or bottle. Tongue moves in a forward-backward plane of movement when transporting fluids.	No mastication required
Pureed foods (e.g., rice cereal, yoghurt, pureed fruit, vegetables, and meats)	Bolus taken from a spoon. Tongue moves in a forward-backward plane of movement when transporting purees.	
Mashed foods (e.g., mashed potato, squash, pumpkin, banana, and avocado)	Bolus taken from a spoon, fork, or fingers. Tongue moves in a forward-backward plane of movement when transporting mashed foods; upwards tongue pressure is often used to compress foods between the tongue and palate.	Food is masticated by the tongue
Soft pieces (e.g., pieces of banana and avocado, cooked pieces of potato and squash)	Bolus taken from fingers, spoon, or fork. Tongue moves in a forward-backward plane of movement when transporting soft pieces of food; upwards tongue pressure is often used to compress foods between the tongue and palate.	
Soft mechanicals* (e.g., cheese, roast chicken, meatballs, boiled vegetables, pasta)	Bolus is cut up or broken then taken from a fork, chopsticks, or fingers. Sideways tongue movement (tongue lateralization) is required to move food onto the chewing surfaces.	Food is masticated by the teeth
Hard mechanicals* (e.g., beef steak, pork, raw apple, raw carrot)	Bolus is cut up or a bite is taken; the bolus is usually taken from fingers or possibly a fork. Sideways tongue movement (tongue lateralization) is required to move food onto the chewing surfaces.	
Mixed textures (e.g., baked beans in sauce, pieces of cooked chicken and pasta in with mashed vegetables)	Bolus is usually taken from a spoon or fork; components of food are fluid or pureed, and tongue moves in a forward-backward plane of movement; other components of food need to be masticated by the teeth, and tongue lateralization is required to move food onto the chewing surfaces.	

*Mechanical food is another term for food that requires chewing.

At **4 months** of age, most infants are still only consuming fluids (as either breastfeeds or bottle feeds). However, from 4 to 6 months infants begin to display separation of tongue and jaw movements, and transition from a suckle (one dimensional, front to back tongue stripping movements) to a suck (two dimensional, upward and backward tongue movements) pattern while feeding. During this time, infants begin to be able to sit more upright, but still require full postural support (e.g., seated in a baby chair with straps, or on the feeder's lap with the feeder's arm supporting the head and trunk). Most infants will begin to bring their hands to their mouth at this stage for oral self-exploration. This helps to desensitize some of the protective reflexes (e.g., tongue protrusion). Toward the end of this period, many infants will begin to consume beginner (i.e., pureed) solids from a spoon (see Table 12-5).

At **7 to 9 months** of age, the infant diet still consists mostly of fluids, but infants are able to consume a greater volume and variety of solid foods. Infants continue to consume fluids from the breast or bottle, but many begin to be able to drink from a cup. As infants develop the core stability to sit up with less external support, and as many of the protective oral reflexes diminish or are integrated into more sophisticated, voluntary oral skills (e.g., phasic bite transitions to chewing), infants can begin to consume mashed solids and small pieces of soft foods (see Table 12-5). As hand-to-mouth coordination improves, most infants begin some (messy) self-feeding; however, much

TABLE 12-5 Developmental Milestones for Feeding

	0-4 Months	4-6 Months	7-8 Months	9-12 Months	12-18 Months	18-24 Months
Positioning	Fully supported (reclined in caregiver's arms)	Able to maintain supported sitting position (slightly reclined, highchair with straps)	Can sit upright, but need support (highchair with straps, foot rest)	Can sit upright with minimal assistance (highchair, straps not required, short periods on floor)	Can sit upright without support (seated in a chair where feet can touch floor or foot rest)	Can sit upright without support
Self-feeding	n/a	Hands to mouth (bilateral movements) Reduction in gag reflex	Hands to mouth (some unilateral movements) Some (messy) self-feeding	Combination of self-feeding and requiring assistance	Largely self-feeding	Predominately self-feeding
Oral skills for fluids	Breastfed, bottle fed Suckle (forward-backward tongue movements, reflexive)	Breastfed, bottle fed Suck (up-down tongue movements, volitional)	Breastfed, bottle fed Can introduce cup drinks	Breastfed, bottle fed Cup drinks	Cup drinking Often still breastfeeds, bottle feeds	Cup drinking May still breastfeed, bottle feed
Oral skills for solids	None Unable to chew Unable to bite	Sucking Reduction in tongue protrusion *May begin to offer runny pureed solids from spoon* Unable to chew Unable to bite	Early chewing Early tongue lateralization Starting to get teeth (central incisors) *Offer thicker purees Introduce textured (mashed) solids Offer spoonable foods, soft cubes* Unable to bite *Offer teething biscuits, teething toys for chewing and biting practice*	Chewing Improving tongue lateralization Starting to get teeth (lateral incisors) *Offer soft pieces* Not biting through foods Hold food between teeth and use hands to break off pieces *Offer teething biscuits, teething toys for chewing and biting practice*	Chewing Good tongue lateralization More teeth (first molars and canines) Biting through soft foods *Offer soft mechanicals*	Efficient chewing Good tongue lateralization Most teeth through Biting through firm foods *Offer hard mechanicals*

Note: Time frames for introduction of solids and independent feeding may be influenced by social and cultural factors. A full history, including details of solid food exposure and mealtime routines, should be evaluated before concluding that a child has delayed feeding skills.

assistance from caregivers is still required during mealtimes at this age.

At **9 to 12 months** of age, infants are generally consuming a mixed diet of fluids and solids. During the day, an increasing proportion of fluids may be taken from a cup, although infants still require breastfeeds or bottle feeds to meet their nutritional requirements. Most infants can sit without support at this age, and most are beginning to stand and walk. However, infants generally continue to be fed in a baby chair or on a caregiver's lap to provide postural support while they continue to develop their fine motor skills. Self-feeding is more common at this age, and improved jaw stability and tongue lateralization skills allow infants to bite and chew soft-mechanical foods (see Table 12-5).

From **12 to 24 months** of age, toddlers' oral feeding skills continue to improve and become more refined and coordinated, which results in improved efficiency of mealtimes and a greater variety of foods consumed. Children gradually learn to bite through hard-mechanical foods (see Table 12-5) during this period. Toddlers also become more competent at using utensils to assist with eating. This process occurs in parallel with improvements in general motor development and sensory integration, as well as with maturation of cognitive processes. Toddlers continue to require assistance from their caregivers in offering appropriate foods in manageable size portions, and should be supervised while eating any foods that pose a choking risk. Note: See Box 15-4 in Chapter 15 regarding choking (see Clinical Corner 12-1, 12-2).

TRANSITION TO MATURE MEALTIME BEHAVIOR

Beyond the initial period of first learning to eat solid foods, young children must learn to make another transition toward mature mealtime behavior. Throughout childhood,

children undergo immense development of their cerebral cortex and subsequent improvements in their cognitive skills. Piaget described four major stages of cognitive development, which are summarized in Table 12-6. Implications of each of these stages for feeding are also detailed.

NUTRITION AND GROWTH CONSIDERATIONS IN INFANTS AND CHILDREN

During the first months after birth, an infant's nutritional needs are met by a diet of breast milk or infant formula. Later in infancy, solid foods are introduced to supplement milk feeds. The transition from a liquid-based diet to a diet consisting of solids and liquids is an important developmental process that allows infants to consume a larger volume and variety of nutrients, which is important in meeting their expanding dietary requirements as they grow.[13]

From birth to 12 months of age, healthy infants generally experience a 50% increase in their length (mean length for boys at birth = 50 cm, mean length at 12 months = 76 cm) and a 200% increase in their weight (mean weight for boys at birth = 3.5 kg, mean weight at 12 months = 10.5 kg).[20,21] Clinically, a child's growth is used as a crude indicator of nutritional intake and feeding skills, such that, if the child is growing well, it is generally assumed that dietary intake must be sufficient to meet nutritional requirements and, if exclusively orally fed (versus tube fed), that feeding skills are sufficient to allow them to consume the required dietary intake.

CLINICAL CORNER 12-1: INTRODUCTION OF SOLIDS

You have been asked to prepare a 45-minute talk for daycare staff regarding introduction of solid foods.

Critical Thinking
Consider how you would explain the following:
1. Signs that an infant is ready to start beginner (pureed solids)
2. Why some infants get stuck on pureed and mashed foods and have difficulty transitioning to more solid foods
3. The importance of supportive positioning for feeding

CLINICAL CORNER 12-2: DELAYED INTRODUCTION OF SOLIDS

While you are at the daycare, you are stopped by a mother who has some questions about feeding. The mother has a daughter called Tara. She reports that Tara is 16 months old, was born term age, and has no significant medical history. She refuses to eat most solid foods, unless they are blended or mashed. Her mother wants her to start eating finger foods to increase lunch options for Tara to bring to daycare.

Critical Thinking
1. Describe the normal oral intake of a child of this age (texture of food, method of delivering food and fluids, position for feeds).
2. Consider possible reasons for Tara's feeding difficulties.
3. Consider possible steps in Tara's feeding therapy program.

TABLE 12-6 Stages of Cognitive Development (Based on Work of Piaget) and Implications for Feeding

Stage	Age	Characteristics	Developmental Changes	Implications for Feeding
Sensorimotor	Birth to 2 years	The infant knows the world through movements and sensations.	During this time infants learn: • Things continue to exist even though they cannot be seen (object permanence). • They are separate beings from the people and objects around them. • Their actions can cause things to happen in the world around them. Learning occurs through assimilation and accommodation.	Infants trust their caregivers to give them "safe" foods. Infants learn from observing their caregivers' reactions to foods and their behavior. Children may refuse foods if they can't manage the texture from a sensory or motor perspective. Older infants and toddlers may refuse foods because it gets them attention.
Preoperational	2 to 7 years	Children begin to think symbolically and learn to use words and pictures to represent objects. Children tend to be egocentric, and see things only from their point of view.	During this time children tend to struggle to see things from the perspective of others. While they are rapidly developing language and thought processes, they still tend to think about things in very literal terms.	Children may form phobias (fear or emotional responses) to foods that are paired in time with an adverse event. Children often like food prepared in a very specific way. If it is changed, they may perceive it as a different food and display neophobia (fear of new things).
Concrete operations	7 to 11 years	Children begin to think logically about concrete events.	During this time children begin to understand the concept of conservation (e.g., the amount of liquid in a short, wide cup is equal to that in a tall, skinny glass). Thinking becomes more logical and organized, but still very concrete. Children begin to use inductive logic and reasoning from specific information to a general principle.	Children begin to understand that they can alter foods to suit their preferences (e.g., cutting up, adding sauces). Children learn best with clear rules and basic explanations (e.g., "doctors and scientists say that we need to eat fruit and vegetables every day to be fully healthy").[19]
Formal operations	12 and older	At this stage, the adolescent or young adult begins to think abstractly and reason about hypothetical problems.	During this time abstract thought emerges. Teenagers begin to think more about moral, ethical, social, philosophical, and political issues that require theoretical and abstract reasoning. Those in this stage begin to use deductive logic and reasoning from a general principle to specific information.	Adolescents begin to learn that there are some things that we don't like, but we do them because they are good for us (e.g., eating spinach).

Current Infant Feeding Guidelines

Health professionals working in the area of pediatric feeding and dysphagia management should be familiar with current feeding and nutrition guidelines for infants, which cover topics such as recommended duration of breastfeeding, the use of infant formula, and the recommended age for introduction of solids. One should regularly check the websites of government and leading nongovernment organizations for up-to-date information. Examples include:

- WHO: http://www.who.int/nutrition/topics/infantfeeding _recommendation/en/
- AAP: http://www.aap.org/en-us/advocacy-and-policy/ aap-health-initiatives/HALF-Implementation-Guide/ Age-Specific-Content/Pages/Infant-Food-and-Feeding .aspx
- ESPHGAN: http://espghan.med.up.pt/index.php?option =com_content&task=view&id=37&Itemid=119
- Australian National Health and Medical Research Committee: https://www.nhmrc.gov.au/guidelines/publications/n20

Currently, most international infant feeding guidelines recommend that infants should be exclusively breastfed until 6 months of age (6 months corrected age for preterm infants) and should continue to receive breastfeeds until at least 12 to 24 months.[12,14,15,18] The benefits of breast milk for young infants are well documented, and include both nutritional and immunologic advantages.[12-18] In cases in which a young infant cannot, or does not, receive exclusive breast-milk feeds, an appropriate human milk substitute (i.e., infant formula) should be offered until at least 12 months of age.[12-18]

There is some variation in current international guidelines regarding the age at which solids should be introduced, with some guidelines suggesting introduction of solids at 4 to 6 months of age and others at (or approximately) 6 months of age.[13,22] However, there is general consensus from international bodies that solid foods should not be introduced before 4 months of age. This recommendation is based on the fact that the gut is unable to effectively digest solid foods before 4 months of age, and exposure to solid foods before this time increases the risk of developing allergy.[12-18,22] In addition, oral skills do not support the introduction of solids before this time. Beyond this particular milestone, however, it is recognized that infants should be gradually introduced to a range of nutritious solid foods, to assist them in meeting their dietary requirements,[12-18,22] as well as to assist them in developing and practicing the oral skills needed for managing a mature diet.

Nutrition Guidelines for Children

Health professionals working in the area of pediatric feeding and dysphagia management should be familiar with current feeding and nutrition guidelines for children, which cover topics such as energy, nutrient, and fluid requirements for children of various ages and methods for monitoring growth. One should regularly check the websites of government and leading nongovernment organizations for up-to-date information. Examples include:

- WHO: http://www.who.int/publications/guidelines/nutri tion/en/
- AAP: http://pediatrics.aappublications.org/content/117/ 2/544.full
- ESPHGAN: http://espghan.med.up.pt/index.php?option =com_content&task=view&id=37&Itemid=119

Energy Requirements

Information regarding average **energy** requirements of children of different ages and sexes are widely available and are summarized in Tables 12-7 and 12-8. In general, energy requirements are provided as the amount of energy (or amount of fluid of a known energy concentration) required per unit of body weight of the child per day. Information regarding the energy content of common fluids and foods can be obtained from food packaging or from freely or commercially available energy calculators.

Individuals with health or medical complications and those who are very under- or overweight may have energy requirements that are different from the average requirements of those of the same age and sex.

Dietitians have specialist knowledge and skills in assessing individual energy requirements of individuals and in making individualized recommendations and diet plans to meet needs. It is recommended that referral to a pediatric dietitian be made whenever concerns regarding energy intake or growth are suspected.

TABLE 12-7 Average Breast Milk and Formula Requirements for Infants and Toddlers per Unit of Body Weight per Day

Day 1-4	30-120 mL/kg/day	<2 oz/lb/day
Day 5 to 3 months	150 mL/kg/day	2.5 oz/lb/day
Preterm and other high-risk neonates	Up to 180-200 mL/ kg/day	3 oz/lb/day
3 to 6 months	120 mL/kg/day	2 oz/lb/day
6 to 12 months	90 mL/kg/day (+ food)	1.5 oz/lb/day
1 to 2 years	Up to 90 mL/kg/ day (+ food)	1.5 oz/lb/day

Note: Average breast milk and standard formula contains 67 kcal per 100 mL (20 kcal/oz).
From World Health Organization: Human energy requirements: report of a joint FAO/WHO/UNU Expert Consultation. *Food Nutr Bull* 26(1):166, 2005.

TABLE 12-8 Average Energy Requirements for Infants and Toddlers

Boys			
		Daily Energy Requirement	
Age (years)	Average weight (kg)	kcal/day	kcal/kg/day
1-2	11.5	948	82.4
2-3	13.5	1129	83.6
3-4	15.7	1252	79.7
4-5	17.7	1360	76.8
Girls			
		Daily Energy Requirement	
Age (years)	Average weight (kg)	kcal/day	kcal/kg/day
1-2	10.8	865	80.1
2-3	13.0	1047	80.6
3-4	15.1	1156	76.5
4-5	16.8	1241	73.9

(Note: See energy calculators for energy content of common food and drinks per unit weight.)
From World Health Organization: Human energy requirements: report of a joint FAO/WHO/UNU Expert Consultation. *Food Nutr Bull* 26(1):166, 2005.

TABLE 12-9 Holliday-Segar Fluid Requirement Calculation

Child Weight	Minimum Daily Fluid Requirement
1-10 kg	100 mL/kg
10-20 kg	1000 mL + 50 mL/kg over 10 kg
>20 kg	1500 mL + 20 mL/kg over 20 kg

From Holliday MA, Segar WE: The maintenance need for water in parenteral fluid therapy. *Pediatrics* 19:823, 1957.

Macronutrient, Micronutrient, and Fluid Requirements

Information regarding average **nutrient** requirements of children of different ages and sexes are widely available. Recommendations are available regarding macronutrient intake (protein, fat, carbohydrate—the main sources of energy in the diet) and micronutrient intake (essential vitamins and minerals, including iron, calcium, zinc, and fiber among others). In general, nutrient requirements are provided as recommended daily intake (RDI)—an average amount of intake per day for that nutrient for a child of a given age. Basic information regarding the key nutrient content of common fluids and foods can often be obtained from food packaging, but more detailed information may need to be obtained directly from the manufacturer or from free or commercial nutritional calculators.

Information regarding average **fluid** requirements can be derived from equations based on the child's weight (Table 12-9). Fluids are primarily derived from drinks, but can also be derived from fluid-containing foods. Signs that a child is not getting enough fluid can include the presence of dry eyes, mouth, or skin, infrequent urination or wet diapers, urine that has a strong color or smell, constipation, lethargy, and irritability.[2]

It is recommended that referral to a pediatric dietitian be made whenever concerns regarding a child's fluid or nutrient intake, absorption, or growth are suspected.

Food Servings and Serving Size

Information regarding both the recommended relative amount of dietary intake across the various food groups (fruit, vegetables, grains, dairy, protein) as well as food serving size for children of different ages is available from a number of different government and nongovernment organizations, often in the form of food plate or food pyramid guidelines. Examples include:

- United States Department of Agriculture: www .choosemyplate.gov/
- European Food Information Council: www.eufic.org/
- UK National Health Service: http://www.nhs.uk/ Livewell/Goodfood/Pages/eatwell-plate.aspx
- Nutrition Australia: http://www.nutritionaustralia.org/

Food Handling and Hygiene

Those involved in the handling of food in any way need to be aware of food handling and hygiene guidelines. These guidelines generally provide suggestions for suitable foods and food preparation, hand washing, food storage (suitable containers and temperature), and food heating and reheating.

Food handling and hygiene guidelines for the general community are usually provided as part of national infant and child nutrition guidelines. Guidelines for daycare and school environments, where foods are provided or served, are often regulated by national or state education policy, and those working in this area should be aware of these guidelines. Guidelines for hospitals and health care facilities, which care for immune-compromised and other medically and nutritionally vulnerable groups, are guided by national or state health policy. Site-specific guidelines may also be enforced. Those working in this area should be aware of these government and site regulations, as well as **universal health precautions**, and use particular caution in the case of children who fall into any of the following groups:

- Immunocompromised patients (e.g., newborns, those on chemotherapy, those who have had organ transplants, those on steroids, or those with human immunodeficiency virus): Fluid or foods prone to carrying contaminants and unhygienic handling process can pose an infection threat to this vulnerable group.

- Children with food allergy or intolerance: Fluids or foods known or suspected to cause an allergic response should be completely avoided. Foods thought to cause an intolerance should be minimized.
- Children with metabolic conditions (e.g., galactosemia, phenylketonuria): Fluids or foods that cannot be metabolized effectively should be completely avoided.
- Patients with transmittable diseases (e.g., herpes simplex virus, hepatitis A): Particular attention should be paid when handling food utensils, equipment, and food scraps that may contain saliva or other bodily fluids that may pose an infection risk to others.

Growth Charts

Growth charts for children of different ages, sex, and nationality are widely available. In general, separate charts are made for children aged 0 to 2 years and 2 to 18 years. Most growth series include charts for weight and height (or length in children younger than 2 years of age), as well as for head circumference. Growth charts can be used to estimate a child's growth percentile relative to a normative sample of typical children (where being at or greater than the fiftieth percentile indicates that a child is the same size or greater than 50% of typical children the same age). Most growth charts provide growth percentiles for the third, fifth, tenth, twenty-fifth, fiftieth, seventy-fifth, ninetieth, ninety-fifth, and ninety-seventh percentiles). In general, growth patterns are more important than single growth measurements in monitoring a child's health and development. Hence, several growth measurements are generally required to determine if a child is moving away from the growth trajectory.

See Box 12-3 for a discussion of different infant growth charts. Specific growth charts exist for some specific populations (e.g., children with Down syndrome, Turner syndrome). There are also equations available for estimating total height from knee height in children who are unable to stand up straight for measurements (e.g., children with cerebral palsy).

Ideal body weight (IBW) is generally calculated by applying an equation based on height. IBW is age and sex specific, and free calculators are widely available. Many growth series provide charts for body mass index (BMI) or weight-for-height charts. It should be noted that standard adult BMI cut-offs for healthy, underweight, and overweight criteria do not apply to children because of changing body proportions as they grow.

Information regarding typical weight gain (in terms of expected weight gain per day or year) of children of

---

BOX 12-3 INFANT GROWTH CHARTS

In 2006 the World Health Organization (WHO) released a set of international growth charts for children aged up to 5 years, based on growth *standards* from a population of children living in what it considers to be ideal circumstances (i.e., exclusively breastfed for at least 4 months, receiving some breast milk until at least 12 months, no smoking in the household[21]). These charts vary from traditional growth charts (such as the American Centers for Disease Control and Prevention [CDC] growth charts)[20] that are based on growth *reference* from the general population. Whereas traditional growth charts document how typical children *do* grow, the WHO charts were developed to provide an indication of how children *should* grow under optimal conditions.

   WHO growth charts can be found at http://www.who.int/childgrowth/en/.
   CDC growth charts can be found at http://www.cdc.gov/growthcharts/cdc_charts.htm.
   UK growth charts can be found at http://www.rcpch.ac.uk/child-health/research-projects/uk-who-growth-charts/uk-growth-chart-resources-2-18-years/school-age.
   Ideally, a child's growth should be plotted on the same chart over time. As discussed earlier in this chapter, growth patterns are more meaningful than individual growth measurements; therefore, regardless of which growth chart is used, deviation away from a growth curve generally indicates growth faltering.

TABLE 12-10 Average Weight Gain of Children 1-5 Years

Age (Years)	Boys		Girls	
	kg/year	*g/day*	*kg/year*	*g/day*
1-2	2.4	6.6	2.4	6.6
2-3	2.0	5.5	2.2	6.0
3-4	2.1	5.8	1.9	5.2
4-5	2.0	5.5	1.7	4.7

From World Health Organization: Human energy requirements: report of a joint FAO/WHO/UNU Expert Consultation. *Food Nutr Bull* 26(1):166, 2005.

---

different ages and sex are widely available and are summarized in Table 12-10. In clinical practice, body weight (or calculations involving weight, such as BMI or IBW) is often used as a crude indicator of nutrition. However, body composition measures that allow calculation of fat versus lean (fat-free) mass (e.g., bioelectrical impedance analysis, air-displacement plethysmography, total body potassium, dual-energy x-ray absorptiometry) and blood chemistry measures (e.g., iron, glucose, electrolytes, such as sodium and potassium) are generally more accurate indicators of nutritional status.

TAKE HOME NOTES

1. It is important to remember that infants aren't just smaller versions of adults. There are a number of differences in head and neck structure and function in infants relative to adults that affect feeding.
2. The relative size and function of the head and neck region of infants differ somewhat from that of older children and adults, which offers some level of protection to neonates and infants while they are developing their oral feeding skills.
3. In neonates and young infants, all four components of feeding are involuntary (oral phase, triggering of the swallowing reflex, pharyngeal phase, and esophageal phase), and it is only later in infancy that the oral phase comes under voluntary control.
4. Infants display a number of brainstem-mediated oral reflexes that assist them with oral feeding. The purpose of these reflexes may be adaptive (i.e., assist to get feed into gut), protective (i.e., assist to keep feed out of the airway), or both.
5. It is important to understand that there are different types of "sucking." The term *suckling* refers to the reflexive oral pattern used by young infants to feed from the breast or bottle and to soothe themselves. The term *sucking* refers to the volitional oral pattern used by older infants, children, and adults to draw fluids into the mouth. Nutritive suckling is the type of suckling used for feeding (i.e., fluid is drawn into the mouth), whereas nonnutritive suckling is the type of suckling used during soothing (i.e., no fluid is drawn into the mouth).
6. Feeding therapists work with children who are breast-fed and bottle fed and need to be able to support the needs of both populations.
7. Breastfeeding is the natural and ideal method for infants to feed. Many infants receive expressed breast milk or formula from a bottle for a variety of reasons, including maternal difficulty breastfeeding, infant difficulty breastfeeding, infant-mother separation (as occurs during prolonged hospitalization of the infant or maternal return to work), or family choice. There are a number of benefits of breast milk and breastfeeding for infants.
8. During suckling or sucking at the breast or bottle, most infants use a combination of positive pressure (compression) and negative pressure (suction) to obtain milk from the nipple.
9. It is important to understand that the transition to solid foods is an important developmental process.

10. Postural support is an important prerequisite for the introduction of solids, as gross motor control of the trunk and neck is needed to support the fine motor skills involved in chewing and biting.
11. Increasing levels of oral motor skill are required to progress from breastfeeding and bottle feeding on to beginner (pureed) solid foods that are taken from a spoon, and then on to mashed and soft solid pieces that can be broken with the tongue, and later soft- and hard-mechanical food textures that require biting and chewing. Increasing oral motor skills are also required to move from drinking from the breast or bottle on to drinking via a spout or straw cup and then an open cup.
12. During infancy, a child progresses from being fully dependent on a feeder through a period of semidependence, during which they begin to take on some responsibility and make some choices related to feeding. Later still, children learn to feed themselves with complete independence.
13. Health professionals working in the area of pediatric feeding and dysphagia management should be familiar with current feeding and nutrition guidelines for infants and older children.

REFERENCES

1. Morris SE, Klein MD: *Pre-feeding skills: a comprehensive resource for feeding development*, ed 2, Tucson, AZ, 2000, Therapy Skill Builders.
2. Kliegman R, Stanton R, Geme J, et al: *Nelson textbook of pediatrics*, ed 19, Philadelphia, 2011, Elsevier Saunders.
3. Kenner C, McGrath JM, editors: *Developmental care of newborns and infants: a guide for health professionals*, ed 2, St Louis, 2010, Mosby.
4. Gardner S, Merenstein G: *Handbook of neonatal intensive care*, St Louis, 2002, Mosby.
5. Stiles J, Jernigan T: The basics of brain development. *Neuropsychol Rev* 20(4):327, 2010.
6. Wolf LS, Glass RP: *Feeding and swallowing disorders in infancy: assessment and management*, Tucson, AZ, 1992, Therapy Skill Builders.
7. Dodrill P: Infant feeding development and dysphagia. *J Gastroenterol Hepatol Res* 2014. [Epub ahead of print].
8. Logemann J: *Evaluation and treatment of swallowing disorders*, ed 2, Austin, TX, 1998, PRO-ED.
9. Thach BT: Maturation of cough and other reflexes that protect the fetal and neonatal airway. *Pulm Pharmacol Ther* 20(4):365, 2007.
10. Wilson-Pauwels L, Akesson EJ, Stewart PA, et al: *Cranial nerves in health and disease*, ed 2, Hamilton, Ontario, 2002, BC Decker Inc.
11. Delaney AL, Arvedson JC: Development of swallowing and feeding: prenatal through first year of life. *Dev Disabil Res Rev* 14(2):105, 2008.
12. Section on Breastfeeding: Breastfeeding and the use of human milk. *Pediatrics* 129(3):e827, 2012.

13. Agostoni C, Decsi T, Fewtrell M, et al: Complementary feeding: a commentary by the ESPGHAN Committee on Nutrition. *J Pediatr Gastroenterol Nutr* 46(1):99, 2008.

14. World Health Organization: *The optimal duration of exclusive breast-feeding*, Geneva, 2001, World Health Organization.

15. World Health Organization: *Global strategy for infant and young child feeding*, Geneva, 2003, World Health Organization.

16. World Health Organization: *Acceptable medical reasons for use of breast milk substitutes*, Geneva, 2003, World Health Organization.

17. World Health Organization: *Infant and young child feeding: model chapter for textbooks for medical students and allied health professionals*, Geneva, 2009, World Health Organization.

18. World Health Organization, UNICEF: *Baby-Friendly Hospital Initiative*. Revised, updated and expanded for integrated care, 2009. <http://www.who.int/nutrition/publications/infantfeeding/bfhi_trainingcourse/en/>.

19. SOS Approach to Feeding: <http://www.sosapproach-conferences.com/>.

20. Centers for Disease Control: Growth charts for infants, <http://www.cdc.gov/growthcharts/>.

21. World Health Organization: *WHO child growth standards: methods and development*, Geneva, 2006, World Health Organization.

22. Australian Society for Clinical Immunology and Allergy: Infant feeding guidelines, <http://www.allergy.org.au/images/stories/aer/infobulletins/2010pdf/ASCIA_Infant_Feeding_Advice_2010.pdf>.

23. World Health Organization: Human energy requirements: report of a joint FAO/WHO/UNU Expert Consultation. *Food Nutr Bull* 26(1):166, 2005.

24. Holliday MA, Segar WE: The maintenance need for water in parenteral fluid therapy. *Pediatrics* 19:823, 1957.

CHAPTER 13

Disorders Affecting Feeding and Swallowing in Infants and Children

Pamela Dodrill

To view additional case videos and content, please visit the evolve website.

CHAPTER OUTLINE

OBJECTIVES

1. Describe key terms related to swallowing and dysphagia in children, such as *laryngeal penetration, aspiration, choking,* and *apnea.*
2. List key indicators of childhood feeding difficulties and behavioral feeding issues.
3. Discuss the potential effect of interruptions to early feeding on ongoing feeding development.
4. Demonstrate an understanding of common medical conditions that may that may affect feeding and swallowing in children.
5. Describe the potential effect of prematurity on feeding and swallowing, and list common feeding problems seen in the preterm population.
6. Demonstrate an understanding of different tube feeding options commonly used for children with feeding or swallowing complications.
7. Describe different types of respiratory support used in children.
8. Discuss other factors that may potentially affect feeding and swallowing in children, such as tonsillitis and tongue-tie, oral motor impairments, sensory processing disorders, and autism.

Like adults, infants and older children can present with swallowing and feeding difficulties. Unlike adults, children have rapidly developing body systems, and even short-term problems with swallowing or feeding can interrupt normal development and cause serious long-term sequelae. For a child to reach his or her physical and cognitive growth potential, sufficient energy and nutrients must be consumed. Feeding difficulties can have a detrimental effect on dietary intake and hence growth and development.

SWALLOWING AND DYSPHAGIA

As described in previous chapters, during normal swallowing, the bolus is propelled from the oral cavity through the pharynx and into the esophagus (Figure 13-1). **Dysphagia** occurs when there is a problem with bolus containment or propulsion, and may occur at the oral, pharyngeal, or esophageal phases of swallowing. Common disorders in children that can affect the various stages of swallowing are presented in Table 13-1.

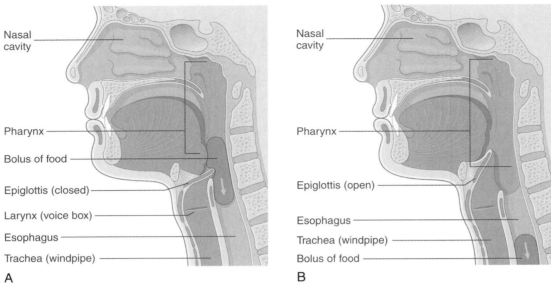

FIGURE 13-1 **A,** Epiglottis closes over the trachea as the bolus of food passes down the pharynx toward the esophagus. **B,** Epiglottis opens as the bolus moves down the esophagus. (From Chabner DE: *The language of medicine,* ed 10, Saunders, 2014, St Louis.)

TABLE 13-1 Common Presentations and Causes of Dysphagia in Children

Oral phase (sucking, drinking, chewing, biting)	Absent oral reflexes, primitive/neurologic oral reflexes, weak suck, uncoordinated suck, immature biting and chewing, oral apraxia Cleft lip or palate, tongue-tie, micro- and macroglossia, micro- and retrognathia, cranial nerve damage (V, VII, XII), developmental or acquired brain injury
Pharyngeal phase (swallowing)	Poor suck-swallow-breath coordination, delayed triggering of the swallow, poor pharyngeal clearance Respiratory disease, prematurity, enlarged tonsils, laryngeal cleft, ingestional injuries, cranial nerve damage (IX, X, XI), recurrent laryngeal nerve damage, developmental or acquired brain injury
Esophageal phase	Impaired UES or LES opening, LES relaxation causing reflux, poor motility Esophageal atresia, tracheoesophageal fistula, esophagitis, esophageal strictures, achalasia, developmental or acquired brain injury

LES, Lower esophageal sphincter; *UES,* upper esophageal sphincter.

BOX 13-1 PRIMARY AND SECONDARY ASPIRATION

Primary aspiration: Aspiration on a bolus that comes from above the airway. Aspirated material is usually saliva, fluid, or food.
Secondary aspiration: Aspiration on a bolus that comes from below the airway. Aspirated material has usually been refluxed or vomited up from the gut (**emesis**), or has built up above a stricture or hold up in the esophagus.

Airway Protection, Aspiration, and Apnea

During normal swallowing, the vocal folds close and a brief deglutition apnea occurs, along with superior and anterior laryngeal excursion and epiglottic deflection. This helps to protect the airway and ensure the bolus ends up in the gut and not in the airway. **Laryngeal penetration** occurs when the bolus (liquid or solid) enters the laryngeal vestibule. **Aspiration** occurs when the bolus enters the airway below the level of the vocal folds, and may be primary or secondary to swallowing (Box 13-1). A prolonged **apnea** event occurs when the airway closes over and fails to reopen in time for regular breathing to continue after a swallow.[1] In young infants, apnea events may occur in response to the presence of a material in or near the entrance to the laryngeal vestibule (see Chapter 12). This reflex is often referred to as the **laryngeal chemoreflex.**[2] In this situation, the vocal folds close for a prolonged period before opening again, presumably to protect the lungs from the potential damage of aspirated material. **Choking** occurs when a solid

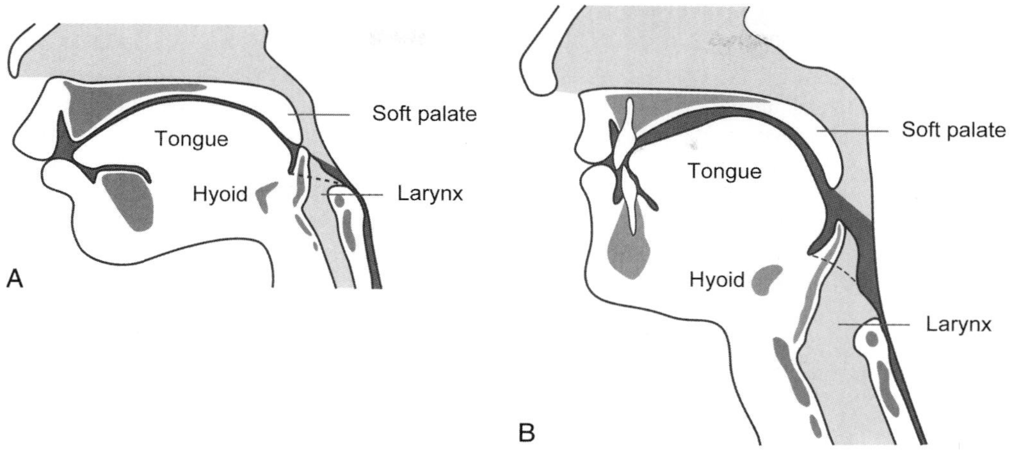

FIGURE 13-2 Sagittal section of the head and neck in an infant (*A*) and an adult (*B*). (From Matsuo K, Palmer JD: Anatomy and physiology of feeding and swallowing: normal and abnormal, *Phys Med Rehabil Clin North Am* 19(4):691, 2008.)

bolus physically blocks the airway.[3] Because the child cannot breathe, choking events can be immediately life threatening. See Box 15-4 in Chapter 15 for further discussion of choking risks and management.

Within the pharynx, swallowing and breathing share a common space (Figure 13-2). Problems in either of these processes, or lack synchronization between processes, can affect a child's ability to ingest fluid and food safely.

MEALTIME BEHAVIOR AND FEEDING DIFFICULTIES

Mealtime behavior disturbances or learned **fluid** or **food aversion** arise in association with dysphagia, aspiration, or a choking event. At other times, there is no apparent physical reason for feeding issues, although aversive experiences in or around the mouth (e.g., tube feeding, suctioning), undetected pain (e.g., as associated with teething, tonsillitis, pharyngitis, or mucositis), or sensory disturbances (e.g., oral hypersensitivity) are usually involved at some level.[4-7]

Several studies have shown that most children presenting to feeding clinics with mealtime behavior disturbances also present with other **feeding difficulties** (such as oral motor or oral sensory processing disorders) that must be managed in conjunction with behavioral issues for therapy to be effective.[4-7]

Childhood feeding difficulties or behavioral feeding issues should not be confused with eating disorders such as anorexia nervosa, which are associated with distorted body self-perception and are more common in adolescence and adulthood. Childhood feeding difficulties or behavioral feeding issues occur when an infant or child is *unable or unwilling* to eat a range of age-appropriate food (and sometimes any food), as a result of poorly developed feeding

---

BOX 13-2 KEY INDICATORS OF CHILDHOOD FEEDING DIFFICULTIES AND BEHAVIORAL FEEDING ISSUES

1. Restricted volume of oral intake (insufficient intake of energy, nutrients, or fluid)
2. Limited range of food in the diet
3. Limited range of textures in the diet (often a reliance on "easy to eat foods," which are pureed, soft, or dissolvable)
4. Prolonged mealtime duration (>30 minutes at mealtimes, >2 hours a day spent trying to feed a child)
5. Battles or problematic behavior at mealtimes
6. Family stress related to the child's eating patterns

---

skills (e.g., delayed oral motor skills affecting his or her ability to chew and bite) or a fear of trying new foods (often as a result of hypersensitivity to smell, taste, or texture of foods). See Box 13-2 for a list of key indicators of childhood feeding difficulties and behavioral feeding issues.

Childhood feeding difficulties and behavioral feeding issues affect approximately 85% of children with disabilities[8] and up to 5% of typically developing children.[9-11] In more severe cases, children will require full or partial nutritional support via artificial tube feeding as a result of their restrictive dietary intake. As a consequence, this further restricts the child's opportunities to develop the motor, sensory, and cognitive skills required to eat a variety of healthy fresh foods. Childhood feeding difficulties and behavioral feeding issues can also adversely affect a child's quality of life and that of the child's family.[9,12,13] These children often struggle to meet their basic nutritional requirements, usually taking significantly longer to eat or feed each day,[9] which limits their time to participate in other developmentally appropriate activities (i.e., play) and their

BOX 13-3 NUTRITIONAL CONSIDERATIONS RELATED TO CHILDHOOD FEEDING DIFFICULTIES AND BEHAVIORAL FEEDING ISSUES

Early nutrition effect on lifelong health: It is universally recognized that a wide range of dietary intake is essential for optimal childhood growth and development. Many government bodies focus their childhood nutrition campaigns on encouraging a wide range of intake (e.g., www.choosemyplate.gov). However, little information is available for parents on *how* to get their children to eat a wide variety of foods. It is well reported that many children aren't meeting the goals set out for them by these health campaigns, and parents frequently report growth, nutrition, and mealtime behavior as their biggest concerns for their children.

Feeding difficulties and behavioral feeding issues are an increasing problem: The prevalence of these feeding issues is increasing. There are two main reasons for this trend:

1. More high-risk children are surviving severe infant and childhood illnesses: Feeding difficulties and behavioral feeding issues occur in approximately 85% of medically complex children[7] (because of medical condition, invasive medical procedures, and time spent in hospital).
2. Lifestyles have changed: Parents are often isolated from other family members and are unsure how to feed their child, fewer families are eating together (so children have less opportunity to see parents model appropriate mealtime behaviors), and more families are relying on convenience food (so children aren't exposed to a wide variety of healthy, fresh foods).

Poor nutritional management can put a child at increased health risk: In children with feeding difficulties or behavioral feeding issues, focusing on weight and not nutrition can promote a diet high in energy and low in nutrients. If children do not learn the physical skills and cognitive behaviors to eat a wide variety of food, it will be difficult for them to meet their nutritional requirements through their oral diet. Unfortunately, parents of many children with feeding issues receive variable advice from a variety of sources, which can be confusing and sometimes misleading.

Clinical experience indicates that well-intentioned parents of children with diet and growth concerns often try to get "weight" onto their child any way they can, and to particularly focus on high-energy foods, such as foods high in fats and carbohydrates. This focus on weight and not nutrition often results in children gaining fat, but not lean or fat-free mass, and does not address their malnutrition. Further, the practice of feeding children high-energy, low-nutrient foods (which are often highly processed and easy to eat and swallow—i.e., "junk" foods) denies the child the opportunity to learn the skills required to eat a variety of healthy, fresh foods, such as fruit and vegetables and protein-rich foods (which often require more time and effort to bite and chew). In clinical practice, we see that this usually results in children being fussy and inefficient eaters (leading to prolonged mealtimes and increased mealtime battles) and being fearful of healthy foods (which are often less predictable in terms of taste, temperature, and texture than junk foods).

parents' time to do the other activities they need to do in a day (e.g., paid work, housework, time with other family members).

Children with **mild** feeding difficulties or behavioral feeding issues may have a problem in one or more of the areas listed in Box 13-3, but generally grow sufficiently. Children with **moderate** feeding difficulties or behavioral feeding issues generally have problems across several of these areas, and would not grow sufficiently without *nutritional supplementation* in the form of formula feeds or energy and nutritional supplements. Children with **severe** feeding difficulties or behavioral feeding issues generally have problems across all of the areas listed in Box 13-3, are unable to meet their fluid, energy, and nutritional requirements from an oral diet, and require *tube feeding*.

INTERRUPTIONS TO EARLY FEEDING DEVELOPMENT

Given the interrelationship between anatomic and neurologic maturation in early development, as well as between sensory, motor, and cognitive development, there is a potential for difficulties to occur if any or all of these processes are interrupted during the developmental process.

The normal developmental process can be interrupted by illness, medical treatments required to manage the illness, as well as time spent in the hospital. Children with major illnesses are often exposed to abnormal or adverse experiences (e.g., surgery, blood tests, tube feeding or hospital food, as well as frequent feeling of pain and nausea), while at the same time missing out on normal experiences (e.g., playing outside, interacting with friends, attending a mainstream school, eating regular food) (Figure 13-3).

Box 13-4 contains a list of medical conditions that are commonly associated with swallowing and feeding difficulties. It should be noted that some of these medical conditions have the potential to affect oral feeding *directly* (i.e., they may affect sucking strength, suck-swallow-breath coordination, or the ability to bite and chew effectively), and others affect oral feeding *indirectly* (i.e., they may not directly affect the oral or pharyngeal phases of swallowing, but may cause pain, discomfort, or fatigue with feeds, or limit the volume the child can consume by mouth). However,

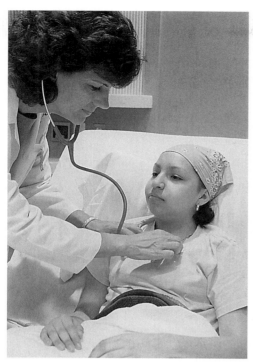

FIGURE 13-3 Children with major illnesses are often exposed to abnormal or adverse experiences, while at the same time missing out on normal childhood experiences. (From Hockenberry MJ, Wilson D: *Wong's essential of pediatric nursing,* ed 9, St Louis, 2013, Mosby.)

during the time when young children are developing their oral feeding skills, any feeding disturbances can potentially affect later feeding skills through interruption of the normal developmental process.

Children need adequate energy balance for growth and development. If their energy intake exceeds their requirements, they will display a **positive energy balance** and excess fat storage. If their energy intake is less than their requirements, they will display a **negative energy balance** and growth faltering (usually weight loss; if this persists, height gain and head size may be affected also).[14]

The three main contributors to negative energy balance in children[14] are summarized in Box 13-5. As can be seen, children with feeding difficulties are at risk across all of these areas.

RESPIRATORY AND CARDIAC DISORDERS THAT MAY AFFECT FEEDING AND SWALLOWING

Apnea of the newborn (or apnea of prematurity) is defined as cessation of breathing that lasts for more than 10 seconds or is accompanied by hypoxia or bradycardia.[15] Apnea is traditionally classified as either *obstructive,*

central, or *mixed.* See Box 13-6 for an overview of these conditions.

Pulmonary hypoplasia is incomplete development of the lungs, resulting in a reduced number of bronchopulmonary segments or alveoli. It most often occurs secondary to other fetal abnormalities that interfere with normal development of the lungs.

Respiratory distress syndrome (RDS, also known as *infant respiratory distress syndrome,* **hyaline membrane disease** or *surfactant deficiency disorder*), is a condition caused by insufficient surfactant production. Surfactant is a lipid-protein compound that increases surface tension of the terminal air-spaces (alveoli) and helps prevent collapse during exhalation. RDS is generally related to premature birth but can also occur as a specific genetic condition in cases in which surfactant proteins are deficient.

Bronchopulmonary dysplasia (BPD) (also known as *chronic neonatal lung disease (CNLD)*) is a chronic lung condition characterized by inflammation and scarring in the lungs. BPD is most common among children who were born prematurely, specifically those who received prolonged assisted ventilation to treat RDS.[16] Barotrauma, oxygen (O_2)-related injury, and infection are the main causes of BPD.[16] Box 13-7 describes the different degrees of severity of BPD.[16]

Laryngotracheobronchomalacia (*malacia* = "soft tissue") is a condition in which the larynx (and/or trachea and bronchi) are softer and less rigid than usual. **Laryngomalacia** is the most common cause of inspiratory stridor in early infancy[16] because the soft cartilage of the airway collapses inward during inhalation, causing upper airway obstruction.

Heart Defects

See Box 13-8 for a description of blood flow through the heart.

Cyanotic heart defects are a group of heart conditions that allow deoxygenated (blue) blood to bypass the lungs and enter the systemic circulation (causing low O_2 saturation and **cyanosis**). They are usually caused by structural defects of the heart that allow right-to-left shunting. Examples of defects that can cause cyanosis include tricuspid valve atresia, transposition of the great arteries, tetralogy of Fallot, and pulmonary atresia.

Acyanotic heart defects are a group of heart conditions that allow oxygenated (red) blood to mix with deoxygenated blood or obstruct outflow from the left heart. They do not cause cyanosis initially, but do place stress on the heart, which has to pump more oxygenated blood through to keep up with any losses. They are usually caused by structural defects of the heart that allow **left-to-right shunting** resulting from the higher pressure in the left side of the heart. Examples of acyanotic defects include patent ductus arteriosus, ventricular septal defects (VSD), and coarctation of the aorta.

BOX 13-4 DISORDERS COMMONLY AFFECTING FEEDING AND SWALLOWING IN INFANTS AND CHILDREN

Prematurity
- Low gestational age at birth
- Low birth weight
- Comorbidities associated with prematurity

Respiratory and Cardiac Disorders
- Apnea of the newborn
- Pulmonary dysplasia
- Respiratory distress syndrome
- Bronchopulmonary dysplasia and chronic neonatal lung disease
- Laryngotracheobronchomalacia
- Cyanotic and acyanotic heart defects

Gastrointestinal Disorders
- Necrotizing enterocolitis
- Hirschsprung's disease
- Gastroschisis
- Tracheoesophageal fistula and esophageal atresia
- Congenital diaphragmatic hernia
- Gastroesophageal reflux
- Eosinophilic esophagitis
- Food allergies and intolerances

Neurological Disorders
- Microcephaly
- Hydrocephalus
- Intraventricular hemorrhage

- Periventricular leukomalacia
- Birth asphyxia and cerebral palsy
- Acquired brain injuries
- Seizures

Congenital Abnormalities
- Cleft lip and palate
- Moebius syndrome
- Down syndrome

Maternal and Perinatal Issues
- Jaundice
- Diabetes
- Fetal alcohol syndrome
- Neonatal abstinence syndrome

Iatrogenic Complications
- Tube feeding
- Respiratory support
- Tracheostomy
- Medication

Miscellaneous Complications
- Ingestional injuries (e.g., detergents, battery)
- Tonsillitis and tongue-tie
- Autism spectrum disorders, sensory processing disorders
- Parent-child interaction difficulties

NOTE: An overview of conditions that are commonly associated with swallowing and feeding difficulties is provided in the following sections. Please note this overview is not exhaustive.

BOX 13-5 POTENTIAL CONTRIBUTORS TO NEGATIVE ENERGY IMBALANCE AND GROWTH FALTERING

Energy Imbalance
Energy is required for maintenance and growth in children.
- Negative energy imbalance results in growth faltering (weight first, then height, then head circumference)
- Positive energy imbalance results in excess weight storage (overweight or obesity)

Potential Contributors to Negative Energy Imbalance
Reduced energy intake:
- Inability to feed because of medical treatments
- Reduced stamina for the work of feeding because of illness and poor energy reserves
- Inefficient feeding skills

- Feed refusal
Increased energy requirements:
- Physiologic demands of illnesses may result in increased energy expenditure
Increased energy losses:
- Loss of feeds because of emesis
- Ineffective digestion or absorption of feeds
In determining whether a child needs energy supplementation in the form of nutritional formula or tube feeding, the following questions need to be considered:
- Can the child consume enough foods and fluids to meet energy, nutrition, and fluid needs and grow?
- Can the child consume foods and fluids safely?

See Box 13-9 for a description of common respiratory and cardiac signs and symptoms that may be observed during feeding assessment on therapy sessions.

Aspiration pneumonia can occur when there is primary aspiration of saliva, fluids, or foods, or secondary aspiration of esophageal or stomach contents into the airway. The degree of infection depends on how much bacteria is in the aspirated material, the pH of the aspirated material,[17,18] as well as the individual's ability to clear the airway (through coughing and movement), his or her general health, and whether the individual is on antibiotics.[17,18] Individuals particularly at risk of aspiration are those who are bedbound

BOX 13-6   TYPES OF APNEA

Obstructive apnea can occur as a result of low pharyngeal muscle tone or to inflammation of the soft tissues, which can block the flow of air though the pharynx and larynx. It may also occur when the infant's neck is hyperflexed or hyperextended.

Central apnea occurs when there is a lack of respiratory effort. This may result from central nervous system immaturity, or from the effects of medications or illness. Respiratory drive primarily depends on response to increased levels of carbon dioxide and acid in the blood (hypercapnea and hypercarbia). A secondary stimulus is low levels of oxygen in the blood (**hypoxemia**). Responses to these

stimuli are impaired in premature infants because of immaturity in regions of the brainstem that sense these changes. In addition, premature infants generally have an exaggerated response to laryngeal stimulation, which may induce apnea. Touch-pressure receptors within the pharynx can be stimulated by the presence of nasogastric tubes. Stretch receptors may be stimulated by a large bolus. Chemoreceptors can be stimulated by aspiration of food or by reflux of gastric content.

Many episodes of apnea of prematurity may start as either central or obstructive, but then involve elements of both, becoming *mixed* in nature.

BOX 13-7   DEGREES OF BRONCHOPULMONARY DYSPLASIA AND CHRONIC NEONATAL LUNG DISEASE

Mild: Need for supplemental oxygen for ≥28 days, but not at 36 weeks' GA or discharge
Moderate: Need for supplemental oxygen for ≥28 days plus treatment with <30% O_2 at 36 weeks' GA
Severe: Need for supplemental oxygen for ≥28 days plus treatment with ≥30% O_2 or positive pressure ventilation at 36 weeks' GA

GA, Gestational age; O_2, oxygen.

BOX 13-8   BLOOD FLOW THROUGH THE HEART

Ex utero, deoxygenated (blue) blood flows into the right side of the heart from the superior and inferior vena cava veins. It travels through the right atrium and ventricle, and then travels via the pulmonary artery to the lungs, where it is reoxygenated. This oxygenated (red) blood travels through the pulmonary veins to the left side of the heart. It then travels through the left atrium and ventricle and leaves the heart via the aorta.

In utero, the placenta does the work of breathing (providing oxygen and removing carbon dioxide) instead of the lungs. As a result, only a small amount of the blood needs to pass through the lungs. Most of the rest of the blood is bypassed or shunted away from the lungs through the ductus arteriosus to the aorta.

At birth, the newborn needs to transition from the fluid-filled environment of the amniotic sac to the outside air-filled environment, and to commence breathing for himself or herself. Normally, the ductus arteriosus closes over within the first hours after birth, directing all blood entering the heart to pass through the lungs before exiting the heart.

or have reduced mobility, those with preexisting lung conditions, and those with compromised immune systems.

Box 13-10 provides an overview of potential contributors to negative energy imbalance and growth faltering in children with respiratory and cardiac disease.

GASTROINTESTINAL DISORDERS THAT MAY AFFECT FEEDING AND SWALLOWING

Necrotizing enterocolitis (NEC) is a condition in which portions of the bowel undergo necrosis (tissue death). NEC occurs most frequently in very preterm infants. Surgical correction usually requires removing a section of the bowel, which results in a shortening of the gut length and reduced absorptive area (short gut syndrome).

Hirschsprung's disease is a condition in which part or all of the large intestines have no nerves and therefore cannot function. Surgical management often involves removing the affected area or creating a colostomy for removal of fecal matter.

Gastroschisis is a defect in the abdominal wall that allows the abdominal contents to protrude through the anterior abdominal wall. Surgical treatment is required to reposition the affected organs back in the abdominal cavity and to close the abdominal wall.

Tracheoesophageal fistula (TEF) is an abnormal connection (fistula) between the esophagus and the trachea. Fistulae can occur in various anatomic locations throughout the trachea and esophagus. Usually, but not always, TEF co-occurs with **esophageal atresia,** in which part of the esophagus is not fully formed (Table 13-2 and Figure 13-4). Surgical correction is required to close any openings between the airway and esophagus, as well as to connect disjointed sections of the esophagus into a continuous tube.

BOX 13-9 COMMON SIGNS AND SYMPTOMS OBSERVED IN PATIENTS WITH RESPIRATORY AND CARDIAC DISORDERS

Tachypnea: Increased respiratory rate (see Table 14-5 in Chapter 14 for normal respiratory parameters for children of various ages)

Apnea: Cessation of breathing. An apnea event is the cessation of breathing for >10 seconds

Dyspnea: Shortness of breath

Tachycardia: Increased heart rate (see Table 14-5 in Chapter 14 for normal cardiac parameters for children of various ages)

Bradycardia: Reduced heart rate

Cardiac arrest: Cessation of functional blood circulation resulting from failure of the heart to contract effectively

Cardiac arrest is accompanied by loss of consciousness, and may progress to causing brain damage or death if untreated (or untreatable).

Hypercapnia (also known as hypercarbia or respiratory acidosis): Increased carbon dioxide (CO_2) in the blood

Usually, a blood gas carbon dioxide level of more than 45 mm Hg is considered to indicate hypercapnia.[16]

Hypoxemia: Reduced O_2 in the blood

Usually, hypoxemia is defined as an O_2 saturation <95%. However, in preterm infants <34 weeks' GA, who are usually anemic, an O_2 saturation <88% is generally considered to indicate hypoxemia.[16]

Cyanosis: Blue tinge to skin or mucous membranes associated with hypoxemia

Stertor: Coarse sound originating in the pharynx by a narrow or obstructed airway

Stridor: High-pitched sound originating in the larynx, trachea, or bronchi, caused by a narrow or obstructed airway

Can be inspiratory, expiratory, or biphasic.

Wheezing: Continuous, coarse, whistling sound caused by narrowing or obstruction of part of the respiratory tree or heightened airflow velocity within the respiratory tree

Rhonchi: Coarse, rattling sounds caused by secretions in the bronchi

Fremitus: Vibration caused by partial airway obstruction (often secretions) that can be felt from outside the body

Rales (also known as crackles or crepitations): Crackling noises made by one of both lungs on inspiration

Often only heard with a stethoscope (auscultation).

Atelectasis: Collapse of one of more lung segments, preventing gas exchange in that area

Pneumothorax: Collapse of one of more lung segments, accompanied by air escape from the lung

The escaped air builds up in the pleural space between the lung and chest wall, putting pressure on the lung from the outside, making breathing more difficult.

Increased work of breathing: Physical presentation of respiratory distress

Signs include nostril flaring, neck extension, head bobbing, tracheal tug, subcostal recession, accessory chest muscle use, and grunting.

Upper respiratory tract infection: An infection of the larynx, pharynx, sinuses, or middle ear

Examples include laryngitis, pharyngitis, tonsillitis, epiglottitis, sinusitis, rhinitis (infection of nasal mucosa), and otitis media (middle ear infection).

Lower respiratory tract infection: An infection of the trachea, bronchi, or lungs that is often accompanied by coughing and shortness of breath

Examples include bronchitis and pneumonia.

Pneumonia: Inflammatory condition of the lungs, usually caused by bacteria, viruses, or fungi

Pneumonia is generally associated with productive cough, fatigue, fever, shortness of breath, and chest pain.

GA, Gestational age; *O_2,* oxygen.

Congenital diaphragmatic hernia (CDH) is a congenital defect of the diaphragm (the muscle that separates the chest and the abdomen). A hole in the diaphragm allows abdominal organs (the stomach, intestines, or liver) to herniate (migrate) into the chest. This occupies space in the chest, which can affect growth of the lungs (i.e., pulmonary hypoplasia) and restrict blood flow to the lungs (causing pulmonary hypertension). In addition, altered pressure in the chest and abdominal cavity can cause gastroesophageal reflux (GER). Surgical correction is required to return abdominal organs to the abdominal cavity.

Gastroesophageal reflux (GER) is the return of stomach contents into the esophagus (+/− pharynx and mouth).

Gastroesophageal reflux disease (GERD) is a chronic symptom of mucosal damage caused by stomach acid in the esophagus. GER is usually caused by abnormal relaxation of the lower esophageal sphincter that normally holds the top of the stomach closed, reduced gastric emptying, or abnormal pressure in the abdomen. Treatment is generally via feed manipulations (e.g., smaller, more frequent feeds; slow bolus feeds into the stomach; or continuous feeds into the stomach or into the small intestines, also known as *transpyloric feeds* or *jejunal feeds*), proton pump inhibitors (PPI), histamine receptor antagonists (H2RA), and antacids (often delivered in alginate rafts that produce a protective layer above stomach contents). Surgery

BOX 13-10 POTENTIAL CONTRIBUTORS TO NEGATIVE ENERGY IMBALANCE AND GROWTH FALTERING IN CHILDREN WITH RESPIRATORY AND CARDIAC DISEASE

Reduced Energy Intake

- Inefficient feeding skills may be a component of the cardiorespiratory medical condition or result from lack of opportunity to practice oral skills.
- Poor suck-swallow-breath coordination may occur because of high respiratory rate and increased work of breathing, which may result in mistiming of a swallow to occur at the same time as a breath or drawing the bolus into airway on inspiration.
- Inability to feed (or feed safely) may occur as a result of effects of medical treatments, such as:
  - CPAP/BiPAP mask (which can obstruct the nose and face)
  - Intubation (which can obstruct the pharynx and make airway closure difficult)
  - Tracheostomy (which can anchor the larynx and reduce laryngeal excursion during swallowing)
  - High airflow ventilation support from high-flow oxygen treatment or CPAP/BiPAP (which can make airway closure difficult against the effects of the airflow, potentially transfer material from the pharynx into the airway, or desensitize sensory receptors in the pharynx from effects of airflow)
- Some surgical procedure for cardiac disease may cause damage to the recurrent laryngeal nerve (the branch of CN X that supplies the intrinsic muscles of the larynx and provides sensation to the larynx below the vocal folds).

- Patients may display reduced stamina for the work of feeding because of poor energy reserves.
- Feed refusal may occur because of nausea, lack of appetite, pain, or learned aversion.
- Frequent fasting for medical procedures may result in periods of reduced intake.

Increased Energy Requirements

- Physiologic demands of respiratory and cardiac illnesses may result in increased energy expenditure (increased work of breathing, increased work of circulation).
- Patients with pulmonary edema or edema of the limbs and abdomen from the effects of cardiac or respiratory disease may need to be put on fluid restrictions and thus may need to be given high-concentration energy feeds to meet their energy requirements. These feeds are not always palatable and may interfere with regular appetite regulation.

Increased Energy Losses

- Vomiting and reflux are more common in children with respiratory disease than in the general population,[16] presumably because of the downward pressure on the diaphragm and stomach caused by effortful breathing. This may result in loss of feeds.

BiPAP, Bi-level positive airway pressure; *CN,* cranial nerve; *CPAP,* continuous positive airway pressure.

TABLE 13-2 Classification of Tracheoesophageal Fistula

Type	Description	TEF	EA
Type A	Proximal and distal esophageal buds (i.e., missing midsegment of esophagus), but no tracheal fistula	No	Yes
Type B	Proximal esophageal termination on the lower trachea (causing fistula) with distal esophageal bud	Yes	Yes
Type C	Proximal esophageal atresia (esophagus continuous with the mouth ending in a blind loop) with a distal esophagus arising from the lower trachea or carina (via fistula); most common variant	Yes	Yes
Type D	Proximal esophageal termination on the lower trachea or carina (causing a fistula) with distal esophagus arising from the carina (via fistula)	Yes	Yes
Type E (or H-Type)	A variant of type D: TEF without EA. If the esophagus is continuous, this is sometimes termed an *H-type fistula* because of its resemblance to the letter H.	Yes	No

EA, Esophageal atresia; *TEF,* tracheoesophageal fistula.
From Gross RE: *The surgery of infancy and childhood* Philadelphia, 1953, WB Saunders.

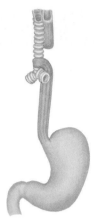

**Esophageal Atresia
With Distal TEF**

Incidence: 85%–88%
Clinical Manifestations: Feeding causes regurgitation and coughing. Constant flow of saliva. Gastric distention.
Diagnostic Findings: Contrast reveals blind pouch. Air on abdominal x ray.
Surgical Treatment: One-stage surgical repair to ligate fistula and anastomose esophagus.

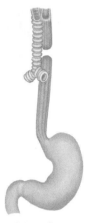

**Esophageal Atresia
Without Fistula**

Incidence: 6%–8%
Clinical Manifestations: Excess oral secretions. Regurgitation of feedings.
Diagnostic Findings: Blind pouch. No air in abdomen.
Surgical Treatment: Two-stage repair: (1) Gastrostomy and cervical esophagostomy; (2) colon interposition to create patent esophagus.

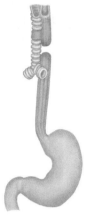

Proximal Esophageal Fistula With Trachea; Distal Segment Has No Communication

Incidence: 1%
Clinical Manifestations: Excessive oral secretions. Immediate respiratory distress with oral intake.
Diagnostic Findings: PO contrast outlines tracheal tree. No air in abdomen.
Surgical Treatment: One- or two-stage repair depending on length of separation.

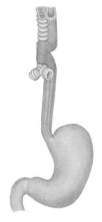

**Proximal and Distal Esophageal
Fistulas With Trachea**

Incidence: 1%
Clinical Manifestations: Excessive secretions. Respiratory distress with feedings.
Diagnostic Findings: PO contrast outlines tracheal tree. Air in abdomen.
Surgical Treatment: Ligation of fistulas and anastomosis of esophagus.

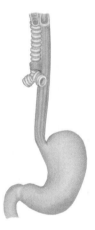

**TEF Without Atresia
(Also Called "H Type")**

Incidence: 4%
Clinical Manifestations: Minimal symptoms unless regurgitation occurs. Choking, coughing. Abdominal distention.
Diagnostic Findings: Bronchoscopy demonstrates fistula.
Surgical Treatment: Ligation of fistula.

FIGURE 13-4 Variations of tracheoesophageal fistula, as defined by Gross. (From James S, Nelson K, Ashwill J: *Nursing care of children,* ed 4, St Louis, 2013, Saunders.)

BOX 13-11 POTENTIAL CONTRIBUTORS TO NEGATIVE ENERGY IMBALANCE AND GROWTH FALTERING IN CHILDREN WITH GASTROINTESTINAL CONDITIONS

Reduced Energy Intake
- Inability for the gut to tolerate large volumes of feed can affect volume of intake.
- Continuous feeds or bolus feeds delivered slowly over time may interfere with normal appetite regulation and suppress hunger.
- Reduced gut motility and constipation may cause discomfort and affect appetite.
- Feed refusal may occur because of nausea, lack of appetite, pain, or learned aversion.
- Patients who are tube fed may develop inefficient oral feeding skills because of lack of practice.
- Some patients may need to be given special feeds, such as elemental formula. These feeds are not always palatable and may lead to feed refusal.

Increased Energy Losses
- Loss of feeds may occur because of vomiting or reflux.
- Ineffective digestion of feeds can mean that not all the energy and nutrition from the feed is absorbed.

Increased Energy Requirements
- Patients may need to replace feeds lost to vomiting, reflux, or ineffective absorption.

(e.g., fundoplication) may be an option in those who do not improve with other interventions (see Chapter 5 for full discussion of esophageal-related disorders) (see Clinical Corner 13-1).

Eosinophilic esophagitis (EE) (also known as *allergic esophagitis*) is an inflammatory condition of the esophagus caused by an allergic reaction to ingested foods. EE is characterized by dense eosinophilic infiltrate into the epithelium of the esophagus. Eosinophils are white blood cells (leukocytes) that release cytokines that inflame the surrounding tissue. EE is generally diagnosed on endoscopy and by biopsy confirmation. EE generally causes pain and difficulty swallowing and often results in strictures and food impaction. It is more common in males than females.[14] Treatment may involve diet modification, elimination of the offending allergen, topical corticosteroids (usually delivered via steroid slurries that are swallowed), and dilatation of strictures where necessary.

Food allergies occur when a person's immune system reacts to normally harmless substances in his or her diet. These reactions are predictable and rapid. In extreme cases, food allergies can cause **anaphylaxis**, a potentially life-threatening condition characterized by swelling of tongue, swelling/tightness in throat, difficulty breathing, and loss of consciousness.[14] A wide variety of foods can cause allergic reactions, but 90% of food allergies are caused by cow's milk, soy, eggs, wheat, peanuts, tree nuts, fish, and shellfish.[14,20,21] Food allergies often can be detected through blood or skin tests and can be triggered by exposure to very small amounts of the allergen. Food allergies are managed by completely eliminating the allergen from the diet. In addition, steroids may be used to suppress the immune response to the allergen, and gradual desensitization may be used to build up a resistance to the allergen.[21] In cases in which anaphylaxis occurs, epinephrine and adrenalin are usually administered to manage the acute symptoms.[21]

Food intolerances occur as a result of adverse, nonimmune responses to components of the diet. The reactions are often less predictable and less severe than allergic responses, and are often proportionate to the amount of the irritant consumed. Food intolerances are generally diagnosed by removing potential irritants from the diet and then reintroducing them by way of **food challenges** to determine if symptoms return. Food intolerances are managed by reducing exposure to the irritant in the diet. Differences between food allergy and food intolerance are summarized in Table 13-3.

Box 13-11 provides an overview of potential contributors to negative energy imbalance and growth faltering in children with gastrointestinal (GI) disorders.

NEUROLOGIC DISORDERS THAT MAY AFFECT FEEDING AND SWALLOWING

Microcephaly is usually defined as a head circumference more than two standard deviations below the mean for age and gender.[14,16] Microcephaly may be congenital or it may

TABLE 13-3 Comparison of Food Allergies and Food Intolerances

Feature	Food Allergy	Food Intolerance
Age of onset	Infants and toddlers (mostly)	Any age
Family history	Atopic: asthma, eczema, hay fever	Commonly irritable bowel, hives, headaches, mouth ulcers
Reaction timing	Immediate (minutes through to 1-2 h)	Hours through days
Reaction reproducibility	Reproducible	Variable
Mechanism	Immune (IgE antibodies)	Nonimmune (irritation of nerve endings)
Food triggers	Specific food proteins: most often cow's milk, soy, eggs, wheat, peanuts, tree nuts, fish, and shellfish	Natural food chemicals (salicylates, amines, glutamates), food additives, highly fermentable foods, components of dairy foods (e.g., lactose), components of some cereals (e.g., gluten)
Tests	Skin prick tests Blood tests (RAST): measure IgE to specific allergens	Elimination diet Food challenges
Dietary management	Complete avoidance of single foods	Comprehensive dietary modification: maintain overall chemical intake below reaction threshold
Outcomes	Egg, milk: usually outgrown Peanut, tree nuts, seafood: often persist (70-80%)	Lifelong susceptibility Variable tolerance Symptoms can come and go

IgE, Immunoglobulin E; *RAST,* radioallergosorbent test.
Adapted from Hodge L, Swain A, Faulkner-Hogg K: Food allergy and intolerance. *Aust Fam Physician* 38(9):705, 2009.

develop in the first few years of life. The disorder may stem from a wide variety of conditions that cause abnormal growth of the brain, or from syndromes associated with chromosomal abnormalities.

Hydrocephalus is a condition in which there is an abnormal accumulation of cerebrospinal fluid (CSF) in the ventricles of the brain. This may cause increased intracranial pressure inside the skull and progressive enlargement of the head. Hydrocephalus can also cause seizures, intellectual impairment, or death as a result of damage to brain structures from compression. Management of hydrocephalus often involves inserting a shunt to allow drainage of CSF.

Hypoxic ischemic encephalopathy (HIE) results from hypoxia or ischemia to the cerebral circulation, resulting in variable inflammation, injury, or death of neural tissues of the brain.

Intraventricular hemorrhage (IVH) is a bleeding into the fluid-filled areas (ventricles) of the brain. It commonly occurs in preterm infants of less than 34 weeks' gestational age (GA) because of vulnerability of the blood vessels of the germinal matrix in the floor of the lateral ventricles.[16] IVH is graded into four categories[16] (Box 13-12).

IVH grades I and II are most common, and usually resolve without permanent complications.[16] IVH grades III and IV are the most serious and may result in long-term brain injury to the infant.[16] After a grade III or IV IVH,

---

BOX 13-12 GRADES OF INTRAVENTRICULAR HEMORRHAGE

Grade I: Bleeding occurs only in the germinal matrix (in the floor of the lateral ventricle).
Grade II: Bleeding occurs inside the ventricles, but they are not enlarged.
Grade III: Ventricles are enlarged by accumulated blood.
Grade IV: Bleeding extends into the brain tissue around the ventricles.

---

blood clots may form, which can block the flow of CSF, leading to increased fluid in the brain (posthemorrhagic hydrocephalus).

Periventricular leukomalacia (PVL) is a brain injury characterized by the death of white matter (*leuko* = "white," *malacia* = "soft") near the lateral ventricles. Preterm infants are at the greatest risk of this condition. Because of the location of the injury, affected individuals may exhibit motor control problems and other developmental delays, and they often develop cerebral palsy (CP) or epilepsy.[16]

Birth asphyxia (also known as *perinatal asphyxia* or *neonatal asphyxia*) results from deprivation of O_2 to a newborn infant that lasts long enough to cause physical harm. Hypoxic damage can occur to any of the infant's organs (e.g., heart, lungs, gut, liver, kidneys), but brain damage generally has the most detrimental and long-lasting effects. Birth asphyxia can occur because of impaired respiratory effort, inadequate ventilation, or inadequate circulation or perfusion in utero or immediately following birth.[14,16] An infant suffering severe birth asphyxia usually appears cyanotic and has poor muscle tone and responsiveness (as reflected in a low 5-minute **Apgar score**). Extreme degrees of asphyxia can cause cardiac arrest and death. Some children who experience birth asphyxia develop intellectual impairment or learning difficulties, and some develop sensory and motor impairments such as CP.[14,16]

Cerebral palsy (CP) is a general term for a group of permanent, nonprogressive movement disorders that cause physical disability. CP is caused by damage to the motor control centers of the developing brain, which can occur in utero, during birth, or after birth (up to 3 years of age). The etiologic factors of the majority of CP remains unknown, but a smaller proportion (approximately 10%) is associated with HIE or bilirubin encephalopathy (**kernicterus**).[16,22,23] Although the central feature of CP is a disorder with movement, it also likely affects the sensory system. Many children with CP have problems with their vision, communication, and learning disabilities.[22,23] Epilepsy is also common in this population.[22,23]

CP is classified by the types of motor impairment and by restrictions to the activities an affected person may perform (Boxes 13-13 and 13-14).

The "Gross Motor Function Classification System" (GMFCS) is a clinical classification system that describes the gross motor function of people with CP on the basis of self-initiated movement abilities (see Box 13-14).[24] Distinctions between levels are based on functional abilities (e.g., the need for walkers, crutches, wheelchairs) and, to a lesser extent, the actual quality of movement.

Benfer et al.[25] studied children with various levels of CP and found that swallowing impairment or dysphagia was prevalent in 85% of children with CP. Although dysphagia was present across all levels of gross motor severity, there was a stepwise relationship between swallowing impairment and GMFCS level. This study found a significant increase in odds of having dysphagia in children who were nonambulant (GMFCS V) compared with those who were ambulant (GMFCS I) (odds ratio = 17.9).

Acquired brain injury (ABI) is brain damage caused by events any time after birth. CP is a form of ABI. However, ABI does not include brain damage caused as part of a genetic or congenital disorder, or damage resulting from progressive neurodegenerative disorders. ABIs are caused by either traumatic brain injury (TBI) (e.g., physical trauma caused by head injury from accidents, assault, surgery) or nontraumatic injury (e.g., hypoxia, infection, encephalopathy, brain tumors, stroke, substance exposure, poisoning). ABI usually results in some degree of physical, cognitive,

---

BOX 13-13 TYPES OF CEREBRAL PALSY

Spastic CP
Spasticity (muscle tightness) is the main type of impairment present. Muscles are hypertonic, resulting from an upper motor neuron lesion (occurring in the motor cortex or pyramidal tracts). Muscle spasms are common, resulting from the pain or stress of the tightness experienced. Therapy regimens consisting of stretching and strengthening muscles and functional tasks are usually the main approach to management for spastic CP. Medical treatments may also be considered, such as antispasmodic medications, botox, or baclofen. This is the most common type of CP, occurring in more than 70% of all cases.

Choreoathetoid CP (or Dyskinetic CP)
Mixed muscle tone (hypotonia and hypertonia) and involuntary motions are present. This type of CP results from damage to the extrapyramidal system (the basal ganglia or extrapyramidal tracts, which control involuntary reflexes and movement, as well as modulation of movement [i.e., coordination]). People with dyskinetic CP show involuntary motions and have trouble holding themselves in an upright, steady position for sitting or walking. Therapy and drug treatments (used to treat spasms and chorea) have some effectiveness. Approximately 10% of individuals with CP have choreoathetoid CP.

Ataxic CP
Ataxia (lack of muscle control during voluntary movements) is present, caused by damage to the cerebellum. Most noticeably, ataxia can affect balance while walking (leading to an awkward gait) and affect speech (leading to dysarthria). Ataxia generally results in an intention (movement) tremor, as well as difficulty with fine motor control (e.g., writing). Ataxia usually results in muscle weakness. Ataxia is the least common type of cerebral palsy, occurring in 5% to 10% of all cases.

Mixed CP
Mixed symptoms of spastic, athetoid, and ataxic CP appear simultaneously, each to varying degrees. Mixed CP is the rarest and most difficult type of CP to treat, as it is extremely heterogeneous and sometimes unpredictable in its symptoms and development over the lifespan.

CP, Cerebral palsy.
From Rosenbaum P, Paneth N, Leviton A, et al: A report: the definition and classification of cerebral palsy, April 2006. *Dev Med Child Neurol Suppl* 109:8, 2007.
Cerebral Palsy Association: http://cerebralpalsy.org/about-cerebral-palsy/types-and-forms/#cm.

---

or behavioral impairments that lead to temporary or permanent changes in functioning.

In the acute period, the severity of ABI is scored using the Glasgow Coma Scale (GCS; Table 13-4) (25%). The scale is composed of three tests: eye, verbal, and motor

---

BOX 13-14 GROSS MOTOR FUNCTIONING CLASSIFICATION SYSTEM

GMFCS Level I
- Has decreased speed, balance, and coordination.
- Can walk indoors and outdoors, and climb stairs without using hands for support.
- Can perform usual activities, such as running and jumping.

GMFCS Level II
- Has difficulty with uneven surfaces, inclines, or in crowds.
- Has only minimal ability to run or jump.
- Has the ability to walk indoors and outdoors, and climb stairs with a railing.

GMFCS Level III
- Walks with assistive mobility devices indoors and outdoors on level surfaces.
- May be able to climb stairs using a railing.
- May propel a manual wheelchair, but need assistance for long distances or uneven surfaces.

GMFCS Level IV
- Walking ability severely limited, even with assistive devices.
- Uses wheelchairs most of the time, and may propel own power wheelchair.
- Can make standing transfers, but may need assistance.

GMFCS Level V
- Has physical impairments that restrict voluntary control of movement.
- Impaired in all areas of motor function.
- Cannot sit or stand independently, even with adaptive equipment.
- Cannot independently walk, but may be able to use powered mobility.
- Restricted ability to maintain head and neck position against gravity.

GMFCS, Gross Motor Functioning Classification System.

---

responses. The three values are often reported separately, in addition to the total score. The highest total GCS is 15 (fully awake and alert) and the lowest possible GCS is 3 (deep coma or deceased). A GCS of 8 or less is considered to indicate severe ABI, GCS 9 to 12 is moderate, and a GCS of 13 or more indicates mild injury.[26]

An individual's recovery from ABI depends on factors such as the location, type, and severity of brain injury, any coexisting physical injuries, the individual's premorbid developmental skills, his or her current cognitive skills for applying therapy techniques and compensatory strategies, and other factors that may affect his or her ability to participate in rehabilitative therapy (e.g., level of alertness, ongoing seizures, and effects of medications).

A literature review by Morgan[27] indicated that acute dysphagia incidence is high (68%-76%) for children with severe TBI, but less for children with milder injury. This review suggests that a GCS of 8 or less and a ventilation period of 1.5 days or longer are specific risk factors for developing dysphagia. In addition, this review indicates that resolution of dysphagia is typically achieved by 12 weeks in children with cortical injury, although some children with TBI will continue to display dysphagia and require modified food or fluids or tube feeding beyond this time.

Seizures are brief episodes of abnormal or excessive neuronal activity in the brain. The syndrome of recurrent, unprovoked seizures is termed **epilepsy,** but seizures can occur in people who do not have epilepsy.[28] The signs and symptoms of seizures vary depending on the type. There are two main types of seizures: focal and generalized (Box 13-15).

Most seizures last less than 2 minutes.[14,28] After the active portion of a seizure, there is typically a period of confusion referred to as the **postictal** period before a normal level of consciousness returns. This usually lasts 3 to 15 minutes, but may last for hours.[14] Common symptoms include feeling tired, headache, difficulty speaking, and abnormal behavior.[14]

TABLE 13-4 Glasgow Coma Scale

	1	2	3	4	5	6
Eye	Does not open eyes	Opens eyes in response to painful stimuli	Opens eyes in response to voice	Opens eyes spontaneously	N/A	N/A
Verbal	Makes no sounds	Incomprehensible sounds	Utters inappropriate words	Confused, disoriented	Oriented, converses normally	N/A
Motor	Makes no movements	Extension to painful stimuli	Abnormal flexion to painful stimuli	Flexion, withdrawal to painful stimuli	Localizes painful stimuli	Obeys command

N/A, Not applicable.

BOX 13-15 TYPES OF SEIZURES

Focal (partial) seizures can often be subtle or unusual and may go unnoticed, or may be mistaken for intoxication or daydreaming. Seizure activity starts in one area of the brain and may spread to other regions of the brain. There are three main types of focal seizures:

- **Focal seizure: awareness retained** (formerly known as *simple partial seizures*). Often proceeded by certain experiences, known as an *aura*. These may include visual, olfactory, or motor phenomena.
- **Focal dyscognitive seizures: awareness altered** (formerly known as *complex partial seizures*). The person may appear confused or dazed, and may not be able to respond to questions or directions.
- **Focal seizures evolving to a bilateral convulsive seizure** (formerly known as *secondarily generalized tonic clonic seizures*). Jerking activity may start in a specific muscle group and spread to surrounding muscle groups. Unusual activities may occur that are not under conscious control, such as lip smacking or other repetitive movements.

Generalized seizures are the result of abnormal activity in both hemispheres of the brain simultaneously. They all involve a loss of consciousness, and typically happen without warning. There are six main types of generalized seizures:

- **Tonic seizures** produce a sustained contraction of the muscles of the limbs followed by their extension, along with arching of the back. The individual often stops breathing during the seizure.
- **Clonic seizures** involve shaking of the limbs.
- **Tonic-clonic seizures** involve a tonic component followed by a clonic component.
- **Myoclonic seizures** involve spasms of muscle groups.
- **Atonic seizures** involve loss of muscle activity.
- **Absence seizures** are often subtle, with a minor activity, such as eye blinking or a turn of the neck.

From Fisher RS, van Emde Boas W, Blume W, et al: Epileptic seizures and epilepsy: definitions proposed by the International League Against Epilepsy (ILAE) and the International Bureau for Epilepsy (IBE). *Epilepsia* 46(4):470, 2005.

BOX 13-16 POTENTIAL CONTRIBUTORS TO NEGATIVE ENERGY IMBALANCE AND GROWTH FALTERING IN CHILDREN WITH NEUROLOGIC DISORDERS

Reduced Energy Intake

- Oral, pharyngeal, and esophageal dysphagia may be present resulting from neurologic damage or medications used to treat symptoms.
- Altered consciousness can affect the ability to swallow safely.
- Lethargy caused by injury or sedative drugs can reduce stamina for the work of feeding or limit opportunities to feed.
- Feed refusal may occur as a result of irritability or behavioral issues.
- Physical impairments and altered movement patterns can affect the ability to self-feed.
- Fasting for medical procedures may result in periods of reduced intake.

Increased Energy Requirements

- Physiologic demands of condition (e.g. high tone, seizures) may result in increased energy expenditure. Conversely, in some cases (e.g. those with low tone) energy needs may be reduced.

Increased Energy Losses

- Altered tone can make reflux more common, which can result in loss of feeds.

---

worsening of preexisting dysphagia occurred in an additional 15% of patients. There was no association found between swallow function and seizure freedom or postoperative hydrocephalus.

Box 13-16 provides an overview of potential contributors to negative energy imbalance and growth faltering in children with neurologic disorders.

CONGENITAL ABNORMALITIES THAT MAY AFFECT FEEDING AND SWALLOWING

Cleft lip, cleft palate, and **cleft lip and palate** are variations of a congenital deformity caused by abnormal facial development during the first trimester of gestation. Approximately 1 in 1000 children have a cleft lip or a cleft palate or both.[30] A cleft lip or palate can almost always be successfully repaired with surgery, especially if conducted in early childhood. However, ongoing therapy is usually required to achieve functional feeding and speech.

Cleft lip or palate can occur as a one-sided (unilateral) or two-sided (bilateral) condition (Figure 13-5). Cleft lip occurs because of the failure of fusion of the maxillary and medial nasal processes. Cleft palate can affect the hard palate, soft palate, or both the hard and soft palate (see

Seizures can arise from a number of causes, including epilepsy. Other causes common in children include fever related to infection (febrile seizures), metabolic disorders, as well as HIE.[14] Benzodiazepine drugs are often used to treat active seizures[14] and have a sedative effect. A variety of antiepileptic drugs (AEDs) are used to try to provide preventative control of seizures.

In cases of medically intractable seizures, surgical options, such as functional hemispherectomy, may be considered. Buckley et al.[29] studied the swallowing outcomes of a group of children with epilepsy who underwent hemispherectomy. They reported that new-onset, transient dysphagia occurred in 26% of patients after surgery and that

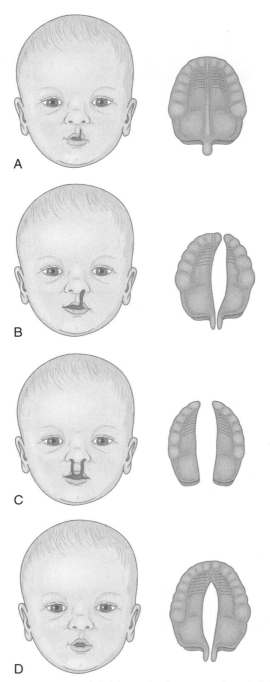

FIGURE 13-5 Types of cleft lip and palate. **A,** Unilateral cleft lip; **B,** Unilateral cleft lip and palate; **C,** Bilateral cleft lip and palate; **D,** Mildline cleft palate. (From McCance K, Huether S: *Pathophysiology: the biologic basis for disease in adults and children,* ed 6, St Louis, 2010, Mosby.)

Figure 13-5). A cleft of the hard palate occurs as a result of the failure of fusion of the lateral palatine processes, the nasal septum, or the median palatine processes. When a cleft of the soft palate occurs, the uvula is often split (bifurcated). In some cases, the mucosa of the palate appears

---

BOX 13-17   FEEDING DIFFICULTIES COMMONLY ASSOCIATED WITH CLEFT LIP AND PALATE

Cleft lip: Poor anterior seal, inability to form sufficient negative pressure (suction) to draw fluid from the breast or bottle effectively

Cleft palate and VPI: Inability to form sufficient negative pressure (suction) to draw fluid from the breast or bottle effectively, nasal regurgitation, increased swallowing of air

Micrognathia and glossoptosis: Inability to form sufficient positive pressure (compression) to draw fluid from the breast or bottle effectively, airway obstruction during feeding

VPI, Velopharyngeal insufficiency.

---

intact, but the muscles below are not fully formed, which is known as a **submucous cleft.**

Velopharyngeal insufficiency (or velopharyngeal inadequacy) (VPI) occurs when the soft palate (velum) is unable to close off the nasal cavity from the oral cavity because of structural deficiencies (e.g., open cleft) or functional restrictions (e.g., inadequate movement of the velum).

There appears to be a genetic component to cleft lip and palate, as some families have multiple members with clefts, although the exact genes involved are often unable to be identified.[30] Genetic factors contributing to cleft lip and palate formation have been identified for some syndromes.[30] Pierre Robin sequence (PRS), Treacher Collins, Stickler, Goldenhar, Van der Woude, and Di George and velo-cardio-facial syndrome[VCFS] (both types of 22q11 micro-deletion) syndromes all have cleft lip or palate as one of their defining features, in addition to a range of other anomalies.

Pierre Robin sequence (PRS) (also known as *Robin sequence*) is characterized by a cleft of the soft palate (often described as a wide, U-shaped cleft) in addition to micrognathia (small mandible or jaw) (Figure 13-6). In addition, PRS often involves posterior displacement or retraction of the tongue (glossoptosis), which can lead to airway obstruction. Many children with PRS require artificial airway support, such as a nasopharyngeal (NP) tube (NP airway) or tracheostomy, to achieve sufficient ventilation. Some children undergo mandibular advancement surgery for airway or aesthetic reasons.

The degree of feeding impairment that occurs as a result of cleft lip or palate depends of the type of impairment to oral structures (cleft lip, cleft palate, micrognathia), the degree of impairment (unilateral, bilateral, incomplete cleft, complete cleft), function (presence of absence of VPI), any airway issues (presence or absence of glossoptosis), as well as any other medical complications (e.g., cardiac issues) (see Box 13-7). See Box 13-17 for an overview of feeding difficulties in this population.

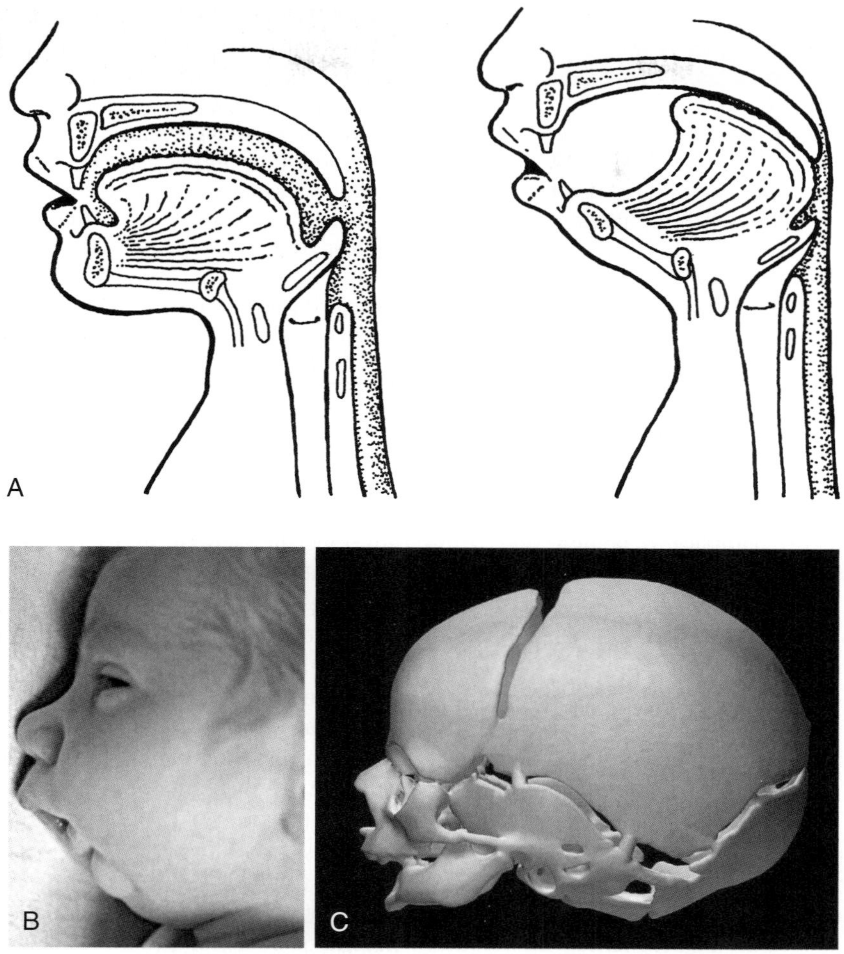

FIGURE 13-6 **A,** Schematic features of Pierre Robin Syndrome. **B,** Lateral view of a child with Pierre Robin sequence, characterized by severe micrognathia and cleft palate. **C,** Lateral view of the craniofacial skeleton of a child with Pierre Robin sequence. Note the small, retruded mandible. (**A** from Allen PJ, Vessey J, Schapiro N: *Primary care of the child with a chronic condition,* ed 5, St Louis, 2010, Mosby. **B** from Clark DA: Atlas of neonatology, ed 7, Philadelphia, 2000, WB Saunders. **C** Courtesy Wolfgang Losken, M.D. IN Zitelli B, McIntire S, Nowalk A: Zitelli and Davis' Atlas of Pediatric Physical Diagnosis, ed 6, Saunders, St. Louis, 2012.)

Strategies, such as the use of special feeding equipment and positioning, may be used to assist feeding efficiency in children with cleft lip or palate (see Chapter 15). Different considerations apply for feeding presurgery, immediately postsurgery (when oral sutures are still in place), and later on after surgery, and are often facility or surgeon specific.

Moebius (or Möbius) **syndrome** results from the underdevelopment of cranial nerve (CN) VI, which controls lateral eye movement and CN VII, which controls the facial muscles. Other cranial nerves may also be affected in addition to CN VI and VII.[31] Most children with Moebius syndrome have some degree of difficulty with the oral phase of feeding, in addition to speech impairments.[31]

Down syndrome (also known as *trisomy 21*), is a genetic disorder caused by the presence of an additional (third) copy of chromosome 21. Down syndrome is typically associated with short stature, low muscle tone, characteristic facial features (including large tongue and narrow roof of mouth), and mild to moderate intellectual impairment.[32] Approximately 40% of children with Down syndrome have a congenital heart defect.[32] Feeding difficulties are common in children with Down syndrome as a result of oral anatomy, as well as low muscle tone and comorbid cardiac issues.[32]

Box 13-18 provides an overview of potential contributors to negative energy imbalance and growth faltering in children with congenital abnormalities.

MATERNAL AND PERINATAL CONDITIONS THAT MAY AFFECT CHILD FEEDING AND SWALLOWING

Jaundice (or hyperbilirubinemia or icterus) is a yellowing of the skin and other tissues (e.g., sclera of eyes) caused by

---

BOX 13-18 POTENTIAL CONTRIBUTORS TO NEGATIVE ENERGY IMBALANCE AND GROWTH FALTERING IN CHILDREN WITH CONGENITAL DISORDERS

Reduced Energy Intake
- Inefficient feeding skills result from structural impairments of oral structures.
- Surgical procedures to repair structural defects (e.g., cleft repair) can result in periods of difficulty feeding during wound recovery.
- If other comorbidities exist (e.g., cardiac defects), the individual may have reduced stamina for the work of feeding as a result of illness and poor energy reserves.

Increased Energy Requirements
- Inefficient feeding skills may lead to excess energy expenditure during feeds.
- Physiologic demands of comorbid illnesses (e.g., cardiac conditions) may result in increased energy expenditure.

Increased Energy Losses
- Low tone or increased swallowing of air can make reflux more common, which can result in loss of feeds.

---

increased levels of bilirubin. In neonates, a bilirubin level of more than 5 mg/dL (85 μmol/L) manifests as clinical jaundice.[14,16] In most cases, jaundice is benign, and will resolve within 2 to 3 weeks after birth, or sooner with light treatment (phototherapy).[14,16] Adverse symptoms to be alert for include lethargy, poor feeding, and high-pitched (irritable) cries. Prolonged high levels of bilirubin can put a baby at risk of neurologic injury (kernicterus).[14,16]

Diabetes is a group of metabolic diseases in which there are high blood glucose levels during a prolonged period. Diabetes is caused by either (1) the pancreas not producing enough insulin or (2) the cells of the body not responding properly to the insulin produced (insulin resistance). Increased health risk has been found for infants of mothers with gestational diabetes (a temporary form of diabetes caused by hormonal changes during pregnancy), as well as those of mothers with prepregnancy type I (insulin-dependent) and type II (non–insulin-dependent or insulin-resistant) diabetes.[33] The main risks to infants of diabetic mothers are fetal obesity (macrosomia) and low blood sugar levels (leading to lethargy, irritability, and potential neurologic injury).[33] Infants of diabetic mothers are also at increased risk of RDS (because of reduced surfactant production), hyperbilirubinemia, and mild neurologic deficits including impaired fine and gross motor skills, impaired memory, and increased symptoms of attention deficit hyperactivity disorder (ADHD).[33]

Fetal alcohol syndrome (FAS) is a group of problems that can occur in a newborn who was exposed to alcohol while in utero. Alcohol passes through the placenta to the fetus during pregnancy and hence can affect the child's development. The degree and type of complications experienced by an infant with FAS depend on how much alcohol the mother consumed, how long and at what stage of pregnancy she drank (alcohol use appears to be the most harmful during the first 3 months of pregnancy), how the mother's body breaks down alcohol, and the mother's general health.[34]

Common symptoms of FAS include poor growth in utero and after birth; decreased muscle tone; poor coordination; a characteristic facial profile including small and narrow eyes with large epicanthal folds, smooth and thin upper lip (absent philtrum), small maxilla, and small head circumference; heart defects (e.g., VSD and atrial septal defect), and delayed development affecting cognition, speech, social skills, or motor skills.[34] The outcome for infants with FAS varies, although few have normal brain development.[34]

Neonatal abstinence syndrome (NAS) is a group of problems that occur in a newborn who was exposed to addictive drugs (illicit or prescription) while in utero. NAS is likely to occur if the pregnant mother takes drugs such as opiates (narcotics e.g., heroin, methadone, codeine), barbiturates (often used as sedatives or anticonvulsant medication), or benzodiazepines (often used as antianxiety medication).[35] These and other substances pass through the placenta to the fetus during pregnancy; hence the child becomes dependent. At birth, given the infant no longer is exposed to the drug, symptoms of abstinence or withdrawal may occur.

The degree and type of symptoms experienced by an infant with NAS depend on the type of drug the mother used, how much of the drug she was taking, how long and at what stage of pregnancy she used the drug, how the mother's body breaks down the drug, and whether the baby was born preterm or full-term.[35] Symptoms of NAS may be present at birth or may take days to appear. They may include hyperactive reflexes, increased muscle tone, irritability, excessive or high-pitched crying, seizures, vomiting, sweating, rapid breathing, tremors, and sleep problems. Poor feeding and slow weight gain are also frequently reported as common symptoms.[35]

Treatment depends on the symptoms experienced by the infant and the drug involved. Careful observation over days to weeks may be required. Infants with poor feeding and those who vomit or who are dehydrated may require intravenous (IV) fluids or tube feeding. Infants with NAS are often irritable and hard to calm, and thus an assessment of the caregiver's ability to interact with the child and meet his or her needs is required. In addition, given that use of illegal drugs (particularly those administered intravenously) is associated with a range of other health issues (including bloodborne diseases), the general health of the mother and the infant must be assessed.

NAS symptoms can last from 1 week to 6 months.[35] Some infants with severe NAS need medications to treat withdrawal symptoms, such as morphine or methadone. The physician will usually prescribe a drug similar to the one the mother used during pregnancy and slowly decrease the dose over time. This helps wean the baby off the drug and relieve some withdrawal symptoms. In addition to withdrawal symptoms, infants exposed to addictive drugs in utero are at risk of low birth weight (BW) and premature delivery, sudden infant death syndrome (SIDS), and ADHD.[35]

Box 13-19 provides an overview of potential contributors to negative energy imbalance and growth faltering in children affected by adverse perinatal conditions.

BOX 13-19 POTENTIAL CONTRIBUTORS TO NEGATIVE ENERGY IMBALANCE AND GROWTH FALTERING IN CHILDREN WITH MATERNAL OR PERINATAL RISK FACTORS

Reduced Energy Intake
- Lethargy can reduce stamina for the work of feeding or limit opportunities to feed.
- Feed refusal may occur because of irritability or behavioral issues.
- In situations of maternal substance abuse, the caregiver's ability to provide and prepare feeds and meals safely must be considered, as well as the caregiver's ability to respond to the child's hunger cues and provide any assistance the child may require with feeds and meals.

Increased Energy Requirements
- Inefficient feeding skills may lead to excess energy expenditure during feeds.
- Physiologic demands of any illnesses that may result from substance exposure (e.g., seizures) may result in increased energy expenditure.

Increased Energy Losses
- Altered insulin control and blood sugar metabolism can result in ineffective digestion of feeds.

PREMATURITY

Normal gestation in humans is 37 to 42 weeks. Infants born prior to 37 weeks are considered preterm (Figure 13-7). Table 13-5 describes the degrees of prematurity based on GA and BW. Box 13-20 lists common terms used in relation to preterm infants.

By virtue of their premature delivery, early development is interrupted in preterm infants. Premature exposure to the ex utero environment forces preterm infants to breathe and feed for themselves at a time when O_2 and nutrients would have been provided to them by the placenta had they remained in utero. In addition, preterm infants are forced to support their body against the effects of gravity, rather than have the support of amniotic fluid and the uterine wall around them. Further, either as a direct result of their premature birth or as a coinciding event, many preterm infants present with severe morbidities.[36] Both the impairments themselves, as well as the interventions required to treat them, have the potential to further interrupt feeding development in these infants.[36,37] In addition, prolonged hospitalization can affect the family's ability to interact and bond with their child, which has the potential to affect feeding interactions (see Clinical Corner 13-2).[37]

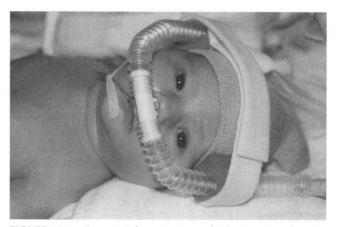

FIGURE 13-7 Preterm infant. (From Hockenberry MJ, Wilson D: *Wong's essential of pediatric nursing*, ed 9, St Louis, 2013, Mosby.)

TABLE 13-5 Degrees of Prematurity Based on Gestational Age and Birth Weight

	Extremely Low	Very Low	Low	Term
Gestational age	<28;0 weeks	28;0-31;6 weeks	32;0-36;6 weeks	37;0-41;6 weeks
Birth weight	<1000 g	<1500 g	<2500 g	3500 g (average)

BOX 13-20 COMMON TERMS USED IN RELATION TO PRETERM INFANTS

Postmenstrual age (PMA): Age of infant based on time since the date at start of the mother's last menstrual cycle. This is the most common method for estimating the age of a fetus and calculating estimated due date (estimated due date = 280 days [40 weeks] from date at start of the mother's last menstrual cycle).

Postconceptional age (PCA): Age of infant based on time since known conception date. PCA is generally 14 days less than PMA.

Gestational age (GA): Often used interchangeably with PMA. "Term" age is 40 weeks' GA. GA is often written in the format of *34/40* or *34;0* to signify 34 weeks' GA, or *34⁴/40* or *34;4* to signify 34 weeks and 4 days.

    GA at birth is aged based on the time between date at start of the mother's last menstrual cycle and birth.

    Corrected GA (CGA) is an infant's current age calculated from date of mother's last menstrual cycle (e.g., a child who was born at 28 weeks' GA who is now 4 weeks old, is 32/40 weeks' CGA)

Chronological age (ChA): Age of infant based on time since birth. Chronological age does not take into consideration degree of prematurity.

Corrected age (CA): Age of the infant relative to his or her expected delivery date (term age) (e.g., a child

who was born 12 weeks early at 28 weeks' PMA, who is now 20 weeks old, is 8 weeks' CA).

Appropriate for gestational age (AGA): An infant born at a weight between the tenth and ninetieth percentile expected for his or her GA.

Small for gestational age (SGA): An infant born smaller than expected for his or her GA (generally defined as birth weight less than the tenth percentile for GA).

Intrauterine growth restriction or retardation (IUGR) (also known as *pathological* SGA): This term describes a fetus that has not reached its growth potential because of genetic or environmental factors in utero.

Neonatal intensive care unit (NICU): Intensive care unit for medically unstable infants who require life-sustaining treatments (e.g., mechanical ventilation) or surgery. Generally 1:1 or 1:2 nurse to patient ratio.

Special care nursery (SCN): Step-down unit for infants who require medical supervision or interventions such as tube feeds, but who are generally medically stable. SCNs have fewer nurses to patients than NICUs. Note: Different countries use different systems to define the various levels (and sublevels) of care for high-risk infants. NICU and SCN are two of the more common terms used to describe the two main levels, but these terms are not used universally.

CLINICAL CORNER 13-2: FEEDING DIFFICULTIES IN MEDICALLY COMPLEX CHILDREN

Conor is a 2-year-old boy. He was born preterm at 30/40 weeks, and has a history of tracheomalacia and chronic neonatal lung disease. He was ventilated until 2 months corrected age, and required O₂ therapy at night while he slept until 12 months corrected age. Conor has been tube fed since birth, initially via a nasogastric tube until 6 months corrected age, and then via a G-tube. He currently is able to manage small amounts of pureed solids from a spoon.

Critical Thinking

1. Describe the normal oral intake of a child of this age (texture of food, method of delivering food and fluids, position for feeds).
2. List the various issues in Conor's case history that have the potential to affect his oral feeding skills, and discuss how each of these issues may possibly have affected his feeding.

Summary of Factors That Can Affect Feeding in Preterm Infants

State control: Different levels (or states) of consciousness occur on a continuum, ranging from sedation and deep sleep though awake states to crying and

extreme irritability (See Box 14-7 in Chapter 14 for a list of various states). The optimal state for suckle feeding is an awake-alert or awake-active state. State control difficulties may be components of a variety of medical conditions common in preterm infants and may affect the ability to feed well.

Stress: The suckle feeding process places many demands on the high-risk infant. These may be *feeding related* (liquid flowing too fast or slow, distracting movements of the feeder), caused by *internal discomfort* (e.g., increased work of breathing and digestion during feeds), or caused by *external or environmental stimuli* (e.g., bright lights, noise, distracting movements of others in the room). If these demands are beyond the infant's adaptive capacities, the infant may respond with behaviors that reflect stress (see Box 14-8 in Chapter 14 for description of stress cues). If stress cues are noted before, during, or after a suckle feed, the source of the stress needs to be identified and modified if possible for the infant to feed well.

Postural control: Premature infants have less muscle bulk and less body fat than full-term infants. They also display reduced flexor tone through the head and neck, often resulting in neck hyperextension and decreased contact between the tongue and palate. Lack of positional stability may lead to difficulty positioning the infant for suckle feeds. Swaddling (firmly wrapping the infant in a sheet or blanket) often assists to provide appropriate support and positioning for feeding.

Oral motor control: Many preterm infants display absent or abnormal oral reflexes because of prematurity or general lethargy, as well as the effects of invasive medical intervention (e.g., intubation, tube feeding). In addition, oral motor difficulties (such as weak or uncoordinated suckling) may be observed in preterm infants. Many problems are due to a lack of positional stability, and lack of oral feeding practice.

Gut maturity and health: Feeding intolerance is a common complication of preterm birth. The immature GI tract has difficulty digesting feeds. Extremely premature infants initially require parenteral nutrition, as they are unable to tolerate sufficient enteral feeds. In addition, the preterm infant's GI tract is fragile, and stresses (infections, altered gut flora, and insufficient O_2 or blood flow) can injure it.[14] Infants with perforated intestines require surgery for removal of dead or dying bowel, and often cannot be fed until the GI tract recovers, and so also require parenteral nutrition. In some cases, removal of large portions of the bowel (short gut syndrome) can leave insufficient area for absorption of feeds and thus long-term parenteral nutrition may be required. In cases in which an infant's gut cannot tolerate enteral feeds, suckle feeding is usually not possible. In some cases, the infant may be able to tolerate small volumes of feed enterally (i.e., trophic feeds). In this circumstance, small suckle feeds may be possible.

Physiologic control: The infant will have physiologic responses to the work of feeding (e.g., increased respiratory rate, increased heart rate). If a high-risk infant is not able to cope with these responses, stress reactions and poor endurance may result, which can affect the infant's ability to feed well.

Respiratory rate: During the early part of suckle feeding, when the infant is sucking eagerly, the respiratory rate usually decreases from baseline values. As the suckle feeding progresses and the infant sucks less eagerly, taking more pauses to breathe, the respiratory rate usually increases back toward baseline. In infants with respiratory compromise, respiratory rate can be significantly elevated. Infants who have a high respiratory rate at rest may not be able to tolerate the suppression in respiration that occurs in the early part of suckle feeding and may fatigue easily. If respiratory rate is more than 60 breaths per minute, the infant may not have time to swallow between breaths and may be at risk of aspiration as he or she tries to gasp for air.

Heart rate: It is not uncommon to see small heart rate increases during suckle feeding. Larger increases (tachycardia) may indicate that suckle feeding is placing excessive demands on the infant. Bradycardia (decreased heart rate) may also be observed during suckle feeding in the preterm infant and is a potentially life-threatening event. Bradycardia may be triggered via a vagally-mediated response to stimulation of sensory receptors in the pharyngeal-laryngeal area. Stretch receptors may be stimulated by a large bolus. Touch receptors can also be stimulated by the presence of nasogastric tubes. Chemoreceptors can be stimulated by aspiration of feeds or by reflux. Decreases in O_2 saturation can also lead to bradycardia. Physiologic instability during feeds is an indicator that the infant is not ready for full (or perhaps any) oral intake.

Endurance: Poor endurance may result in the infant ending the suckle feeding before taking the required volume. Endurance is a reflection of the infant's cardiopulmonary reserve, the work to maintain physiologic stability and homeostasis, and work for other activity (such as suckle feeding). Endurance is compromised by many disease processes that are more common in preterm infants, which can affect the infant's ability to feed well.

Sucking, swallowing, and breathing: In young infants, all of these life-sustaining reflexes are driven by control centers in the brainstem (Box 13-21). Many preterm infants are born before these control centers have developed fully, which can affect the initiation, timing, and coordination of these related reflexes. Difficulties in any of these functions, or lack of coordination between them, can affect airway safety during feeding, as well as volume of intake.

Suckle feeding interactions: Preterm infants and their families are at risk of problems in feeding interactions because of long periods of hospitalization and separation, which can limit opportunities for bonding. Physiologic instability and illness can affect the infant's ability to tolerate handling. Lack of state control can result in the infant spending a large amount of time in either a sleep or irritable state, and not in a state suitable for feeding or other interaction. Noxious environmental stimuli (bright lights, loud noises, painful procedures) can cause the preterm infant's developing sensory system to react and show signs of distress or go into shut down. Motor delays and disorders can affect the infant's ability to interact normally to stimulation and input.

Parental shock and grief at premature delivery and the infant's compromised health condition can affect their interaction skills. In some cases, the mother's health is compromised as well, and so she may be in pain or need medical treatment herself. Approximately 60% of twins, more than 90% of triplets, and essentially all quadruplets

---

BOX 13-21   SUCKLING, SWALLOWING, AND BREATHING COORDINATION AND THE ROLE OF CENTRAL PATTERN GENERATORS

Central pattern generators (CPGs) are neural networks that, when activated, can produce rhythmic patterned outputs without sensory feedback.

Both breathing and swallowing are rhythmical activities driven by CPGs.[38,39] In young infants, suckling is also driven by a CPG. During nutritive sucking, each suck draws in fluid that needs to be swallowed. Therefore the timing of sucking and swallowing needs to be coordinated. Breathing and swallowing occur in a shared space and both cannot occur safely at the same time. Thus the timing of swallowing and breathing also needs to be coordinated. Neural control centers responsible for coordination of sucking, swallowing, and breathing are contained in the dorsomedial and ventrolateral regions of the medulla in the brainstem.

As infants mature, cortical structures play an increasing role in facilitating and modulating the actions of the CPGs and the coordination of sucking (and later mastication), swallowing, and breathing. As a result, infants can learn to adapt and adjust their sucking style if bolus volume changes (e.g., infants generally show weaker, slower sucks with a faster flowing nipple that delivers a larger bolus, to slow the milk flow[40-43]) or if their work of breathing changes (e.g., infants with respiratory infections generally show

weaker, slower sucks when they are working harder to breathe, to allow themselves time to breathe[44,45]). Eventually, when they start to eat solid foods, infants need to be able to alter their degree of mouth opening, direction of tongue movement, and degree of biting and chewing force depending on the size, firmness, and cohesiveness of the bolus they consume.

In premature infants, the various CPGs that control sucking, swallowing, and breathing are often not fully developed at birth, and mature at different times in the weeks leading up to term age.[38] In addition, the target areas controlled by the CPGs can be affected by disease processes (e.g., lung disease) or absent or adverse sensory experiences (e.g., intubation, tube feeding). Thus preterm infants often lack the ability to adapt and may not be able to adjust their sucking style if bolus volume changes or if their work of breathing changes. As a result, during feeding, preterm infants often display oxygen desaturation events[44] (caused by reduced respiratory rate or reduced respiratory depth [i.e., shallow breathing]) or apnea events (the cessation of breathing). This is presumably the reason why it has been shown that reduced milk flow can assist with coordination of swallowing and breathing in preterm infants.

From Mathew OP, Belan M, Thoppil CK: Sucking patterns of neonates during bottle feeding: comparison of different nipple units. *Am J Perinatol* 9(4):265, 1992.
Mathew OP: Breathing patterns of preterm infants during bottle feeding: role of milk flow. *J Pediatr* 119(6):960, 1991.
Chang YJ, Lin CP, Lin YJ, et al: Effects of single-hole and cross-cut nipple unit on feeding efficiency and physiological parameters in premature infants. *J Nurs Res* 15:215, 2007.
Conway AE: Young infants' feeding patterns when sick and well. *Matern Child Nurs J* 18(4):1, 1989.

---

and higher-order multiples are born preterm.[46] Parents of multiple birth sets have the additional job of spreading their time and support between children.

Box 13-22 provides an overview of potential contributors to negative energy imbalance and growth faltering in premature infants.

IATROGENIC COMPLICATIONS THAT MAY AFFECT FEEDING AND SWALLOWING

Tube Feeding

Often, prematurity or illness can result in periods during which children cannot feed by mouth. Even if a child is well enough to attempt some oral feeds, he or she may not have sufficient skill or endurance to support full, independent oral feeding. During the period when medically complex children are unable to feed exclusively by mouth, they require some form of artificial tube feeding to meet their energy, nutrition, and fluid requirements (Figure 13-8). Box 13-23 provides an outline of the various types of tube feeding.

Reasons for commencing tube feeds include dysphagia, failure to gain weight (e.g., related to cardiorespiratory disease or GER), and digestive disorders (e.g., inflammatory bowel disease, cystic fibrosis, intestinal malabsorption).[47] Each of these groups accounts for approximately one third of children who require long-term tube feeding.[48]

In the short term, tube feeding (as well as other invasive procedures that occur in and around the mouth, such as suctioning and intubation) may cause obstruction or irritation of the structures involved in feeding (Table 13-6). In the longer term, the iatrogenic effects of medical interventions affecting the mouth and associated structures, as well as lack of oral feeding practice, may contribute to the development of altered oral sensitivity or oral aversion, as well as inefficient feeding patterns.[49] In addition, any coinciding developmental delays in motor skills or alterations to muscle tone may result in poor postural support and reduced control of the muscles of the mouth involved in oral feeding.[49] Further, because of the effects of prematurity or illness, many medically complex infants display poor nutritional and energy reserves, which may result in low endurance levels for the work of feeding[49] (see Table 13-6).

Reduced Energy Intake

- Inefficient feeding skills may be related to prematurity, comorbid medical conditions, or result from a lack of opportunity to practice oral skills.
- Poor suck-swallow-breath coordination may occur because of brainstem immaturity or respiratory complications, which may put the infant at risk of aspiration or apnea.
- Inability to feed (or feed safely) may occur because of effects of medical treatments, such as respiratory support (mechanical ventilation, CPAP, BiPAP, high-flow oxygen therapy).
- Patients may display reduced stamina for the work of feeding because of poor energy reserves.
- Feed refusal may occur because of nausea, lack of appetite, pain, or learned aversion.
- Frequent fasting for medical procedures may result in periods of reduced intake.

Increased Energy Requirements

- Physiologic demands of comorbid illnesses may result in increased energy expenditure (increased work of breathing, increased work of circulation).
- "Catch-up" growth requires the infant to consume additional energy to grow rapidly to make up for small size at birth.

Increased Energy Losses

- Ineffective digestion of feeds can mean that not all the energy and nutrition from the feed is absorbed.
- Vomiting and reflux are more common in preterm infants than in the general population because of low tone in the lower esophageal sphincter and respiratory issues. This may result in loss of feeds.

BiPAP, Bilevel positive airway pressure; *CPAP,* continuous positive airway pressure.

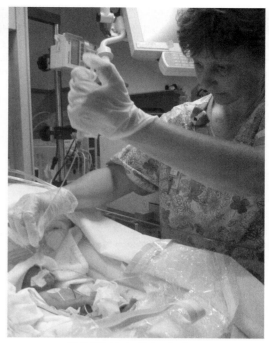

FIGURE 13-8   Tube feeding.

diet. Although tube feeding is useful and appropriate when a child is medically unstable or if there is a chronic condition affecting the ability to swallow or to digest feeds, it is not the method of choice if oral feeding is possible. Consensus among health professionals suggests that the transition from tube feeding to oral feeding should be established as soon as tube feeding is no longer required. However, in many cases children refuse to eat even when the feeding tube is removed. At this point, a tube weaning program may be required (see Chapter 15).

Respiratory Support

Ventilation (breathing) is the movement of air between the environment and the lungs via inhalation and exhalation (Figure 13-9). Ventilation is necessary to allow cellular respiration (gas exchange of O_2 and carbon dioxide). Box 13-24 provides an overview of the stages of breathing.

Spontaneous breathing can be interrupted by neurologic, anatomic, or physiologic changes.

Mechanical ventilation is a method to mechanically assist or replace spontaneous breathing. There are two main types of mechanical ventilation: positive pressure ventilation and negative pressure ventilation. **Negative pressure ventilation** involves generating negative pressure outside the patient's chest, which is used to expand the lungs and allow air to flow in. Negative pressure ventilation machines are large and require the patient to be positioned inside. They are generally only used with paralyzed patients.

Because of advances in medical treatment, an increasing number of medically complex children are surviving infancy, which may result in **tube dependency.** As discussed previously, many medically complex children require some period of tube feeding to assist them in meeting their nutritional requirements. Unfortunately, even once their acute medical and nutritional needs are addressed, many refuse oral feeds and remain dependent on prolonged tube feeding. Unnecessary tube feeding can hinder a child from developing age-appropriate feeding skills, prevent participation in social activities, and cause considerable family stress.

Long-term tube feeding is not an acceptable option for children who are capable of eating and digesting a regular

---

BOX 13-23 COMMON TYPES OF TUBE FEEDING

Enteral nutrition (gavage feeds) are delivered into the gut.
- **Nasogastric (NG)** tubes are inserted via the nose and end in the stomach. They are usually secured to the face with tape.
- **Orogastric (OG)** tubes are inserted via the mouth and end in the stomach. They may or may not be secured to the face with tape.
- **Gastrostomy (G)** tubes are inserted directly into the stomach surgically and stitched into place.
- **Percutaneous endoscopic gastrostomy (PEG)** tubes are inserted directly into the stomach via endoscopically guided "key-hole" surgery. A small "button" is visible on the surface, which is connected to a removable tube for feeds.
- **Nasojejunal (NJ)** tubes are inserted via the nose and end in the jejunum. Because they pass though the stomach and into the small intestine via the pyloric sphincter, they are also referred to as *transpyloric tubes (TPT)*.
- **Gastrojejunal (GJ)** tubes are inserted directly into the stomach. A TPT is then extended from the stomach into the jejunum.
- **Jejunostomy (J)** tubes are inserted directly into the jejunum.

Parenteral nutrition feeds bypass the gut and are delivered into the bloodstream.
- **Intravenous (IV)** fluids such as dextrose or saline are provided into the bloodstream, usually via a peripheral vein.
- **Total parenteral nutrition (TPN)** provides full nutrition (protein, lipids, carbohydrates, electrolytes, and trace elements) directly into the bloodstream, usually via a central vein.

TABLE 13-6 Possible Interruptions to Oral Feeding Development Associated with Illness and Medical Treatment

Primary Condition	Intervention	Outcomes
PREMATURITY	ARTIFICIAL FEEDING	PRIMARY CONDITION PERSISTS TO
Premature:	Enteral nutrition (gavage	SOME DEGREE
Anatomic and physiologic development	feeds)	Ongoing morbidity
(cardiac, respiratory, gastrointestinal	NG	Energy imbalance
systems)	OG	EFFECTS OF INTERVENTION
Neurologic development (reflexes,	Gastrostomy, PEG	Immediate
tone, coordination)	TP	Local irritation of swallowing
ILLNESS/MORBIDITY	Jejunostomy	mechanism
Impairment of:	Parenteral nutrition	Obstruction of swallowing
Major body systems (neurologic,	OTHER INTERVENTIONS	mechanism
cardiac, respiratory, gastrointestinal	Intubation (or suctioning)	Injury to swallow mechanism
systems)	Orotracheal	Altered breathing
Swallowing mechanism (oral region,	Nasotracheal	Delayed
pharynx, larynx, esophagus)	Via NP airway	Disuse of muscles involved in
OTHER ISSUES	Via tracheostomy	swallowing
Physiologic instability	VARIABLES	Altered sensitivity in swallowing
Altered alertness, state	Age when intervention	mechanism
Poor endurance	started	INTERRUPTED DEVELOPMENT FOR
Altered appetite (medication, reduced	Duration of intervention	INFANTS
gastric emptying, constipation)	Frequency of intervention	Delayed development of oral motor
Altered nutritional and energy	Total vs. supplemental tube	skills
requirements	feeding (i.e., opportunity	Defensive oral behavior, food
Increased energy requirements	for any oral experience)	aversion
(morbidity, such as cardiac and	Route for tube feeding (via	Reduced association between
respiratory disease)	oral or nasal cavity or	feeding and reduction of hunger
Increased energy losses (poor	directly into gut)	Lack of mealtime routines
absorption, gastroesophageal reflux)	Rate of tube feeding (bolus	Limited exposure to tastes, textures,
Low nutritional stores	or continuous)	feeding utensils
REASONS FOR COMMENCING	Type of feed offered	Altered bonding opportunities with
INTERVENTION	Positioning during feeds	parents
Risk of aspiration		Reduced parental confidence in
Risk of inadequate growth		feeding infant
Delivery of medication (e.g.,		
chemotherapy)		

NG, Nasogastric; *NP,* nasopharyngeal; *OG,* orogastric; *PEG,* percutaneous endoscopic gastrostomy; *TP,* transpyloric.

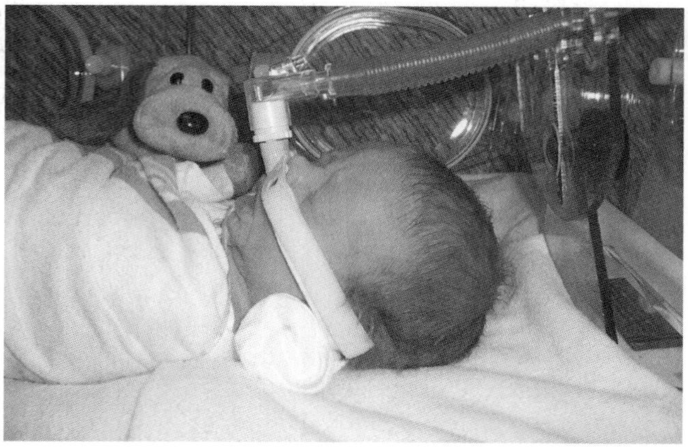

FIGURE 13-9 Respiratory support. (From Hockenberry MJ, Wilson D: *Wong's essential of pediatric nursing,* ed 9, St Louis, 2013, Mosby.)

BOX 13-24 STAGES OF SPONTANEOUS BREATHING

1. The medulla's inspiratory center sends a nervous impulse to the diaphragm (via the phrenic nerve, originating at C3-5) and intercostal muscles (via the intercostal nerves, originating T1-11) to contract causing expansion of the thoracic cavity. Impulses are also sent to the medulla to inhibit the expiratory center.
2. Air enters the lungs because of the negative pressure in the expanded thoracic cavity.
3. When the lungs are inflated, stretch receptors send nervous impulses back to the medulla (via the vagus nerve, CN X) to inhibit the inspiratory center.
4. The expiratory center is no longer inhibited and sends nervous impulses to muscles to relax. The lungs deflate, expelling air.
5. When the lungs are deflated, the stretch receptors become inactive, and the inspiratory center is no longer inhibited. This allows the cycle to start again.

CN, *Cranial nerve.*

Positive pressure ventilation involves delivering air into the airways and lungs under positive pressure, producing positive airway pressure during inspiration (blowing the lungs open, like inflating a balloon). Positive pressure ventilation machines are smaller and more portable than negative pressure machines.

Mechanical ventilation strategy involves attempting to achieve an adequate airflow volume with the lowest possible airway pressure (high pressure at the level of the alveoli can cause lung damage, such as atelectasis). The rate, pattern, and duration of gas flow control the interplay between volume and pressure. In addition, airway compliance and resistance can affect the pressure and volume that can be achieved.

Compliance is the distensibility of a system. The higher the compliance of the respiratory system, the easier it is to inflate the lungs. Compliance can be affected by conditions such as RDS (insufficient surfactant) and pneumonia.[16]

Resistance causes an impediment to airflow. The higher the resistance, the harder it is to inflate the lungs. Resistance can be affected by size (smaller airways are harder to inflate) and by conditions such as laryngotracheobronchomalacia, asthma, and subglottal stenosis.[16]

Mechanical ventilation can be adjusted by the medical team using a number of variables.

Cycle: *Ventilator cycling* refers to the mechanism by which the phase of breathing switches from inspiration to expiration. The respiratory cycle can either be set with volume control or pressure control (Box 13-25).

Strategy: *Ventilation strategy* relates to the fact that the frequency of breaths (respiratory rate) may be controlled by the ventilator or the patient. The ventilator can be set to provide mandatory ventilation or allow for spontaneous ventilation (Box 13-26).

Mechanical ventilation is termed **invasive** if it involves any instrument entering the lower airway (below the vocal cords).[16,50] This can be achieved by passing a tube into the airway via the pharynx (e.g., endotracheal tube [ETT]) or via the skin and cartilage below the vocal folds (e.g.. tracheostomy tube). In a patient with a functioning brainstem, sedation is generally required for the patient to tolerate an ETT passing through the upper airway and vocal folds because of normal airway protection reflexes. Tracheostomy insertion is a surgical procedure. Note: Cuffed tubes may be required to prevent air "leak" around the tube.

Noninvasive forms of ventilation support can be effectively delivered via mask or nasal prongs and include continuous positive airway pressure (CPAP) and variable positive airway pressure (VPAP) or bilevel positive airway pressure (BiPAP) support, as well as O_2 supplementation and vaporized high-flow therapy. See Box 13-27 for an overview of noninvasive methods of ventilation support.

A number of factors can potentially affect feeding and swallowing safety in patients requiring mechanical ventilation or other respiratory support. These include:
- Neurologic injury and absent oral reflexes (suckle, swallow, gag, cough)
- Decreased level of alertness caused by sedation
- Obstruction to swallowing mechanism caused by ventilation tubes
- Desensitization caused by presence of ventilation tubes or high airflow
- Positional restrictions
- Increased work of breathing

BOX 13-25 VENTILATOR CYCLE CONTROL

Volume control (VC): Any mode that relies on airflow volume to trigger or cycle a breath is in the VC category. Airflow volume can be measured by the tidal volume (volume of each breath) or the minute ventilation (total tidal volume over 1 minute). Once the ventilator detects that the set volume has been achieved, the inspiratory flow stops. Patient complications can occur if airway pressure generated is higher than is desirable.

Volume-related terms and acronyms:
- V_t **(tidal volume):** Volume of each breath, usually measured on expiration
- $V_t x$ **(breaths per minute):** Number of breaths per minute
- MV_e **(minute ventilation):** Total volume of ventilation per minute
- **I:E ratio (inspiratory to expiratory ratio):** The relative time in the ventilation cycle allocated to inspiration and expiration

Pressure control (PC): Any mode that relies on a set pressure to cycle or trigger a breath is in the PC category. Pressure is measured at the patient end of the ventilator circuit. Once the ventilator detects that the set pressure has been achieved, inspiratory flow stops. Patient complications can occur if flow volume is lower or higher than is desirable.

Pressure-related terms and acronyms:
- M_{paw} **(mean airway pressure):** The mean pressure applied to the lungs during ventilation

- P_{ip} **(peak inspiratory pressure):** The highest level of pressure applied to the lungs during inhalation. This can be increased by increased secretions, bronchospasm, or decreased lung compliance.
- **PEEP (positive end-expiratory pressure):** Pressure present in the airways at the end of expiration.
  - Extrinsic (applied) PEEP is set on the ventilator. A small amount of applied PEEP (3-5 cm H_2O) is used in most mechanically ventilated patients to mitigate end-expiratory alveolar collapse.[16]
  - Intrinsic (auto) PEEP occurs when there is incomplete expiration prior to the initiation of the next breath, which causes progressive air trapping (breath stacking) leading to lung hyperinflation. Auto-PEEP commonly develops when there is high minute ventilation (hyperventilation) or expiratory resistance (narrow airway, obstructed airway).
- **CPAP (continuous positive airway pressure):** Pressure support applied to the airways throughout inspiration and expiration.
- **VPAP or BiPAP (variable or bilevel positive airway pressure):** Provides two levels of pressure to the airways: IPAP (inspiratory positive airway pressure) and a lower EPAP (expiratory positive airway pressure) for easier exhalation.

From Gardner S, Merenstein G: *Handbook of neonatal intensive care*, St Louis, 2002, Mosby.
Chatburn RL, Volsko TA, Hazy J, et al: Determining the basis for a taxonomy of mechanical ventilation. *Respir Care* 57(4):514, 2012.

BOX 13-26 VENTILATOR STRATEGY

Continuous mandatory ventilation (CMV): Every breath is mandatory (i.e., inspiration is patient or machine triggered, but machine cycled).

Intermittent mandatory ventilation (IMV): Spontaneous breaths (i.e., inspiration that is patient triggered and patient cycled) can exist between mandatory breaths.

Continuous spontaneous ventilation (CSV): Every breath is spontaneous (i.e., patient triggered and patient cycled).

From Gardner S, Merenstein G: *Handbook of neonatal intensive care*, St Louis, 2002, Mosby.
Chatburn RL, Volsko TA, Hazy J, et al: Determining the basis for a taxonomy of mechanical ventilation. *Respir Care* 57(4):514, 2012.

In general, most pediatric patients are able to be weaned off ventilation or other respiratory assistance after days, weeks, or months of treatment, as their underlying medical condition improves and other medical treatments can be withdrawn. It most situations, a step-down approach is used to wean the patient from the respiratory support. A list of common criteria that are considered in determining whether a patient no longer requires respiratory support is presented in Box 13-28.

Tracheostomy

A **tracheostomy** is a surgically created incision through the front of the neck and into the trachea, below the cricoid cartilage. The resulting stoma (hole) can be used independently as an airway or as a site for a tracheostomy tube to be inserted (Figure 13-10).

A tracheostomy is used for three main reasons in children:
- **Airway patency:** When the usual route for breathing is somehow impaired or obstructed (e.g., subglottic stenosis, laryngomalacia), a tracheostomy tube can provide a patent airway.
- **Airway protection:** When there is frank aspiration risk (e.g., brainstem tumor, stroke), a cuffed tracheostomy tube can be used to protect the lower airway from soiling, while providing a patent airway.

BOX 13-27 TYPES OF NONINVASIVE VENTILATION SUPPORT

CPAP support: Continuous positive airway pressure applied to a patient who is spontaneously ventilating.

VPAP or BiPAP support: Variable or biphasic positive airway pressure applied to a patient who is spontaneously ventilating.

Nasal intermittent positive pressure ventilation (NIPPV): Continuous positive airway pressure applied to a patient who is spontaneously ventilating. In addition, periodic additional flow is triggered, known as *sighs*. The sighs occur on a time schedule and are mandatory. The aim of NIPPV is to help offload the work of diaphragm and accessory muscles, decreasing the infant's work of breathing.

Oxygen (O$_2$) supplementation: Additional oxygen mixed with room air (of varying concentration) applied to a patient who is spontaneously ventilating (note: O$_2$ supplementation can also be used on top of mechanical ventilation).

Humidified high-flow therapy (also known as *transnasal insufflation*): Room air with or without additional oxygen is humidified to allow higher flow rates than can be delivered via traditional nasal prongs. This allows the delivery of flow rates that meet or exceed the patient's inspiratory flow rate, and may avoid the need for invasive mechanical ventilation.

From Gardner S, Merenstein G: *Handbook of neonatal intensive care*, St Louis, 2002, Mosby.
Chatburn RL, Volsko TA, Hazy J, et al: Determining the basis for a taxonomy of mechanical ventilation. *Respir Care* 57(4):514, 2012.

BOX 13-28 COMMON WEANING CRITERIA FOR PATIENTS WHO REQUIRE RESPIRATORY SUPPORT

Neurologic
- Spontaneous breaths (no apnea, low level of sedation)
- Sufficient spontaneous tidal volume (adequate muscle strength)
- Airway protection (e.g., cough, gag, swallow reflexes)

Pulmonary
- Patent airway
- Pulmonary compliance and resistance within normal limits
- Normal work of breathing
- Normal blood gas

Cardiovascular
- Hemodynamically stable
- Able to meet work of spontaneous breathing

From Gardner S, Merenstein G: *Handbook of neonatal intensive care*, St Louis, 2002, Mosby.

- **Mechanical ventilation:** When a long-term route for invasive mechanical ventilation is required (e.g., severe lung disease, cervical spinal injury), a tracheostomy provides a means for ventilation that does not involve passing a tube through the upper airway and vocal folds or require ongoing sedation (as occurs with an ETT).

For some children, a tracheostomy is permanent. In cases in which the underlying medical condition improves and a tracheostomy is no longer needed, the stoma is surgically closed or allowed to heal over. A list of common criteria that are considered in determining whether a patient can be **extubated** are summarized in Box 13-29.

Speaking valves are designed to assist with vocalization in patients with tracheostomies. Speaking valves are one-way valves that are connected to the outer hub of the tracheostomy tube. They allow airflow in through the tracheostomy tube during inhalation, but close to prevent airflow out through the tracheostomy tube during exhalation. Ideally, airflow is then directed up past the tracheostomy tube (this is commonly referred to as *leak*), through

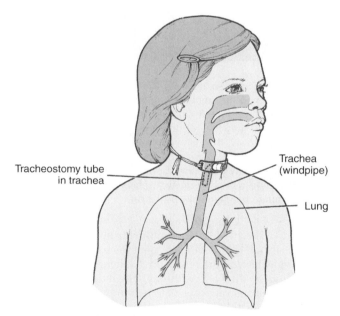

FIGURE 13-10 Tracheostomy tube in place. (From Hockenberry MJ, Wilson D: *Wong's essential of pediatric nursing*, ed 9, St Louis, 2013, Mosby.)

the vocal cords, and out through the upper airway, thus enabling vocalization, as well as clearing of secretions from the upper airway. If a patient cannot get sufficient leak to allow expiratory airflow while wearing a speaking valve, he or she will not be able to vocalize and (more dangerously) will be at risk of respiratory compromise. See Box 13-30 for a list of some of the factors that can affect whether a child can tolerate use of a speaking valve.

BOX 13-29 COMMON EXTUBATION CRITERIA FOR PATIENTS WHO ARE TRACHEOSTOMIZED

Airway Patency
- Does the patient have a patent airway?
- Can the patient produce sufficient expiratory airflow for voicing and coughing?

Airway Protection
- Can the patient protect the airway from soiling (i.e., aspiration of saliva, food and fluids, or stomach contents)?
- Can the patient swallow secretions?
- Can the patient swallow fluid and food, or does he or she have a nonoral method of nutrition?

Mechanical Ventilation
- Can the patient ventilate through noninvasive means?
- Does the patient have spontaneous breaths?
- Can the patient achieve sufficient tidal volume?

From Gardner S, Merenstein G: *Handbook of neonatal intensive care*, St Louis, 2002, Mosby.

BOX 13-30 FACTORS TO CONSIDER WHEN DETERMINING WHETHER A CHILD CAN TOLERATE USE OF A SPEAKING VALVE

Leak Space
- Children have smaller airways than adults, and hence even the smallest available tracheostomy tube (2.5 or 3 mm inner cannula, 4 or 4.7 mm outer diameter) may take up the full space of a young child's airway, thus preventing leak.
- Leak is not possible if a patient has a cuffed tracheostomy that cannot be deflated (because of aspiration risk or because a seal is required to allow adequate mechanical ventilation).

Patency of the Upper Airway
- Even if there is leak around the tracheostomy, exhalation is not complete until the expiratory airflow has left the respiratory system. If airflow cannot exit the airway through the mouth or nose, the speaking valve needs to be removed to allow the airflow to exit via the tracheostomy.
- Speech requires airflow through functional vocal folds, as well as through functional articulators. If there is dysfunction in the larynx or pharynx, speech may not be possible.

The presence of a tracheostomy tube has the potential to affect both swallowing and communication development in children. The degree of impact can be affected by factors such as:
- Age when tracheostomized
- Duration of tracheostomization

- Any ventilation or O_2 therapy delivered via tracheostomy
- Frequency of suctioning
- Time spent as inpatient

In addition, swallowing skills can potentially be affected by factors such as whether the child had any oral intake or received any oral stimulation while tracheostomized. Factors such as whether the child had any leak around the tracheostomy to allow coughing with or without the use of a speaking valve can potentially affect the child's laryngeal and pharyngeal sensation and the integrity of airway protection reflexes.

Ingestional Injuries

Chemical ingestion can cause serious and sometimes life-threatening complications to the swallowing mechanism, airway, and gut. In children, the main causes of serious ingestional injuries are household chemicals, such as cleaning products (e.g., bleach, ammonia, dishwashing powder, laundry powder and liquids) and batteries (e.g., button batteries).[51] These chemicals often corrode (burn) the tissues with which they come in contact, and may cause pain, swelling, necrosis, and fistulas. Surgery is often required to repair damaged structures. On healing, scar tissue and **strictures** may form, which can further complicate healing and compromise oral feeding. Common feeding complications in children with ingestional injuries include impaired airway protection, swallowing difficulties, and bolus impaction, as well as food aversion and fear of choking.[51] Some of these children will require a tracheostomy for a time. Many display aspiration and need to be put **nil per os (NPO)** (also referred to as **nil by mouth (NBM)**) and receive all feeds via tube feeding, or may require thickened fluids or modified diets. Many of these children will require months or years of monitoring, as they heal and gradually learn to eat again.

OTHER FACTORS THAT MAY POTENTIALLY AFFECT FEEDING AND SWALLOWING IN CHILDREN

Tonsillitis and Tongue-Tie

Tonsillitis is an inflammation of the palatine tonsils, most commonly caused by viral or bacterial infection.[14] Symptoms may include sore throat and fever. Most people suffer tonsillitis at some point in life, and most people recover completely, with or without medication. In chronic or recurrent cases, or in acute cases in which the tonsils become so swollen that swallowing or breathing is impaired, a tonsillectomy can be performed to remove the tonsils.

Tongue-tie (ankyloglossia) is a congenital condition characterized by a tight lingual frenulum (the membrane connecting the underside of the tongue to the floor of the mouth), which may decrease mobility of the tongue tip. Tongue-tie varies in degree of severity from mild cases to complete tethering of the tongue to the floor of the mouth. Rating scales, such as the Hazelbaker scale,[52] can be used to grade the degree of tongue-tie.

It is widely recognized that tongue-tie can affect breast-feeding success, causing inefficient feeding for the infant and pain for the mother. Several studies have shown that early tongue-tie surgery (frenulotomy) early on can improve breastfeeding.[53,54] There is less information about the effect of tongue-tie on bottle feeding or eating of solids, or about the effectiveness of tongue-tie surgery beyond infancy. Many families report significant improvements in their child's feeding and speech after tongue-tie surgery. Some families and individuals choose not to have tongue-tie surgery and report functional feeding and speech regardless.

Oral Motor Impairments

Children who experience feeding difficulties may have some degree of oral motor impairment that affects their ability to suck, chew, or bite. This may be caused by a developmental delay, disordered motor patterns (e.g., low or high tone, the presence of primitive oral reflexes), or a motor planning problem (i.e., apraxia). These motor issues may be general or specific to the oral region, and may or may not affect speech in addition to feeding. It is the role of the feeding therapist to identify any oral motor impairment, to determine its effect on the child's feeding ability, and to develop a treatment plan to address these issues or provide compensations to assist with feeding, if possible (see Chapter 15).

Sensory Processing Disorders

Winnie Dunn, an occupational therapist who has pioneered much of the clinical research around the issue of sensory processing in children, described different individual variation in perception and response to the same sensory stimuli as a result of being positioned on a different part of the sensitivity spectrum for that particular type of sensory input.[55] According to this model, the middle of the sensory spectrum is normal sensitivity, in which individuals display a "normal" threshold for registering sensory input and a "typical" response to the sensory stimulation. On one side of the spectrum is hypersensitivity, in which individuals display a reduced threshold for registering sensory input and an increased response to normal stimulation. On the other side of the spectrum is hyposensitivity, in which individuals display an increased threshold for registering sensory input and a reduced response to normal stimulation. Dunn's model also allows for a range of sensory responses between both ends of the spectrum and the central normal response[55] (Figure 13-11 and Box 13-31).

Through her research in this area, Dunn has shown that severe alterations in sensory processing abilities may be a

Neurological thresholds	Self-regulation strategies/behavioral responses	
	Passive	Active
High threshold	Low Registration	Sensation Seeking
Low threshold	Sensory Sensitivity	Sensation Avoiding

FIGURE 13-11 Sensory profile. (Adapted from "The Impact of Sensory Processing Abilities on the Daily Lives of Young Children and Families: A Conceptual Model" by W. Dunn 1997, Infants and Young Children 9(4):23–25, 1997. IN Dunn W: The sensations of everyday life: theoretical, conceptual and progmatic considerations, Am J Occup Ther 55(6):608, 2001.)

> **BOX 13-31** HIGH AND LOW SENSORY THRESHOLDS
>
> **Hypersensitivity:** The child has a low threshold for the stimulus, leading to high registration. When exposed to the stimulus, the child may show a heightened response (sensory sensitivity) or may actively avoid the stimulus (sensation avoiding).
> **Hyposensitivity:** The child has a high threshold for the stimulus, causing low registration. When exposed to the stimulus, the child may show a lowered response (low registration) or may actively seek more of the stimulus (sensation seeking).

> **BOX 13-32** PAIN, SENSORY SENSITIVITY, AND FOOD AVERSION
>
> **Pain:** Painful sensory stimulus, associated with actual tissue damage
> **Sensory sensitivity:** Abnormally high response to (even normal) sensory stimulus
> **Food aversion:** Behavioral response to a stimulus or anticipation of a stimulus, which may persist beyond initial pain or sensory processing problem

key component of many developmental disorders (e.g., autistic spectrum disorder and ADHD).[56-58] There is also support in the literature to suggest that altered sensory processing may result from repeated exposure to adverse sensory stimulation or the absence of normal sensory stimulation.[59-61] Also, it is understood that individuals without developmental disorders or a history of any apparent traumatic experiences display some degree of variation in how they perceive and respond to sensory input.[62-63]

Oral Sensitivity

As part of their medical management, many children who have required hospitalization or frequent medical interventions are exposed to a range of invasive procedures involving their oral, pharyngeal, and facial regions, such as tube feeding, intubation, and suctioning. In addition, hospitalized children may go through periods during which they are unable to engage in oral feeding and other normal, pleasurable oral stimulation. It has been shown that such experiences can affect the oral sensory processing abilities of children.[63] Clearly, this is a concern, as altered oral sensitivity may have the potential to affect oral feeding ability.[64]

Dunn's classification system allows for the fact that individuals may be positioned at one point on the sensory spectrum for one type of sensory input and another part of the sensory spectrum for another type of input (e.g., the individual who displays a normal response to auditory input but a low threshold for tactile input and a hypersensitive response to touch).[55] It is also understood that sensitivity integration disorders may affect the whole body or specific regions of the body (e.g., the mouth).[55] Feeding therapists are generally most interested in investigating a child's ability to process sensory information related to oral feeding (i.e., sensitivity to touch, taste, and temperature within the mouth).

It is important to note that although they may be related, oral sensitivity is not the same as oral aversion or pain. See Box 13-32 for an overview. Oral aversion often follows

from pain or altered sensitivity, but that aversion may endure beyond the original sensory processing problem. Behavioral feeding therapy may help to address oral aversion but is unlikely to be effective if there is still underlying pain or sensory sensitivity. These must be addressed first (see Chapter 15).

Autism Spectrum Disorder

Autism spectrum disorder (ASD) is a group of neurodevelopmental disorders that affect typical childhood development. The most current diagnostic criteria for ASD, as defined in the American Psychiatric Association's *Diagnostic and Statistical Manual of Mental Disorders, 5th Edition* includes markedly abnormal or impaired developments in social interaction and communication and markedly restricted and stereotyped patterns of behavior and interests.[65] Although ASD is a spectrum disorder, and the presentation of shared features in this group is quite variable, many children with ASD present with concomitant developmental delays in the areas of sensory processing disturbances and motor development.[66,67]

Feeding difficulties have been observed in children with ASD since the disorder was first described by Kanner in 1943.[68] It has been reported that between 46% and 89% of children with ASD have feeding difficulties.[69] In the social media there is frequent reference to the "white food diet" common in children with ASD. Nutritional literature often focuses on the implications of poor diet on subsequent behavior. It seems likely that behavior and features of ASD may in turn affect nutrition, given that oral motor delay, sensory sensitivity, and desire for "sameness" may contribute to a preference for bland foods lacking in color, taste, and temperature that are easy to eat (e.g., bread, potato, crackers, cookies, milk). These foods also tend to be high in energy, but low in nutrients.

Marshall et al.[70] performed a literature review that identified more than 40 research studies describing feeding difficulties and nutritional issues in children with ASD. The study identified that restricted dietary variety, food neophobia, food refusal, limiting diet based on texture, and a propensity toward being overweight were frequently reported.

It was identified that poor nutrition can affect health outcomes, and that the feeding issues described can cause significant parental concern and can affect family dynamics.[70]

Parent-Child Interaction

It is widely recognized that parents who are attentive to their child's needs and development tend to have children who are better able to regulate their own emotions and interact well with others.[71,72] The premise of **cue-based care** (also known as *developmentally supportive care*) is to observe the child's behavior and to provide support when needed, as well as encouragement.[73]

Given the potential effect of feeding difficulties on parent-child interaction, it is important for feeding therapists to be aware of any parenting styles or strategies that are not supportive of the child's needs, and help to facilitate family support as needed. Feeding therapists may participate in advanced training in this area or may work alongside other health professionals who specialize in supporting parent-child relationships (e.g., family counselors, psychologists, and other mental health experts).

Several different methods for describing parent-child interaction exist. Cooper, Hoffman, and Powell, who developed the *Circle of Security* model (www.circleofsecurity.net), use the model shown in Figure 13-12 to describe ideal parenting methods to support child development.

This model explains parenting attachment strategies, summarized in Box 13-33, and parenting styles, summarized in Box 13-34.

TAKE HOME NOTES

1. Feeding difficulties can have a detrimental effect on dietary intake and hence growth and development. Children need adequate energy balance for growth and development. If their energy intake is less than their requirements, they will display a negative energy balance and growth faltering (usually weight loss; if this persists, height gain and head size may be affected also).
2. Feeding therapists are trained to identify the signs of aspiration. Aspiration occurs when the bolus enters the airway below the level of the vocal folds, and may be primary or secondary to swallowing.

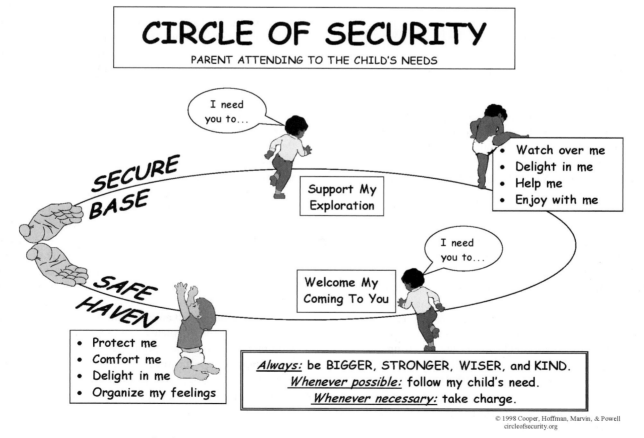

© 1998 Cooper, Hoffman, Marvin, & Powell
circleofsecurity.org

FIGURE 13-12 Circle of Security Model. (Copyright Cooper, Hoffman, Marvin, and Powell. Circleofsecurity.org.)

BOX 13-33 ATTACHMENT STRATEGIES

Attachment Strategies

Secure: A secure relationship creates confidence in the availability of a specific protective caregiver if needed and supports exploration when it is safe to do so. The child does not need to focus on the needs of the caregiver but can simply attend to what she or he wants, needs, thinks, and feels and make that known all the way around the Circle.

Ambivalent: An *ambivalent attachment* refers to an organized strategy of attachment that overemphasizes the demonstration of closeness and proximity (safe haven/bottom half of Circle) while underemphasizing the exploratory aspects of the relationship (secure base/top half of Circle). The child seeks to keep an inconsistent caregiver available through a heightened display of emotionality and dependence. This attachment strategy is not considered a risk for significant psychopathology.

Avoidant: Avoidance is an organized strategy of attachment that overemphasizes the exploratory aspects of the relationship (secure base/top half of Circle) while underemphasizing the need for emotional closeness and comfort to stay as close as possible to the caregiver while expressing a minimum of emotional need. This attachment strategy is not considered a risk for significant psychopathology.

Disorganized: Disorganized refers to attachment of a child to a caregiver who is either frightened of the child or frightening to the child (or both); a breakdown in organized behavior by the child occurs when needing to seek comfort and protection from the attachment figure, particularly when under stress. This attachment style is considered to be at risk of significant psychopathology.

© Cooper.Hoffman, Marvin, and Powell, www.circleofsecurity.org The Ainsworth Attachment Clinic and The Circle of Security. Http://theattachment clinic.org/AboutUs/terminology.html.

BOX 13-34 ATTACHMENT STRATEGIES

Parenting Styles

Authoritarian: A parenting style that has a high level of control and a low level of warmth and affection. Children from these families tend to have lower self-esteem, be less trusting, and more withdrawn.

"Bigger, stronger, wiser, and kind": A parenting style with a high level of the caregiver being "in charge" matched with a high level of caregiver warmth and affection. Children from these families tend to be more mature, independent, and academically successful. "Bigger, stronger, wiser, and kind" becomes a central parenting focus/goal (repeated often) within the COS [circle of security] protocol.

Permissive: A parenting style that has a low level of control and a high level of warmth and affection. Children from these families tend to be low in self-reliance and self-control and have trouble adjusting to school.

Reflective Capacity: The ability to stand back, observe, and understand one's own behavior, motivation, and needs and to observe and understand the behavior, motivation, and needs of others; the ability to "turn one's self in"; to see in a genuine way how one may be a part of any given problem within a relationship, while simultaneously recognizing that the other may also have responsibility.

© Cooper.Hoffman, Marvin, and Powell, www.circleofsecurity.org The Ainsworth Attachment Clinic and The Circle of Security. Http://theattachmentclinic.org/AboutUs/terminology.html.

3. Aspiration isn't the only adverse event that can occur as a result of swallowing difficulties. A prolonged apnea event occurs when the airway closes over and fails to reopen in time for regular breathing to continue after a swallow. In young infants, apnea events may occur in response to the presence of a material in or near the entrance to the laryngeal vestibule, presumably to protect the lungs from the potential damage of aspirated material. Choking occurs when a solid bolus physically blocks the airway and, because the child cannot breathe, can be immediately life threatening.

4. Pediatric feeding therapists often work with children who have mealtime behavior disturbances or learned fluid or food aversion. Feeding difficulties and mealtime disturbances often arise in association with dysphagia, aspiration, or a choking event. At other times, there is no apparent physical reason for feeding issues, although aversive experiences in or around the mouth, undetected pain, or sensory disturbances are usually involved at some level.

5. It is important for feeding therapists to have an awareness of common medical conditions that may affect feeding and swallowing. Some medical conditions have the potential to affect oral feeding *directly* and other conditions may affect oral feeding *indirectly*.

6. During the time when young children are developing their oral feeding skills, any feeding disturbances can potentially affect later feeding skills through interruption of the normal developmental process.

7. It is important to recognize that preterm infants (i.e., those born before 37 weeks' GA) are at high risk of developing feeding and swallowing difficulties. By virtue of their premature delivery, early development is interrupted in preterm infants. Further, either as a direct result of their premature birth or as a coinciding event, many preterm infants present with severe morbidities. Both the impairments themselves, as well as the interventions required to treat them, have the potential to further interrupt feeding development in these infants. Prolonged hospitalization can also affect the family's ability to interact and bond with their child, which has the potential to affect feeding interactions.

8. Feeding therapists need to be aware of various tube feeding options. Parenteral feeds bypass the gut and are delivered into the bloodstream. Enteral (gavage) feeds are delivered into the gut, either as bolus feeds or continuous feeds. Enteral feeds may be given via a tube that is inserted in the nose or mouth (e.g., nasogastric, nasojejunal, orogastric) or may be given directly into the gut via a surgical incision (e.g., G-tube, J-tube). Reasons for commencing tube feeds include dysphagia, failure to gain weight (e.g., related to cardiorespiratory disease, GER, or nonorganic failure to thrive), and digestive disorders (e.g., inflammatory bowel disease, cystic fibrosis, intestinal malabsorption).

9. Feeding therapists also need to be aware of various types of ventilation support. Ventilation support may be invasive (e.g., mechanical ventilation) or noninvasive (CPAP, humidified high-flow therapy, and O_2 supplementation).

REFERENCES

1. Tutor JD, Gosa MM: Dysphagia and aspiration in children. *Pediatr Pulmonol* 47(4):321, 2012.
2. Thach BT: Maturation of cough and other reflexes that protect the fetal and neonatal airway. *Pulm Pharmacol Ther* 20(4):365, 2007.
3. St John Ambulance: Managing choking, http://www.sja.org.uk/sja/first-aid-advice/breathing-problems/choking.aspx.
4. Field D, Garland M, Williams K: Correlates of specific childhood feeding problems. *J Paed Child Health* 39:299, 2003.
5. Rudolph CD: Feeding disorders in infants and children. *J Ped* 125:S116, 1994.
6. Burklow KA, Phelps AN, Shultz JR, et al: Classifying complex pediatric feeding disorders. *J Ped Gastroent Nutr* 27:143, 1998.
7. Rommel N, De Meyer AM, Feenstra L, et al: The complexity of feeding problems in 700 infants and young children presenting to a tertiary care institution. *J Pediatr Gastroenterol Nutr* 37(1):75, 2003.
8. Reilly S, Skuse D, Poblete X: Prevalence of feeding problems and oral motor dysfunction in children with cerebral palsy: a community survey. *J Pediatr* 1996.
9. Reau NR, Senturia YD, Lebailly SA, et al: Infant and toddler feeding patterns and problems: normative data and a new direction, Pediatric Practice Research Group. *J Dev Behav Pediatr* 17(3):149, 1996.
10. Mathisen B, Skuse D, Wolke D, et al: Oral-motor dysfunction and failure to thrive among inner-city infants. *Dev Med Child Neurol* 31(3):293, 1989.
11. Carruth BR, Skinner JD: Feeding behaviors and other motor development in healthy children (2-24 months). *J Am Coll Nutr* 21(2):88, 2002.
12. Carruth BR, Skinner JD: Mothers' sources of information about feeding their children ages 2 months to 54 months. *J Nutr Educ* 33(3):143, 2001.
13. Satter E: Children, the feeding relationship, and weight. *Md Med* 5:26, 2004.
14. Kliegman R, Stanton R, Geme J, et al: *Nelson textbook of pediatrics*, ed 19, Philadelphia, 2011, Elsevier Saunders.
15. Committee on Fetus and Newborn, American Academy of Pediatrics: Apnea, sudden infant death syndrome, and home monitoring. *Pediatrics* 111(4 Pt 1):914, 2003.
16. Gardner S, Merenstein G: *Handbook of neonatal intensive care*, St Louis, 2002, Mosby.
17. Weir K, McMahon S, Barry L, et al: Oropharyngeal aspiration and pneumonia in children. *Pediatr Pulmonol* 42(11):1024, 2007.
18. Karim RM, Momin IA, Lalani II, et al: Aspiration pneumonia in pediatric age group: etiology, predisposing factors and clinical outcome. *J Pak Med Assoc* 49(4):105, 1999.
19. Gross RE: *The surgery of infancy and childhood Philadelphia*, 1953, WB Saunders.
20. Hodge L, Swain A, Faulkner-Hogg K: Food allergy and intolerance. *Aust Fam Physician* 38(9):705, 2009.
21. Boyce JA, Assa'ad A, Burks AW, et al: Guidelines for the diagnosis and management of food allergy in the United States: summary of the NIAID-sponsored expert panel report. *Nutr Res* 31(1):61, 2011.
22. Rosenbaum P, Paneth N, Leviton A, et al: A report: the definition and classification of cerebral palsy, April 2006. *Dev Med Child Neurol Suppl* 109:8, 2007.
23. Cerebral Palsy Association: http://cerebralpalsy.org/about-cerebral-palsy/types-and-forms/#cm.
24. Palisano R, Rosenbaum P, Walter S, et al: Development and reliability of a system to classify gross motor function in children with cerebral palsy. *Dev Med Child Neurol* 39:214, 1997.
25. Benfer KA, Weir KA, Bell KL, et al: Oropharyngeal dysphagia and gross motor skills in children with cerebral palsy. *Pediatrics* 131(5):e1553, 2013.
26. Teasdale G, Jennett B: Assessment of coma and impaired consciousness: a practical scale. *Lancet* 2(7872):81, 1974.
27. Morgan AT: Dysphagia in childhood traumatic brain injury: a reflection on the evidence and its implications for practice. *Dev Neurorehabil* 13(3):192, 2010.
28. Fisher RS, van Emde Boas W, Blume W, et al: Epileptic seizures and epilepsy: definitions proposed by the International League Against Epilepsy (ILAE) and the International Bureau for Epilepsy (IBE). *Epilepsia* 46(4):470, 2005.
29. Buckley RT, Morgan T, Saneto RP, et al: Dysphagia after pediatric functional hemispherectomy. *J Neurosurg Pediatr* 13(1):95, 2014.
30. The American Academy of Otolaryngology—Head and Neck Surgery: http://www.entnet.org/content/cleft-lip-and-cleft-palate.
31. Moebius Syndrome Foundation: http://www.moebiussyndrome.com/.
32. National Down Syndrome Society: http://www.ndss.org/Down-Syndrome/What-Is-Down-Syndrome/.

33. American Diabetes Association: http://www.diabetes.org/diabetes-basics/gestational/what-is-gestational-diabetes.html.

34. National Association on Fetal Alcohol Syndrome: http://www.nofas.org/.

35. Kocherlakota P: Neonatal abstinence syndrome. *Pediatrics* 134(2):e547, 2014.

36. Dodrill P, Donovan T, Cleghorn G, et al: Attainment of early feeding milestones in preterm neonates. *J Perinatol* 28(8):549, 2008.

37. Dodrill P: Feeding difficulties in preterm neonates. *Infant Child Adolesc Nutr* 3(6):324, 2011.

38. Mistry S, Hamdy S: Neural control of feeding and swallowing. *Phys Med Rehabil Clin N Am* 19:709, 2008.

39. Barlow SM: Central pattern generation involved in oral and respiratory control for feeding in the term infant. *Curr Opin Otolaryngol Head Neck Surg* 17(3):187, 2009.

40. Mathew OP, Belan M, Thoppil CK: Sucking patterns of neonates during bottle feeding: comparison of different nipple units. *Am J Perinatol* 9(4):265, 1992.

41. Mathew OP: Breathing patterns of preterm infants during bottle feeding: role of milk flow. *J Pediatr* 119(6):960, 1991.

42. Chang YJ, Lin CP, Lin YJ, et al: Effects of single-hole and cross-cut nipple unit on feeding efficiency and physiological parameters in premature infants. *J Nurs Res* 15:215, 2007.

43. Conway AE: Young infants' feeding patterns when sick and well. *Matern Child Nurs J* 18(4):1, 1989.

44. Thoyre SM, Carlson JR: Preterm infants' behavioural indicators of oxygen decline during bottle feeding. *J Adv Nurs* 43(6):631, 2003.

45. Thoyre SM, Shaker CS, Pridham KF: The early feeding skills assessment for preterm infants. *Neonatal Netw* 24(3):7, 2005.

46. March of Dimes: http://www.marchofdimes.org/.

47. British Association for Parenteral and Enteral Nutrition, 2006. http://www.bapen.org.uk/bans_report_07.pdf.

48. Davelay W, Guimer D, Uhlen S, et al: Dramatic changes in home-based enteral nutrition practices in children during an 11-year period. *J Pediatr Gastroenterol Nutr* 43(2):240, 2006.

49. Dodrill P: Infant feeding development and dysphagia. *J Gastroenterol Hepatol Res* 2014. [Epub ahead of print].

50. Chatburn RL, Volsko TA, Hazy J, et al: Determining the basis for a taxonomy of mechanical ventilation. *Respir Care* 57(4):514, 2012.

51. Lupa M, Magne J, Guarisco JL, et al: Update on the diagnosis and treatment of caustic ingestion. *Ochsner J* 9:54, 2009.

52. Hazelbaker AK: *The Assessment Tool for Lingual Frenulum Function (ATLFF): use in a lactation consultant private practice*, Pasadena, CA, 1993, Pacific Oaks College. unpublished thesis.

53. Hogan M, Westcott C, Griffiths M: Randomized, controlled trial of division of tongue-tie in infants with feeding problems. *J Paediatr Child Health* 41(5–6):246, 2005.

54. Dolberg S, Botzer E, Grunis E, et al: A randomized, prospective, blinded clinical trial with cross-over of frenotomy in ankyloglossia: effect on breast-feeding difficulties. *Ped Res* 52:822, 2002.

55. Dunn W: The sensations of everyday life: theoretical, conceptual and pragmatic considerations. *Am J Occup Ther* 55(6):608, 2001.

56. Ermer J, Dunn W: The sensory profile: a discriminant analysis of children with and without disabilities. *Am J Occup Ther* 52(4):283, 1998.

57. Kientz MA, Dunn W: A comparison of the performance of children with and without autism on the Sensory Profile. *Am J Occup Ther* 51(7):530, 1997.

58. Dunn W, Bennett D: Patterns of sensory processing in children with attention deficit hyperactivity disorder. *Occ Thy J Res* 22(1):4, 2002.

59. Hellerud BC, Storm H: Skin conductance and behaviour during sensory stimulation of preterm and term infants. *Early Hum Dev* 70(1–2):35, 2002.

60. Anderson J: Sensory intervention with the preterm infant in the neonatal intensive care unit. *Am J Occup Ther* 40(1):19, 1986.

61. Dodrill P, McMahon S, Ward E, et al: Long-term oral sensitivity and feeding skills of low-risk pre-term infants. *Early Hum Dev* 76(1):23, 2004.

62. Dunn W, Brown C: Factor analysis on the Sensory Profile from a national sample of children without disabilities. *Am J Occup Ther* 51:490, 1997.

63. Dunn W, Westman K: The sensory profile: the performance of a national sample of children without disabilities. *Am J Occup Ther* 51(1):25, 1997.

64. Davis AM, Bruce AS, Khasawneh R, et al: Sensory processing issues in young children presenting to an outpatient feeding clinic. *J Pediatr Gastroenterol Nutr* 56(2):156, 2013.

65. American Psychiatric Association: *Diagnostic and statistical manual of mental disorders: DSM-5*, Washington, DC, 2013, American Psychiatric Association.

66. Watling RL, Deitz J, White O: Comparison of Sensory Profile scores of young children with and without autism spectrum disorders. *Am J Occup Ther* 55(4):416, 2001.

67. Fournier KA, Hass CJ, Naik SK, et al: Motor coordination in autism spectrum disorders: a synthesis and meta-analysis. *J Autism Dev Disord* 40(10):1227, 2010.

68. Volkmar FR, McPartland JC: From Kanner to DSM-5: autism as an evolving diagnostic concept. *Annu Rev Clin Psychol* 10:193, 2014.

69. Ledford JR, Gast DL: Feeding problems in children with autism spectrum disorders: a review. *Focus Autism Other Dev Disabl* 21(3):153, 2006.

70. Marshall J, Hill RJ, Ziviani J, et al: Features of feeding difficulty in children with Autism Spectrum Disorder. *Int J Speech Lang Pathol* 16(2):151, 2014.

71. Davies WH, Satter E, Berlin KS, et al: Reconceptualizing feeding and feeding disorders in interpersonal context: the case for a relational disorder. *J Fam Psychol* 20(3):409, 2006.

72. Satter E: Eating competence: definition and evidence for the Satter Eating Competence model. *J Nutr Educ Behav* 39(5 Suppl):S142, 2007.

73. Kenner C, McGrath JM, editors: *Developmental care of newborns and infants: a guide for health professionals*, ed 2, St Louis, 2010, Mosby.

74. Circle of Security: http://circleofsecurity.net/.

CHAPTER 14

Evaluating Feeding and Swallowing in Infants and Children

Pamela Dodrill

To view additional case videos and content, please visit the evolve website.

CHAPTER OVERVIEW

OBJECTIVES

1. Describe the common role of various members of the feeding and swallowing team.
2. Demonstrate an understanding of the various models of teamwork.
3. Discuss how the International Classification of Functioning, Disability, and Health model can be used to map the various areas that need to be considered when performing an assessment of a child's feeding and swallowing skills.
4. List essential areas to be covered in a case history.
5. Describe key components of a clinical feeding evaluation.
6. Discuss factors that need to be considered when assessing hospitalized children with acute health issues

and children in the community with chronic health issues or developmental delay.
7. Demonstrate an understanding of assessment considerations for infants and for older children.
8. Discuss pediatric-specific issues that need to be considered when performing imaging studies.

MEMBERS OF THE FEEDING AND SWALLOWING TEAM

A number of health professionals may be involved in the process of assessing and treating children with feeding difficulties. Some regional differences exist in professional

TABLE 14-1 Members of the Pediatric Feeding Team

Role	Typical Health Professional
Primary care for children	Primary care provider, general practitioner, child health nurse, pediatrician
Specialist medical care	Specialist physicians (e.g., otorhinolaryngologist, pulmonologist, gastroenterologist, neurologist, surgeon, radiologist), nurse practitioners
Nutrition	Registered dietitian
Swallowing, feeding	Speech-language pathologist
Breastfeeding	Lactation consultant, midwife, pediatric or child-health nurse
General development (motor and sensory skills)	Occupational therapist, physical therapist
Cognition, learning, behavior	Psychologist, counselor, behavior therapist

training degrees and qualification required to work in this area. Some differences in facility practices also occur because of staffing levels and availability of various health professionals, as well as historical practices.

Table 14-1 provides a summary of the various roles in a pediatric feeding team, and the most common health professionals who fulfill those roles.

For information regarding the role of speech-language pathologists in assessing and managing swallowing and feeding difficulties in children, see the American Speech-Language-Hearing Association website: http://www.asha.org/ (search *pediatric dysphagia*, then *roles and responsibilities*).

For information regarding the role of lactation consultants in assisting mothers and their infants who are struggling with breastfeeding, see the International Lactation Consultant Association: http://www.ilca.org/ (search *roles and responsibilities*).

For information regarding the role of registered dietitians, see the Academy of Nutrition and Dietetics website: www.eatright.org (search *roles and responsibilities*).

For additional information regarding the role of other health professionals in managing children with feeding difficulties, see their professional association websites (search *pediatric feeding, dysphagia,* and *roles and responsibilities*).

MODELS OF TEAMWORK

Various models of teamwork may be used in feeding and swallowing teams during the assessment and treatment process. In general, the terms *multidisciplinary, interdisciplinary,* and *transdisciplinary* are used to describe various models. Although no fixed definition of these terms exists, the most common features of these various models of teamwork are described in this section.

Multidisciplinary Team

The multidisciplinary team consists of a number of health professionals working individually within their specific professional boundaries, with some level of interaction or coordination. Often each team member assesses and manages the child separately, focusing of the aspect of the feeding difficulty traditionally managed by his or her profession. Team members usually share reports or contribute to a common report for the patient. Team members are usually aware of each others' goals for the patient, but may not actively try to incorporate those goals into their own management of the patient.

Interdisciplinary Team

The interdisciplinary team consists of a number of health professionals working together within their specific professional boundaries. Often team members assess and manage the child together, with each focusing of the aspect of the feeding difficulty traditionally managed by his or her profession. Team members usually contribute to a common report for the patient. Team members are aware of each others' goals for the patient and usually try to incorporate those goals into their own management of the patient.

Transdisciplinary Team

The transdisciplinary team consists of a number of health professionals working together across their specific professional boundaries. Usually, team members have worked together for some time and may have undertaken advanced training together. Team members are all aware of the aspects of the feeding difficulty traditionally managed by other members of the team. Often one team member is delegated to assess or manage the child, with input from and feedback to other members of the team as necessary. The primary team member for the child incorporates the goals of all the various team members into the assessment and management process.

Separate to the role of health professionals in a child's feeding assessment and management team, parent involvement is essential in assessment, setting therapy goals, delivering intervention, and monitoring progress to ensure that any intervention is meaningful for the child and family, and to assist with the generalization of therapy gains to the home environment (this is often referred to as **family-centered practice**).

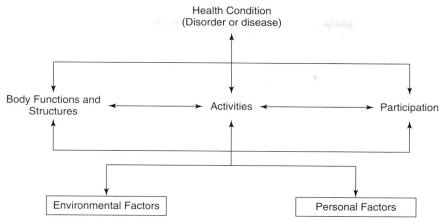

FIGURE 14-1   International Classification of Functioning, Disability, and Health model.

TABLE 14-2 Application of the ICF Model to Feeding and Swallowing in Children

Area of ICF Model	Examples in Relation to Feeding and Swallowing
Body structures	Anatomy, physiology, and neurology of oral and pharyngeal structures, larynx and other airway structures, esophagus and other gut structures
Body functions	Swallowing, sucking, biting, and chewing skills; physiologic stability; cognitive skills; motor skills; sensory perception
Activity versus disability	Ability to eat a meal, self-feed, drink a bottle, drink from a cup Determine, where necessary, whether use of modified food and fluids, special utensils, altered positioning, or special feeding strategies can prevent activity limitations or disability
Participation versus handicap	Participation in family mealtimes, participation in social and educational settings where food and fluid is consumed Determine, where necessary, whether social inclusiveness policies and strategies can prevent participation limitations or handicap for children on tube feeds and those who cannot eat developmentally appropriate foods and fluids (and their families)
Personal and environmental factors	Other factors that need to be considered include: The family's understanding of the child's feeding difficulties The family's access to appropriate and hygienic food, fluids, utensils, seating equipment Where necessary, the family's ability and willingness to prepare modified food and fluids, use special feeding utensils and seating equipment, and apply special feeding strategies Societal and cultural judgment of families (particularly mothers) who have a child with feeding difficulties

INTERNATIONAL CLASSIFICATION OF FUNCTIONING, DISABILITY, AND HEALTH

The World Health Organization's (WHO) International Classification of Functioning, Disability, and Health (ICF) model[1] is a classification of health conditions and their effects on the individual, as well as factors that can affect health. The ICF model is the WHO framework for measuring health and disability at both individual and population levels (Figure 14-1). The ICF model was officially endorsed in 2001 as the international standard to describe and measure health and disability.[2]

Table 14-2 gives examples of how the ICF model can be used to map the various areas that need to be considered when performing an assessment of a child's feeding and swallowing skills.

CASE HISTORY

Case history information is usually collected in writing (from the patient's medical chart, reports from other health professionals, and often a parent-completed form) and verbally (from discussions with other health professionals or an interview with the parent), and generally involves collecting information across multiple areas that may have the

---

BOX 14-1 AREAS TYPICALLY ASSESSED WHEN COLLECTING A ROUTINE CASE HISTORY

Medical history:
- Pregnancy and birth complications
- Medical conditions
- Medical investigations, surgeries, medications

Growth:
- Any known growth measurements
- Weight, weight-for-age percentile
- Height, height-for-age percentile
- Weight-for-height percentile, BMI, BMI-for-age percentile
- Any changes in pattern of growth

Diet:
- Foods and fluids taken by mouth
- Details of any oral nutritional supplements
- Details of any tube feeds
- Typical pattern of intake, volume and frequency of meals/feeds

Early feeding history:
- Breastfeeding, bottle feeding
- Transition to solids

General development

Cognitive skills

Onset of feeding difficulties

Current eating and drinking ability:
- Foods and fluids consumed
- Positioning for feeding
- Utensils used for feeding
- Self-feeding skills
- Mealtime duration and frequency

Behavior during mealtimes

Parent stress associated with mealtimes

Details of any specific concerns regarding child's eating and drinking abilities

---

BMI, Body mass index.

---

potential to affect feeding. See Box 14-1 for an outline of areas typically assessed when collecting a case history.

The following webpages contain specific examples of combined case history and clinical assessment forms for infants and for older children.

http://www.asha.org/uploadedFiles/Infant-Feeding
-History-and-Clinical-Assessment-Form.pdf
http://www.asha.org/uploadedFiles/Pediatric-Feeding
-History-and-Clinical-Assessment-Form.pdf

After gathering a basic case history, it is essential for a feeding therapist to confirm reported issues through additional interviews with the parent and observation of the child. In addition to the factors listed previously, feeding therapists should try to gather information from the parents about environmental factors such as the following:
- Family arrangement and primary caregiver for mealtimes
- Daycare and schooling arrangements and ability of educational staff to manage child's needs at mealtimes
- Any cultural issues that need to be considered in relation to feeding and eating
- Family access to safe food and food storage, access to necessary feeding equipment, and ability to modify food and fluids to meet child's needs

CLINICAL FEEDING EVALUATION

The clinical assessment is largely guided by information collected as part of the case history.

See Box 14-2 for an outline of areas typically assessed by feeding therapists during a standard clinical feeding evaluation for children with feeding or swallowing difficulties, and Box 14-3 for areas typically assessed by a dietitian during a routine nutrition assessment.

When observing a child feeding, the feeding therapist needs to make an assessment of the child's **swallowing safety** during mealtimes, as well as his or her **feeding competence.**

To assess **swallow safety,** the feeding therapist needs to observe and evaluate whether the child can protect the airway during feeds or mealtimes. This usually requires the feeding therapist to offer fluid or food trials and observe for any adverse clinical signs suggestive of laryngeal penetration or aspiration (Box 14-4). If present, the therapist should note the timing of any adverse clinical signs. If adverse signs are observed to occur during oral preparation or swallowing, they may indicate that material is entering the airway on descent through the pharynx (i.e., **primary aspiration**). If adverse clinical signs are observed during pauses in feeding or after feeds, they may indicate that material (reflux) is ascending into the pharynx or larynx from the gut (i.e., **secondary aspiration**).

Imaging studies (as detailed later in this chapter) are used to confirm or allay clinical suspicions of aspiration and guide management practices.

For young infants who are breastfed or bottle fed, the **coordination of suckling, swallowing, and breathing** is assessed by observing and listening to the ratio of sucks to swallows, as well as the timing and adequacy of respiratory efforts throughout the feed. The normal rhythmic suckling pattern during breastfeeding or bottle feeding consists of a series of bursts and pauses. Normally, full recovery in all respiratory parameters occurs within the suckling pauses. Even if the infant does not show clinical signs of aspiration during feeding, other adverse physiologic events during feeding (Box 14-5) can indicate a

---

BOX 14-2 AREAS TYPICALLY ASSESSED DURING ROUTINE CLINICAL FEEDING AND SWALLOWING EVALUATION

Examination of oral anatomy

Testing of oral reflexes

Observation of oral sensory processing

Assessments of oral-motor skills for nonfeeding tasks

Observation of oral-motor skills in feeding tasks

Observation of swallowing skills and airway protection during swallowing

Observation of physiological stability during feeding

Trials of modified food and fluids, where necessary

Trials of different feeding equipment, where necessary

Trials of different feeding strategies, where necessary

Observation of child behavior and parent-child interaction during meals

---

BOX 14-3 AREAS TYPICALLY ASSESSED DURING ROUTINE NUTRITION ASSESSMENT

Perform growth measurements (anthropometry):
- Weight (used to determine weight-for-age percentile)
- Height (used to determine weight-for-height percentile and to calculate BMI and BMI-for-age percentile)
- Head circumference (used to determine size-for-age percentile)
- Waist circumference and midarm circumference (used to determine size-for-age percentiles)

Determine any changes in patterns of growth.

Determine energy and nutrient requirements based on:
- Gender
- Age
- Height and weight
- Presence of specific medical conditions
- Need for "catch-up" growth

Collect dietary recall and record for analysis in relation to:
- Dietary adequacy (energy, nutrition, fluid)
- Mealtime patterns (volume and frequency of feeds, duration of feeds)
- Type of foods (variety across food groups)

Determine degree of nutritional risk and needs for supplementation:
- Oral supplementation
- Supplementation via tube
- Supplementation of energy +/− nutrients

BMI, Body mass index.

BOX 14-4 ADVERSE CLINICAL SIGNS DURING AND AFTER FEEDS SUGGESTIVE OF POSSIBLE ASPIRATION IN CHILDREN

Wet voice, cry

Wet, rattly chest (rales, fremitus)

Coughing

Color change, cyanosis

Stress cues, such as eye tearing, furrowing of the forehead, finger splaying, hypervigilance (staring)

Weir K, McMahon S, Barry L, et al: Clinical signs and symptoms of oropharyngeal aspiration and dysphagia in children. *Eur Respir J* 33(3):604–611, 2009.

BOX 14-5 ADVERSE CLINICAL SIGNS DURING AND AFTER FEEDS SUGGESTIVE OF RESPIRATORY COMPROMISE DURING FEEDING

Increased work of breathing (nostril flaring, head bobbing, neck extension, tracheal tug, subcostal recession)

Increased stridor

Altered respiratory rate or heart rate

Decreased oxygen saturation

Apnea

Color change, cyanosis

Stress cues, such as eye tearing, furrowing of the forehead, finger splaying, hypervigilance (staring)

From Weir K, McMahon S, Barry L, et al: Clinical signs and symptoms of oropharyngeal aspiration and dysphagia in children. *Eur Respir J* 33(3):604–611, 2009.
Weir KA, McMahon S, Taylor S, et al: Oropharyngeal aspiration and silent aspiration in children. *Chest* 140(3):589–597, 2011.
Thoyre SM, Carlson JR: Preterm infants' behavioural indicators of oxygen decline during bottle feeding. *J Adv Nurs* 43(6):631–641, 2003.

---

problem with swallowing or with suck-swallow-breath coordination.

To assess **feeding competence,** the feeding therapist needs to observe the child's oral skills to determine whether he or she has the ability and competence to consume enough fluids and food to meet dietary requirements (Box 14-6). To start, a brief assessment should be performed of oral anatomy, oral reflexes, oral sensory processing, and oral motor control (see Box 14-6). Then the feeding therapist should try to observe how the child feeds at a **typical meal.** Wherever possible, it is useful to ask the parent to bring in the child's usual feeding equipment and samples from the child's usual diet. In addition, clinicians should have a range of developmentally appropriate feeding equipment (e.g., bottles, spoons, trainer cups, high chair or other

---

BOX 14-6 COMMON COMPONENTS OF CLINICAL ASSESSMENT OF ORAL STRUCTURES AND FUNCTIONS

Oral Anatomy

Structures to be assessed: Lips, palate, tongue, jaw, teeth (if present), cheeks

Features to observe: Whether structures are intact, symmetrical, appropriate size, tone, range of motion

Oral Reflexes

The presence of both adaptive and protective reflexes should be noted.

- Adaptive reflexes (assist in getting feeds into gut): Rooting, suckling
- Protective reflexes (assist in keeping feeds out of airway): Phasic bite, tongue protrusion, tongue lateralization, gag, cough

Note: Expression of oral reflexes can change depending on infant's level of hunger or state of alertness, so assessment should take this into account.

Reflex	Stimulus	Expect until
Rooting	Stroke cheek, lips	3-4 months (rooting may diminish earlier in bottle-fed infants)
Suckling	Stroke center of tongue, palate	4-6 months (sucking may be elicited after this age, but is not reflexive)
Tongue protrusion	Touch tongue tip	4-6 months
Tongue lateralization	Stroke side of tongue, gums	6-9 months
Phasic bite	Apply firm pressure to gums	9-12 months
Gag	Touch back of tongue	Adulthood

Oral Motor Control

- Offer age-appropriate nonnutritive tasks (e.g., sucking on a pacifier or gloved finger, chewing on a teething toy) to assess use of oral structures.
- Where possible, observe oral-motor skills in nutritive (feeding) tasks. Note symmetry, strength, coordination, and efficiency (i.e., time taken to perform task).
- Ensure the child is positioned appropriately before making an assessment of oral motor skills, as postural (gross motor) stability can affect the fine motor skills involved in feeding.

Oral Sensory Processing

- Note response to touch in and around the mouth (light, firm), texture of foods, temperature of foods.
- Responses should be categorized as *typical, hypersensitive,* or *hyposensitive.*
- Where possible, observe oral sensitivity in feeding tasks. Note type of response, degree of response, and any change in response with repeated exposure.
- Also note general response to visual stimuli, auditory stimuli, movement (vestibular and proprioceptive input).

---

seating option), fluids, and foods to allow a functional assessment of a child's oral skills in the context of a meal.

It should be noted that, although there are a number of formal feeding assessment tools available, most were developed to assist in classifying the feeding skills of children with cerebral palsy and other neurodevelopmental disorders. In clinical practice, many clinicians do not routinely use formal assessment tools when assessing children with feeding difficulties, but rather rely on informal checklists based on normal feeding development to guide their evaluation.[6]

In addition to observing oral skills and swallowing, it is important for the feeding therapist to observe the child's **mealtime behavior** and, where possible, **parent-child interaction** during the meal (see Table 14-3 for an example of a mealtime interaction rating scale). One of the main objectives of a pediatric feeding assessment is to determine how much of a child's feeding issues are related to **skill deficits versus learned behaviors** that may or may not be reinforced by the family. It often helps to videotape the session to allow later playback for further analysis and parent training.

In cases in which primary aspiration or respiratory compromise during feeding is suspected or in which the child is struggling to consume enough fluid or food, a number of different **feeding therapy techniques and compensations** may be trialed by the feeding therapist as part of the assessment process. Examples are detailed in Table 14-4.

ASSESSING HOSPITALIZED CHILDREN WITH ACUTE HEALTH ISSUES

In addition to factors that have to be considered as part of a standard feeding assessment, a range of issues needs to be considered when assessing children with acute health issues (Figure 14-2). A summary of key issues is outlined in this section.

TABLE 14-3 Checklist of Parent-Child Mealtime Interaction

Antecedent		
Check if any of the following strategies are being used by the caregiver when presenting food:		
Verbal	Questions (e.g., "Would you like a bite?")	
	Begging/ pleading (e.g., "Please take a bite for Mommy, please")	
	Bargaining/coaxing (e.g., "You can play games on my phone if you take a bite")	
	Raised voice (e.g., "Take a bite, now!")	
	Threats (e.g., "Take a bite, or I'll take all your toys away")	
Physical	Restraining the child (e.g., Holding down the child's arms)	
	Force feeding (e.g., Holding the spoon to the child's mouth until he or she accepts it; forcing the food into the child's mouth)	
Behavior		
Check if the child is demonstrating any of the following behaviors when presented with food:		
Verbal	Verbal protest (e.g., "No, I don't like it")	
Physical	Physical protest (e.g., tantrums, crying, throwing food)	
Escape	Leaves the table, runs away, pulls away from the feeder	
Withdrawal	Shut-down response (e.g., unresponsive, not engaging)	
Consequence		
If the child demonstrates undesirable behavior, check if the caregiver is using any of the following responses:		
Verbal	Verbal punishment (e.g., "You are a naughty boy for not eating that")	
Physical	Restraining the child until he or she eats	
	Force feeding	
Escape	Allowing escape from the situation (e.g., Letting the child leave the table without doing what was requested)	
Withdraw	Withdrawing from the interaction (e.g., Giving up and ignoring the child)	

(Adapted by Marshall J & Dodrill P (2014) from Eyberg et al.[7])

TABLE 14-4 Feeding Therapy Techniques That May Be Trialed as Part of Feeding Assessment

Modified fluids	Adding thickening agent to regular fluids; trialing naturally thick fluids
Modified foods	Altering the texture or size of solid foods by boiling, baking, blending, mashing, chopping, etc.; offering naturally easier to eat foods
Special feeding equipment	Offering different bottles and nipples, spoons, cups, etc.
Special feeding strategies	Altering positioning or seating equipment; altering pace of delivery (pacing); trialing swallowing maneuvers (e.g., chin tuck)

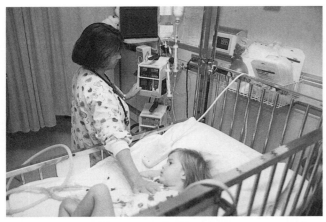

FIGURE 14-2 In addition to standard feeding assessment considerations, additional factors need to be considered for a child who is hospitalized. (From Price D, Gwin J: Pediatric Nursing, ed 10, Saunders, St. Louis, 2008.)

Medical Stability

The feeding therapist needs to have a general awareness and understanding of the variety of health issues that may present in children with feeding difficulties and be sensitive in their interactions with patients, their family members, and other health professionals. In medically complex children, there are times when the greatest focus for medical staff and the family needs to be managing acute health complications. Feeding assessment and intervention may not be appropriate or a priority. In contrast, there are times when care can become focused on supporting developmentally appropriate activities, such as feeding. In between these events, there are often times when feeding assessment and intervention can start to be introduced, provided they do not interfere with other essential health care activities (this is something that needs to be discussed and agreed on by medical and therapy staff). Some medically complex children undergo multiple cycles of acute illness and medical treatment, and frequent monitoring of feeding skills is required to track any progress or regression in these cycles.

Nutritional Stability

When an unwell child is nutritionally compromised, the primary focus of nutrition and feeding management has to be ensuring the child consumes enough energy, nutrition, and hydration to meet basic requirements. At these times, this focus supersedes considerations for promoting an oral diet or a developmentally appropriate diet. This may mean using parenteral feeds or using enteral feeds that are delivered continuously to the stomach or intestines. Some children may require special feeds or supplements that are

unpleasant tasting and are better tolerated if given via nonoral means. During this time, the role of the feeding therapist is to assess whether it is possible to introduce activities that can promote normal oral experiences (e.g., suckling on a pacifier, chewing on teething toys) and minimize adverse oral experiences while the child is not consuming a typical oral diet.

Once the child's nutritional status has stabilized, there is often a sudden push for oral feeding assessment and intervention to be prioritized when a patient is preparing for discharge home. The feeding therapist plays an important role during this time. However, the therapist must resist pressure to clear a child for full oral feeding and discharge if the child or the family is not fully competent in the tasks that will be required for the child to manage full oral feeds at home.

Limitations Caused by Medical Treatments and the Hospital Environment

The feeding therapist working in an acute health environment must be considerate of a range of factors when assessing and providing assessment and intervention. For example, fragile infants may not tolerate the handling required for feeding, and older children who are unwell may not tolerate sitting upright for meals. In addition, feed schedules may need to be interrupted if the patient displays nausea, pain, irritability, or fatigue related to his or her illness, medications, or other interventions. Children who need frequent surgeries often have to have their feeding schedules interrupted by the need to fast before, during, and in the time immediately following surgery. Feeding therapists need to be considerate of these issues when scheduling feeding assessments and therapy sessions.

In general, it is often hard to replicate normal mealtime experiences in the hospital environment. Patients are often confined to their beds and may not have access to normal seating or positioning options for meals or the ability to participate in social mealtimes with others. Hospital food is notorious for being bland and lacking variety and appeal. Many hospitals offer children meals from an adult menu and supply adult-sized utensils—neither of which are developmentally appropriate for children. The sights and sounds of the hospital environment are often anxiety producing, and the variety of smells in the hospital environment are often unpleasant when eating. Again, the feeding therapist must be considerate of these factors when assessing hospitalized children. The feeding therapist also has a role in advocating for developmentally supportive practices, such as the provision of age-appropriate food and feeding equipment, to assist in promoting normal feeding development.

Despite general improvements in hospital policies regarding family visits, which allow greater visitation access than in previous decades, parents of hospitalized children may still often have to leave their children for hours or days at a time because of other responsibilities such as caring for other children or work. As a result, many patients end up with multiple caregivers who all might have somewhat different approaches to supporting feeding. Wherever possible, the feeding therapist should advocate for a family member to be present for feeds and meals so that the child has a consistent feeder and the family can assist with the assessment process and any interventions.

All of the factors mentioned previously need to be considered when assessing feeding in a hospitalized child with acute health issues. In addition, a number of specific parameters should be monitored during feeding assessments in any acutely unwell child.

State Control

Levels (states) of consciousness exist on a continuum (Box 14-7). Assessment of state should start by noting the child's state before, during, and after feeds. If at any point the child is not in an appropriate state for feeding, the feeding therapist should note if the child can be brought into an appropriate state (through calming or arousing techniques),

as well as what techniques are successful and how much assistance the child needed to maintain an appropriate state for feeding.

Stress Cues

Children may display stress in a number of different ways. Careful observation by the feeder is needed to notice and interpret these stress cues. Stress may be indicated by changes in state or attention (e.g., irritability, lethargy, fluctuations in state), motor patterns (e.g., change in tone, flexion, and extension patterns), and autonomic responses (e.g., respiratory and heart rate changes, color changes, sweating, sneezing, hiccoughing). See Box 14-8 for examples of stress cues.

Physiologic Control

Assessment of physiologic control during feeding should start by assessing **respiratory rate** and **heart rate** at baseline, during feeding, and after feeding. See Table 14-5 for normal physiologic parameters for children of various ages. Many hospitalized children have vital signs monitors in place (or available nearby), which makes observing parameters easy. However, the most basic method of measuring heart rate is to take the pulse at the neck or wrist, and the simplest way to measure respiratory rate is counting the child's breaths.

Particular attention must be paid to respiratory rate in infants who are breastfeeding or bottle feeding. Suckle feeds require the infant to coordinate sucking, swallowing, and breathing cycles that occur approximately once per second. If the infant's respiratory rate is more than 60 breaths per minute (i.e., more than once per second) the infant is unlikely to be able to suck and swallow between breaths without either occasionally suppressing

BOX 14-7 INFANT STATES OF CONSCIOUSNESS	
Asleep states	Sedated
	Quiet sleep
	Active sleep
Awake states	Drowsy
	Quiet alert
	Active alert
	Mild irritability, crying
	Extreme irritability

BOX 14-8 STRESS CUES		
State and Attention	**Motor**	**Autonomic**
• Irritability	• Motoric flaccidity	• Sighing, yawning
• Crying	• Motoric hypertonicity	• Sweating
• Silent crying	• Hyperextension	• Sneezing
• Frenzy, inconsolability	• Hyperflexion (tucking, fisting)	• Hiccups
• Rapid state changes	• Facial grimacing	• Startling
• Hypervigilance	• Frantic, diffuse activity	• Tremor
• Gaze aversion	• Frequent twitching	• Frequent or prolonged coughing
• Strained alertness		• Gagging, choking
		• Vomiting
		• Color changes, cyanosis
		• Respiratory pauses
		• Irregular respirations

From Kenner C, McGrath J (Eds): *Developmental Care of Newborns and Infants: A Guide for Health Professionals*, St Louise, 2010, Mosby.

TABLE 14-5 Normal Ranges for Heart Rate and Respiratory Rate (Vital Signs) in Children

	Newborn and Young Infants	Older Infants and Toddlers	Preschool Children	School Children	Adolescents
Respiratory rate (breaths per minute)	30 to 50 BPM	25 to 35 BPM	25 to 30 BPM	20 to 25 BPM	15 to 20 BPM
Heart rate (beats per minute)	110 to 160 BPM	110 to 160 BPM	110 to 160 BPM	80 to 120 BPM	60 to 100 BPM

BPM, Beats per minute.
Note: Brady = slow; tachy = fast (tachycardia = fast heart rate, tachypnea = fast respiratory rate; bradycardia = slow heart rate, bradypnea = slowed breathing).

breathing or inadvertently inhaling some of the feed during breaths.

Respiratory effort (work of breathing) should be evaluated before, during, and after feeding. Increased respiratory effort is indicated by retractions at the neck, trunk, or rib cage, chin tugging, grunting, or forced exhalation. The feeding therapist should also take note of any changes to the child's **sounds of respirations** during feeding. Abnormal respiratory sounds (e.g., stertor, stridor, wheeze, rales, cough) feeds may indicate airway obstruction or alteration in airway patency. In addition, the feeding therapist should observe for any changes in **respiratory pattern** during feeding (e.g., increased or decreased rate, cessation of breathing or apnea). Short respiratory pauses of less than 10 seconds are often normal, but longer periods (i.e., apnea events) or those associated with a loss of color (pallor), change of color (cyanosis), or slowed heart rate (bradycardia) are abnormal and potentially life threatening.

If **oxygen desaturation** is observed during feeding evaluation, the pattern of desaturation should be noted. Sudden dips below 95% may be associated with apnea or bradycardic episodes, whereas a gradual decline may indicate inadequate respiratory support for feeding. During feeding assessment without oximetry, attention should be focused on the child's color around the mouth and eyes. If cyanosis is noted, it is recommended that the child be fed with an oximeter in place. A lack of color change with feeding, however, does not necessarily imply that oxygen saturation is normal. Many children can have relatively low oxygen saturation without external evidence such as cyanosis.

Assessment of Feeding Interactions

The feeding observation should include an assessment of how the caregiver and infant work together as a team during feeding. Children who have experienced pain or discomfort with feeds may learn to dislike and avoid feeds and may also show aversion toward the caregiver as part of a classically conditioned response. Unfortunately, caregivers may unintentionally reinforce food refusal behaviors by giving in when the child protests.

Long periods of hospitalization and separation can affect the normal bonding process. Children who have been acutely unwell may not know how to interpret the feelings of hunger and fullness and may give mixed or unclear cues to their feeders, which can make the caregivers nervous or apprehensive about feeding the child. Parents of children who have been acutely unwell or who are medically complex are often stressed and fatigued, which can affect their coping mechanisms. Many of these children have prolonged mealtimes and need much support and encouragement to feed, which puts a lot of extra responsibility on already stressed caregivers.

ASSESSING CHILDREN IN THE COMMUNITY WITH CHRONIC HEALTH ISSUES OR DEVELOPMENTAL DELAY

In addition to factors considered as part of a standard feeding assessment, a number of issues must be considered when assessing children with chronic health issues or developmental delay. A summary of these issues follows.

Developmental Level and Potential

To perform a meaningful assessment, the feeding therapist needs to consider the child's age and developmental level. Young children are developing their feeding skills, so there are very different expectations for children at different ages. In addition, feeding is part of a larger developmental process. Interruptions to feeding development caused by illness or injury or general developmental delays in cognitive skills or in gross or fine motor skills all have the potential to affect feeding development and alter expected feeding skills.

Nature of the Condition (Stable, Resolving, Deteriorating, or Progressive)

Depending on the status of the child's underlying medical or developmental condition, the appropriate assessment and treatment plan may be quite different. For some children, the long-term goal is cure of dysphagia or age-appropriate feeding skills. For others the goal may be to achieve developmentally appropriate feeding skills (knowing they may not achieve age-appropriate skills) or to achieve functional feeding and swallowing skills with the use of modified food or fluids, special feeding equipment, or other compensations. For some children, the best goal may be to try to slow the decline in their feeding or swallowing skills, or to minimize the risk of aspiration or malnutrition by having small oral feeds and tube top-ups, or to have all feeds via a tube and have a nonoral stimulation program. For many children, feeding goals change at different points in their medical and developmental course. Regular assessment and reassessment is needed to set meaningful goals and to monitor outcomes against those goals. Either the intervention or the goals need to be changed if progress toward the goals is not being achieved.

Transition from Acute Care

Families of children who have spent a long time in the hospital often form strong relationships and trust with hospital staff who helped them though their child's acute illness. These staff members usually know the child's medical history well, often specialize in managing the child's condition, and have spent a long time in the child's company. Also, families get used to the high level of support and safety measures in place in a hospital environment. Thus it can be challenging for families when they then have to transition from the hospital environment to home.

Often different health care providers are involved in providing acute and hospital-based health care versus community-based services for children with chronic, subacute health issues or developmental delay. Ideally, a coordinated transition process needs to occur for patients who are transitioning from acute care to community-based services (or vice versa). For this to occur, staff members from both services should work together to help the family of the patient to assess the patient's current needs and set goals for this new stage in the child's care. In reality, this can be difficult to coordinate, but should always be encouraged.

Parent Involvement in Assessment and Treatment Planning

At home in the community, parents generally do not have the day-to-day assistance of health professionals to assist with feeding their child, as occurs in an inpatient facility. Thus it is especially important for parents to be involved in the goal-setting process and for them to be trained in how to implement therapy strategies themselves. Parents should also be taught how to monitor feeding outcomes so that they can determine if their child's progress is on track with goals or if further input from health professionals is required.

Social Aspects of Eating

Mealtimes are supposed to be social. For infants, more of their awake and interaction time is spent feeding and eating than on any other activity. Much of early parent-child bonding occurs at mealtimes, and children learn early turn-taking and a lot of other communication skills from mealtime interactions. For older children, many important family events (e.g., birthdays, holidays) are celebrated with meals. In addition, many friendship-building activities are based around sharing meals (e.g., play-dates, lunch-time discussions, social outings to restaurants). Thus assessment needs to take into consideration the effect the child's feeding difficulties have on his or her social participation in meals.

Burden on Family

Childhood feeding difficulties can be very stressful for families. In addition to long and difficult mealtimes, families often spend much time at appointments with health professionals. Not all community feeding services have the whole health care team on one site or as part of one practice or network, and often parents may have to go to several community health care providers for a full team approach. It is important for the various health professionals involved in the child's care to strive to communicate well with each other to minimize the chance of overlooking important issues or of different professionals giving parents contradictory advice.

Health care bills can cause considerable financial strain for families. In addition, loss of income because of frequent medical and therapy appointments can cause financial burden, as can loss of income when a parent is unable to return to work when paid caregivers (e.g., daycare staff) are unable to look after the child because of feeding difficulties. All of these factors need to be considered when assessing a patient and setting therapy goals. As mentioned earlier, it is essential that goals are meaningful for families and that outcome measures are collected to determine the effectiveness of intervention in achieving these goals.

ASSESSMENT CONSIDERATIONS FOR INFANTS

The following factors need to be considered when performing feeding assessments in infants, in addition to general assessment consideration detailed earlier.

Timing of Assessment

During the first few months of life, young infants rely on oral reflexes to assist them with feeding. These reflexes are affected by alertness and hunger and thus young infants generally feed when they are awake and hungry, but not at other times. Therefore feeding assessments need to be scheduled to coincide with feed and sleep times for this population. Older infants and toddlers can be hard to persuade to eat when they are not interested. Thus feeding assessments need to be scheduled to coincide with feed and sleep times for this population too.

Breastfeeding

Breastfeeding is a dual task for the infant and his or her mother. Certain issues, both maternal and infant, may challenge the establishment or maintenance of successful breastfeeding. Some women will decide not to breastfeed, whereas others may be unable to breastfeed. All mothers and babies should be supported by health professionals, regardless of their choice or ability to breastfeed.

Feeding success can be affected by infants' feeding skills, their attachment at the breast, and maternal milk supply. In cases in which feeding concerns arise in a breastfed infant, it is recommended that the feeding therapist work with a lactation consultant to ensure that assessment considers both infant and maternal factors, and that recommendations work for both mother and child.

At-risk groups for breastfeeding difficulties include:
- Children with cleft palate and other craniofacial conditions
- Children with severe pathologic conditions of the neurologic, cardiorespiratory, or gut systems
- Children with allergy, intolerance, or metabolic conditions

A number of breastfeeding assessment tools are available that assist in determining the effectiveness of a particular breastfeed. See Hill[9] for an overview and comparison. Some examples are the following:
- LATCH tool (Jensen et al.[10])
- Systematic Assessment of the Infant at the Breast (Shrago et al.[11])
- Infant Breastfeeding Assessment Tool (Mathews[12])

See Figure 14-3 for images of effective attachment during breastfeeding.

Bottle Feeding

Young infants are unable to feed themselves from a bottle. Thus bottle feeding must be seen as a joint task

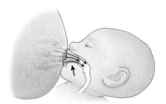 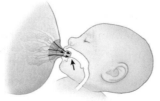

Good attachment   Poor attachment
FIGURE 14-3 Attachment for breastfeeding.

CLINICAL CORNER 14-1: INFANT CASE HISTORY

Ciara is a 3-month-old girl who presented to the hospital 3 days ago with stridor, shortness of breath, and barking cough. Her mother reported that she drank a total of 5 ounces of formula in the 24 hours prior to admission. She was found to be dehydrated and an intravenous line was placed to deliver fluids. She was tested for respiratory viruses, and has had a positive result for the respiratory syncytial virus (RSV). She has refused most bottles since admission to hospital. You have been requested to consult and assess her feeding skills.

Critical Thinking
1. Consider what additional information you should try to obtain from Ciara's medical chart and discussion with her nurse.
2. Determine what kind of information you should obtain from her mother.
3. Consider how her mother will be feeling when you meet her and how this will affect your interaction with her.
4. Think about how you should explain to Ciara's mother why respiratory illness may affect oral feeding.

between the feeder and the child. Certain feeder behaviors and strategies may affect how the infant feeds. These include the feeder's positioning and handling of the infant (e.g., whether appropriate head support is offered), equipment used (e.g., various bottles and nipples), as well as other things the feeder may do without necessarily thinking about it (e.g., rocking or patting the infant during feeds, making eye contact with the infant, jiggling the nipple in the infant's mouth). Thus assessment needs to include a judgment about both the infant's and feeder's skills. Many feeding therapists like to offer a bottle feed to the infant themselves so that they can observe the infant's skills in isolation from the feeder. Although this may provide useful clinical information, it is also important to observe a regular caregiver feeding the infant to see how the infant feeds at a regular feed and strategies used by the caregiver.

Bottle feeding assessments often involve a trial of different bottles and nipples. See Box 15-7 in Chapter 15 for a description of the main variables that differ between common bottle feeding equipment (see Clinical Corner 14-1).

ASSESSMENT CONSIDERATIONS FOR OLDER CHILDREN

The following factors need to be considered when performing feeding assessments in older children, in addition to general assessment considerations.

Developmental Level

In cases of developmental delay, a child's developmental level may be different from his or her chronological age, and this needs to be considered when planning assessment tasks and interpreting results.

Food Preferences

When performing a swallow assessment, it is important to realize that most children will refuse or struggle to eat a food (or drink a fluid) that is disliked or unfamiliar to them. Wherever possible, it is preferable to use familiar foods when assessing oral skills and swallowing ability.

Interest and Motivation

In general, a child's willingness to perform a requested task and his or her performance of the task can be affected by the child's level of interest and motivation to perform the task. Often a child can be encouraged to perform a task by using play (e.g., playing hide and seek with food and modeling "hiding" food in your mouth), competition (e.g., suggesting, "Let's see who can drink their milk the fastest!"), or by using reward for trying or finishing the task (e.g., providing verbal praise or use of object reinforcement, such as sticker or turn at a toy) (see Clinical Corner 14-2).

> **CLINICAL CORNER 14-2: CASE HISTORY IN AN OLDER CHILD**
>
> Patrick is a 7-year-old boy with cerebral palsy. He has been referred to the feeding and dietetic services at your center because of concerns regarding weight and volume of oral intake.
>
> **Critical Thinking**
> 1. Consider the type of information that you, as the feeding therapist, and the dietitian should collect.
> 2. Discuss the possible benefits and limitations of performing a joint-assessment session.
> 3. Without knowing anything else about Patrick, consider what kinds of foods and feeding utensils you should have available for the feeding assessment session.
> 4. List any other health professionals who may need to be involved in Patrick's care, and what their role would be.
> 5. Consider the possible effects (desirable and undesirable) of having multiple professions involved in the management of children with complex medical conditions.
> 6. How can some of the undesirable effects be addressed?
> 7. Discuss some of the factors that need to be considered when planning therapy with children of Patrick's age.

IMAGING STUDIES

Following clinical assessment, **imaging studies** (also known as *instrumental assessments*) provide important additional information that cannot be gathered from the clinical feeding evaluation alone. In particular, imaging studies are essential for evaluating pharyngeal and esophageal stages of swallowing, which cannot be directly viewed during a clinical examination. In addition, other imaging studies can provide information about the structure and function of the airway and gut that needs to be considered in feeding and swallowing management.

Note: Given that the imaging studies discussed in this section are described in detail in Chapter 10 of this text, this section focuses on the pediatric-specific issues that need to be considered when performing and interpreting these assessments.

Videofluoroscopic Swallow Study

A videofluoroscopic swallow study (VFSS; also known as *modified barium swallow [MBS]*) is a radiographic procedure that provides a dynamic view of the feeding mechanism during swallowing. Fluid and food samples need to contain barium to allow them to be visualized on the x-ray image. The VFSS is generally considered to be the "gold standard" for detecting laryngeal penetration and aspiration during swallowing. A radiologist and feeding therapist work together to plan and conduct the study.

Pediatric-Specific Issues Relating to VFSS Studies

Fluid and Food Samples

The types of fluid and food to be tested during the VFSS are based on the child's age and results of a clinical feeding evaluation. Standard barium test samples are available in the United States for thin, nectar-thick, honey-thick, and pudding-thick consistencies. Alternatively, powder or liquid barium can be mixed with thickening agents or food to create radioopaque test samples (note: if developing barium test samples, the feeding therapist must test that the samples match the desired thickness using some objective measure—see Box 15-3 in Chapter 15 for an example). It is important for barium test samples to be of the same thickness as fluids and foods that would be used in the child's diet; otherwise the VFSS test results will not be a reflection of how the child performs in reality when eating his or her regular diet.

It is standard practice during pediatric VFSS procedures to offer approximately 3 teaspoons of any solid consistencies and approximately three sips of any drinks that are offered via a cup.[13] For infants who drink from a bottle, 10- to 20-second samples of sucking are usually observed. Where there is concern that the child's feeding skills fluctuate or deteriorate over the duration of a bottle feed, **fatigue testing** is performed. During fatigue testing, fluoroscopy is turned off and the child is allowed to keep feeding for a time (often 5-10 minutes). Subsequently, fluoroscopy is turned back on and another 10- to 20-second sample is taken.[13]

Seating and Feeding Equipment

Developmentally appropriate seating and feeding equipment needs to be used during the VFSS. This depends on the child's age and physical skills and should be established ahead of the procedure during the clinical feeding evaluation. Any seating support needs to be radiotranslucent (i.e., should not contain any metal in the part of the seat that will be in the x-ray field) so that it does not obscure anatomic structures during the procedure. Often pediatric seats are positioned on top of the standard seat used for adult VFSS procedures and need to be secured safely. For children with severe physical impairments, a specialized wheelchair may need to be used.

Feeding equipment used during VFSS procedures should be reflective of what the child would usually use or have access to, otherwise the VFSS test results will not necessarily be a reflection of how the child would perform in reality when feeding at home.

Strategies That May Be Trialed during the Study

If the child displays laryngeal penetration or aspiration on regular fluids or food during the study, the feeding therapist may trial certain strategies during the procedure to see if they assist swallowing and airway protection. Many of the therapeutic strategies that are trialed with adults (e.g., super-supraglottic swallow) may not be achievable with young children who do not have the cognitive skills to understand or follow detailed instructions, or the self-awareness to voluntarily control movement of anatomic structures. Some therapeutic strategies may be elicited with positioning changes or modeling (e.g., chin tuck, head turn), but these may be difficult to implement in reality. Thus the most common interventions trialed during pediatric VFSS procedures include trials of modified fluids and food (i.e., trialing thickened fluids, different textures of solids) and trials of compensatory strategies, such as use of different feeding equipment (e.g., different nipples or cups) and implementation of specific feeding strategies (e.g., offering pacing or frequent breaks in feeding to catch breath).[13,14]

Breastfeeding Infants

It is not possible to assess an infant breastfeeding via VFSS because of logistical issues (i.e., it is not possible to position a breastfeeding infant in such a way that the swallowing structures can be easily viewed within the x-ray field, and because it is not possible to introduce barium to milk as it comes from the breast). Thus if aspiration is suspected in a breastfeeding infant, swallowing skills can only be assessed during a VFSS using a bottle. Where possible, the infant should be positioned similarly to the way he or she is positioned during breastfeeds. This may require changing the position of the C-arm from upright position used during most VFSS procedures to the traditional horizontal position used for gastrointestinal (GI) barium series, and feeding the child on his or her side, as this position may be closer to the position used for breastfeeding.

Compliance Issues

In general, children are not as compliant with testing procedures as adults. Some children are frightened by the radiology equipment and sight of hospital staff (particularly when the child has had painful and distressing procedures previously). Thus every effort needs to be made to maintain the child in a calm-alert state during testing. Toys may be needed to distract the child, and can also be used to capture the child's attention and motivate him or her to participate in required tasks. If possible, children should be fed by a familiar family member or caregiver.

Safety Concerns

Acceptable radiation exposure levels are set by the hospital Radiology Department and are controlled by the radiologist. It should be noted that acceptable radiation doses are much lower in children than in adults because of a number of factors. Specifically, children's developing organs are more susceptible to the effects of radiation than adults, and their head makes up a greater proportion of their total body size, resulting in a greater proportion of their body being in the x-ray field during swallow studies. The radiologist and feeding therapist work together to ensure that the VFSS is completed within the dosage limits for the child's age. Dosage amount is as low as reasonably achievable (ALARA), without affecting the accuracy of the swallowing assessment, as recommended by the International Commission on Radiological Protection.[15]

Strategies that can be used to reduce radiation exposure include reducing fluoroscopy time (most radiology departments limit pediatric VFSS to a maximum of 2 minutes of active fluoroscopy time), collimate the x-ray beam to the area of interest (i.e., limit the field to the pharynx and larynx), avoid the use of magnification (this increases the radiation dose), remove the antiscatter grid (this is generally not needed in children or other small patients), and consider using pulsed fluoroscopy (e.g., switching to 15 frames per second versus the 30 frames per second provided during continuous fluoroscopy) (see Practice Note 14-1).[16,17]

PRACTICE NOTE 14-1

The issue of acceptable pulse rate during VFSS procedures is controversial (see Bonilha et al.,[17] Cohen,[18] and Hiorns and Ryan[19] for different opinions on this issue). Each facility needs to make its own decision regarding acceptable pulse rate, weighing radiation dose against quality of the image. Many argue that, if the feeding therapist performing the procedure doesn't feel confident in his or her ability to visualize aspiration events during the procedure because of poor quality of the fluoroscopy image, then it would be better not to do the procedure at all and avoid exposing the patient to any radiation.

Adults in the fluoroscopy suite wear a lead apron to minimize their exposure to scattered radiation. Pregnant women are generally not permitted in the examining room during the study. This practice may affect which family member accompanies the child for the procedure.

Facilities and Access to Experienced Staff

Outside of major cities, many children are seen in facilities that care for both children and adults. If a VFSS is performed on a child at a facility that usually sees adult patients, clinicians must ensure that the room is set up appropriately, with appropriate seating and feeding equipment, as noted previously. In addition, staff may need to be familiarized with the pediatric VFSS procedure and how to interpret images of pediatric anatomy.

Following a VFSS procedure, an assessment report is generated by the feeding therapist and radiologist outlining the findings of the study. At minimum, the report should detail what materials were tested during the procedure, whether laryngeal penetration or aspiration was seen with each sample, and whether airway compromise was consistent or inconsistent with the samples tested. In addition, recommendations should be provided for which fluids and foods (if any) can be safely consumed, as well as whether any special feeding equipment or compensatory strategies are recommended to improve swallow safety and airway protection.

Two scales that can be useful to summarize information gained from VFSS and the functional implications of these findings are detailed in the following sections.

Penetration-Aspiration (PA) Scale

The eight-point "Penetration-Aspiration" (PA) scale was developed by Rosenbec et al.[20] to describe the degree of laryngeal penetration and aspiration seen, as well as the patient's response to the event (i.e., this is a measure of swallowing impairment) (Table 14-6). A PA score can be

TABLE 14-6 Penetration-Aspiration Scale

Score	Description
1	Material does not enter airway.
2	Material enters the airway, remains above the vocal folds, and is ejected from the airway.
3	Material enters the airway, remains above the vocal folds, and is not ejected from the airway.
4	Material enters the airway, contacts the vocal folds, and is ejected from the airway.
5	Material enters the airway, contacts the vocal folds, and is not ejected from the airway.
6	Material enters the airway, passes below the vocal folds, and is ejected into the larynx or out of the airway.
7	Material enters the airway, passes below the vocal folds, and is not ejected from the trachea despite effort.
8	Material enters the airway, passes below the vocal folds, and no effort is made to eject.

TABLE 14-7 Functional Oral Intake Scale (Original)

1	Nothing by mouth
2	Tube dependent, with minimal attempts at food, fluid
3	Tube dependent, with consistent intake of food, fluid
4	Total oral diet, of a single consistency
5	Total oral diet, with multiple consistencies, but requiring special preparation or compensations
6	Total oral diet, with multiple consistencies, without special preparation, but with specific food limitations or compensations
7	Total oral diet, with no restrictions

assigned to each swallow, or the worst PA score for each consistency trialed can be reported. This tool has been shown to have good reliability for use with infants and children.[21,22] It should be noted, however, that, although this scale may be useful in describing aspiration events, it is not a dysphagia severity scale. See Chapter 8 for further discussion of this scale.

Functional Oral Intake Scale (FOIS)

The original Functional Oral Intake Scale (FOIS) was developed by Crary et al.[23] to describe the degree of functional dietary limitation (i.e., swallowing disability) caused by a patient's swallowing impairment (Table 14-7). The original version of this scale was designed for use with adults but can also be used with children who would be expected to be on a full adult diet (i.e., those older than 2

TABLE 14-8 Functional Oral Intake Scale (Suckle Feeds and Transitional Feeds)

1	Nothing by mouth
2	Tube dependent, with minimal attempts at liquids, foods
3	Tube dependent, with consistent intake of liquids, foods
4	Total oral diet, but requiring special preparation of liquids (i.e., thickened liquids) +/– compensations (e.g., special feeding equipment, feeder uses special strategies)
4.5	*Total oral diet, but requiring special preparation of solids (e.g., liquid supplements or foods of different texture than those required by peers)* +/– compensations (e.g., special feeding equipment, feeder uses special strategies)
5	Total oral diet, without special preparation (i.e., regular thin fluids, *foods of same texture as peers, no additional liquid supplements*), but with compensations (e.g., special feeding equipment, feeder uses special strategies)
6	Total oral diet, with no restrictions relative to peers

Note: Italicized items only apply to children older than 6 months of age who would be expected to have solids in their diet.

years of age). Patients are scored between 1 (minimum) and 7 (maximum).

Recently, we have developed an adapted version of this tool for use with young children who are suckle feeding or in the transitional feeding period[24] (Table 14-8). Patients are scored between 1 (minimum) and 6 (maximum). This adapted scale has not been formally validated, but our clinical experiences indicate that it is appropriate for use with younger children and adds to the information obtained from the clinical evaluation.

Fiberoptic Endoscopic Examination of Swallowing

Fiberoptic endoscopic examination of swallowing (FEES) involves using a flexible fiberoptic endoscope to provide a direct, dynamic view of the feeding mechanism during feeding. The endoscope is passed transnasally and positioned within the pharynx. Fluid and food samples are usually dyed a nonbiological color (most often green) to allow them to be viewed more easily as they pass through the pharynx. In addition, this helps to detect material that has penetrated the airway or has been aspirated below the vocal folds.

Generally, an otorhinolaryngologist and a feeding therapist work together to perform a pediatric FEES procedure. Although FEES can provide useful information about swallowing function, it is used much less commonly than VFSS in children for a variety of reasons.

Pediatric-Specific Issues Relating to FEES Studies

Infants

Young infants are often described as "obligate nasal breathers." This is because (1) their anatomic configuration is such that their oral cavity is smaller and their tongue rests high in their mouth against their palate at rest, which makes oral breathing difficult; and (2) when suckle feeding, infants' lips form a seal around the breast or bottle, which they generally maintain for several minutes at a time during sucking bursts, thus precluding oral breathing during this time. Both of these factors result in infants primarily relying on their nasal airway during breathing.

Because the endoscope is passed through the nasal cavity during FEES, it precludes much of the infant's available pathway for respiration. This may cause additional work of breathing, which in turn can affect suck-swallow-breath coordination and swallow safety. Therefore it is possible that FEES may give a worse impression of the infant's ability to protect the airway than would be observed without a nasal tube in place.

Pediatric Anatomy

As mentioned previously, infant swallowing anatomy is configured somewhat differently from adults. Therefore if FEES is performed by staff who are more familiar with working with adult patients, some time may need to be spent familiarizing them with what to expect during a pediatric FEES procedure and how to interpret images of pediatric anatomy.

In general, it is harder to view the infant larynx via FEES because of its higher placement in the neck. In addition, the continuous sucking and swallowing pattern seen during breastfeeding and bottle feeding make visualization of the larynx (and hence detection of laryngeal penetration and aspiration) more difficult than in adult studies. Older children can be prompted to take discrete sips and swallows (or bites and swallows), which makes visually tracking the bolus easier.

Compliance Issues

As discussed previously, children are generally not as compliant with testing procedures as adults. Compliance is generally worse for FEES than VFSS, as the presence of the scope is irritating. Some children cry or struggle, which can make passing the endoscope and maintaining its position difficult. However, many children tolerate FEES with minimal fuss.

Safety Concerns

Unlike VFSS, FEES does not involve radiation exposure. Therefore the procedure doesn't have the same time restrictions occur during VFSS procedures. In addition, because barium does not have to be added to fluid and food samples, children can be assessed using real fluids and foods from their diet in an unaltered form, and assessment of breast-feeding is possible.

Sensory Testing

When performing FEES on adult patients, some clinicians incorporate laryngeal sensory testing by delivering an air puff via a third (working) channel on the laryngoscope.[13] Because of size restrictions in the pediatric airway, most pediatric-sized laryngoscopes only have the two basic channels (light source and fiberoptics for viewing the airway) and so do not allow air puffs to be delivered. Some clinicians will attempt to assess laryngeal sensitivity by tapping the scope to the laryngeal wall to test the laryngeal adductor reflex.[13] However, given that taps cannot be standardized the way air puffs can, any judgment based on this technique is subjective.

In addition to VFSS and FEES studies, which provide images of the swallowing process, a number of other instrumental assessments can provide useful information that needs to be considered by feeding therapists.

ENDOSCOPIES

An **upper-airway endoscopy** involves passing an endoscope through the nose or mouth into the pharynx or larynx for evaluation. Endoscopies are generally performed by an otorhinolaryngologist. This procedure can provide important information relating to swallowing, such as identifying structural impairments (e.g., laryngeal cleft) and detecting evidence of laryngeal changes from aspiration. The patient generally is given topical anesthetic for the procedure.

Bronchoscopy (or lower-airway examination) involves passing an endoscope through the upper airways into the lower airway for evaluation. Bronchoscopies are generally performed by a pulmonologist or otorhinolaryngologist. This procedure can provide important information relating to swallowing, such as identifying structural impairments (e.g., tracheoesophageal fistula), identifying the cause of increased respiratory effort (e.g., tracheomalacia), and detecting evidence of lung changes from aspiration. Because the endoscope is passed below the vocal folds, the patient is fully anaesthetized for the procedure. Therefore the examination cannot directly assess swallow function but can provide useful information about structures involved in breathing and swallowing.

An upper-gastrointestinal (GI) endoscopy involves passing an endoscope through the pharynx and into the gut for evaluation. GI endoscopies are generally performed by a gastroenterologist. This procedure can provide important information relating to swallowing, such as identifying structural impairments (e.g., esophageal strictures), and detecting evidence of esophageal changes

from reflux or allergies. Because the endoscope is passed through the upper esophageal sphincter, the patient is generally anaesthetized for the procedure. Therefore the examination cannot directly assess swallow function, but can provide useful information about structures involved in swallowing.

Manometry, Impedance, and pH Testing

Esophageal manometry measures peristalsis and bolus flow in the esophagus via a series of pressure transducers. Esophageal impedance measures bolus flow in the esophagus via a series of electrical transducers. pH probes detect the presence of acid in the esophagus. These studies are generally performed by a gastroenterologist. Manometry and impedance provide information about the esophageal phase of swallowing. pH probes and impedance can provide information about the presence of acidic and nonacidic reflux respectively. Although none of these studies directly assess the oral or pharyngeal swallow function, they can provide useful information about other aspects of swallowing function.

CERVICAL AUSCULTATION

Cervical auscultation (CA) involves placing a stethoscope or microphone on the outside of the larynx to listen for swallowing and breath sounds during eating and drinking.

Debate exists in the literature regarding the usefulness of CA for detecting aspiration,[25-29] mostly because of concerns regarding reliability and validity of swallow assessments based on auditory information alone. Currently, CA is seen by many as a tool that may augment a clinical feeding evaluation, providing amplification of clinical signs that are suggestive of possible aspiration (e.g., wet voice following swallow, throat clearing). However, sounds heard via CA may be affected by stethoscope or microphone placement, the nature of the bolus being swallowed (e.g., saliva, thin fluid, thickened fluid, pureed food, solid food), features of the individual's anatomy (e.g., size of larynx, presence of scar tissue, subcutaneous fat stores), and background sounds in the airway (e.g., stertor, stridor, wheeze, rales).[28,29] Thus information gathered from CA is only used as part of a clinical feeding evaluation and must be combined with visual information gathered at the time of assessment (e.g., observation of laryngeal elevation during swallowing, work of breathing, oxygen saturation levels on pulse oximetry). Where concerns exist regarding airway protection during swallowing, this should be confirmed with an imaging study, such as VFSS or FEES.

Aside from aspiration concerns, in pediatric practice, CA is used by many as a useful tool to provide information about suck-swallow-breath coordination during breastfeeding and bottle feeding.[30] Because sucking infants feed in bursts for an average of approximately 20 minutes per feed, versus taking discrete sips of drinks like adults do, much of the swallow assessment is focused on the infant's ability to coordinate the activities of sucking, swallowing, and breathing over the duration of a feed. Even if an infant doesn't aspirate during a feed, he or she is still considered to have swallow difficulties if swallowing was observed to adversely affect breathing patterns (e.g., decreased respiratory rate while feeding or apnea) or respiratory effort (e.g., increased work of breathing during feeds).

Because infants need to be positioned closely to the feeder during breastfeeds and bottle feeds, and because of their anatomic configuration (i.e., large stores of fat in face and neck, larynx positioned higher and more anteriorly than in adults), it can be hard for the feeding therapist to view external signs of movement of swallowing structures during feeds. Thus auditory information from CA can help augment the clinical feeding evaluation. Again, because of the subjective nature of swallow assessments based on auditory information, information gathered from CA should only be described as being "suggestive of possible aspiration" or "suggestive of poor suck-swallow-breath coordination." In cases in which concerns exist regarding airway protection during swallowing, this should be confirmed with an imaging study such as VFSS or FEES.

In reality, implementation of CA with infants and young children requires the use of either a stethoscope with a pediatric bell or a small microphone taped in place (e.g., lapel microphone). An advantage of using a microphone is that it can be plugged into an amplifier so that all in the room can hear the swallow and breath sounds live, or into a camera so that the sounds and image can be reviewed later. In contrast, only the user can hear sounds via a stethoscope, which makes interpretation more subjective and limits the ability for parents or other staff to use sounds from CA to guide therapy strategies, such as pacing.

See Appendix B on Evolve for an example of equipment used for pediatric CA.

TAKE HOME NOTES

1. It is important to remember that feeding therapists generally work as part of a team. A number of health professionals may be involved in the process of assessing and treating children with feeding difficulties.
2. Various models of teamwork may be used in feeding and swallowing teams during the assessment and treatment process. In general, the terms *multidisciplinary, interdisciplinary,* and *transdisciplinary* are used to describe various models.
3. It is important for a child with feeding or swallowing difficulties to undergo a thorough assessment.
4. The WHO's ICF model can be used to map the various areas that need to be considered when performing an assessment of a child's feeding and swallowing skills.
5. Case history information is usually collected in writing or verbally, and generally involves collecting information across multiple areas that may have the potential to affect feeding.
6. Areas typically assessed during routine clinical feeding and swallowing evaluation include examination of oral anatomy; observation of oral-motor skills during feeding, as well as observation of swallowing skills, airway protection, and physiologic stability during feeding; trials of modified food and fluids, different feeding equipment, or feeding strategies, as needed; and observation of child behavior and parent-child interaction during meals.
7. When observing a child feeding, the feeding therapist needs to make an assessment of the child's swallowing safety during mealtimes, as well as of the feeding competence.
8. Imaging studies are used to confirm or allay clinical suspicions of aspiration and guide management practices.
9. In addition to observing oral skills and swallowing, it is important for the feeding therapist to observe the child's mealtime behavior and, as possible, parent-child interaction during the meal.
10. One of the main objectives of a pediatric feeding assessment is to determine how much of a child's feeding issues are related to skill deficits versus learned behaviors that may or may not be reinforced by the family.

REFERENCES

1. World Health Organization: International Classification of Functioning, 2001. http://www.who.int/classifications/icf/icf_more/en/.
2. World Health Organization: *Fifty-fourth World Health Assembly,* 22 May 2001. (resolution WHA 54.21).
3. Weir K, McMahon S, Barry L, et al: Clinical signs and symptoms of oropharyngeal aspiration and dysphagia in children. *Eur Respir J* 33(3):604–611, 2009.
4. Weir KA, McMahon S, Taylor S, et al: Oropharyngeal aspiration and silent aspiration in children. *Chest* 140(3):589–597, 2011.
5. Thoyre SM, Carlson JR: Preterm infants' behavioural indicators of oxygen decline during bottle feeding. *J Adv Nurs* 43(6):631–641, 2003.
6. Benfer KA, Weir KA, Boyd RN: Clinimetrics of measures of oropharyngeal dysphagia for preschool children with cerebral palsy and neurodevelopmental disabilities: a systematic review. *Dev Med Child Neurol* 54(9):784–795, 2012.
7. Eyberg S, Bessmer J, Newcomb K, et al: *Dyadic Parent-Child Interaction Coding System—II: A Manual, in Social and Behavioural Sciences Documents,* 1994.
8. Kenner C, McGrath J (Eds): *Developmental Care of Newborns and Infants: A Guide for Health Professionals,* St Louise, 2010, Mosby.

9. Hill PD, Johnson TS: Assessment of breastfeeding and infant growth. *J Midwifery Womens Health* 52(6):571–578, 2007.

10. Jensen D, Wallace S, Kelsay P: LATCH: A breastfeeding charting system and documentation tool. *J Obstet Gynecol Neonatal Nurs* 23:27–32, 1994.

11. Shrago LC, Bocar DL: The infant's contribution to breastfeeding. *J Obstet Gynecol Neonatal Nurs* 19:209–215, 1990.

12. Matthews MK: Developing an instrument to assess infant breastfeeding behaviour in the early neonatal period. *Midwifery* 4:154–165, 1988.

13. Guidelines for Speech-Language Pathologists Performing Videofluoroscopic Swallowing Studies. ASHA Special Interest Division 13, Swallowing and Swallowing Disorders (Dysphagia), http://www.asha.org/policy/gl2004-00050.htm.

14. Arvedson JC, Lefton-Greif MA: *Pediatric Videofluoroscopic Swallow Studies: A Professional Manual With Caregiver Guidelines*, San Antonio, TX, 1998, Communication Skill Builders.

15. Willis CE, Slovis TL: The ALARA concept in pediatric CR and DR: dose reduction in pediatric radiographic exams—a white paper conference executive summary. *Pediatr Radiol* 34(Suppl 3):162–164, 2004.

16. Pediatric Dysphagia: Assessment. American Speech-Language-Hearing Association. http://www.asha.org/PRPSpecificTopic.aspx?folderid=8589934965&section=Assessment.

17. Bonilha HS, Humphries K, Blair J, et al: Radiation exposure time during MBSS: influence of swallowing impairment severity, medical diagnosis, clinician experience, and standardized protocol use. *Dysphagia* 28(1):77–85, 2013.

18. Cohen MD: Can we use pulsed fluoroscopy to decrease the radiation dose during videofluoroscopic feeding studies in children? *Clin Radiol* 64(1):70–73, 2009.

19. Hiorns MP, Ryan MM: Current practice in paediatric videofluoroscopy. *Pediatr Radiol* 36(9):911–919, 2006. [Epub 2006 Mar 22]; Review. PubMed PMID: 16552584.

20. Rosenbek JC, Robbins J, Roecker EV, et al: A Penetration-Aspiration Scale. *Dysphagia* 11:93–98, 1996.

21. Gosa M, Powers L, Temple C, et al: *Reliability of the Penetration-Aspiration Scale for Use with Infants and Young Children. Proceedings of the Dysphagia Research Society Meeting*, Vancouver, Canada, March, 2007.

22. Gosa M, Suiter D: *Reliability of the Penetration-Aspiration Scale for Use with Infants and Young Children. Proceedings of the Dysphagia Research Society Meeting*, San Antonio, March, 2011.

23. Crary MA, Mann GD, Groher ME: Initial psychometric assessment of a functional oral intake scale for dysphagia in stroke patients. *Arch Phys Med Rehabil* 86(8):1516–1520, 2005.

24. Crary MA, Dodrill P, Mann GD, et al: *A functional oral intake scale for dysphagia in infants and toddlers*, 2014.

25. Stroud AE, Lawrie BW, Wiles CM: Inter- and intra-rater reliability of cervical auscultation to detect aspiration in patients with dysphagia. *Clin Rehabil* 16(6):640–645, 2002.

26. Leslie P, Drinnan MJ, Finn P, et al: Reliability and validity of cervical auscultation: a controlled comparison using videofluoroscopy. *Dysphagia* 19(4):231–240, 2004.

27. Borr C, Hielscher-Fastabend M, Lücking A: Reliability and validity of cervical auscultation. *Dysphagia* 22(3):225–234, 2007.

28. Reynolds EW, Vice FL, Gewolb IH: Variability of swallow-associated sounds in adults and infants. *Dysphagia* 24(1):13–19, 2009.

29. Bergström L, Svensson P, Hartelius L: Cervical auscultation as an adjunct to the clinical swallow examination: a comparison with fibreoptic endoscopic evaluation of swallowing. *Int J Speech Lang Pathol* 16(5):517–528, 2014.

30. Comrie JD, Helm JM: Common feeding problems in the intensive care nursery: maturation, organization, evaluation, and management strategies. *Semin SpeechLang* 18(3):239–260, quiz 261, 1997.

CHAPTER 15

Treatment of Feeding and Swallowing Difficulties in Infants and Children

Pamela Dodrill

To view additional case videos and content, please visit the evolve website.

CHAPTER OVERVIEW

OBJECTIVES

1. Demonstrate an understanding of the importance of using assessment findings to guide therapy goals.
2. Describe the different models of service delivery.
3. Outline therapy strategies aimed at improving swallowing and airway protection (thickened fluids, modified foods, swallowing maneuvers).
4. Outline therapy strategies aimed at addressing feeding difficulties and mealtime behavior (oral sensory-motor [OSM] therapy, feeding utensils and equipment, mealtime positioning, behavioral feeding therapy, feeding therapy as part of nutritional supplement weaning).

5. Discuss therapy consideration for infants and for older children.
6. Detail factors that need to be considered when working with hospitalized children with acute health issues and with children living in the community.
7. List methods of measuring therapy outcomes.

SETTING THERAPY GOALS

Effective interventions for feeding and swallowing difficulties need to target the cause of the problem. For this reason, a thorough assessment is required to guide intervention.

Once the nature and any possible factors contributing to the feeding or swallowing difficulty have been established, the treatment plan can be developed.

See Table 14-2 in Chapter 14 for an overview of how the International Classification of Functioning, Disability, and Health model can be used to map the various areas for consideration during assessment and treatment planning for children with feeding and swallowing difficulties.

MODELS OF SERVICE DELIVERY

Different facilities and providers may use different models of service delivery when providing therapy services to children with feeding and swallowing difficulties. These differences may exist as a result of patient variables (e.g., severity of feeding or swallowing difficulty) or as a result of professional variables (e.g., staffing levels, staff experience or preference, limitations imposed by health insurance providers, historical factors at the facility) or as a result of a combination of these. In general, different models of service delivery for pediatric feeding and swallowing difficulties can be categorized according to the variables listed in Table 15-1.

Inpatient services are delivered while the child is an inpatient at a hospital. Often the child is admitted because of an acute health issue or for a medical or surgical procedure. Sometimes the child is admitted specifically because of feeding or swallowing difficulties.

Outpatient services occur when a child is living in the community. Services may take place at a hospital or clinic, or at the child's home or educational setting. The therapist may be at the same location as the child or may communicate with the child via telehealth.

Child-focused intervention involves the feeding therapist working directly with the child to improve swallowing and feeding function. A caregiver may be present, but the primary focus of the therapist's time is with the child. For young infants, therapy often involves the use of compensations (e.g., using modified fluids or foods or changing positioning, utensils, or feeder strategies). With older children, compensations may be used, but therapy often also incorporates skill-building activities to assist the child to gain or regain the skills necessary for independent feeding. Further discussion of specific therapy techniques is included in the following sections (see Practice Note 15-1).

Parent-focused intervention involves the feeding therapist working with a parent or caregiver to teach the caregiver how to work with the child to improve the child's swallowing and feeding function. The child may or may not be present, but the primary focus of the therapist's time is with the adult.

- Parent-focused intervention may involve the therapist providing the caregiver with general or individualized **information** (verbal or written educational material).
- Parent-focused intervention may also incorporate individualized **commentary** regarding the child's feeding performance and discussion of therapy strategies that do or do not assist the child. In some situations this can be done live (e.g., when watching the child via a one-way mirror or closed-circuit TV) or later (e.g., while watching a playback of a recording of the child).
- Parent-focused intervention may also involve providing the parent with opportunities to **practice** using therapy strategies with his or her child with guidance and feedback from the therapist, as needed. Again, this can be done live (e.g., via a microphone in the ear or baby monitor) or later (e.g., during a debriefing session, which may or may not involve watching a playback of a recorded interaction) (see Practice Note 15-2).

PRACTICE NOTE 15-1

A potential criticism of using a child-focused approach on its own is that there may not be generalization of therapy gains to other situations (i.e., that the child would not feed as well with others, either because others are not able to support the child the same way the therapist does or because the child becomes classically conditioned to feeding only when the therapist or certain environmental stimuli are present).

PRACTICE NOTE 15-2

A potential criticism of using a parent-focused approach is that a lot of parents find delivering therapy difficult or confronting ("You're the therapist, can't you just fix them?"). The primary goals of parent-focused intervention should be to improve parent understanding of the child's swallowing or feeding difficulties, and to improve his or her competence and confidence in assisting the child at mealtimes. In doing so, the parent becomes empowered to help address the child's needs.

TABLE 15-1 Models of Service Delivery

Location of services	Inpatient
	Outpatient
Primary recipient of input	Child
	Parent or caregiver
	Staff (e.g., hospital, daycare, school)
Numbers involved in sessions	Individual
	Group
Frequency of sessions	Weekly or intermittently
	Intensive
	Consult only

Staff-focused intervention involves the feeding therapist working with other health or educational staff (e.g., nurses, other therapists, daycare staff, school support staff). The primary focus of the therapist's time is with the adult (or group of adults). Staff-focused intervention usually involves the therapist providing either general information about feeding and swallowing intervention (verbal and written educational material) or information specific to a particular patient (e.g., verbal and written therapy recommendations). Staff-focused intervention may also involve participating in joint sessions with the patient to allow the feeding therapist to point out features of the child's feeding performance and to demonstrate therapy strategies that do or do not assist the child (see Practice Note 15-3).

Individual sessions involve the feeding therapists working one-on-one with the child (or the child's parent or another staff member). This type of input allows the therapist to directly observe the individual he or she is working with and provide immediate, specific feedback, changes, and reinforcement contingent on the individual's behavior. Individual therapy blocks may be offered as an outpatient service at a hospital or clinic, or at the child's home or educational setting. Individual sessions are the most time-intensive for the feeding therapist.

Group sessions involve the feeding therapists working with several children (or working with several parents or other staff members) (see Practice Note 15-4). Group

members benefit from input from the therapist, as well as other group members through social modeling and social reinforcement. Group therapy is often run in educational settings or may be offered as an outpatient service at a clinic.

Weekly or intermittent therapy blocks involve providing therapy sessions regularly over time (e.g., one session per week for 10 weeks). Weekly therapy blocks are usually offered as an outpatient service. Weekly therapy is often seen as the "standard" approach.[1] (see Practice Note 15-5).

Intensive therapy blocks involve providing frequent therapy sessions over a short period (e.g., two to three sessions per day for 1-2 weeks) (see Practice Note 15-6). Intensive blocks may be offered as part of an inpatient stay or as an outpatient service (e.g., with the patient staying near the clinic). These types of blocks may suit families who are traveling a long distance to receive therapy (i.e., those who live outside major cities or those who

---

PRACTICE NOTE 15-3

A potential criticism of staff-focused intervention from feeding therapists is that, once other staff are trained in therapy strategies, they may attempt to manage children with feeding difficulties without involving the feeding therapist. Moreover, other staff may overgeneralize therapy strategies to other children with different underlying issues and therapy needs. It is important to maintain working relationships with staff members from other professions to ensure that appropriate and timely referrals for feeding therapy services are made, when appropriate.

PRACTICE NOTE 15-4

Groups can be more time-efficient for the feeding therapist than individual sessions. However, for this form of intervention to be successful, the individuals have to be well matched so that the input is relevant to all. For children, this means matching based on age ranges and developmental level, as well as specifically considering types of feeding issues for those in the group. Safety issues, such as hygiene and the presence of food allergies and intolerances, need to be considered when children are sharing food.

PRACTICE NOTE 15-5

Families can sometimes lose interest if they don't perceive change happening fast enough. In addition, families may struggle to attend sessions if they have a lot of other commitments (e.g., other therapy sessions, medical appointments, parental work responsibilities). Weekly therapy should not run indefinitely. Blocks should be scheduled for a finite period, with specific goals and regular monitoring of progress. Some children require multiple blocks of therapy, and the goals need to be reviewed for each block to ensure they are relevant and meaningful for the child and family.

PRACTICE NOTE 15-6

It is important to consider that intensive blocks require a lot of therapist time during the block (often 3 hours or more per child per day). These time demands must be considered when scheduling multiple patients. If the child or therapist happens to get sick or injured, the entire block may need to be rescheduled (which can be difficult if the family has made travel and accommodation plans, and arranged time off work, school, etc.).

A potential criticism of intensive programs is that the child and parent don't get the opportunity to gradually incorporate therapy strategies at home. As a result, it is often argued that there may be poor maintenance of therapy gains and a high level of recidivism. Providing parent-focused education, commentary, and practice concurrent with child-focused intervention can help to address this issue and help facilitate carryover of gains made to the home environment. Phone, e-mail, or telehealth follow-up may assist where additional input is needed after attending the intensive block.

PRACTICE NOTE 15-7

Whenever providing information to a parent via a consult session, it is important to check the parent's understanding of information provided and to provide information in multiple formats to assist parents in understanding and retaining the key pieces of information. Ideally, information and advice should be given verbally and in writing (e.g., a report and handouts, or a report and home therapy package). Phone or e-mail follow-up may assist if additional input is needed, or another session may need to be scheduled.

specifically travel to a particular center to receive a specialist service) or those who want to see rapid change.

Consult-only intervention generally involves the feeding therapist providing information and advice over a single time point (or series of time points). Often the therapist assesses the child and consults with the parent in the same session (see Practice Note 15-7).

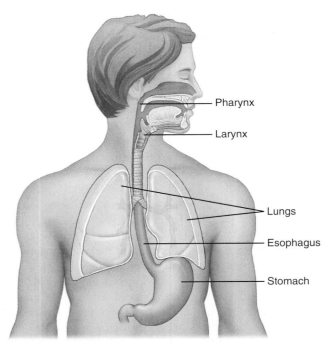

FIGURE 15-1 During normal swallowing, the bolus is transported through the pharynx and ends up in the gut.

THERAPY FOCUSED ON SWALLOWING AND AIRWAY PROTECTION

During normal swallowing, through a series of coordinated actions (detailed in previous chapters), the bolus is transported through the pharynx and ends up in the gut and not in the airway (Figure 15-1). Dysphagia occurs when there is a problem with bolus containment or propulsion, and may occur at the oral, pharyngeal, or esophageal phases of swallowing. Laryngeal penetration, aspiration, or choking may occur if there is insufficient airway protection during the swallowing process. Interruption to breathing or apnea may occur if there is excessive airway protection during the swallowing process.

INTERVENTIONS FOR SWALLOWING DIFFICULTIES

For children with **oral phase** swallowing problems, treatment generally involves working on improving the sensory and motor skills required for drinking and eating.[2] An outline of these interventions is provided later in this chapter.

For children with swallowing problems affecting the **pharyngeal phase,** treatment generally involves teaching the child to modify the swallowing strategy or for the feeder to modify the bolus.[2] A summary of interventions reported to be used with infants with poor suck-swallow-breath coordination and older children with poor swallowing

and breathing coordination are detailed in Tables 15-2 and 15-3.

Note: A few studies have reported these strategies to be effective in improving physiologic stability during feeds and improving volume of intake in preterm infants.[2] Further research is required to evaluate the effectiveness of treatment strategies in both infants and older children.

THICKENED FLUIDS

The use of thickened fluids is routinely recommended by health professions for two main pediatric populations: (1) children with swallowing problems (i.e., dysphagia), and (2) infants who display regurgitation. Note: Some families commence thickening infant feeds themselves (often with infant cereal) based on the belief that this will help the infant to settle and sleep better or may assist with weight gain. Hence if a family reports that the child has been on thickened fluids, the feeding therapist should ask why and who recommended that the child start thickened feeds before making any assumptions about swallowing skills.

Use of Thickened Fluid for Dysphagia

Children suspected of dysphagia should be assessed by a feeding therapist, who will perform a clinical feeding evaluation and possibly an imaging study. As previously discussed, the main aim of a swallowing assessment is to

TABLE 15-2 Summary of Interventions Reported for Infants with Poor Suck-Swallow-Breath Coordination

EVENT	Child can't control bolus	Child actively controls bolus	Feeder actively controls bolus
EVENT DETAILS	Aspiration Prolonged apnea	Gag or cough to clear bolus from airway Slower sucking Weaker sucking Stop sucking	The infant is positioned in a side-lying position or semiupright position to slow the flow of milk in the mouth. The feeder uses pacing, giving the child intermittent breaks from sucking. The mother expresses some breast milk to slow flow before offering breastfeed. Slow-flow nipple is used on bottle (or a nondrip nipple). Milk is thickened to slow flow.
POSSIBLE CONSEQUENCE	Lung damage Hypoxia	Child may not finish feed Reduced risk of lung damage or hypoxia	Feeds may take longer. Greater input is required from the feeder. Reduced risk of lung damage or hypoxia.

From Dodrill P: Infant feeding development and dysphagia. *J Gastroenterol Hepatol Res* 3(5) 2014. [Epub ahead of print].

TABLE 15-3 Summary of Interventions Reported for Older Children with Poor Swallow-Breath Coordination

EVENT	Child can't control bolus	Child actively controls bolus	Feeder actively controls bolus
EVENT DETAILS	Aspiration Choke	Gag or cough to clear Smaller sips or bites Increased chewing (oral motor exercises may be used to increase chewing strength, chewing speed, chewing effort) Improved sensory awareness (oral sensory exercises may be used to increase sensory awareness) Protective swallowing maneuvers (strategies such as chin tuck may be taught)	Fluids are offered via a straw or cut-out cup to minimize neck extension while drinking. Fluids are thickened to slow flow. Feeder offers softer or more processed food. Feeder offers smaller pieces of food. Feeder assists child and offers fluid and food at slower pace.
POSSIBLE CONSEQUENCE	Lung damage Hypoxia	Child may not finish meal Feeds may take longer Reduced risk of lung damage or hypoxia	Meals may take longer. Greater input is required from the feeder. Risk of lung damage or hypoxia is reduced.

From Dodrill P: Infant feeding development and dysphagia. *J Gastroenterol Hepatol Res* 3(5) 2014. [Epub ahead of print].

establish whether the child is able to maintain sufficient coordination of swallowing and breathing to allow safe oral intake. If a child demonstrates that he or she is not able to swallow regular (thin) liquids safely, then alternative means of hydration must be provided. Historically, this has been accomplished by either making liquids thicker (by adding a thickening agent) or by providing fluids directly into the stomach (e.g., via nasogastric tube or gastrostomy feeding). Thickening liquids is the less invasive method of these two options and so is generally the first option attempted. Other potential therapy strategies may also be trialed as alternatives (or adjuncts) to thickening fluids for children with poor airway protection during swallowing. These are described in a later section of this chapter.

The rationale behind thickening fluids for this population is to slow the rate of fluid flow, thereby allowing more time to close the airway prior to the swallow. In addition, thickened fluids "hold together" better than thin fluids so are easier to control in the mouth and are generally less likely to penetrate into the airway entrance before or during the swallow. However, it should be noted that the use of thickened fluids has been shown to result in increased pharyngeal residue,[5] which may potentially increase the risk of aspiration after the swallow.

The effectiveness of thickened fluids in preventing primary aspiration can be evaluated objectively during videofluoroscopic swallowing studies or empirically by a reduction of clinical symptoms. Depending on the severity of their dysphagia, children may require fluids to be thickened to different degrees to be able to swallow safely, without primary aspiration. Some children may not be able to swallow any consistencies of fluids safely and therefore require all fluids to be given via tube feeding.

Use of Thickened Feeds for Regurgitation

Infants suspected of demonstrating regurgitation of feeds should see a primary care provider or pediatrician as a first step, and may require referral to a gastroenterologist if concerns regarding acid reflux exist. In some cases, infants who regurgitate feeds will be commenced on thickened bottle feeds (either formula or expressed breast milk) as part of their medical treatment.

The rationale behind thickening bottle feeds for this population is that thickened feeds may be less likely to be regurgitated from the stomach back into the esophagus. The effectiveness of thickened bottle feeds in reducing regurgitation can be evaluated objectively using videofluoroscopy (i.e., barium swallow). However, effectiveness is usually rated subjectively, by parental report of reduction of symptoms of regurgitation (i.e., less vomiting, less irritability).

Thickening Fluids

As discussed, the goal of using thickened fluids in children is to assist in the safe swallowing of fluids or to reduce regurgitation of feeds, thereby optimizing nutritional status and preventing dehydration. Therefore it is important that thickened fluids are prepared correctly. If thickened fluids are too thin, they may not assist in managing the underlying problem (i.e., aspiration during swallowing or regurgitation). Conversely, if thickened fluids are too thick, they may cause additional problems (e.g., increased work of breathing, reduced intake resulting from fatigue).

Feeding therapists need to be aware that different types of fluid (milk, juice, etc.) can react differently with the same thickening agent and that different types of thickening agents can react differently with the same fluid (Box 15-1). Thus clinicians need to ascertain that the recipe being used makes the correct thickness. The goal is to avoid giving the child liquids that are more or less viscous than identified during assessment. In addition, caregivers should be educated to recognize clinical signs of fatigue and aspiration demonstrated during feeding (e.g., coughing, wet vocalizations, increased work of breathing), as these signs may indicate the need to adjust fluid thickness.

BOX 15-1 FACTORS AFFECTING THE THICKNESS OF THICKENED FLUIDS

The thickness of thickened fluids can be affected by:
- **Type of thickening agent:** Thickening agents used to thicken fluids for those with dysphagia are generally starch-based, gum-based, or a combination of starch- and gum-based. Thickeners are not all consistent in how they react to different types of fluids.
  - Smaller or larger amounts of different thickening agents may be required to produce the same level of thickness for a particular fluid.
  - Be aware that companies that manufacture thickening agents may change their recipes in their thickening products or may change the provided measuring utensil. These changes can affect the recipe you use for preparing thickened fluids.
- **Type of base fluid:** More or less thickening agent may be required when thickening different fluids (milk, juice, water, soda).
- **Amount of base fluid:** The relationship between amount of base fluid and amount of thickening agent may not be linear (e.g., the amount of thickening agent that needs to be added to thicken 1000 mL of a fluid may be more or less than 10 times the amount that needs to be added to thicken 100 mL).
- **Temperature:** Fluids generally get thicker when cooler and thinner when warmer.
- **Standing time:** Fluids generally get thicker with time.

From Gosa M, Dodrill P: Effects of time and temperature on thickened fluids. In *Proceedings of the American Speech Hearing Association Conference,* New Orleans, November 2009.

Thickened Infant Feeds

For bottle-fed infants, bottle feeds provide both nutrition and hydration. Bottle-fed infants should be able to suck the feed through a nipple on a bottle in 20 to 30 minutes. The amount of feed consumed must meet their nutritional and fluid requirements without expending excess energy. If a bottle-fed infant requires thickened fluids, he or she may need to be switched to a faster flowing nipple to accommodate the thicker fluid. In addition, the temperature of the bottle is important. Thickened bottle feeds are generally served warmed but will cool over the duration of a feed and will likely get thicker. If the feed is reheated, it may get somewhat thinner.

If a bottle-fed infant is on formula and is able to tolerate a standard cow's milk–based formula, he or she may be able to have a prethickened infant formula. These are generally sold as *antiregurgitation (AR)* formula. Be aware that some AR formulas are designed to be thick when prepared and others are designed to be thin when prepared and thicken

BOX 15-2 CAUTIONS REGARDING THE USE OF THICKENING AGENTS WITH INFANTS

The United Stated Food and Drug Administration issued cautions in 2011 and 2013 regarding the use of commercial, gum-based thickening agents with infants prior to term age. See

http://www.fda.gov/NewsEvents/newsroom/Press Announcements/ucm256253.htm.

The main concern was triggered by a series of preterm infants who developed necrotizing enterocolitis following the use of a particular thickening agent. At this stage it is unclear if the adverse events were caused by the thickening agent itself (a product made from xanthan gum) or from bacterial contamination in the product.

Feeding therapists should be aware of these cautions and should adhere to their facility guidelines for using thickening agents with infants.

---

in the stomach. If an infant requires thickened fluids because of a swallowing problem, the fluid must be thick when it is swallowed. Bottle-fed infants receiving expressed milk or a special (nonstandard) formula can have their feed hand-thickened with a thickening agent.

Which Thickening Agent to Use?

Thickening agents used for children with dysphagia should be labeled as suitable for use with patients with dysphagia and suitable for use with children (Box 15-2). In addition, the packaging should contain clear instructions on how much thickening agent is required to prepare fluids that are consistent with the levels set out in national diet standards or to thicken infant bottle feeds.

In addition to feeding therapists, dietetic, pharmacy, and medical staff should be involved in deciding which types of thickening agents are suitable for use with children. Feeding therapists need to be aware that some thickening agents may contain allergens and take particular care if a child has an allergy or intolerance to corn, wheat, or gluten (as these are common ingredients in thickening agents), or if the child has eosinophilic esophagitis (these children often need to remove all grains from their diet). Feeding therapists also need to be aware that most suppliers of thickening agents do not recommend the use of their products with infants prior to term age (i.e., preterm neonates) or if the child has been diagnosed with certain pathologic conditions of the gut. This is because some thickening agents may not be digested by the premature or damaged gut, and may possibly cause gut complications. To be cautious, some facilities do not allow thickening agents to be used with infants aged less than 12 months, and some manufacturing companies do not recommend their thickening product be used with any children younger than 3 years of age (see Practice Note 15-8).

PRACTICE NOTE 15-8

Given concerns regarding the safety of using some commercial thickening agents with infants, many therapists have turned to using infant cereal (e.g., rice, oat) to thicken infant feeds. Prior to using these materials to thicken infant feeds, a number of precautions must be considered.

Thickness

A variety of companies make a number of infant cereal products, and no standard recipes are available for making thickened fluids with the various cereal products. Thus it remains unclear what volume of different cereals is required to be added to breast milk or formula to make the "standard" thickness levels (e.g., AR thick, nectar-thick, honey-thick). Many facilities have developed their own recipes but, anecdotally, much variation exists across facilities. In addition, infant cereals are not manufactured for the purpose of thickening fluids and tend to separate from the fluid with time. If an infant requires thickened fluids because of a swallowing problem, he or she will need the fluid to remain thick throughout the feed.

Energy Content

Unlike most commercial thickening agents, infant cereal adds significantly to the energy content of the feed.

Standard formula and breast milk: Average energy content = 67 Kcal/100 mL (20 cal/oz)

Rice and oat cereal: Average energy content = 4 Kcal/g, 5 Kcal/tsp (teaspoon = 5mL)

Average infant energy requirements = 100 Kcal/kg/day (50 Kcal/lb/day)

Average infant formula and breast milk requirements = 150 mL/kg/day (2.5 oz/lb/day)

Energy Calculations

- Adding 1 teaspoon of cereal to 1 oz of breast milk or formula increases the energy content of each oz from 20 to 25 Kcal (25% increase). Adding 3 teaspoons (1 US tablespoon) of cereal to 1 oz of formula increases the energy content from 20 to 35 Kcal (75% increase).
- If an infant is on 30 oz of breast milk or formula per day, adding 3 teaspoons of cereal per ounce of fluid adds 450 Kcal per day (increasing energy intake from 600 Kcal to 1050 Kcal). In some cases, this can cause excess weight gain.

Allergy Risk

It should be noted that rice and oat cereals are technically "food." It is generally not recommended to introduce foods into an infant's diet until the child is at least 4 months (more than 16 weeks) old because of allergy risk from early exposure to potential allergens. In addition to rice and oats, many infant cereals contain soy and wheat, all of which are potential allergens.

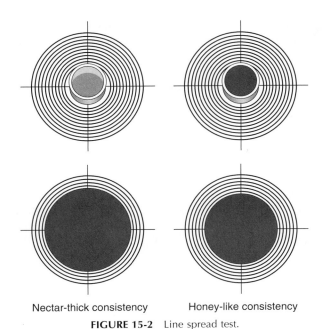

Nectar-thick consistency   Honey-like consistency

FIGURE 15-2 Line spread test.

Testing the Thickness of Thickened Fluids

It is important that feeding therapists test the thickness of thickened fluids (and liquid barium used in videofluoroscopic swallow studies) to ascertain the appropriate level of thickness. Tests will need to be repeated if the manufacturers change their products in any way.

A number of methods are available to test the thickness of fluids. Viscometers provide the most accurate and reliable measurements,[4,5] but the costs and training required to use them make them unavailable to most clinical settings. The most reliable method available in most clinical facilities is the line spread test (LST)[6] (Figure 15-2). Information on how to interpret LST values is detailed in Box 15-3 and Table 15-4. Although it has its limitations, the LST is more reliable than other clinical methods used for judging the thickness of fluids, such as by eye, with a fork, or by mouth feel.[5]

ALTERNATIVES TO THICKENING FLUIDS

Given some of the potential issues regarding the use of thickened fluids (as detailed previously), many therapists and families are keen to try other approaches to avoid or reduce the need to thicken fluids for children with swallowing impairments. These approaches include changes to positioning, use of special feeding equipment, and active pacing. The goal of these strategies is to slow the fluid flow during feeding or to interrupt the feeding process intermittently to allow the child to regain physiologic stability.

BOX 15-3   LINE SPREAD TEST MEASUREMENTS

Methodology as per Mann and Wong[7]:
- Use LST with 1-cm concentric circles.
- Place LST on flat surface with Perspex/Plexiglass sheet over the top.
- Place pipe with 2.5-cm radius/5-cm diameter on top of center of LST.
- Prepare 200 mL of thickened liquid, as per instructions.
- Place 50 mL thickened liquid into pipe or tube at center of LST.
- Lift pipe and allow liquid to spread for 1 minute.
- Measure spread of liquid on north, south, east, and west radius axes of LST. Estimate spread to the nearest 0.5 cm.
- Take the mean of the four radius measurements (i.e., total/4).
- Repeat measurement three times for each sample.
- Clean Perspex/Plexiglass between each test using water and a soft cloth. Do not use detergent. Dry surface well.

LST, Line spread test.

TABLE 15-4 Expected Spread of 50 mL of Various Fluids on Line Spread Teat

Thickened Fluids	Radius (Mean)
Extremely thick (pudding)	2.2 cm
Moderately thick (honey)	3.2 cm
Mildly thick (nectar)	4.2 cm
Infant thick (AR)	6.0 cm
Infant formula	9.7 cm

AR, Antiregurgitation.

Positioning

Because of the effects of gravity, fluids flow faster vertically than horizontally.

- Positioning an infant in a more **upright position** versus a reclined supine position can slow the flow of feeds. In this position, the milk flow is horizontal versus vertical.
- During bottle feeding, the feeder can position the infant in an upright position by adjusting the position of his or her arm, or by having the infant sit in a supportive chair for feeds.
- During breastfeeds, this can be achieved by having the mother recline so that the infant is positioned above her, or by having the infant sitting upright on her lap.
- Positioning an infant in a **side-lying position** versus a supine position may also slow the flow of feeds. Again, in this position, the milk flow is horizontal versus

vertical. This position also makes it easier for excess milk to dribble out of the side of the infant's mouth (versus having to be swallowed).

- Most mothers will naturally place a child in side-lying for breastfeeds.
- It can be harder to get infants in this position during bottle feeds. Infants may need to be positioned along the length of their feeder's lap or on a pillow placed on the feeder's lap (with the infant facing the feeder to allow the feeder to monitor the infant).
- If an infant is unable to tolerate handling, he or she can be placed in a side-lying position in the crib for feeds. The bottle may need to be angled slightly upward to prevent air from entering the nipple and causing wind (alternatively, an angled bottle may be used, or a bottle with a one-way valve that keeps milk in the nipple).
- For older children, encouraging a **chin-tuck position** for airway protection and **avoiding neck extension** while drinking can slow the flow of drinks. Older children can often be taught these strategies, but younger children often need assistance, as well as the use of special feeding equipment.

Feeding Equipment

Different feeding equipment can be used to slow the flow of fluids.
- For infants, the use of **slow-flow** nipples (i.e., nipples with smaller or fewer holes) and **nondrip** nipples (i.e., nipples that do not deliver milk flow without active compression) can assist in managing fluid flow.
- For older children, use of **straws** or **cut-out cups** can assist the child to drink fluid without having to tip the head backward (creating neck extension and reducing airway protection), as often occurs when drinking from an open cup, spout cut, or pop-top bottle.

Pacing

Pacing involves imposing breaks during feeding and drinking to interrupt the flow of fluid.
- For infants, the feeder may actively impose breaks to allow the child to swallow and catch his or her breath.
- During breastfeeds, this can be achieved by having the mother pull her breast away or insert her finger in the side of the infant's mouth to break the seal on the breast intermittently.
- During bottle feeding, the feeder can tip the bottle to stop milk flow or remove the nipple from the child's mouth intermittently.
- Pacing can be done based on **infant cues** (e.g., when the child needs to take a breath or starts to show stress cues) or on a **schedule** (e.g., every three sucks).
- For older children, the feeder may prompt the child to take a break from drinking by using verbal cues (e.g.,

"stop, take a breath") or by manually controlling the cup. Some older children can be taught to pace drinking themselves.

SWALLOWING MANEUVERS

As noted in Chapter 14, many of the therapeutic strategies used with adults with swallowing impairment (e.g., super-supraglottic swallow) may not be possible with young children. Children do not have the cognitive skills to understand or follow detailed instructions or the self-awareness to voluntarily control movement of anatomic structures. With children, some therapeutic strategies may be possible to elicit with positioning changes or modeling (e.g., chin tuck, head turn), but in reality these may be difficult to implement.

MODIFIED FOODS

By 2 to 3 years of age, most children have the oral skills to eat most solid foods (see Chapter 12). However, developmental delay and neurologic impairment can result in some children requiring modified food textures beyond this age. Depending on the degree of impairment or delay, different levels of food modification may be required. Documents outlining the various levels of food modification (i.e., **dysphagia diets**) exist in most countries. See the following websites for examples:

> http://www.asha.org/SLP/clinical/dysphagia/Dysphagia -Diets/
> http://www.speechpathologyaustralia.org.au/resources/ terminology-for-modified-foods-and-fluids
> http://www.thenacc.co.uk/assets/downloads/170/Food %20Descriptors%20for%20Industry%20Final%20 -%20USE.pdf

Additional precautions regarding swallowing safety exist for children regardless of their oral skills. These concerns exist because of **developing motor skills** (e.g., self-feeding skills, coordination when walking and running) and **developing cognitive ability** (e.g., visual perception, attention, risk assessment) in children (see Chapter 12). Furthermore, children have smaller airways, which, in addition to the factors mentioned previously, predispose them to choking risk. See Box 15-4 for information on choking risk in children.

THERAPY FOCUSED ON FEEDING DIFFICULTIES AND MEALTIME BEHAVIOR

One of the main purposes of an assessment is to guide intervention. It is therefore vital during assessment to establish whether the child's feeding difficulties are caused by a skill deficit, learned behavior, or both.

BOX 15-4 CHOKING RISK IN CHILDREN

Young children often put pieces of food that are too big into their mouth or try to swallow pieces of food that have not been thoroughly chewed. In addition, if children are playing or running while eating, they are prone to getting distracted. In either case, gagging or choking may occur. **Gagging and choking are not the same thing.** Gagging is usually noisy. Choking is usually silent—and very dangerous!

Gagging occasionally on foods is normal in young infants. Gagging is a reflex that pushes objects from the back of the throat to the front of the mouth. Gagging helps to stop objects from blocking the airway and is usually noisy (i.e., the child will often vocalize, splutter, or cough). Gagging on food is the infant's way of getting rid of a piece of food that is too big to swallow. Sometimes gagging will also occur if a child is too full.

Choking is not normal during meals and is potentially life threatening. Choking occurs when food gets stuck in the airway. A child who is choking will struggle to breathe and usually be unable to make any noise with his or her voice. **If a child looks like he or she is choking, he or she needs help immediately.**

Call emergency services if a child is choking (dial 9-1-1 in the United States) and follow their directions.

In general:
- Check the child's mouth to see if there is anything visibly blocking the airway.
- Sit down and position the child facedown across your lap. The child's head needs to be below his or her chest.
- Use the heel of your hand to give a firm blow to the back between the child's shoulder blades.
- Check the mouth again to see if anything has dislodged.
- Continue for up to five firm blows to the back, checking each time to see if the obstruction has been dislodged.

- If the obstruction is dislodged but the child is still not breathing, position the child on his or her back and perform cardiopulmonary resuscitation (CPR).
- Do not leave the child until help has arrived or he or she has fully recovered.

For more information about managing choking or performing CPR see:

Infant younger than 1: http://www.nlm.nih.gov/ medlineplus/ency/article/000048.htm

Child older than 1 or adult: http://www.nlm.nih.gov/ medlineplus/ency/article/000049.htm

Minimize Choking Risk
- Always supervise young children while they are eating.
- Infants need to be in an appropriate baby seat while eating. Older children should sit down while eating. Slumping over or moving around while eating food increases the risk of choking.
- Avoid distractions while eating, such as watching the TV.
- Avoid access to foods that could block a child's airway, such as the following:
  - Hard candy
  - Nuts
  - Popcorn
  - Corn chips
  - Chewy pieces of meat
  - Hot dogs (remove the skin and cut them into small pieces)
  - Whole grapes (cut them in half)
  - Raw carrot, apple, celery (grate or cook these foods if offering them)
  - Any hard food that can break off into pieces

Intervention aimed at improving mealtime behavior is unlikely to be effective unless the underlying cause of the feeding difficulty (i.e., pain or discomfort with feeding, skill deficit) is addressed.

ORAL SENSORY-MOTOR THERAPY

OSM therapy is a broad term, encompassing many different therapy techniques aimed at improving the functioning of the structures involved in the skills of eating (and speaking). Feeding therapists are often taught the basic principles of OSM therapy as part of their training programs. However, feeding therapists need to be aware of the range of new OSM therapy texts, equipment resources, and therapy programs that become available each year.

The basic premise of most OSM therapy programs is to modify the child's current oral motor skills and sensory processing ability in relation to eating and drinking. A series of therapy exercises is applied to move the children from their current functional level toward the intended outcome of intervention.

Although OSM is commonly used in clinical practice, only a few small, randomized controlled trials (RCTs) have evaluated the effectiveness of OSM techniques. These were specifically focused on preterm infants.[8,9] A recent Cochrane systematic review investigating the use of OSM techniques in children with neurologic impairments[10] determined there is currently insufficient high-quality evidence to provide conclusive results about the effectiveness of any particular type of therapy technique for older children. Thus further research is required to evaluate OSM treatment strategies in children of different ages.

A number of commercial OSM programs are available (including, but not limited to the MORE program, the Beckman protocol, and the Talk Tools approach). To date, none of these programs have been compared with other programs or a control protocol (i.e., not receiving any intervention) in a clinical trial. However, many pediatric therapists use these programs and believe them to help their patients. In the absence of research data, clinicians need to use their own knowledge and experience to guide practice, and should be scientific in their approach (Box 15-5).

A common criticism of OSM therapy is that performing sensory and motor exercises in isolation rarely leads to functional changes in feeding or swallow skills. These criticisms can be addressed by setting functional goals and recording outcome measures (Box 15-6) (see Practice Note 15-9).

FEEDING UTENSILS AND EQUIPMENT

A variety of feeding utensils and equipment are available commercially and via specialty therapy suppliers. Common **feeding utensils** include spoons, forks, knives, chopsticks,

---

BOX 15-5 PRINCIPLES OF SCIENTIFIC THERAPY PRACTICE

- Set specific and measurable goals for the patient (ideally, goals should be functional).
- Determine which specific therapy techniques to use to assist in achieving goals, based on best available evidence (this may be clinical experience, if no published studies exist).
- Implement the therapy techniques.
- Monitor relevant outcomes.
- Modify therapy techniques as necessary to achieve goals.

BOX 15-6 OVERVIEW OF ORAL SENSORY-MOTOR THERAPY

Common Aims of OSM Therapy
Main Aim
- To achieve an individual's maximal functional capacity for feeding (and speech)

Target Areas
- Oral structures (lips, tongue, cheeks, jaw, palate)
- Neck, chest, posture, respiration

Common Overall Goals of OSM Therapy
Depending on the individual, goals may be to achieve:
- Skills appropriate to age
- Skills appropriate to level of development or physical capacity
  At different times during therapy specific goals may be to:
- Acquire new skills
- Develop existing skills
- "Normalize" skills the individual already demonstrates

Examples of Goals for a Child Undergoing OSM Therapy
- Appropriate levels of arousal and preparation for oral-motor tasks
- Increased or decreased oral sensitivity to touch, taste, and temperature
- Increased awareness of oral structures and movements
- Coordinated oral movement sequences

Examples of Individual Impairment-Focused Goals for OSM Therapy
- Increased or decreased oral muscle tone
- Increased or decreased range of movement of oral structures
- Increased oral muscle strength
- Increased rate of movement of oral structures

- Increased precision of oral movements
- Facilitating appropriate oral reflexes, integrating or inhibiting any abnormal oral reflexes
- Establishing functional oral movement patterns by guiding or facilitating oral movements

Individual Functional (Activity or Participation) Goals for OSM Therapy
- Improved oral sensory integration for feeding (acceptance of new or different tastes)
- Improved oral motor skills for feeding (sucking, chewing, biting)
- Safe swallowing
- Improved saliva control
- Facilitate transition from nonoral to oral feeding
- Improve mealtime participation

Specific OSM Therapy Techniques
- Utilizing equipment (purpose-specific equipment or adapting nonspecific equipment)
- Using taught therapy exercises and strategies
- Prompting (tactile, visual, auditory)
- Reinforcement (verbal praise, object reinforcement)
- Games to make the task more appealing to children

Features Essential to the Success of OSM Therapy
- Individualized program
- Graded tasks
- Direct hands-on intervention
- Repetitive practice
- Intensive short-term therapy blocks
- Only forms part of an overall therapy plan
- Skills targeted during OSM therapy must be necessary and relevant to functional activities important to the individual's life
  See Appendix D for examples of oral toys.

PRACTICE NOTE 15-9

A common goal of feeding therapy is for a child to transition from pureed and mashed foods onto solid food pieces. Pureed and mashed foods can be masticated using a forward-backward tongue pattern, as is used during suckling. However, to sufficiently masticate firmer, solid pieces, the tongue has to move sideways (tongue lateralization) to transport the food pieces onto the chewing surfaces and hold them there to be broken down before being swallowed. If a child tries to swallow solid food pieces without chewing them, the child will often gag and may choke.

To encourage tongue lateralization, a range of OSM techniques may be used. A series of step-wise therapy tasks follow:

- Present stick-shaped oral toy (then a stick-shaped teething cracker and stick-shaped pieces of food) to the child's lateral chewing surface (use flavorful food or dip oral toy in a flavor to encourage tongue movement toward stimulus).
- Prompt the child to hold stick-shaped oral toy, teething cracker, or food between side teeth to encourage tongue movement toward stimulus (model desired behavior if required or encourage the child to look at himself or herself in the mirror).
- Prompt the child to chew on stick-shaped oral toy, teething cracker, or food to encourage tongue support to hold the stimulus on the chewing surface (model if required).
- Present a piece of solid food to child's side teeth in a food net and prompt the child to chew the food (model if required).
- Present a piece of solid food to child's side teeth and prompt the child to chew the food (model if required).
- Hand the child a piece of solid food, prompt him or her to put it in the mouth, then use the child's finger to move it onto the side teeth for chewing (model or provide a mirror if required).
- Hand the child a piece of solid food, prompt him or her to put it in the mouth, then use the child's tongue to move it onto the side teeth for chewing (model or provide a mirror if required).

The ultimate goal in this case is for the child to be able to independently use tongue lateralization effectively while eating solid food pieces, and to safely swallow these foods. Thus all earlier steps in therapy should progress toward this skill.

cups, bowls, and plates. In addition, a variety of **special feeding equipment** exists, such as teething toys and other oral stimulation toys (e.g., pacifiers, teething rings, gum brushes, vibrating oral toys, food nets), as well as mouth toys aimed at improving strength and coordination of oral structures (e.g., tubing for chewing, bite blocks, tongue depressors, oral blow toys). Feeding therapists often incorporate these utensils and equipment into their therapy sessions or provide advice to parents about their use. See Appendixs A, C-F for examples of feeding utensils and equipment.

Bottle Feeding Equipment

In addition to the other feeding equipment mentioned previously, feeding therapists spend much time providing advice about **artificial bottle nipples** for infants who are bottle fed. When going into any grocery store, drug store, or baby shop, parents are confronted with numerous options (often taking up an entire aisle of the store) and various claims to superiority. In reality, many infants can accommodate different types of nipples. Those who can't, or who struggle with feeds in any way (e.g., difficulty finishing feeds, concerns regarding swallow safety during feeds), should have a feeding assessment and receive individualized advice regarding the type of nipple to use. See Box 15-7 for an outline of different nipple types and factors that need to be considered when recommending nipples.

Breastfeeding Equipment

Accredited lactation consultants, midwives, and maternity and child health nurses generally provide specialist advice and assistance to mothers who are having difficulty with breastfeeding. However, all pediatric feeding therapists should have an awareness of common breastfeeding issues and commonly used equipment, such as those detailed in Box 15-8.

See Practice Note 15-10 for a discussion of the use of pacifiers with infants.

MEALTIME POSITIONING

As discussed in Chapter 12, postural support is important during feeding, as control of the trunk and neck is needed to support skills involved in sucking, chewing, and biting. An optimal feeding position is characterized by orientation around midline, neutral anterior-posterior alignment of the head and neck, neutral alignment of the trunk, and flexed hips and knees. Infants and young children all need some degree of postural support to achieve an appropriate position for feeding. Some children (particularly those with altered muscle tone) will continue to require postural support during mealtimes beyond the infancy-toddler period.

For **infants** who are having breastfeeds or bottle feeds, postural support during feeding is provided by the feeder's arm and trunk. Some infants benefit from the extra support given when swaddled (i.e., when the infant is

BOX 15-7 OVERVIEW OF ISSUES TO CONSIDER WHEN CHOOSING ARTIFICIAL NIPPLES FOR BOTTLE FEEDING

A "standard" nipple for bottle feeding is a straight nipple, with a round hole at its tip. They are generally made from silicone. Hole sizes usually come in small, medium, and large (or the nipple may have one, two, or three small holes). Standard nipples deliver an unrestricted milk flow (i.e., they drip even if the infant isn't sucking).

Variations in nipple design include:

- Shape of the nipple (e.g., orthodontic or wide necked)
- Length of the nipple (e.g., short or long)
- Pliability of the nipple (e.g., latex vs. silicone, soft cleft palate nipples, stretchable or "peristaltic" nipples)
- Flow rate (e.g., variable flow, where the same nipple can be turned to create a different flow rate)
- Flow type (e.g., restricted flow or nondrip, where fluid only flows when the nipple is compressed. These nipples are often labeled *x-cut* or *y-cut*)
- Pressure release valves (e.g., one-way valves/tube or air release holes)

It is important to consider both the infant's sucking and swallowing skills when deciding which nipple to use for bottle feeds.

- Nipples that deliver large volumes of milk quickly and easily may assist in compensating for weak sucking skills; however, they may produce a bolus that is too large to be swallowed safely.
- Nipples that require the infant to suck very hard or frequently to draw milk may cause the infant to become fatigued quickly. This can affect the volume consumed and can also affect suck-swallow-breath coordination and swallow safety.

Other factors to consider when choosing a nipple for bottle feeds include:

- Structure of child's mouth (e.g., cleft lip or palate, high arched palate, tongue-tie)
- Size of the infant's mouth (e.g., micrognathia, premature infant)
- Oral reflexes (e.g., increased gag reflex, reduced suck reflex)
- Oral motor skills (e.g., bunched tongue movements, tongue thrust, weak lip seal, weak tongue and cheek movements)
- Respiratory control (e.g., increased respiratory rate)
- Endurance (e.g., cardiorespiratory problems leading to early fatigue)
- Other (e.g., gastroesophageal reflux, infants on limited oral intake)
- Financial (e.g., cost of nipple, access to replacement parts, ability to use other nipples with same bottle)

Outcomes to consider when comparing bottle nipples include:

- Volume taken during bottle feed (mL or oz)
- Duration of bottle feed (minutes)
- Rate of bottle feed intake (mL per minute or oz per minute)
- Incidence of physiologic abnormalities during bottle feeds (e.g., apnea, bradycardia, or tachycardia)
- Number of breaks needed during bottle feeds
- Infant fussing or refusal behaviors during feeds
- Number of bottle feeds taken per day
- Time taken to transition from first oral bottle feed to exclusive oral feeding

---

wrapped in a blanket). See Appendix G for images of various infant feeding positions.

For **older children,** postural support during feeding is generally provided by the chair. Most children benefit from **back support** during meals. Most children also benefit from being seated in a chair that allows their **feet to reach the floor** or a foot-plate attached to their chair (or a stool placed under their feet if no other option is available). Stable foot contact helps children stabilize themselves in their chair. Some children require **side support** in the form of armrests or side cushioning to help them keep their trunk in the midline. Some children also require **head support** to help them keep their head in the midline. In addition, some older children continue to require a **support harness** or **seat belt** or for their chair to be reclined (**tilted in space**) to help them stay upright and not slump over while eating.

When performing a seating evaluation, it is important to consider the effect of the child's position on his or her oral skills and swallow safety, as well as the effect of his or her position on the ability to bring the hands to the mouth for self-feeding (Figure 15-3).[17] Also, see Appendix H for examples of feeding chairs.

Occupational therapists and physical therapists have specialized knowledge and skills to assess individual seating requirements and to make recommendations to meet positioning needs. Referral to a pediatric occupational therapist or physical therapist is recommended whenever concerns exist regarding positioning for meals or self-feeding.

BEHAVIORAL FEEDING THERAPY

The primary goals of feeding therapy are to **increase desirable mealtime behavior** and **decrease undesirable mealtime behavior.** Table 15-5 provides examples of behaviors generally considered to be "desirable" or "undesirable."

Other goals of behavioral feeding therapy generally include:

- Improving adequacy of dietary intake from food versus supplements (i.e., total energy intake, macronutrient and micronutrient intake)

BOX 15-8 COMMON BREASTFEEDING EQUIPMENT

Breast pumps are used to assist with expressing milk from the breast. Electronic pumps are generally easy to use and can typically be set to different expression rates and strength. Manual pumps are more portable than electronic pumps but require more effort for the mother during pumping. With all pumps, milk is expressed into a bottle for storage. Regular pumping can assist with maintaining milk supply even if the infant isn't feeding at the breast.

Breast shields are sometimes used when an infant is having difficulty attaching or staying attached at the breast for feeds. Breast shields are generally made of clear silicone and fit over the mother's nipple and areola.

Line feeders can be used to supplement breast feeds. They consist of a fine tube (similar to a nasogastric [NG] tube) that is attached to a bottle filled with milk. The tube is placed along the mother's nipple and the infant is held to the breast. When the infant is suckling, he or she receives additional milk from the tube. At the same time, the stimulation from the infant's suckling can help stimulate additional maternal milk supply. Flow rate from the line feeder can be altered by altering the position of the bottle (lower position leads to slower flow).

Finger feeders can also be used to supplement breast feeds. They consist of a fine tube (similar to an NG tube) that is attached to a bottle that is filled with milk. The tube is placed along a caregiver's finger and the infant is encouraged to suckle. Finger feeders are generally used when a mother is unable to breastfeed (e.g., because of pain caused by mastitis or cracked nipples) but does not want her child to receive feeds from an artificial nipple.

Cup feeders are an alternative way to supplement breastfeeds. They are generally used when a mother is unable to breastfeed but does not want her child to receive feeds from an artificial nipple (or does not have access to artificial nipples or the ability to clean and store them safely). Custom-made cup feeders are available commercially, but often a regular cup is used. Close attention must be paid to the flow of milk coming out of the cup, so as not to flood the infant's mouth. A Cochrane review[11] concluded that cup feeding cannot be routinely recommended over bottle feeding as a supplement to breastfeeding because it confers no significant benefit in maintaining breastfeeding beyond hospital discharge and carries the consequence of a longer stay in hospital.

PRACTICE NOTE 15-10

Pacifiers (also known as *dummies* and *soothers*) are commonly provided to infants to assist with self-calming. Some infants habitually suckle their thumb or fingers, others prefer pacifiers, and some infants prefer neither.

Use of pacifiers in breastfed infants: International guidelines for the promotion of breastfeeding recommend avoiding the use of pacifiers with infants while establishing breastfeeding,[12] especially in the first 6 weeks of life. Arguments against pacifier use include the observation that infant pacifier use may make it hard for the mother to identify cues for hunger, indicating the need to feed the infant,[12] as well as the possibility that the infant may develop a preference for the firm artificial nipple on the pacifier over the breast (this is sometimes referred to as "nipple confusion").[12] However, a Cochrane review concluded that pacifier use in healthy breastfeeding infants had no significant effect on the proportion of infants exclusively or partially breastfed at 3 or 4 months of age.[13]

Use of pacifiers in infants receiving tube feeds: A Cochrane review concluded that the use of pacifiers in preterm infants receiving tube feeds has been shown to assist with transition from tube to bottle feeds and significantly decrease the length of hospital stay in this population.[14] No negative outcomes were reported in any studies completed to date. Providing a pacifier during tube feeding may help to establish the link between suckling and the feeling of fullness and satiation. Providing a pacifier before a scheduled feed can help an infant learning to feed by mouth to get into the appropriate state for feeding and organize suckling skills in preparation for the feed.[15]

Use of pacifiers in older children: Consensus among health professionals is that pacifiers should not be used beyond the age when children use suckling and sucking to obtain nutrition (i.e., infants generally take breastfeeds or bottle feeds for the first 1-2 years of life and should not use a pacifier beyond this time). As children get older, they develop teeth and begin to talk. Available information suggests that prolonged use of pacifiers is associated with increased incidence of otitis media and can affect dental alignment.[16] As children get older, they should not continue to rely on oral stimulation for calming and should develop more sophisticated emotion regulation strategies, such as using words and language skills to talk about their feelings, express desires, and negotiate outcomes.

- Improving dietary variety (i.e., number of foods consumed, percentage of total intake derived from each of the core food groups—fruit and vegetable, proteins, grains)
- Maintaining or improving growth (i.e., weight for height/ body mass index [BMI] within healthy range)

- Reducing parent stress (i.e., overall stress and mealtime-specific stress)

When planning a behavioral feeding therapy program, it is important to set goals that are **achievable** for the child from a feeding tolerance and feeding skill perspective. In particular, feeding therapists need to consider whether the child is

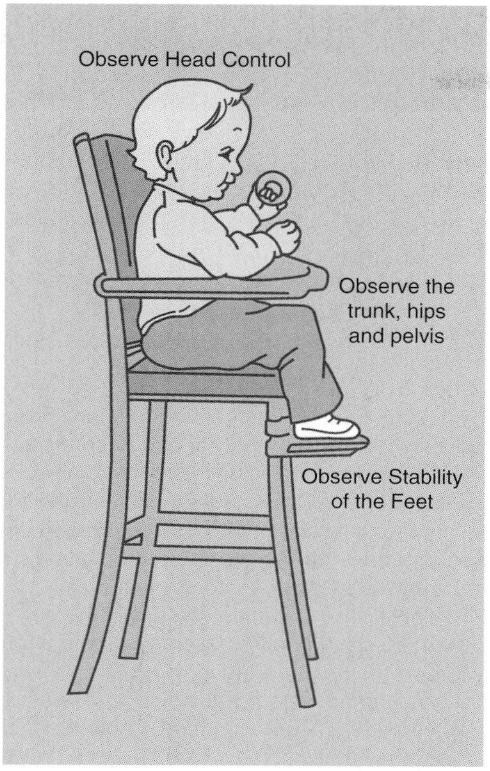

Observe Head Control

Observe the trunk, hips and pelvis

Observe Stability of the Feet

FIGURE 15-3 Seating considerations. (From Mahan LK, Raymond J, Escott-Stump S: Krauses's Food & Nutrition Therapy, ed. 12, Saunders, St. Louis, 2008).

> **BOX 15-9** COMMON BEHAVIORAL FEEDING THERAPY APPROACHES
>
> **Operant conditioning** is designed to improve feeding difficulties and increase oral intake through specific prompted food goals (i.e., externally driven, top-down approach) and a reinforcement system (i.e., operant conditioning, also known as "prompt-and-reward therapy").
>
> **Systematic desensitization** is designed to improve feeding difficulties and increase oral intake by exposing children to a range of foods in play-based activities, which become gradually more challenging (i.e., a bottom-up approach). This approach encourages the child to learn to regulate his or her own intake (i.e., intake is internally driven).

TABLE 15-5 Examples of Desirable and Undesirable Mealtime Behaviors

Desirable Mealtime Behaviors	Undesirable Mealtime Behaviors
Accepting foods offered	Refusing foods offered
Eating an acceptable volume of food	Verbal protest (e.g., "No," "I don't like it," "I don't want to," "I don't eat peas," "I want custard instead.")
Eating an acceptable variety of food types	
Eating an acceptable variety of food textures	Physical protest (e.g., head turning, hand-batting, throwing food, tantrums, staring out window)
Completing meals in an acceptable amount of time	
Staying seated at the dining table for meals	Escape from table
Interacting socially with others involved in the meal	Withdrawal or refusal (as detailed previously)

Note: The definition of *acceptable* varies depending on factors such as the child's age, developmental level, feeding skills, presence of medical issues, culture, and family expectations. These should be assessed and discussed with the family prior to starting therapy.

currently experiencing acute health issues, acute nutritional issues, or has swallowing issues that have not been addressed. If so, it is probably not the right time to move forward with a behavioral feeding program. Addressing these other issues is a higher priority. It is unlikely that any degree of prompting or reinforcement will be able to encourage a child to eat if he or she is in pain, uncomfortable, nauseated, or not hungry, or if the child doesn't have the physical skills to swallow safely the foods and fluids that are offered. For children who have oral motor delays or sensory issues, behavioral feeding therapy either needs to focus on food textures that the child can currently manage or incorporate OSM activities to work on oral skills while also working on behavior.

In general, two main approaches to behavioral feeding therapy been advocated: operant conditioning and systematic desensitization. Both are common forms of behavior management that are widely used across various areas of psychology. See Box 15-9 for an overview.

When planning any behavioral feeding therapy program, it is important for the therapist and parent to discuss the approach that will be used to ensure that the approach fits with the family's expectations and parenting style. In addition, it is important to remember that children generally learn best with **routine** and **predictability.** Thus it is important for the therapist and parent to have a clear plan regarding the therapy approach and strategies that will be used as part of the child's therapy block.

When using any approach based on **behavior management,** it is important for feeding therapists to have a thorough understanding of the key concepts underlying these interventions and correct use of terminology. Many people (including some health professionals) use behavior management terms loosely or incorrectly. This can result in behavior management strategies being used incorrectly or inconsistently as well. See Boxes 15-10 and 15-11 and

---

BOX 15-10 REINFORCEMENT AND PUNISHMENT

Reinforcement is any response to a behavior that causes an *increase* in the probability of that behavior reoccurring in the future.

Positive reinforcement involves responding to a behavior by *adding a desirable stimulus* to increase the probability of that behavior reoccurring in the future.

Negative reinforcement involves responding to a behavior by *removing an undesirable stimulus* to increase the probability of that behavior reoccurring in the future.

Punishment is any consequence following a behavior that causes a *decrease* in the probability of that behavior reoccurring in the future.

Positive punishment involves responding to a behavior by *adding an undesirable stimulus* to decrease the probability of that behavior reoccurring in the future.

Negative punishment involves responding to a behavior by *removing a desirable stimulus* to decrease the probability of that behavior reoccurring in the future.

BOX 15-11 OVERVIEW OF ADDITIONAL BEHAVIOR MANAGEMENT STRATEGIES OFTEN USED IN FEEDING THERAPY

Fading: Initially, when encouraging a new behavior, **prompts** are often used each time the feeding therapist wants the child to perform the desired task (e.g., saying "take a bite" or modeling desired behavior). Ideally, prompts should be gradually reduced (faded) until the child can perform the desired task without prompting.

Thinning: Initially, when encouraging a new behavior, the feeding therapist often provides **reinforcement,** used each time the child performs the desired task (e.g., taking a bite). Ideally, reinforcement should be gradually reduced (thinned) until the child can perform the desired task without reinforcement.

Shaping: While working toward a new behavior, the feeding therapist will often reward successive approximations toward the desired behavior. This is referred to as *shaping.* Examples include:

- Starting with a modified version of the goal food, then offering gradually closer approximations toward the goal food (e.g., apple juice > apple sauce > apple crisp > apple slice, *or* French fry > potato wedge > baked potato > boiled potato)
- Starting with small bites, and gradually increasing the size of bites
- Starting by feeding the child, then moving to loading the spoon or fork for the child and presenting it to the child to feed himself or herself, then to expecting the child to load the spoon or fork and feed himself or herself
- Starting by having the child look at a new food, then having the child touch it (then smell it, touch it to his or her lips, lick it, bite it, chew it, swallow it, etc.)

Table 15-6 for an overview of common therapy terms and techniques.

Both operant conditioning and systematic desensitization are forms of behavior modification. However, the two approaches use somewhat different strategies to reach the therapy goals. A recent RCT found both approaches can be effective in addressing feeding difficulties and expanding oral intake in young children when performed in a structured manner by trained and experienced therapists.[18] An overview of the general feature of both approaches is detailed in Table 15-7.

Many feeding therapists attend specialist training to learn how to apply behavior modification techniques to feeding therapy (e.g., the SOS Approach to Feeding workshops, by Toomey et al.[19,20]). Some feeding therapists prefer to work alongside other health professionals specifically trained in this area (e.g., behavior modification therapists, developmental psychologists) when working with children with behavioral feeding issues.

FEEDING THERAPY AS PART OF NUTRITIONAL SUPPLEMENT WEANING

Thanks to advances in medical treatment, an increasing number of medically complex children are surviving infancy and childhood. Many of these children require some period of nutritional supplementation via the oral route or via tube feeding to meet their nutritional requirements. Unfortunately, even once acute medical and nutritional needs are addressed, many children refuse regular oral feeds (or sometimes any oral feeds) and remain dependent on prolonged nutritional supplementation (Figure 15-4). These children generally require assistance from a feeding therapist. Unnecessary reliance on supplementation can hinder a child from developing age-appropriate feeding skills, prevent participation in social activities, and cause considerable family stress and financial burden.

Reason for Commencing Nutritional Supplementation

The population of children who require nutritional supplementation (via the oral route or tube feeding) have varied and complex underlying medical issues. Some children require nutritional supplementation because they

TABLE 15-6 Overview of Basic Behavior Management Strategies Often Used in Feeding Therapy

Antecedent (strategies used to encourage child)	Verbal prompt (e.g., "Sam, take a bite.")
	Visual prompt (e.g., modeling, cue cards, visual scheduling)
	Physical prompt (e.g., spoonful of food presented)
Behavior (child's behavior)	Desirable response (e.g., child takes a bite)
	Undesirable response (e.g., child turns head and squeals)
Consequence (adult's responses to child's behavior)	Positive reinforcement: Verbal reinforcement (e.g., "good eating," "nice bite") Object reinforcement (e.g., providing turn at a toy or game) Spontaneous social reinforcement (smile, cheer, visual attention)
	Negative reinforcement: Escape (e.g., "You can leave the table now you have finished.") Countdown (e.g., "Yay! Only three more bites to go!")
	Positive punishment: Preventing escape (e.g., "You have to stay at the table for 5 more minutes because you spat that out.") Verbal redirect (e.g., "Stop. Food goes on the plate, not the floor.")
	Negative punishment: Withholding attention (e.g., ignoring the child's behavior, putting the child in "time-out") Withholding reward (e.g., "You're not getting dessert now because you didn't eat your peas.")

TABLE 15-7 Operant Conditioning and Systematic Desensitization Approaches to Feeding

	Operant Conditioning	Systematic Desensitization
Antecedent prompt	Verbal prompt Visual prompt Physical prompts	Modeling
Consequence for desirable behavior	Spontaneous social reinforcement Specific verbal reinforcement Object reinforcement	Spontaneous social reinforcement
Consequence for undesirable behavior	Preventing escape Verbal redirect Withholding attention Withholding reward	Withholding attention Verbal redirect, if needed
Primary outcome measures	Volume consumed Reduction of undesirable behaviors	Variety (number) of foods consumed Level of interaction with food
Size of group	Usually individual, as it is difficult to provide contingent reinforcement to multiple children at once	May be individual, often group—extra participants add to the amount of modeling and spontaneous social reinforcement to which the child is exposed

form an aversion to food after illness. Some children are put on nutritional supplementation because they cannot eat efficiently enough to meet all of their nutritional requirements from an oral diet. Others are put on nutritional supplementation via tube feeds because they cannot swallow safely. Before nutritional supplementation can be stopped (and, if applicable, the tube is removed), the underlying medical condition (and any associated skill deficits and behavioral issues) needs to be managed or resolved.

Feeding Difficulties in Children Who Are on Nutritional Supplementation

Some children are not able to eat efficiently or safely when they start nutritional supplementation; hence a feeding tube is inserted. Others are able to eat well when they start nutritional supplementation but, by virtue of a lack of eating practice or the presence of a feeding tube (or associated issues, such as feed schedules that prevent the child from

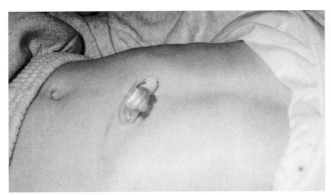

FIGURE 15-4 Child with skin-level gastrostomy device. (From Hockenberry MJ, Wilson D: *Wong's essential of pediatric nursing*, ed 9, St Louis, 2013, Mosby.)

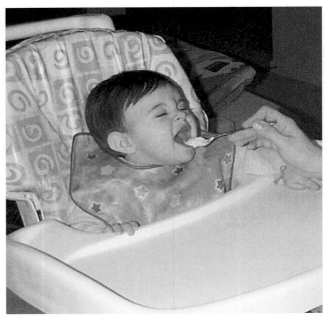

FIGURE 15-5 In addition to standard feeding assessment considerations, there are additional factors that need to be considered for infants. (From Mahan LK, Escott-Stump S, Raymond JL: *Krause's food and the nutrition care process*, ed 13, St Louis, 2012, Saunders.)

feeling hungry or full), they do not progress or may actually regress in their eating skills.

Prerequisites for Regular Oral Feeding

For a child to be able to meet all nutritional and energy needs by mouth, he or she needs to have the skills to eat and drink efficiently and safely. The child also needs to overcome any fear or anxiety regarding food or eating. For a child to have the appetite to eat, he or she first needs to be able to tolerate bolus feeds so that he or she can experience a fullness and hunger cycle. Subsequently, the volume of supplemental feeds should be reduced to induce hunger and allow the child the opportunity to want to eat. This is usually done by reducing the supplemental feed before a meal, although some children may need to miss two or three supplemental feeds to feel hungry enough to eat. It is important that supplement weaning is only done under the supervision of a physician and dietitian. These professionals need to monitor whether the child is still getting sufficient fluid, nutrients, and energy to meet basic requirements.

Often children transition from supplemental feeds on to easy-to-eat foods, such as pureed foods and drinks (Figure 15-5). For children to be able to eat a developmentally appropriate diet, including a wide variety of foods of various textures, they need to have appropriate oral skills (biting, chewing, drinking) and pharyngeal skills (swallowing). This often requires ongoing therapy after the initial supplement weaning. Therapy is usually provided by a feeding therapist.

Therapy Considerations for Children Who Are Ready to Wean from Nutritional Supplements

Whenever a parent is considering bringing a child to a therapy program, he or she should try to find out details about the type of intervention used at the clinic before pursuing therapy. Many feeding clinics use different approaches to assist children who rely on nutritional supplements to transition to regular oral feeds. In addition, clinics set different goals for patients during therapy and use different measures of therapy success. Feeding therapists involved in providing feeding therapy as part of a nutritional supplement weaning program (often referred to as a *tube weaning program*) should be able to provide parents with answers to the questions presented in Box 15-12.

THERAPY CONSIDERATION FOR INFANTS

Breastfeeding

As discussed in previous sections, during breastfeeding, both maternal milk supply and infant feeding and swallowing abilities can influence the infant's feeding performance.

Unless feeding therapists have undergone additional training specifically in breastfeeding management, it is suggested that they work alongside an accredited lactation consultant when working with infants who breastfeed and are displaying signs of swallowing or feeding difficulties.

BOX 15-12 QUESTIONS TO ASSIST DECISION MAKING REGARDING NUTRITIONAL SUPPLEMENT WEANING PROGRAMS

Is the program an inpatient or outpatient program?

How long is the program? How many sessions will the child receive? How frequently are sessions run?

Are there any criteria that would stop some children from being eligible for the program?

Which professions are involved in assessing and providing intervention?

How will any skill-based issues affecting feeding (e.g., sensory or motor problems affecting chewing, biting, drink etc.) be assessed and managed?

How will any fear or anxiety ("behavioral") issues affecting feeding (e.g., reluctance to try new foods) be assessed and managed?

How will the volume of supplement feeds be dropped to encourage appetite for eating?

Does the clinic use appetite stimulants (e.g., antihistamines, corticosteroids), and how are these used?

What will happen if supplement feeds are stopped and the child doesn't eat (i.e., how long will the child be allowed to go without fluids or feeds before a decision is made to top-up the child with supplement feeds)?

What therapy techniques are used to prompt the child to eat (e.g., modeling, verbal instructions, physical prompt, nonremoval of the spoon)?

What therapy techniques are used to reward desirable eating behavior (e.g., praise, turn at toy, reward chart)?

What therapy techniques are used to discourage undesirable eating behavior (e.g., ignoring, verbal instruction, removal of a toy, escape extinction)?

What role do parents play in sessions (i.e., are they in the therapy room, are they feeding the child, are they providing praise for good eating)?

Are parents provided with training about how to implement the therapy program at home?

How is success measured? (See the following.)

Nutrition outcomes:
- Is the goal for the child to no longer require any supplemental feeds? Or is it okay if the child has fewer supplement feeds?
- If child has some nutritional supplements given orally, is that considered okay? Or is it a goal for the child to be taking all energy and nutrition from food?
- If the child eats a narrow range of foods, is that considered okay? Or is it a goal for the child to eat a wide range of foods (e.g., fruit, vegetables, meat, dairy, and other proteins)?

Growth outcomes:
- Is it a goal for the child to maintain (or not lose) weight? Or is it a goal for the child to gain weight? Or is it a goal for the child to display appropriate weight for height and body mass index?

Developmental outcomes:
- If the child is just eating pureed foods, is that okay? Or is it a goal for the child to be eating developmentally appropriate textures?
- Is it a goal for the child to be self-feeding?
- Is it a goal for mealtimes to be of an appropriate length (not too long) and fuss-free?

How long are patients followed up after treatment?

What happens if the patient doesn't maintain gains made after treatment?

Is any outcome data from other patients available?

How much does the program cost (assessments, therapy, any hospital costs, accommodation)?

Where is the program run?

For overseas or interstate programs, what expectations will exist for local health professionals on the child's return home?

How will information about the child's treatment be shared with other members of the child's health care team?

Whenever breastfeeding is compromised, the breastfeeding management priorities are as follows[12]:

1. Feed the baby according to need (this may mean providing tube feeds or bottle feeds if breastfeeding is not possible; if available, expressed breast milk should be offered before formula).

2. Where possible, try to protect the mother's milk supply (this usually involves the mother regularly expressing breast milk, and may involve using medications to increase breast milk supply).

3. Address the issue (this may involve working on the infant's feeding skills or addressing maternal milk restrictions or other health issues in the mother or infant).

4. Where appropriate, try to reestablish breastfeeding.

Health professionals have a responsibility to offer information and education to assist mothers to make informed choices about breastfeeding. Specifically:

- Mothers should be offered information regarding the benefits of breastfeeding, the risks of not breastfeeding, and safe alternatives in their situation.
- Women who are considering a change from breastfeeding need to be aware of the difficulties associated with reversing their decision and reestablishing breastfeeding should they again change their mind.
- Mothers should be supported by health professionals regardless of whether they decide (or are able) to breastfeed.

Common breastfeeding complications include nipple pain or trauma, engorgement, mastitis, and low milk supply.

BOX 15-13 THERAPY CONSIDERATIONS FOR INFANTS WHO ARE BREASTFED

Positioning
The breastfeeding mother should be positioned to enable her baby to have easy access to the breast. Consider:
- Mother's comfort
- Privacy
- Infant's position
  In general, the infant should be held close to the mother's body at the same level of the breast with the infant's:
- Whole body turned toward the mother
- Trunk and head aligned
- Mouth at nipple level
- Head slightly tilted back with support across back and the shoulders, not the head

Attachment
Signs of effective attachment include:
- The infant should look comfortable and relaxed, and not be tense, frowning, or grimacing.
- The infant will generally display the following:
  - Mouth open wide against the breast with the nipple and surrounding breast tissue included in the gape
  - Chin against the breast
  - Observed deep jaw movements
  - Swallowing that can be seen once the milk ejection reflex occurs
- After feeding, nipples will appear slightly longer but should not be flattened, white, or ridged.

Issues that need to be addressed include infant positioning for feeds and attachment at the breast. See Box 15-13 for an overview of issues that need to be considered.

Bottle Feeding

During bottle feeding, both the feeding equipment used and the actions of the feeder can influence the infant's feeding performance.

Principles of **cue-based care** (also known as *developmentally supportive care*) suggest that all caregivers (including health care staff) should observe and respond appropriately to the infant's cues during all caregiving activities, including feeding.[21] This involves observing the infant's level of arousal, physiologic status, muscle tone, and responses to sensory input during and around feed times, in addition to his or her sucking skills and suck-swallow-breath coordination (see Chapter 14).

Principles of the cue-based care approach suggest that bottle feeds should only be offered to infants when they are at an optimal level of arousal and physiologic stability. In addition, although therapeutic techniques may be necessary to facilitate safe and successful oral feeding, they should only be applied when needed.

Therapy techniques applied *prior* to bottle feeds are generally aimed at preparing the infant for the subsequent feed.[15] Specific aims may include:
- Improving the tone and readiness of the oral musculature for feeding (e.g., nonnutritive sucking during tube feeds or prior to oral feeds, oral stimulation, suck training)
- Optimizing the level of arousal for the feed (i.e., some infants are not alert enough for feeds and may need to be stimulated; others are not settled enough and may need to be calmed)

Therapy techniques used *during* bottle feeds often aim to:
- Maintain an appropriate level of arousal for the feed (e.g., rocking, tapping)
- Augment the infant's existing sucking skills (e.g., chin and cheek support)
- Facilitate suck-swallow-breath coordination (e.g., use of slow-flow or nondrip nipples, active pacing, side-lying position for feeds)[15]

The cue-based approach emphasizes that early feeding success for the infant largely depends on the caregiver's attention to the individualized needs of the infant. It is suggested that reciprocity between the infant and the caregiver is important for successful feeding to occur. However, it is often acknowledged that this reciprocity might be difficult to achieve if there is not a consistent care provider. This can be a significant issue for hospitalized children, and parental education and involvement is highly encouraged.

Introduction of Solids

An outline of typical transition onto solids is included in Chapter 12. In summary, children are generally presented with foods in the order listed in Table 15-8.

Recently, an approach toward the introduction of solids referred to as **baby-led weaning**[23] has emerged. The main premise of this approach is that children do not necessarily have to be gradually introduced to solid foods in the order listed previously. Rather, a range of solid foods of various textures are offered to an infant who is learning to eat solids. This approach has strong advocates and opponents, and many newer parenting books and websites give much discussion to this issue. See Practice Note 15-11 for an overview of issues that need to be considered when working with an infant who is learning to eat solid foods.

As discussed, some children display difficulty in the transition period between consuming foods that can be masticated by the tongue and consuming foods that need to be masticated by the teeth. To make this transition, children need to be able to use tongue lateralization to move foods

TABLE 15-8 Typical Transition to Solid Foods

Fluids (e.g., breast milk, formula, water)	No mastication required
Pureed foods (e.g., rice cereal; yogurt; pureed fruit, vegetables, meats; stage I baby foods)	
Mashed foods (e.g., mashed potato, pumpkin, banana, avocado; stage II baby foods)	Food masticated by the tongue
Soft pieces of food (e.g., pieces of banana and avocado, cooked pieces of potato and pumpkin or squash)	
Soft mechanical food (e.g., cooked chicken, pasta, and vegetables, meatballs, cheese)	Food masticated by the teeth
Mixed food textures (e.g., baked beans in sauce, pieces of cooked chicken and pasta with mashed vegetables, stage III baby foods)	
Hard mechanical food (e.g., beef steak, raw apple, raw carrot)	

from the center of the tongue to the lateral chewing surfaces. If they try to swallow these foods without chewing them, they will generally gag and possibly choke. Practice Note 15-12 provides a discussion of the use of dissolvable foods and stick-shaped foods to assist with transition to foods that require mastication by the teeth (see Clinical Corner 15-1).

THERAPY CONSIDERATION FOR OLDER CHILDREN

There are a number of therapy considerations specific to older children with feeding difficulties, some of which are outlined below.

Active Participation in Therapy

Once children are mature enough to realize they have feeding or swallowing difficulties, it is important for the feeding therapist to explain assessment results and therapy plans to children in terms they can understand. This

PRACTICE NOTE 15-11

Baby-led weaning can work for some infants if it is truly "baby-led" (i.e., if the feeder provides cue-based care).

To provide cue-based care for an infant who is learning to eat solid foods means that the feeder (1) always has to be present and attentive during meals (i.e., doesn't walk away; doesn't get distracted by the phone, TV, etc.) and (2) has to make sure that the child is positioned appropriately for meals to provide the positional support they need (i.e., provide back support during meals until at least 12 months of age, and position infant with right angles at hips, knees, and feet for postural stability while eating).

Most children occasionally gag when learning to eat, which is normal. However, gagging can turn into choking (which is not normal, and potentially life-threatening) if they can't get the food out of their mouth. This is much more likely to happen if the food is of a firmer texture, the child isn't positioned appropriately, or there isn't an adult on hand to help him or her remove whatever is causing him or her to gag. (Note: Solid pieces of food should never be given before a child can hold his or her head fully upright while sitting, usually at approximately 6 months of age. If the child is in any kind of reclined position, gravity will make it hard to spit food out if needed).

Another part of cue-based care is observing what works for the child—and changing the approach if it isn't working. Some children like pureed food (many adults do too; common foods in the adult diet, like yogurt and mashed potato, are purees). Most infants struggle if their meal is only solid pieces. The ability to eat solid pieces doesn't mean infants can eat enough pieces efficiently at a meal to meet all of their nutritional needs. This often means mixing things up, so the infant gets a balance of

food textures during a meal. (A lot of adults have steak with some kind of cooked potato because the "easy to eat" potato balances the effort of eating steak. Not every meal has to be a marathon of chewing effort!)

It is important to note that from 6 to 12 months, breast milk and formula alone can't meet a child's iron requirements.[22] Thus it is important to ensure infants are getting additional iron from their food. For this to be effective, the iron-containing food has to be swallowed and get into the gut (not just played with and thrown on the floor). This can be challenging for infants unless caregivers cook and puree meat (commercial baby food containing meat is another option) or give iron-fortified baby cereal.

In all developmental activities, it is the job of the parent to support the child from full dependence through semi-independence to full independence. We do this when helping a child to walk and ride a bike, and we need to do this with eating too. This means pushing children to move forward with their skills, without pushing them too fast. Throughout history and cultures, adults have always recognized that some foods need to be modified for infants while they are learning to eat (whether this was by boiling, mashing, or cutting up food, prechewing food, or, more recently, blending).

Separate to the nutritional and developmental goals of meals, mealtimes are also social events. Parents spend more time with their infants during meals than during any other activity. Mealtimes are important bonding opportunities and are when young children learn much of their early communication skills. If mealtimes aren't enjoyable for the child, the parent, or both, or if any concerns exist about feeding, it is recommended that help be sought from a feeding therapist.

PRACTICE NOTE 15-12

Dissolvable foods are foods that can be easily snapped with the fingers or teeth and can be crushed into a powder. They are generally high in starch and, if held in the mouth, will dissolve quickly in saliva. For this reason, dissolvable foods are often a useful transition and stepping-stone food to assist children to learn to start biting and chewing foods without the choking risk associated with regular solids that do not dissolve in the mouth. A various range of manufactured dissolvable solid foods have become available and are common in most western grocery stores. Examples include varieties of corn puffs (e.g., Cheetos Puffs, Pirate Booty, Cheezels, Gerber Lil Crunchies), rice puffs (e.g., Gerber Puffs, Baby MumMum), "prawn crackers" or "veggie chips" (made from a cassava and tapioca starch with added shrimp or vegetable flavor), freeze dried yogurt drops (e.g., Gerber Melts), and freeze dried or baked fruit and vegetables (e.g., Fruit Crisps, Snap Pea Crisps).

Stick-shaped foods are thin and long in shape and allow the child to hold one end and direct the other end onto the chewing surface. Initially, stick-shaped oral toys and hard stick-shaped foods can be used for nonnutritive chewing practice. Stick-shaped teething crackers are ideal for this purpose. If the child has teeth or a strong bite, care must be taken to avoid toys and foods that could break off into solid pieces that could block the airway (e.g., raw carrot sticks), and full adult supervision should always be provided. As the child's chewing skills improve, softer stick-shaped foods can be offered for nutritive chewing practice. Most solid foods can be easily cut into this shape (e.g., boiled carrots served "julienne" style, roast chicken cut into strips, potato wedges). Many children will learn to eat bread sooner if offered to them in the form of "soldiers" (i.e., cut into sticks that they can easily direct to their chewing surface) than if offered as sandwiches (where they have to bite into the bread and then transfer the bolus from the center of their mouth to the side for chewing).

CLINICAL CORNER 15-1: INFANT THERAPY PLANNING

You have been requested to provide assessment and intervention for a new inpatient. Michaela is a 9-month-old girl with a recent onset of infantile seizures. The neurology team is currently working on establishing a medication schedule that controls Michaela's seizures without making her too drowsy. Michaela is currently tube fed, but the medical team has advised that you can offer her oral feeds if you feel it is appropriate to do so.

Critical Thinking
1. Determine the type of information you need to obtain to determine if Michaela is appropriate for an oral trial.
2. When you do perform an oral trial, what do you think you should offer her first?
3. What feeding equipment should you bring to the session?
4. What strategies might you consider trialing during the session?
5. Consider:
   a. How many health professionals are Michaela's parents likely to meet?
   b. Do you think they will remember everything from the various conversations they have?
   c. How might you assist them to follow through on your recommendations?

often involves using models and diagrams. See Table 12-6 in Chapter 12 for an overview of cognitive development in childhood.

Motivation

It is widely recognized that for older children (and adults), motivation is required to facilitate functional change.[24] Older children generally display more persistence at a therapy task when they are interested and when they experience some level of success. This often involves incorporating play or games into therapy sessions and requires the feeding therapist to break down tasks into manageable steps so that the child can experience mastery motivation as he

or she proceeds through various steps toward the overall goals of feeding and swallowing therapy.

Learning Compensation Strategies

For some children with swallowing or feeding difficulties, considerable time may be required before their skills improve (some children may always have some degree of swallowing or feeding difficulties). Thus once children are mature enough, they should be taught active strategies to improve their swallowing safety and feeding strategies. This can include teaching children to make suitable food choices and modifications (e.g., teach the child strategies regarding how to ask for soft food at the school cafeteria, how to cut up food into small enough pieces, how to use a chin-tuck position to improve swallow safety, how adding ketchup can cover up tastes you don't like) (see Clinical Corner 15-2).

WORKING WITH HOSPITALIZED CHILDREN WITH ACUTE HEALTH ISSUES

Feeding therapists providing therapy to children in a hospital environment need to pay particular attention to **safety issues** such as the following.

CLINICAL CORNER 15-2: THERAPY PLANNING IN AN OLDER CHILD

Joseph is a 4-year-old boy with autism who presents with a BMI on the seventieth percentile but very limited dietary variety. You have been asked to see him for feeding therapy targeting a wider variety of food intake.

Critical Thinking

1. Why do you think Joseph only eats a few foods and refuses most others?
2. What information should you obtain from a clinical feeding evaluation to guide your therapy planning?
3. What other developmental information should you obtain prior to commencing therapy, and where can you get it?
4. Compare and contrast different behavioral feeding therapy approaches.
5. List three goals for Joseph's therapy block.
6. List five possible therapy steps for one of Joseph's therapy goals.

Infection Management

Feeding therapists working in a hospital environment should always adhere to universal health precautions (e.g., regularly wash hands; avoid contact with bodily fluids; and wear personal protective equipment as needed, such as gloves, mask, and face shield). Those working in this area should use particular caution when working with children who fall into the following groups:

- Patients with transmittable diseases (e.g., infections spread by droplets such as influenza and respiratory syncytial virus [RSV] and infections spread by bodily fluids, such as human immunodeficiency virus [HIV], herpes simplex virus, and hepatitis)
- Immunocompromised patients (e.g., newborns, those receiving chemotherapy, those who have had organ transplants, those receiving steroids, or children with HIV)

Guidelines for hospitals and health care facilities are influenced by national or state health regulations. Site-specific guidelines may also be enforced.

Patients Requiring Special Diets

Feeding therapists should review a child's medical notes and, if possible, confirm with the parents the presence of any dietary restrictions before offering fluids or foods as part of a feeding or swallowing evaluation. Therapists should use particular caution in the case of children who fall into the following groups:

- Children with food allergy or intolerance: Fluids and foods known or suspected to cause an allergic response

should be completely avoided. Foods thought to cause an intolerance should be minimized.
- Children with metabolic conditions (e.g., galactosemia, phenylketonuria): Fluids and foods that cannot be metabolized effectively should be completely avoided.

In addition, those involved in the handling of food in any way need to be aware of food handling and hygiene guidelines. These guidelines generally provide suggestions for suitable foods and food preparation, hand washing, food storage (suitable containers and temperature), and food heating and reheating.

Safe Handling of Patients

If feeding therapists are involved in handling patients in any way for feeds or meals (e.g., holding infant for feed, helping older child sit up in bed or transfer to chair for meals) then they should receive training in safe patient handling techniques and precautions. These training programs are generally offered regularly at hospital and other health facilities. Therapists should note that there are some occasions when assistance from another health worker (e.g., nurse, physical therapist, ward staff) may be required.

It is suggested that readers review the issues discussed in Chapter 14 regarding working with hospitalized patients (e.g., medical stability, nutritional stability, limitations caused by medical treatments and the hospital environment).

WORKING WITH CHILDREN LIVING IN THE COMMUNITY

It is suggested that readers review the issues discussed in Chapter 14 regarding working with patients living at home in the community (e.g., considering developmental level and potential, nature of the condition [stable, resolving, deteriorating, progressive], transition from acute care, social aspects of eating, parent involvement in assessment and treatment, planning, burden on family).

MEASURING THERAPY OUTCOMES

A range of key outcomes often reported for feeding and swallowing therapy are outlined in Box 15-14.

In addition, functional assessment tools, such as the Functional Oral Intake Scale (FOIS): Suckle Feeds and Transition Feeds,[25,26] help to document change in overall feeding and swallowing ability and the degree of diet modification and compensation that is required. See Tables 14-7 and 14-8 in Chapter 14.

BOX 15-14 COMMON OUTCOME MEASURES FOR PEDIATRIC FEEDING AND SWALLOWING THERAPY

Feeding Skills
- Oral skills
- Swallow safety
- Variety of food textures consumed
- Variety of food types consumed
- Number of foods and fluids consumed across key food groups
- Self-feeding skills
- Mealtime duration
- Mealtime behavior (proportion of desirable behaviors versus undesirable behaviors)

Diet
- Nutritional adequacy from oral diet (e.g., overall energy intake, intake of key nutrients)

Growth
- Change in weight
- Weight for height and body mass index

Social Factors
- Parent-child interaction
- Parent stress
- Parent satisfaction
- Child satisfaction

From American Speech-Language-Hearing Association: Pediatric dysphagia, http://www.asha.org/Practice-Portal/Clinical-Topics/Pediatric-Dysphagia/.

TABLE 15-9 Goal Attainment Scaling

Outcome relative to goal		Goal 1 (specify details below)	Goal 2	Goal 3
Much more	+2			
Somewhat more	+1			
Expected outcome	0			
Somewhat less	−1			
Much less	−2			

Goal Attainment Scaling

Another tool that is often used to measure therapy outcomes for pediatric swallowing and feeding therapy is referred to as *Goal Attainment Scaling*[27] (Table 15-9). This tool is used to document specific, measurable therapy goals and to measure outcomes against these goals to track progress. Goal Attainment Scaling was initially developed by mental health professionals to measure their patient's progress in therapy,[27] but can be used with patients with various kinds of treatment requirements. This tool specifically measures only those symptoms, skills, or behaviors that the intervention is designed to change.

General guidelines for setting goals using Goal Attainment Scaling are as follows:
- Specify the "most probable" level of goal attainment first (this is assigned a score of 0, the middle level). This should be what you reasonably expect from therapy.
- Specify the "somewhat more" and "somewhat less" than expected (+1 and −1) levels next.
- Specify the "much more" and "much less" than expected (+2 and −2) levels of outcome last.

Progress against goals set out during therapy planning should be monitored regularly and reviewed with families at clinically meaningful times (e.g., midway through a therapy block, at the end of a therapy block).

TAKE HOME NOTES

1. It is important to set functional therapy goals and record outcome measures.
2. Effective interventions for feeding and swallowing difficulties need to target the cause of the problem. For this reason, a thorough assessment is required to guide intervention.
3. Different facilities and providers may use different models of service delivery when providing therapy services to children with feeding and swallowing difficulties. Common variables include location of services (inpatient, outpatient), primary recipient of input (child, parent or caregiver, staff), numbers involved in sessions (individual, group), and frequency of sessions (weekly or intermittently, intensive, consult only).
4. Pediatric feeding therapists are involved in proving treatment for children with swallowing problems. For children with oral phase swallowing problems, treatment generally involves working on improving the sensory and motor skills required for drinking and eating. For children with swallowing problems affecting the pharyngeal phase, treatment generally involves teaching the child to modify the swallowing strategy or for the feeder to modify the bolus.
5. If a child demonstrates that he or she is not able to swallow regular (thin) liquids safely, then alternative means of hydration must be provided. Historically, this has been accomplished by either making liquids thicker (by adding a thickening agent) or by providing fluids directly into the stomach (e.g., via nasogastric tube or gastrostomy feeding). Other potential therapy strategies may also be trialed as alternatives (or adjuncts) to thickening fluids for children with poor airway protection during swallowing. These approaches include changes to positioning, use of special feeding equipment, and active pacing.

6. Many of the therapeutic strategies used with adults with swallowing impairment (e.g., super-supraglottic swallow) may not be possible with young children. Children do not have the cognitive skills to understand or follow detailed instructions, or the self-awareness to voluntarily control movement of anatomic structures. With children, some therapeutic strategies may be possible to elicit with positioning changes or modeling (e.g., chin tuck, head turn), but these may be difficult to implement in reality.

7. If used, it is important that thickened fluids are prepared correctly. If thickened fluids are too thin, they may not assist in managing the underlying problem (i.e., aspiration during swallowing or regurgitation). Conversely, if thickened fluids are too thick, they may cause additional problems (e.g., increased work of breathing, reduced intake because of fatigue).

8. During bottle feeding, both the feeding equipment used and the actions of the feeder can influence the infant's feeding performance. Feeding therapists spend much time providing advice about artificial bottle nipples for infants who are bottle fed, as well is in training parents and caregivers in how to implement therapeutic feeding strategies.

9. Pediatric feeding therapists are also involved in proving treatment for children with feeding difficulties and mealtime behavior problems. Intervention aimed at improving mealtime behavior is unlikely to be effective unless the underlying cause of the feeding difficulty (i.e., pain or discomfort with feeding, skill deficit) is addressed.

10. By 2 to 3 years of age, most children have the oral skills to eat most solid foods. However, developmental delay and neurologic impairment can result in some children requiring modified food textures beyond this age. Depending on their degree of impairment or delay, different levels of food modification may be required.

11. The basic premise of most OSM therapy programs is to modify the child's current oral motor skills and sensory processing ability in relation to eating and drinking. A series of therapy exercises is applied to move the child from his or her current functional level toward the intended outcome of intervention.

12. A variety of feeding utensils and equipment are available commercially and via specialty therapy suppliers, which may assist with developing feeding skills or compensating for skill deficits.

13. The primary goals of behavioral feeding therapy are to increase desirable mealtime behavior and decrease undesirable mealtime behavior. In general, two main approaches to behavioral feeding therapy have been advocated: operant conditioning and systematic desensitization. Both are common forms of behavior management that are widely used across various areas of psychology.

14. An increasing number of medically complex children are surviving infancy and childhood, and many of these children require nutritional supplementation via the oral route or via tube feeding to meet their nutritional requirements. Unfortunately, many of these children become dependent on tube feeds and refuse oral feeds. These children often have to undergo a structured supplement or tube weaning program. Key members of the weaning team include feeding therapists, dietitians, and physicians.

REFERENCES

1. American Speech-Language-Hearing Association: Pediatric dysphagia, http://www.asha.org/Practice-Portal/Clinical-Topics/Pediatric-Dysphagia/.
2. Dodrill P: Infant feeding development and dysphagia. *J Gastroenterol Hepatol Res* 3(5) 2014. [Epub ahead of print].
3. Gosa M, Dodrill P: Effects of time and temperature on thickened fluids. In *Proceedings of the American Speech Hearing Association Conference*, New Orleans, November 2009.
4. Cichero JA, Steele C, Duivestein J, et al: The need for international terminology and definitions for texture-modified foods and thickened liquids used in dysphagia management: foundations of a global initiative. *Curr Phys Med Rehabil Rep* 1:280–291, 2013.
5. Steele CM, Alsanei WA, Ayanikalath S, et al: The Influence of Food Texture and Liquid Consistency Modification on Swallowing Physiology and Function: A Systematic Review. *Dysphagia* 2014. [Epub ahead of print].
6. Lund AM, Garcia JM, Chambers E: Line spread as a visual clinical tool for thickened liquids. *Am J Speech Lang Pathol* 22(3):566, 2013.
7. Mann LL, Wong K: Development of an objective method for assessing viscosity of formulated foods and beverages for the dysphagic diet. *J Am Diet Assoc* 96(6):585, 1996.
8. Fucile S, Gisel EG, Lau C: Effect of an oral stimulation program on sucking skill maturation of preterm infants. *Dev Med Child Neurol* 47(3):158, 2005.
9. Barlow SM, Finan DS, Lee J, et al: Synthetic orocutaneous stimulation entrains preterm infants with feeding difficulties to suck. *J Perinatol* 28:541, 2008.
10. Morgan AT, Dodrill P, Ward EC: Interventions for oropharyngeal dysphagia in children with neurological impairment. *Cochrane Database Syst Rev* (10):CD009456, 2012.
11. Flint A, New K, Davies MW: Cup feeding versus other forms of supplemental enteral feeding for newborn infants unable to fully breastfeed. *Cochrane Database Syst Rev* (2):CD005092, 2007.
12. World Health Organization, UNICEF: Baby-friendly hospital initiative, revised, updated and expanded for integrated care, 2009, http://www.who.int/nutrition/publications/infantfeeding/bfhi_trainingcourse/en/.
13. Jaafar SH, Jahanfar S, Angolkar M, et al: Pacifier use versus no pacifier use in breastfeeding term infants for increasing duration of breastfeeding. *Cochrane Database Syst Rev* (3):CD007202, 2011.
14. Pinelli J, Symington A: Non-nutritive sucking for promoting physiologic stability and nutrition in preterm infants. *Cochrane Database Syst Rev* (4):CD001071, 2005.

15. Dodrill P: Feeding difficulties in preterm neonates. *Infant Child Adoles Nutri* 3(6):324, 2011.

16. Nelson AM: A comprehensive review of evidence and current recommendations related to pacifier usage. *J Pediatr Nurs* 27(6):690, 2012.

17. Morris SE, Klein MD: *Pre-feeding skills: a comprehensive resource for feeding development*, ed 2, Tucson, AZ, 2000, Therapy Skill Builders.

18. Marshall J, Hill R, Ware R, et al: Multidisciplinary intervention for childhood feeding difficulties: a randomized clinical trial. *J Pediatr Gastroenterol Nutr* 2014. [Epub ahead of print].

19. Toomey K, Ross E: SOS approach to feeding, SIG 13 perspectives on swallowing and swallowing disorders. *Dysphagia* 20:82, 2011.

20. SOS Approach to Feeding: http://www.sosapproach-conferences.com/.

21. Kenner C, McGrath JM, editors: *Developmental care of newborns and infants: a guide for health professionals*, ed 2, St Louis, 2010, Mosby.

22. Baker RD, Greer FR, Committee on Nutrition American Academy of Pediatrics: Diagnosis and prevention of iron deficiency and iron-deficiency anemia in infants and young children (0-3 years of age). *Pediatrics* 126(5):1040, 2010.

23. Rapley G: Baby-led weaning, http://www.rapleyweaning.com.

24. Gilmore L, Cuskelly M: Mastery motivating in children with Down syndrome. In Faragher R, Clarke B, editors: *Educating learners with Down syndrome*, Oxon, Great Britain, 2014, Routledge.

25. Crary MA, Dodrill P, Mann GD, et al: *A functional oral intake scale for dysphagia in infants and toddlers*, 2014.

26. Crary MA, Mann GD, Groher ME: Initial psychometric assessment of a functional oral intake scale for dysphagia in stroke patients. *Arch Phys Med Rehabil* 86(8):1516, 2005.

27. Kiresuk TJ, Sherman RE: Goal attainment scaling: a general method for evaluating comprehensive community mental health programs. *Comm Mental Health J* 4(6):443, 1968.

Appendix A

Common bottles

STRAIGHT BOTTLES

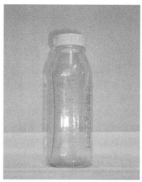

- Fit most standard nipples.
- Easy to clean and store.
- Easy to obtain, cheap, available in supermarkets, drug stores, baby shops.

ANGLED BOTTLES

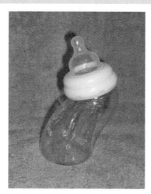

- May minimize air swallowed, especially if feeding child in side-lying position.
- May be difficult to clean and store.
- Generally more expensive than regular bottles, usually only fit the same brand nipple.
- Fairly easy to obtain in baby stores.

OTHER SHAPED BOTTLES

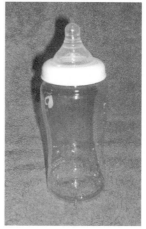

- Consider cost—generally more expensive than regular bottles, usually only fit the same brand nipple.
- May be difficult to clean and store.
- Fairly easy to obtain in supermarkets, drug stores, baby shops.

HABERMAN (SPECIAL NEEDS FEEDER)

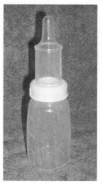

- One-way valve prevents milk from flowing back from nipple into bottle, which minimizes air in nipple.
- Specialist equipment—may be difficult to obtain and expensive.

DR BROWN'S BOTTLES

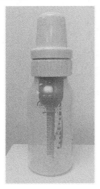

- Internal vent system prevents buildup of air or vacuum, which makes sucking easier.
- Fairly easy to obtain in baby shops.
- Generally more expensive than regular bottles; may only fit the same brand nipple.

BOTTLES WITH COLLAPSABLE BAGS

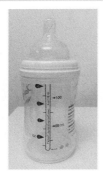

- Collapsible bags prevent buildup of air or vacuum, which makes sucking easier.
- Fairly easy to obtain in baby stores.
- Generally more expensive than regular bottles; usually only fit the same brand nipple.

SQUEEZE BOTTLES

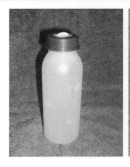 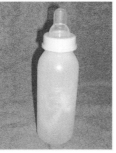

- Made of soft plastic to allow the bottle to be squeezed.
- Often used with soft nipples, which reward minimal sucking effort.
- Used with infants with cleft lip or palate, weak suck.
- Feeder needs to observe and respond to infant's cues to avoid flooding the oral cavity.
- Specialist equipment—may be difficult to obtain and relatively expensive.

MEDICINE DISPENSER NIPPLES

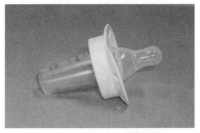

- Good for very small volumes of milk.
- Can be used with regular nipples.
- Often sold in drug stores, may be difficult to obtain.

SYRINGE NIPPLES

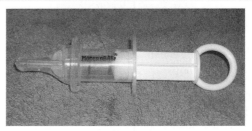

- Good for very small volumes of milk.
- Syringe allows feeder to control the volume of milk delivered.
- Feeder needs to observe and respond to infant's cues to avoid flooding the oral cavity.
- Useful for delivering small volumes of fluid or pureed solids laterally within mouth for children with severe oral hypersensitivity.
- Often sold in drug stores, may be difficult to obtain.

Cervical auscultation equipment

STETHOSCOPE

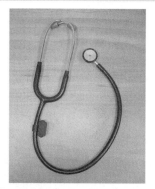

- Allows swallowing and breathing sounds to be heard by an individual listener.
- Neonatal or pediatric bell preferable.
- Relatively easy to obtain around hospitals.
- May be difficult to hold in place while feeding child or for long periods.

LAPEL MICROPHONE

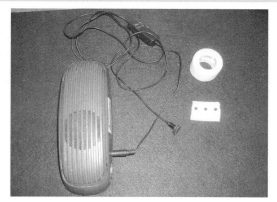

- Available from electronic shops.
- Can be plugged into amplifier or into video camera.

AMPLIFIER

- Allows swallow and breathing sounds to be heard aloud.
- Good for providing biofeedback to parent or feeder; also useful for older children to hear their swallows.

ADHESIVE

- Holds microphone in place during feed to free the feeder's hands.
- Small electrode adhesive disks can be used if a washer is placed around the end of microphone.

Appendix C

Common cups

SPOUT CUPS

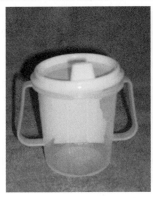
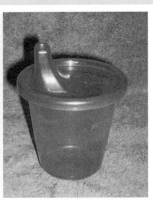

- Many children can drink from spout cup before open cup.
- Variable spout lengths and widths available.
- Variable flow rates available.
- Cups with nondrip valves require stronger suck to create flow; in some cases nondrip valve can be removed.
- Handles may assist with self-feeding.
- Easily accessible, cheap; available in supermarkets, drug stores, baby shops.

STRAW CUPS

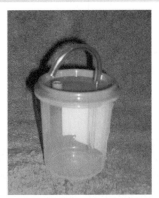

- Many children can drink from straw cup before open cup.
- Minimize neck extension, allow chin tuck.
- Wider straws require less lip control.
- Narrow straws create faster flow.
- Handles may assist with self-feeding.
- Easily accessible, cheap; available in supermarkets, drug stores, baby shops.

REGULAR CUPS

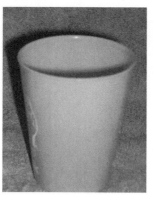

- May require feeder to assist infant to regulate flow at first.
- Handles may assist with self-feeding.
- Consider size and weight of cup if infant is to self-feed.
- Easily accessible, cheap; available in supermarkets, drug stores, baby shops.

CUT-OUT CUPS

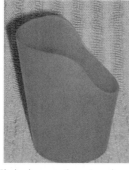 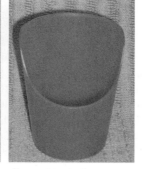

- Minimize neck extension, allow chin tuck.
- Allow feeder to see the fluid as it enters the child's mouth.
- External frame with handles available for self-feeding.
- Specialist equipment—may be difficult to obtain and relatively expensive.

OTHER CUPS

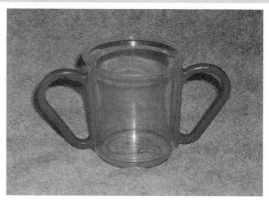

- Small cups suit small volumes and can help with pacing and self-feeding.
- Rim on cup can assist in stabilizing cup position if poor lip and jaw control is apparent.
- Clear cups allow feeder to see the fluid as it enters the child's mouth.
- Handles can assist with self-feeding.
- May be difficult to obtain and can be relatively expensive.

Common pacifier types

CHERRY-SHAPED PACIFIERS

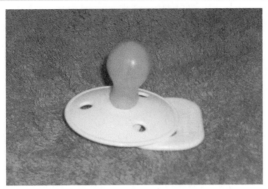

- Traditional shape offered to many infants.
- May be easier for some infants to hold in their mouth.
- Cheap, easy to obtain; available in supermarkets, drug stores, baby shops.

ORTHODONTIC PACIFIERS

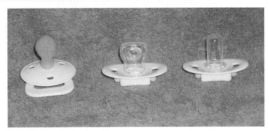

- Wide bulb.
- May be easier for some infants to hold in their mouth.
- Fairly easy to obtain in supermarkets, drug stores, baby shops.

STRAIGHT PACIFIERS

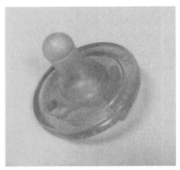

- Closer in shape to bottle nipples, so may help transition to oral feeds.
- Some infants may find difficult to hold in their mouth.
- Available in most baby shops.
- Generally more expensive than traditional pacifiers.

ORAL TOYS

TEETHING TOYS

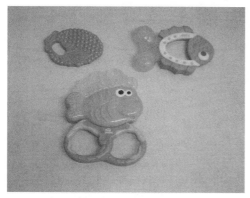

- Promote oral exploration, allow infants to experience a variety of oral sensations.
- Promote chewing and biting.
- Can help establish tongue lateralization.
- Can be used to introduce first tastes.
- Consider weight and whether infants can hold in their mouths themselves.
- Fairly easy to obtain in supermarkets, drug stores, baby shops.

INFADENT FINGER TOOTHBRUSHES

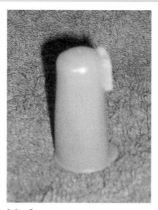

- Worn on adult's finger.
- Allow infants to experience varied oral sensations.
- Can help to establish tongue lateralization.
- Can be used to introduce first tastes.
- Specialist equipment—may be difficult to obtain.

NUK GUM BRUSHES

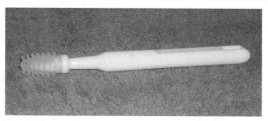

- Allow infants to experience varied oral sensations.
- Promote chewing and biting.
- Can help establish tongue lateralization.
- Can be used to introduce first tastes.
- Older children can hold; promote oral exploration.
- Specialist equipment—may be difficult to obtain.

BABY TOOTHBRUSHES

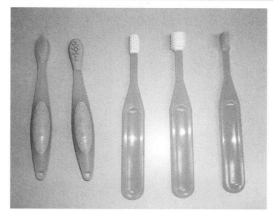

- Available in a variety of textures.
- Allow infants to experience a variety of oral sensations.
- May promote chewing and biting.
- May help establish tongue lateralization.
- Can be used to introduce first tastes.
- Older children can hold; promote oral exploration.
- Often available in baby shops.

THERAPY TUBING

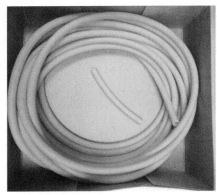

- Available in different thicknesses.
- Can be cut to size.
- Can promote chewing and biting.
- May help establish tongue lateralization.
- Older children can hold; promotes oral exploration.
- Specialist equipment—may be difficult to obtain.

NET FEEDERS

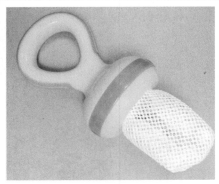

- Food pieces are put in net. The net prevents the child from swallowing the piece of food whole.
- Can be used to introduce first tastes.
- Promote chewing and biting.
- Older children can hold; promote oral exploration.
- Often available in baby shops.

Appendix E

Common spoons

METAL SPOONS

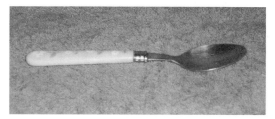

- Traditional spoon.
- Come in different sizes (teaspoon, table, soup, dessert spoon).
- Accepted by many children.
- Cold metal may irritate children with severe oral sensitivity.
- Harness of metal may cause damage to teeth in children with phasic bite.
- Very easy to access.

SILICONE SPOONS

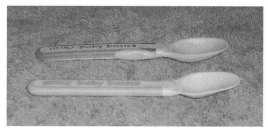

- Won't shatter or damage teeth if bitten.
- Available in different sizes.
- Shallow bowl limits volume offered.
- Deeper bowl promotes development of lip closure around spoon.
- Finger grips and shape of spoon can assist the infant to hold the spoon during self-feeding.
- Fairly easy to obtain in supermarkets, drug stores, baby shops.

MAROON SPOONS

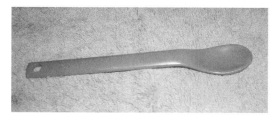

- Hard plastic won't shatter or damage teeth if bitten.
- Available in small and large sizes.
- Flat bowl may make it easier to obtain food with poor lip closure.
- Flat bowl may assist to flatten and depress tongue in children with tongue thrust.
- Specialist equipment—may be difficult to obtain and relatively expensive.

LOOP SPOONS

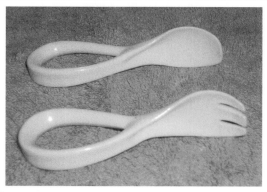

- Shape of spoon assists the infant to turn the spoon ready to enter the mouth during self-feeding.
- Fairly easy to obtain in supermarkets, drug stores, baby shops.

BEGINNER BOWLS

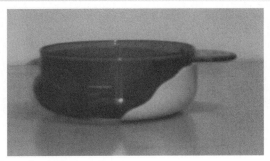

- Come in different sizes.
- Smaller bowls can limit volume.
- Walls of bowl can assist the infant to lift the food from the bottom of the bowl.
- Wide base and rubber grips can assist the bowl to stay in one spot during self-feeding.
- Fairly easy to obtain in supermarkets, drug stores, baby shops.

Artificial nipples for bottle feeding

SLOW FLOW

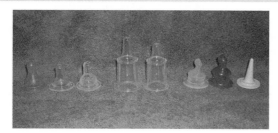

- Generally suitable for infants aged 0-3 months.

MEDIUM FLOW

- Generally suitable for infants 3-6 months.

FAST FLOW

- Generally suitable for infants older than 6 months.
  Note: Definition of *slow, medium,* and *fast* varies between brands, so evaluate on a case-by-case basis.
  Standard nipples are widely available in supermarkets, drug stores, baby shops.

GENERAL RECOMMENDATIONS

- Decrease the flow rate if increased respiratory effort or poor suck-swallow-breath coordination is apparent.
- Increase the flow rate if thickened fluids are required.
- Increase the flow rate if weak suck is apparent; check that the infant is able to swallow safely.

VARIABLE FLOW NIPPLES

- Rotate nipple in infant's mouth to alter flow rate (rotation changes alignment of slit in end of nipple, which changes flow).

- If pacing is required, may be less disturbing for the infant than removing the nipple from his or her mouth.
- Often more expensive than regular flow nipples.
- Fairly easy to obtain in baby stores.

NONDRIP NIPPLES

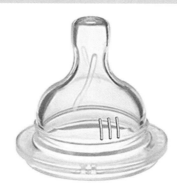

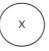

- Do not deliver fluid unless compressed.
- Respond to active compression during sucking.
- Assist the infant to regulate the flow rate; may allow infants to learn to regulate their own suck-swallow-breath pattern.
- May minimize the chance of flooding the oral cavity.
- Often more expensive than regular-flow nipples.
- Fairly easy to obtain in baby stores.

STRAIGHT NIPPLES

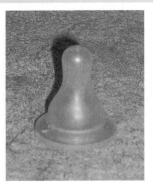

- Suit most infants.
- Easy to obtain, cheap, available in supermarkets, drug stores, baby shops.
- Longer nipples may produce more natural sucking patterns (consider that breast fills more than two thirds of mouth during breast feeding).
- Longer may induce gagging in infants with severe oral hypersensitivity.

WIDE NECK NIPPLES

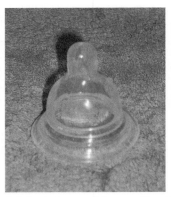

- May be useful for infants with poor lip closure.
- Some argue those with short nipples may encourage strong compression or tongue thrusting.
- Fairly easy to obtain in supermarkets, drug stores, baby shops.
- Generally more expensive than regular nipples.
- Usually only fit the same brand bottle.

ORTHODONTIC NIPPLES

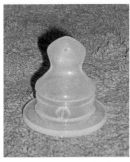 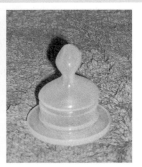

- Preferred by some infants.
- Easy to obtain, cheap, available in supermarkets, drug stores, baby shops.
- Fewer options (i.e., do not come in variable flow or nondrip).
- Once introduced, may be difficult to switch back to straight nipples.
- Some argue they may encourage strong compression or tongue thrusting.

PERISTALTIC NIPPLES

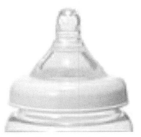

- Stretchable nipple elongates during sucking.
- May be useful if breastfed infant requires complementary bottle feeds.
- Available in regular-neck and wide-neck varieties.
- Often available in baby stores.
- Generally more expensive than regular nipples.
- Usually only fit the same brand bottle.

PIGEON AND CHU CHU NIPPLES

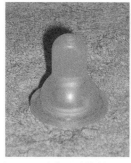 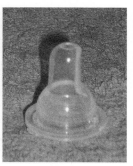

- Often used for children with cleft palate.
- Mostly used along with squeeze bottle.
- Very soft side walls reward even minimal tongue action; can be useful for infants with weak suck.
- Nondrip nipple minimizes the chance of flooding the oral cavity between sucks.
- Specialist equipment—may be difficult to obtain and relatively expensive.

HABERMAN (SPECIAL NEEDS) BOTTLE NIPPLES

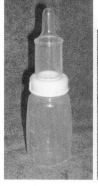 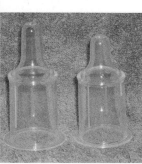

- Only work as part of Haberman set (with Haberman bottle and valve).
- Sold as part of Haberman set, as well as separate replacement parts.
- Nondrip nipple may assist in preventing flooding of the oral cavity.
- Variable flow options (slow, medium, fast) may assist infants who have poor suck-swallow-breath coordination or who fatigue easily.
- Squeezable reservoir allows feeder to assist in delivering milk, if needed.
- Two nipple lengths: Long nipple is standard; shorter nipple may be useful for premature infants, as well as infants with small oral cavities or severe oral hypersensitivity.
- Specialist equipment—may be difficult to obtain and relatively expensive.

Appendix G

Common infant feeding positions

SIDE-LYING FOR BREASTFEED

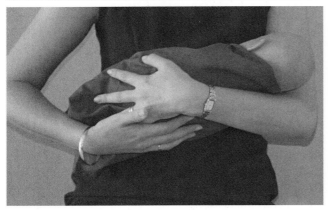

- Infant is generally positioned on his or her side.
- Infant is supported by mother's body and arm.

CRADLE HOLD FOR BOTTLE FEEDING

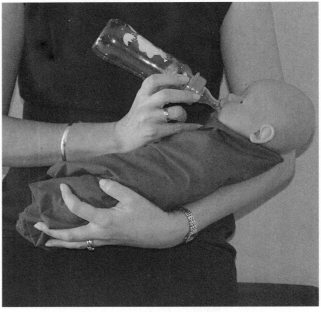

- Infant is generally positioned in supine position and may be somewhat elevated in space.
- Infant is supported by feeder's arm and body.

SIDE-LYING FOR BOTTLE FEED

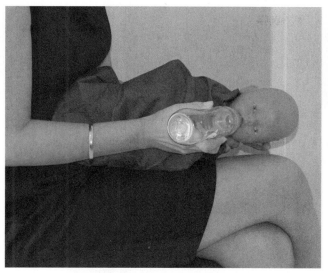

- Infant is positioned on his or her side and may be somewhat elevated in space.
- Infant is supported by feeder's lap (or cushion) and feeder's hand.

SEMIUPRIGHT IN BABY CHAIR

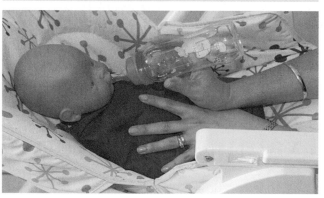

- Infant is positioned in supine but is elevated in space.
- Infant is supported by chair and straps.

SEMIUPRIGHT IN FEEDER'S ARMS (ELEVATED CRADLE HOLD)

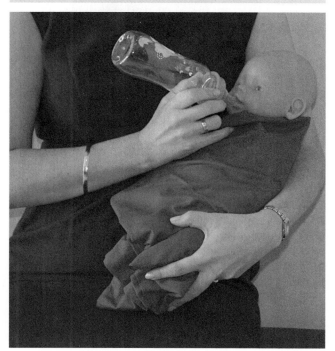

- Infant is positioned in supine but is elevated in space.
- Infant is supported by feeder's arm and body.

Appendix H

Examples of seating options

INFANT SEAT

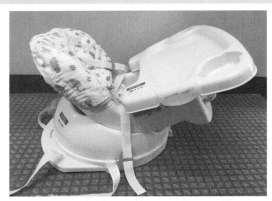

- Appropriate size for most infants.
- Chair can usually be tilted in space and reclined to several different positions (from semiupright to upright), but not always.
- Cushioning and shoulder straps provide additional support.
- Infants with poor postural support may need extra cushioning beside them (to prevent them from falling to the side).
- Tray can help encourage active exploration of food and self-feeding.
- Available in baby stores.

HIGH CHAIRS

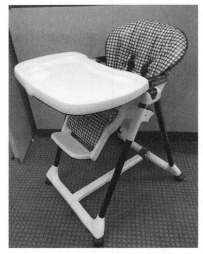

- Appropriate size for most older infants and toddlers.
- Chair can usually be tilted in space and reclined somewhat, but not always.
- Provide some postural support; cushioning and shoulder straps provide additional support.
- Younger children and children with poor postural support may need extra cushioning underneath them so they don't sink into chair or beside them to prevent them from falling to the side.
- Foot plate can assist children to prop themselves up and not fall out, if at the correct height.
- Tray can help encourage active exploration of food and self-feeding.
- Widely available in baby stores and found in most restaurants.

MULTIAGE CHAIRS

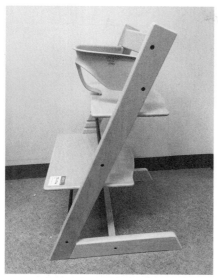

- Seat and footplate can be adjusted to suit children of different ages, from older infants to older children.
- Generally come with straps that can be removed.
- Chair cannot be tilted in space or reclined.
- Younger children and children with poor postural support may struggle to sit up in these chairs.
- Adjustable foot plate can assist children to prop themselves up and not fall out and help with positional stability.
- Often used without tray, so child can be positioned at dining table.
- If used, tray can help encourage active exploration of food and self-feeding.
- Generally more expensive than high chairs.
- Available in baby stores.

TUMBLEFORM SEAT

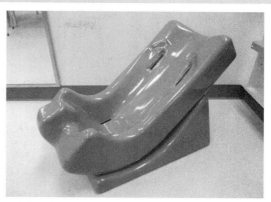

- Specialty therapy seat.
- Available in different sizes for children of different ages.
- Shape and harness provide high level of support.
- Chair can be tilted in space.
- Specialist item, relatively hard to access and expensive.

TOMATO CHAIR

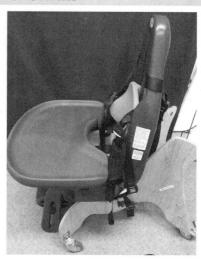

- Specialty therapy seat.
- Can be adjusted to suit children of different ages, from older infants to older children.
- Shape and harness provide high level of support.
- Head rest, seat, and foot plate can all be adjusted.
- Chair can be tilted in space and angle of chair can be adjusted.
- Specialist item, relatively hard to access and expensive.

HOOK ON CHAIR (SASSY SEAT)

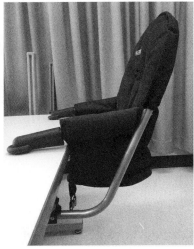

- Appropriate size for most infants.
- Cannot be tilted in space or reclined.
- Cushioning and shoulder straps provide additional support.
- Infants with poor postural support may need extra cushioning beside them (to prevent them from falling to the side).
- Children may need a foot stool to help with positional stability.
- Very portable.
- Available in baby stores.

TODDLER TABLE AND CHAIRS

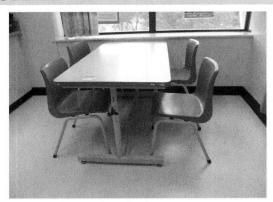

- Appropriate size for most toddlers.
- Cannot be tilted in space or reclined.
- Infants with poor postural support may struggle stabilizing themselves.
- Children should be able to reach the floor with their feet to help with positional stability.
- Widely available in baby stores.

Glossary

24-hour pH monitoring: A timed measurement by specialized sensors that monitors the amount of acid at various levels in a fixed period in the alimentary system.

Abruptio placentae: Premature detachment of the placenta.

Acidosis: Increase of acid in the blood.

Acute care setting: Short-term health care offered in a hospital or emergency room for an illness with severe or rapidly developing symptoms.

Adenocarcinoma: A type of tumor (adenoma) arising from an organ such as the esophagus.

Adjuvant: Additional treatment, typically referring to chemotherapy given after radiation therapy or surgery in the treatment of cancer.

Advanced directive: A legal document prepared by a competent individual that is a statement to guide the health care team in specific medical situations, such as whether the person wants a feeding tube.

Aerodigestive tract: Referring to the common passage connecting the mouth, pharynx, esophagus, and stomach.

Albumin: A soluble protein in the blood that is a long-term marker of nutritional status. Normal values range between 3.8-5 g/dL.

Alimentation: Providing food or fluid.

Amniotic band syndrome: Abnormal collection of fibrotic strands that entangle the fetus resulting in various malformations, usually of the limbs or digits.

Amyotrophic lateral sclerosis: A progressive degeneration of the motoneurons of the spinal cord, brainstem, or cortex.

Aphasia: A multimodal (speak, write, understand) deficit in language ability secondary to brain damage.

Anaphylaxis: An allergic reaction, usually to an injection.

Anastomosis: The point where two tubular parts have been surgically joined.

Ankylosis: Fixed in place, unmovable.

Anorexia: Loss of appetite.

Anterior cingulate gyrus: A region in the limbic cortex just above the corpus callosum.

Apert's syndrome: A congenital syndrome characterized by a peaked head, webbed fingers and toes, and oral structure changes including cleft palate.

Apgar score: A 10-point scale judging an infant's physical condition at birth.

Apraxia: A deficit in the execution of learned, voluntary movements secondary to brain damage.

Aspiration: Swallowed material that has entered the trachea below the level of the true vocal folds.

Aspiration pneumonia: Aspiration of swallowed materials from the pharynx that results in a lung infection.

Aspiration pneumonitis: Aspiration of gastric contents usually seen in patients with depressed consciousness that may result in life-threatening illness.

Ataxia: Loss of coordination of movement, especially voluntary movement, often from damage to the cerebellum.

Autologous: Originating within the individual, especially in tissues or fluids.

Balloon dilatation: A catheter with an uninflated, attached balloon is placed at the level of stenosis wherein the balloon is inflated to gradually open the blockage.

Barrett's esophagitis: Precancerous changes in the mucosa of the lower esophageal sphincter often secondary to chronic gastroesophageal reflux.

Barthel score: A score taken from the Barthel Index of Functional Independence; a reliable and valid measure for measuring disability in chronically ill patients.

Beckwith-Wiedeman syndrome: An autosomal dominant syndrome with variable expressivity, usually seen as a growth-related disorder in infants with risk of the development of hypoglycemia and tumors.

Benign: Not recurrent or progressive; nonmalignant.

Blinding: Technique used in an experimental study in which the researchers are not aware of who is in the experimental group or who is in the control group and during the study have little contact with the participants.

Bolus: Masticated food that is ready to be swallowed.

Brachial nerve plexus: Network of nerves supplying the arm, forearm, and hand.

Brachytherapy: A form of radiotherapy where the radioactive source is placed inside or near the area needing treatment.

Bradycardia: Slow heart rate.

Bradykinesia: Slow movement.

Bronchoscopy: Inspection of the lungs with a light source under anesthesia.

Bulbar musculature: The muscles of the head and neck that are innervated peripherally by the lower part (bulbar region) of the brainstem.

Bulimia: Recurrent binge eating followed by self-induced vomiting and diarrhea.

Cachexia: A state of ill health, malnutrition, and muscle wasting.

Cardia: The part of the stomach surrounding the region where the esophagus meets the stomach.

Cardiomegaly: Enlarged heart.

Centipoise: Unit of measurement that describes the viscosity of liquids.

Cephalohematoma: Collections of blood in the brain.

CHARGE association: C = cranial nerve abnormality; H = heart malformation; A = choanal atresia; R = retardation of growth; G = genital hypoplasia; E = ear malformations.

Chemesthetic (also chemesthesis): Chemical sensibility of skin and mucosa. Examples of chemesthetic sensations include burning from chili peppers, tingling from carbonation, and tearing eyes from onions. These are viewed as chemically induced sensations that do not fit into the traditional categories of taste or smell. Often medicated by the trigeminal nerve, these senses are thought to result by direct chemical activation of sensory fibers.

Chemo-control: Achieving the correct balance between oxygen and carbon monoxide.

Chemodenervation: Using chemicals to interfere with normal nervous system transmission.

Chemotherapy: Treatment of certain types of cancer by the use of intravenous medications.

Chiari-Arnold deformity: Congenital anomaly allowing the cerebellum and medulla to protrude into the spinal canal through the foramen magnum.

Choana: A funnel-shaped opening, as in the space in the posterior nasal cavity behind the septum.

Chronic: A condition that lasts for a prolonged period, showing little change or progression.

Clonic movement: Spasmodic alteration in antagonistic muscles that cause a structure to move rhythmically back and forth.

Collagen-vascular disease: A group of inflammatory disorders that affect the integrity of joints and connective tissue.

Columella: The anterior part of the septum of the nose.

Comorbidity: A disease existing with the primary disease or secondary to it.

Contrast agent: In radiology, a foreign substance used to provide a different density so the tissue can be visualized; positive agents appear black on x-ray to better delineate the adjacent tissue and air space that are lighter.

Cortical plasticity: The ability of the cortex to change or reorganize so that functions may be recovered.

Creatinine: A component in the blood that is important in muscle contraction. Normal levels are less than 1.2 mg/dL.

Cross-cradle: Supporting the child with both arms crossed.

Crossed extension reflex: Extension of the lower extremity on the opposite side in response to a painful stimulus.

Cross-system effect: The effect when functional improvement occurs indirectly when treatment is focused on a related function.

Crown-heel length: From the top of the head to the bottom of the foot.

Cyanosis: Bluish-colored or purple skin from reduced oxygenation.

Cytologic brushing: A method of collecting cells for microscopic analysis of disease.

Cytomegalovirus: A virus related to the herpes family.

Decannulation: The removal of a tube, as in tracheostomy.

Decubitus ulcers: Breakdown in skin layers, also called pressure sores.

Dermatomyositis: An inflammation of the skeletal muscle connective tissue, often associated with skin lesions.

Diffuse esophageal spasm: A condition marked by generalized spasm in the esophagus, usually resulting in retrosternal pain.

Diurnal: Daytime.

Diverticulum: A sac or pouch on the wall of a canal or organ.

Dysarthria: A group of motor speech disorders usually resulting from neurologic disease.

Dyspepsia: Abdominal discomfort after eating.

Dyspnea: Shortness of breath.

Dystocia: Difficult labor during the birth act.

Dystonia: A group of movement disorders characterized by prolonged muscle contractions causing twisting and turning movements or abnormal postures.

Endarterectomy: The surgical removal of the lining of an artery.

Edematous: Swollen.

Edentulous: Without teeth.

Effectiveness study: Treatment applied to a group to achieve a desired outcome with no control group for comparison.

Efficacy study: Treatment applied to a group with a disorder and to another (control) group without the disorder to achieve a desired outcome.

Electromyographic (also surface electromyography; EMG): A record of the electrical activity produced by muscles doing movement or at rest. The EMG signal may be obtained from surface electrodes taped to the skin or from needles or wires inserted into muscles.

Emesis: Vomit.

Emotional lability: Sudden and inappropriate change in emotions secondary to neurologic damage such as crying after hearing a funny joke.

Endoscopy: Using a rigid or flexible scope with a light source to view the alimentary tract or other parts of the body.

Enteral: Being fed using the stomach or duodenum through a tube.

Eosinophils: White blood cells.

Erosive esophagitis: Erosion to the mucosal lining of the esophagus usually from gastroesophageal reflux disease.

Erythema or erythematous: Diffuse redness of an area.

Esophagram: An x-ray study done with large amounts of barium to evaluate the esophagus and lower gastrointestinal tract.

Executive functions: A set of cognitive functions that control other behaviors or abilities. Needed to achieve goal-oriented behaviors such as initiating and stopping actions, monitoring behavior, or planning activities.

Expires: Dies.

Extubated: Removal of a tube such as an endotracheal tube.

fMRI (functional magnetic resonance imaging): A special form of imaging of brain structures that identifies brain activity during functions of interest such as swallowing or speaking.

Fasciculations: Small muscle twitches seen in a muscle at rest or after palpation often seen in patients with lower motoneuron disease.

Fibrosis: An abnormal replacement of fibrotic tissue (as in scarring) often resulting in a change of function of that tissue.

Flexor withdrawal reflex: Flexion of a body part in response to a painful stimulus.

Fontanelles: A soft spot between the cranial bones.

Freeman-Sheldon syndrome: Congenital anomalies affecting the structures of the head and neck, feet, and muscles and joints.

Functional independence measure (FIM): The FIM is a widely used functional assessment measure used in rehabilitation settings to rate communication and motor skills as they relate to daily activity.

Fundoplication: A surgical procedure at the level of the lower esophageal sphincter designed to tighten the sphincter to prevent gastroesophageal reflux.

Galactosemia: A hereditary disorder of galactose metabolism that may lead to multiple medical disorders including poor weight gain and malnutrition in early infancy.

Gastric pull up: A surgical technique in which the stomach is raised into the thorax often with reconnection to the swallowing tract at the level of the hypopharynx.

Gastroesophageal reflux disease (GERD): Excessive acid in the stomach that enters the esophagus, pharynx, or mouth that may or may not be associated with dysphagia.

Gastroparesis: Paralysis of the stomach muscles.

Gastrostomy: Placement of a feeding tube into the stomach.

Gavage: Feeding through a gastrostomy or nasogastric tube.

Glasgow Coma Scale: A neurologic scale documenting the conscious state of the patient in three areas: eye opening, verbal responsiveness, and motor ability.

Globus sensation: Feeling of a lump in the throat, typically during non-swallow activity.

Goldenhar's syndrome: A congenital defect characterized by incomplete development of the ear, nose, velum, lip, and mandible.

Granuloma: A tumor or growth that results when macrophages are unable to destroy foreign bodies.

Halo: The halo vest-brace is a device that fits around the patient's head, stabilized at the shoulders to keep the head from moving, so the spine can heal following surgery.

Holter monitor: Portable device used by a patient to monitor the activity of the heart over a period of 24 hours.

Hematoma: Swelling or mass of blood resulting from the break of a blood vessel.

Hiatal hernia: The protrusion of the stomach into the mediastinal cavity through the esophageal hiatus of the diaphragm pushing the lower esophageal sphincter away from the crual diaphragm.

Hippocampus: A structure in the limbic system of the cortex.

Hirschsprung's disease: An extremely dilated colon that usually is congenital.

Histamine (H₂) receptor agonist: A drug that blocks the stimulation of cells by histamine when controlling stomach acid is frequently referred to as an *H₂ blocker.*

Histopathology: The microscopic evaluation of diseased tissues.

Home health setting: Medical care that is provided by specialists visiting the patient's home.

Hyaline membrane disease: Respiratory distress syndrome usually in a premature infant.

Hydration: Providing adequate amounts of fluid.

Hypercapnia: An increased amount of carbon monoxide in the blood.

Hypernatremia: An excess amount of sodium in the blood.

Hyperoxia: Increased oxygenation of the blood.

Hyperplasia: Excessive proliferation of cells.

Hypertension: High blood pressure.

Hypertrophy: Abnormal enlargement of a structure.

Hypopnea: Shallow breathing or a low respiratory rate; differs from apnea in that some airflow is present.

Hypotensive: Low blood pressure.

Hypothyroidism: A condition caused by deficient thyroid secretion resulting in lowered basal metabolism.

Hypotonia: Reduced or low muscle tone contributing to weakness.

Hypoxemia: Decreased oxygen concentration in the blood.

Hysterical: A mental disorder simulating any type of physical disease.

Idiopathic: Unknown origin.

Incidence: The rate of new occurrences of any outcome of interest during a specified observation, for example, the rate of new pneumonias identified in a patient group during a year. This differs from **prevalence,** which is the rate of any (existing or new) outcomes at a specific time or during a specified period.

Inclusion body myositis: Inflammation of the nuclei of a cell body in a muscle resulting in muscle weakness.

Inferior nasal meatus: The inferior passage from the nasal entrance to the choana, below the inferior turbinate.

Infiltrates: Deposition of material into a cell, tissue, or organ.

Insular cortex: Deep brain region behind the anterior temporal lobe.

Intention tremor: Tremor (phasic movement of a body part) that is seen at the initiation of a movement but not at rest.

Intraluminal: Literally within a lumen (closed, circular structure) such as the esophagus.

Intrapartum: Happening during the birth process.

Intubation: Placement of a tube through the mouth and vocal folds into the trachea to provide air to the lungs.

Irritable bowel disease: Abnormal, painful defecation and abdominal bloating.

Isokinetic: Strength training in which the tension remains the same but the muscle length changes, such as in lifting or a bicep curl.

Isometric: Strength training in which the joint angle and muscle length do not change during the exercise. Basically, exercise done in a static position.

Jejunal transfer: Taking a portion of the jejunum (portion of the small intestine) and replacing part of the esophagus or hypopharynx.

Jejunum: Part of the small intestine.

Kabuki syndrome: Facial anomalies similar to the makeup of traditional Japanese Kabuki dancers; other related problems include hypotonia, feeding difficulty, recurrent infections, congenital heart defects, and cleft palate.

Kernicterus: Abnormal accumulation of bilirubin that may cause brain injury.

Kinematic (also biokinematic): Describes motion or movement such as the movement of the hyoid bone.

Klippel-Feil syndrome: Reduction or fusion of a cervical vertebra resulting in a short neck and limited motion.

Kyphosis: Abnormal convexity in the curvature of the spine.

Laparoscopic: Surgery done through an endoscope.

Laryngeal aditus: The entrance into the upper airway (larynx).

Laryngeal ventricle: Space between the true and the vestibular (false) vocal folds.

Laryngeal vestibule: Space between the laryngeal aditus and the vestibular folds.

Laryngopharyngectomy: Removal of the larynx and pharynx.

Laryngospasm: Spasm of the laryngeal muscles that may contribute to reduced ability to breathe.

Left to right shunting: The left side of the heart is oxygenated blood, and the right side is unoxygenated. The left side may abnormally mix with the right via defects in the heart.

Likelihood ratio: Tells one how likely the statistical result will occur in any given sample.

Limbic cortex: Phylogenetically the oldest part of the cortex located at the edge of the cerebral hemispheres. It is part of the limbic system that is comprised of structures such as the amygdale, hippocampus, and parts of the hypothalamus.

Lordosis: Abnormal anterior concavity in the curvature of the spine.

Lower motoneuron: Peripheral motor nerves that course from the brainstem or spinal cord to muscle. Injury results in flaccid paralysis.

Lumen: The cavity or channel within a tube.

Lymph: A fluid system containing vessels and nodes throughout the body that eventually enters the thoracic area where it enters the bloodstream.

Malacia: An abnormal softening of tissues.

Malignant: Growing worse or resisting treatment; tending or threatening to produce death.

Maloney (bougie) dilators: Mercury-filled tubes of various diameters that are used to open a stricture. Small sizes are used initially, then larger ones until the desired diameter is reached.

Mandibulotomy: A procedure in which a portion of the mandible is split or opened to gain access to other structures it encloses.

Manometry: A test that measures the pressures in the alimentary tract during swallowing.

Mediastinum: The mass of organs and tissues separating the lungs.

Mesenchymal: Layer of cells giving rise to connective tissue.

Metaanalysis: A statistical method to contrast and combine results from different studies to identify patterns across those studies. A metaanalysis provides a thorough summary of several studies and identifies any effects weighted across different studies.

Metastasis: Movement of body cells from one part of the body to another.

Micrognathia: Small jaw.

Micrographia: Writing characterized by small letters often seen in Parkinson's disease.

Morbidity: A state of having a disease or problems associated with a disease.

Moro reflex: A whole-body response to sensation in an infant characterized by abduction and adduction primarily of the arms.

Morphology: Pertaining to the science of structure and form without regard to function.

Mortality: Death.

Multicystic encephalomalacia: Multiple sites of cerebral softening.

Multiple sclerosis: An autoimmune, progressive, inflammatory neurologic disease affecting all parts of the central nervous system.

Multivariate analyses: Testing multiple independent variables against the dependent variable to assess which factors might predict a relationship between the two.

Myasthenia gravis: A progressive disease affecting muscle strength caused by a chemical imbalance at the neuromotor junction.

Myoneural junction: The connection (synapse) between the lower motoneuron and the muscle.

Myopathy: Muscle weakness.

Myopic: Good near sight, but poor sight at a distance.

Myositis: Inflammation of muscle tissue.

Myotomy: The surgical relaxation of a muscle or group of muscles.

Myotonia: A tonic spasm of a muscle after contraction that interferes with normal relaxation.

Nasogastric tube: A feeding tube that is placed through the nose, into the esophagus, and into the stomach to provide nutrition.

Neglect: An impairment in sensory processing in which an individual does not attend to one side of the body.

Neoadjuvant: Before the primary treatment, often referring to chemotherapy given before radiotherapy or surgery.

Neocortex: Phylogenetically the newest part of the cortex that includes the primary motor and sensory cortices and the association cortex.

Neopharynx: Technically meaning "new pharynx," a term referring to the reconstructed pharynx following total laryngectomy.

Neuronal proliferation defect: Insufficient production of neurons during development.

Nodose ganglion: Group of neurons mediating the vagus as the nerve exits the skull base.

Obex: At the level of the fourth ventricle in the medulla of the brainstem.

Odynophagia: Painful swallowing.

Orbitofrontal operculum: Region in the inferior frontal lobe above the eyes.

Ordinal scale: Measurement scale that ranks items based on their relation to one another; distance between items is not considered to be equal.

Organicity: A medical cause.

Osteoradionecrosis: A breakdown in bone or connective tissue caused by the side effects of radiation therapy.

Oxygen desaturation: Sometimes referred to as *hypoxia*, representing a drop in blood oxygen levels below 90%. Often measured by a pulse oximeter on the fingertip.

Paradoxical breathing: Irregular breathing.

Palliative: Relieving symptoms without curing the disease; sometimes refers to reducing symptoms of discomfort in terminal disease.

Paradoxical breathing: Abnormal breathing pattern, sometimes difficult to explain.

Parenteral: Being fed through the venous system, bypassing the stomach.

Parkinson's disease: A progressive neurologic disorder affecting movement caused by damage in the basil ganglia.

Passy-Muir valve: A valve that fits over a tracheotomy tube that allows free flow of air on inhalation but closes on the exhalation cycle.

PECS: Picture exchange communication system.

Pedaling: Involuntary muscle contractions.

Percutaneous endoscopic gastrostomy (PEG): A feeding tube placed in the stomach through an endoscope.

Percutaneous endoscopic jejunostomy (PEJ): A feeding tube placed in the jejunum through an endoscope.

Periventricular white matter: Sheaths of axons that pass close to the cerebral ventricles.

Pierre-Robin sequence: A small jaw associated with cleft palate and a displaced tongue.

Pharyngoesophageal sphincter: The muscular segment between the pharynx and esophagus, sometimes referred to as the *upper esophageal sphincter* or *cricopharyngeus muscle.*

Placenta previa: A placenta abnormally implanted in the lower uterine segment.

Plagiocephaly: Malformation of the head wherein it appears twisted or lopsided.

Plane films: Still x-rays of a particular part of the body taken at varying angles or planes.

Plantar grasp reflex: Closing of the hand in response to stroking the sole of the foot.

Plate guard: A metal barrier that is attached to the side of a plate so that food is not pushed off the edge.

Pneumothorax: A collapsed lung.

Polyhydramnios: An excess of amniotic fluid.

Polymyositis: An inflammation of the skeletal muscle connective tissue particularly affecting the proximal limbs, neck, and pharyngeal muscle.

Popliteal angle: Relationship between the calf and the leg when the calf is flexed.

Postprandial: After the meal.

Predictive value: The predictive value of a test is a measure of the times that the value (finding, positive or negative) is the true value. For instance, the percent of all positive tests that has a true positive is the positive predictive value.

Prokinetic drugs: Drugs used to improve digestive tract motility.

Proprioceptive placing: A normal response of the body to changes in position (maintaining equilibrium).

Prospective data: Experimental design variables are established prior to the beginning of data collection.

Prosthodontist: A dentist trained in making artificial teeth and other maxillofacial structures.

Proton pump inhibitor (PPI): Class of drugs used to control acid secretion in the stomach.

Proximal muscles: Muscles of the body closer to the midline such as pharyngeal muscles.

Ptosis: Drooping of an organ, as in the eyelid.

Pulsion: Moving in any direction by external forces.

Radiation therapy: A controlled radiation beam directed at a specific part of the body, often as an attempt to cure cancer.

Radiopaque: Impenetrable to x-rays or other forms of radiation; opposite of radiolucent or radioparent.

Radiopaque pill: One that can be seen with x-ray.

Rales: Abnormal crackling sounds in the lung.

Rancho Los Amigos Scale: Describes the cognitive level of patients following traumatic brain injury.

Refractory: Does not respond to traditional treatment.

Regurgitation: Swallowed material that is not digested but is retropulsed from the esophagus into the pharynx or mouth.

Rehabilitation setting: A medical facility designed to teach patients how to adapt or compensate for a disability.

Reliability: A measure of consistency of observations between judges (interjudge) or within the same judge (intrajudge).

Renal agenesis: Failure of the kidney to grow.

Resection: "Cutting off"; removing part of a structure.

Resting tremor: Tremor in a body part seen at rest that may diminish during volitional movement.

Retromolar trigone: The area behind the molars.

Rheology: The science that studies the deformation and flow of materials.

Rheumatoid arthritis: An inflammation of the body's joints.

Rigidity: Inability to move or bend, often as a result of excessive muscle tone as in Parkinson's disease.

Satiety: Feeling full after eating.

Scarf sign: The elbow crosses the body without resistance when touching the opposite shoulder.

Scleroderma: A connective tissue disorder that frequently affects the body's smooth muscles like the esophagus.

Setting sun eyes: Eyes that roll down abnormally.

Sialorrhea: Excessive salivation or drooling.

Sign: A physical finding on a clinical evaluation.

Silent aspiration: Swallowed material that goes below the vocal folds that does not produce a cough reflex.

Sjögren's syndrome: A disease of the connective tissue that also affects the lacrimal glands.

Skilled nursing facility: Chronic care facility for patients who require supervised medical care.

Slip-through: A technique used to evaluate an infant's tone. Hold the infant upright under the arms and note if he or she is able to maintain an erect posture by resistance, or if the infant "slips through" the arm support because of low tone.

Smooth muscle: Muscle under control of the autonomic nervous system.

Squamous cell carcinoma: A cancer that affects squamous cells commonly found on epithelium such as in the aerodigestive tract.

Stasis: Lack of movement, stoppage of flow.

Stenosis: A narrowing.

Stent: Material or a device used to support or hold other tissue in place; may be used to open a closed lumen.

Striated muscle: Muscle under control of the central nervous system.

Subacute care setting: A level of health care that is not acute, but is more oriented toward rehabilitation.

Supplementary motor cortex: Superior frontal lobe region anterior to the primary motor cortex.

Supraglottic laryngectomy: A procedure to remove cancer in the laryngeal region that does not sacrifice the true vocal folds but sacrifices the false vocal folds and hyoid bone.

Surfactant: An agent that lowers surface tension.

Surrogate: A substitute, acting on behalf of another especially for emotional purposes.

Symptom: A patient complaint.

Symptom cluster (also symptom complex):   Has been defined in different ways, but all refer to the presence of multiple symptoms in patients. One common definition is the presence of three or more concurrent symptoms that are related but may or may not have a common cause.

Syncope: Light-headedness, fainting, temporary loss of consciousness.

Systematic review: A literature review focused on a research question that identifies, appraises, and synthesizes all high-quality research evidence relevant to that research question. Systematic reviews are important to evaluate evidence-based practice.

Systemic rheumatic disease: Inflammation in the joints and connective tissue throughout the entire body.

Swallowing apnea: The cessation of respiration during a swallowing event.

Tachycardia: Rapid heart rate.

TEACCH: Treatment and education of autistic and related communication-handicapped children.

Tongue-lip adhesion: Temporary surgery joining the tongue and lip to maintain an open airway in children with anomalies of the oral and jaw structures.

Tonic bite reflex: Abnormal muscular tension (biting) elicited by stimulation usually to the dentition.

Torticollis: Shortening of the neck muscles causing the head to tilt toward the affected side.

Toxemia: Poisonous byproduct of bacteria.

Toxoplasmosis: An infectious disease caused by the protozoan toxoplasma gondii.

Tracheoesophageal fistula: An opening in the common wall between the trachea and esophagus.

Tracheostomy: A surgical procedure in which an opening (stoma) is made into the trachea to establish an airway.

Tracheostomy tube: A plastic tube placed through a surgical incision in the neck below the level of the vocal folds to help the patient breathe; it provides a direct access to the lungs for suctioning.

Transnasal: Across the nose, as in passing an endoscope through the nose.

Treacher Collins syndrome: Disorder of the structures of the head and neck including abnormal eyes and eyelids, underdeveloped cheek bones, malformed ears, cleft palate, and hearing loss.

Trismus: Reduced ability to open the mouth secondary to tonic contraction of the muscles.

Truncus arteriosus: Defect in the arterial trunk from the embryonic heart.

Umami: A proposed fifth basic taste; from the Japanese word meaning "savory"; related to the detection of amino acid or glutamates common in protein-heavy foods.

Umbilical cord prolapse: Premature expulsion of the umbilical cord before the fetus is delivered.

Undernutrition: A type of malnutrition in which the body does not have a sufficient amount of food intake or utilizes food intake poorly.

Upper and lower motoneurons: The two major divisions of the pyramidal motor tracts; the upper motoneuron governs voluntary movement, and the lower motoneuron governs reflexive movement.

Validity: Trust that a measurement tool actually measures the variable it is intended to measure.

Vallecular spaces: Depressions at the tongue base, lateral to the epiglottic root.

Vasoconstrictor: A substance that causes constriction of blood vessels, as a vasoconstrictor might be used to "shrink" nasal tissues resulting in a larger passage through which to pass an endoscope.

Vasovagal response: Sudden fainting from stimulation to the vagus nerve accompanied by pallor, sweating, hyperventilation, and bradycardia.

Velocardiofacial syndrome: Congenital abnormality affecting the velum and heart.

Ventilator: A mechanical device used for supporting lung function.

Ventriculoperitoneal shunt: Moving cerebrospinal fluid through tubing from a brain ventricle to the lining of the stomach.

Videofluoroscopy: A moving x-ray of the mouth, pharynx, larynx, and cervical esophagus during swallowing.

Viscosity: Resistance offered by a fluid when force is applied; in simple terms, how thick a fluid is.

Xerostomia: Dry mouth.

Index

Page numbers followed by "*f*" indicate figures, "*t*" indicate tables, and "*b*" indicate boxes.